Encyclopedia of Herbal Medicine

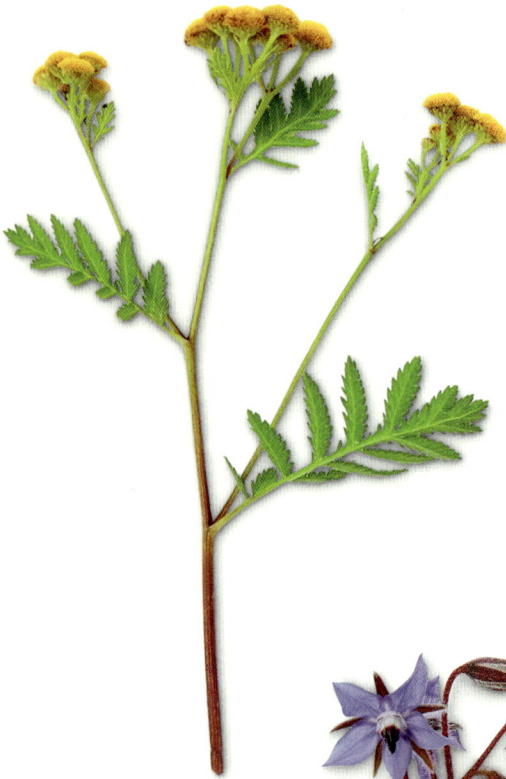

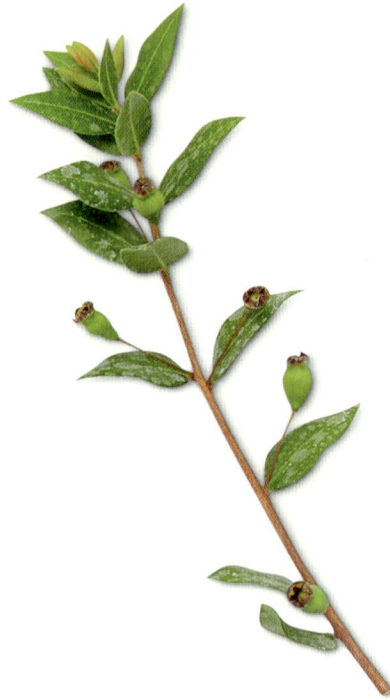

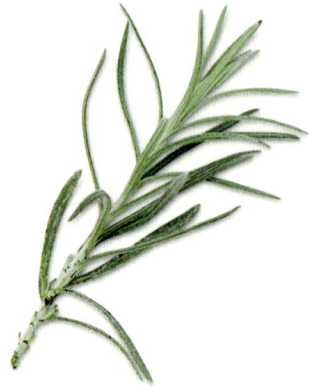

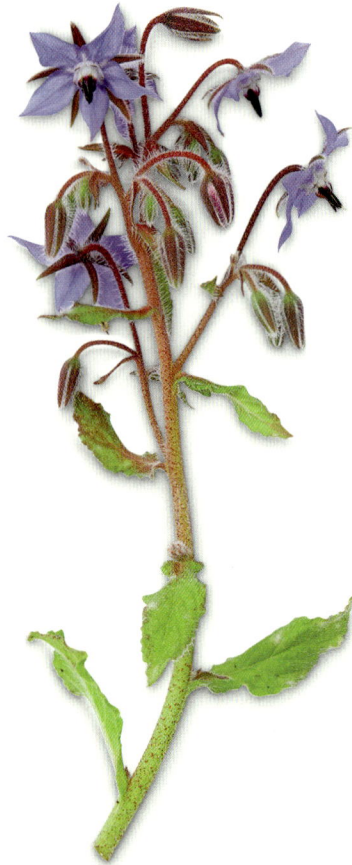

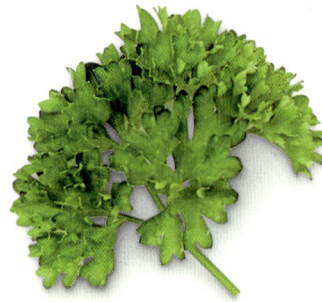

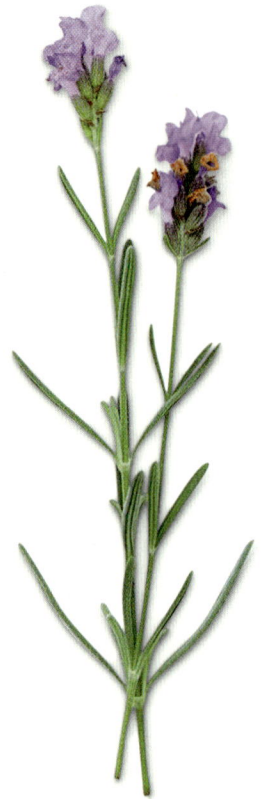

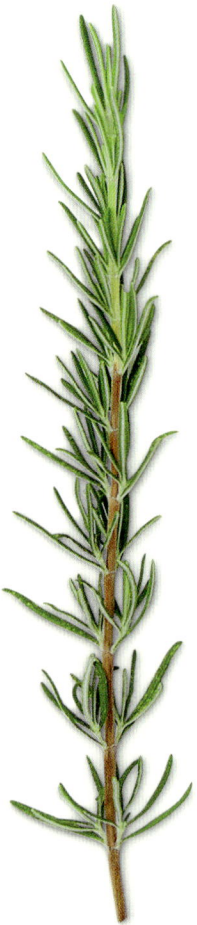

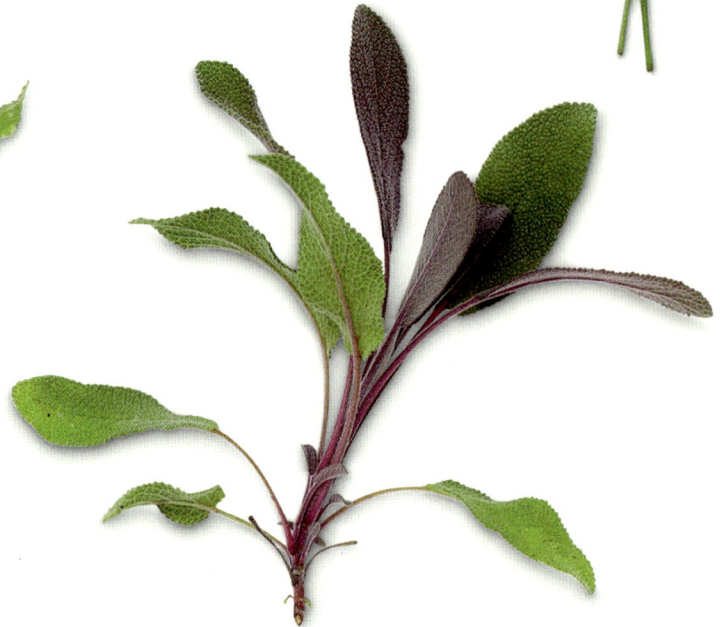

Encyclopedia of Herbal Medicine

Andrew Chevallier, FNIMH

Contents

A visual guide to 100 key herbs from around the world with details of their habitat, constituents, actions, traditional and current uses, and information on the latest research. Also included are key preparations and practical self-help uses.

450 other herbs from different herbal traditions with descriptions of their therapeutic properties and past and present uses.

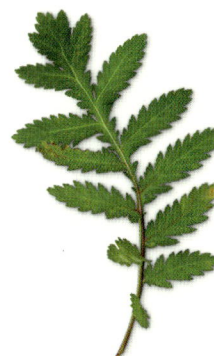

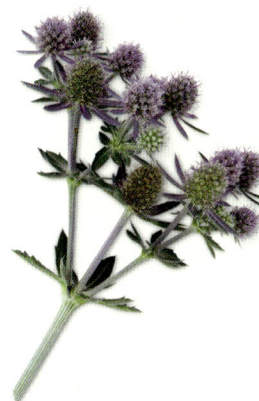

Introduction

In the nearly thirty years since the first edition of this encyclopedia in 1996, herbal medicine has gone through unprecedented change. Herbs, which have always been the principal form of medicine in developing countries, have again become popular in the developed world, as people strive to stay healthy in the face of chronic stress and pollution, and to treat illness with medicines that work in concert with the body's defenses. A quiet revolution has been taking place. Tens of millions of people now take herbs such as ginkgo (*Ginkgo biloba*, p. 104) to help maintain mental and physical health, and increasingly people consult trained herbal professionals and naturopaths for chronic or routine health problems. Increasingly, too, scientific evidence is accumulating to show that herbal medicines can provide treatment that is as effective as conventional medicines but with few side effects. Sales of herbal medicines continue to grow year after year—by over 50 percent in the US in 2020—and several mainstream pharmaceutical companies now manufacture and market herbal medicines.

Plant medicines

The variety and sheer number of plants with therapeutic properties are quite astonishing. Some 50,000 to 70,000 plant species, from lichens to towering trees, have been used at one time or another for medicinal purposes. Today, Western herbal medicine still makes use of hundreds of native European plants, as well as many hundreds of species from other continents. In Ayurveda (traditional Indian medicine) about 2,000 plant species are considered to have medicinal value, while the Chinese *Pharmacopoeia* lists over 5,700 traditional medicines, mostly of plant origin.

About 500 herbs are still employed within conventional medicine, although whole plants are rarely used. In general, the herbs provide the starting material for the isolation or synthesis of conventional drugs. Digoxin, for example, which is used for heart failure, was isolated from common foxglove (*Digitalis purpurea*, p. 207), and the contraceptive pill was synthesized from constituents found in wild yam (*Dioscorea villosa*, p. 95).

Ecological factors

The increased use of medicinal herbs has important environmental implications. Growing herbs as an organic crop offers new opportunities for farmers, and sometimes, especially in developing countries, opportunities for whole communities. In northeastern Brazil, for example, community-run herb gardens grow medicinal herbs that are sold to local hospitals. Doctors at the hospital then prescribe these medicines for their patients.

The rise in popularity of herbal medicines, however, also directly threatens the survival of some wild species. Demand for goldenseal (*Hydrastis canadensis*, p. 109) has become so great that it now fetches up to $115 a pound (£190 a kilo). It was a common plant in the woodlands of northern America two centuries ago, but is now an endangered species, with its survival in the wild threatened by over-collection. This example is by no means unique, and, sadly, many species are similarly threatened across the planet. The extinction of plant species as a result of over-intensive collecting is nothing new. The herb silphion, a member of the carrot family, was used extensively as a contraceptive by the women of ancient Rome. Silphion proved difficult to cultivate and was gathered from the wild in such large quantities that it became extinct during the 3rd century CE.

Today, if herbal medicine continues to grow at its present rate, it is imperative that manufacturers, suppliers, practitioners, and the public use only produce that has been cultivated or wildcrafted in an ecologically sensitive manner.

About this book

In the past, books on herbal medicine have tended to focus either on the traditional and folkloric use of plants or on their active constituents and pharmacology. *The Encyclopedia of Herbal Medicine*, which features over 550 plants, aims to cover both aspects. It discusses each plant's history, traditions, and folklore, and explains in simple terms what is known from scientific research about its active constituents, actions, and potential new uses.

It is easy when concentrating on the scientific aspect of herbal medicine to forget that much, in some cases all, that we currently know about a particular plant results from its traditional use. Moreover, even when a plant has been well researched, herbal medicines are so complex and variable that what is currently known is rarely definitive, but rather a sound pointer as to how it works. Sometimes the traditional use, insofar as it is based on the experience of practitioners, provides an insight into how best to use an herb that is missing from scientific knowledge alone. Herbal medicine is, after all, both a science and an art.

In choosing the plants profiled in the *Encyclopedia*, the aim has been to select herbs that are commonly used in different parts of the world and are considered to have particular health benefits. The index of key medicinal plants (pp. 58–159) contains many herbs that are readily available in health stores and pharmacies, for example St. John's wort (*Hypericum perforatum*, p. 110). It also includes herbs that are more commonly known as foods, such as lemon (*Citrus limon*, p. 86), but which, nonetheless, are valuable medicines. The index of other medicinal plants (pp. 160–293) contains some less commonly known but important medicinal herbs, such as Shatavari (*Shatavari racemosus*, p. 178), a traditional Indian medicinal plant that aids fertility and hormonal balance and supports immune function.

A global overview of the history of herbal medicine puts the development of different herbal traditions from earliest origins to the present day into perspective. This is complemented with features on herbal medicine in Europe, India, China, Africa, Australia, and the Americas, providing a rounded picture of herbal medicine worldwide.

Herbal medicine is nothing if not practical in its approach, and the *Encyclopedia* has a detailed self-help section with advice on preparing and using herbal medicines to treat a range of common health problems.

If more people come to appreciate the immense richness of the world of herbal medicine and are able to benefit from the curative properties of medicinal herbs, this book will have achieved its aim.

Andrew Chevallier, FNIMH MCIPP

Cautions

Throughout the medicinal plant entries, take note of the cautions given concerning using the herb medicinally and about the plant in general. These also state if the plant, its constituents, or its extracts are legally restricted.

There are some plants you should not self-medicate with as they are known to be toxic or unsafe. In certain cases, they may be safely prescribed by experienced health care practitioners within a very narrow dosage range. At a higher dose such plants will be poisonous.

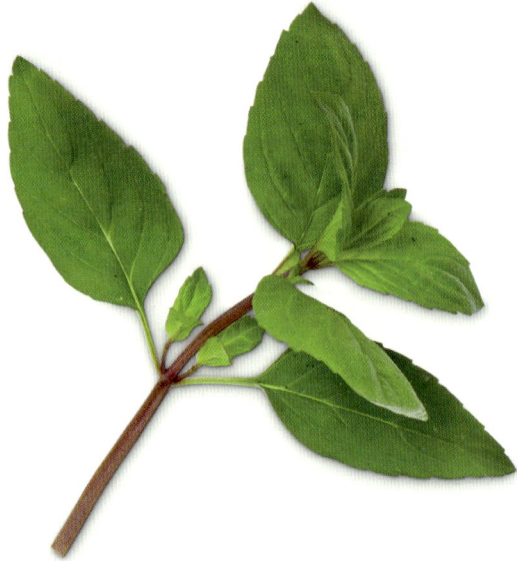

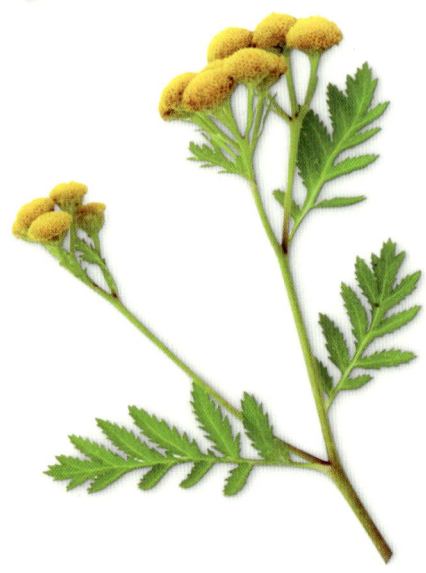

The development of herbal medicine

From the earliest times, herbs have been prized for their pain-relieving and healing abilities, and today we still rely on the curative properties of plants in about 75 percent of our medicines. Over the centuries, societies around the world have developed their own traditions to make sense of medicinal plants and their uses. Some of these traditions and medical practices may seem strange and magical, others appear rational and sensible, but all are attempts to overcome illness and suffering, and to enhance quality of life.

How medicinal plants work

Many of the thousands of plant species growing throughout the world have medicinal uses, containing active constituents that have a direct action on the body. They are used both in herbal and conventional medicine and offer benefits that pharmaceutical drugs can often lack, helping to combat illness and support the body's efforts to regain good health.

There is no doubt that in extreme situations, the treatments devised by modern medicine offer an unparalleled opportunity to relieve symptoms and save lives. A newspaper article in 1993 described the terrible conditions in a hospital in war-torn Sarajevo, the capital of Bosnia-Herzegovina. Deprived of conventional medical supplies and drugs, the doctors were forced to use a well known European herb, valerian (*Valeriana officinalis*, p. 152), as a painkiller for the wounded and as an anesthetic. Valerian is an effective herbal medicine for anxiety and nervous tension, but it is woefully inadequate as an analgesic or anesthetic.

Orthodox pharmaceutical medicines sustain life and counter infections in situations where other types of treatment may have little to offer. Modern surgical techniques, such as laparoscopic surgery and plastic surgery, and the whole range of diagnostics and of life-support machinery now available, can all be used to improve the chances of recovery from serious illness or injury.

The benefits of herbal medicine

Yet despite the dramatic advances and advantages of conventional medicine, or biomedicine as it is also known, it is clear that herbal medicine has much to offer. We tend to forget that in all but the past 70 years or so, humans have relied almost entirely on plants to treat all manner of illnesses, from minor problems such as coughs and colds to life-threatening diseases such as tuberculosis and malaria.

Today, herbal medicine is coming back into prominence for several reasons. There is a growing awareness that a more natural lifestyle improves health and helps to prevent illness. Used thoughtfully, herbal medicines support good health, protect body systems under strain or attack, and provide safe, effective treatment in many contexts, countering infection, inflammation, and allergy. Herbal medicines will also promote healthy bacterial populations within the digestive tract, on the skin and elsewhere within the body, and as natural products, do not stress the environment.

People are more aware that antibiotics and other pharmaceutical medicines carry with them a risk of side effects. Between 10–20% of hospital patients in the West are there due to the side-effects of conventional medical treatment. Pharmaceutical medicines also have an impact on wildlife and the wider environment.

"A stitch in time saves nine" goes the old saying—here it indicates that when used early on, and taken consistently, plant medicines are often able to prevent the onset of health problems that might otherwise require medical intervention. Taking cranberry juice (*Vaccinium macrocarpon* p. 290) and a corn silk (*Zea mays* p. 158) infusion at the first signs of symptoms of cystitis will cleanse the urinary tract and may prevent the need for antibiotics. Where conventional treatment is necessary, selected herbal medicines can be safely taken as complementary treatment alongside prescribed medication. Many chronic health problems such as asthma, arthritis, chronic fatigue, and irritable bowel syndrome benefit from an *integrated* medical approach that combines pharmaceutical and herbal medicines with lifestyle changes and treatments such as acupuncture.

Using herbs wisely

Most commonly used herbs are extremely safe to use. But plants can produce side effects and, like all medicines, herbal remedies must be treated with respect. It is essential to take or use certain plants only under the guidance of a well-trained practitioner, to avoid adverse consequences. Ma huang (*Ephedra sinica*, p. 99), for example, can be extremely toxic at the wrong dosage, and comfrey (*Symphytum officinale*, p. 142), a very popular herb in the past, is thought to cause severe or even fatal liver damage in rare circumstances. When an herbal medicine is used correctly, however, the chances of developing a serious side effect are remote.

Potent plant chemicals

The ability of an herbal medicine to affect body systems depends on the chemical constituents that it contains. Scientists first started extracting and isolating chemicals from plants in the 18th century, and since that time we have grown accustomed to looking at herbs and their effects in terms of the active constituents they contain. This *Encyclopedia* is no exception, providing details of all the main active constituents of the medicinal herbs featured and explaining their actions.

Research into isolated plant constituents is of great importance, for it has given rise to many of the world's most useful drugs. Tubocurarine, the most powerful muscle relaxant in existence, is derived from pareira (*Chondrodendron tomentosum*, p. 193), and the strongest painkiller of all, morphine, comes from opium poppy (*Papaver somniferum*,

p. 251). Many anesthetics are also derived from plants—for example cocaine comes from coca (*Erythroxylum coca*, p. 211).

Today, biomedicine still relies on plants rather than the laboratory for at least 20% of its medicines, and many of these are among the most effective of all conventional drugs. It is hard to think of a world deprived of the key antimalarial properties of quinine (derived from *Cinchona spp.*, p. 84) and artemisinin (from *Artemisia annua*, p. 71); or the heart remedy digoxin (from *Digitalis* spp., p. 207); or the cough-relieving properties of ephedrine (from *Ephedra sinica*, p. 99), which is present in many prescription and over-the-counter cold remedies. These and many other conventional medicines are all derived from isolated plant constituents.

Value of whole plants

Although it is important to understand the actions of individual active constituents, herbal medicine, unlike biomedicine, is ultimately about the use and actions of whole plants—medicines that are literally god- or goddess-given, rather than developed in a laboratory. In the same way that taking a watch apart and identifying its key parts will not show you how it works as a whole, dividing up a medicinal herb into its constituent parts cannot explain exactly how it works in its natural form. The whole herb is worth more than the sum of its parts, and scientific research is increasingly showing that the active constituents of many herbs, for example those in ginkgo (*Ginkgo biloba*, p. 104), interact in complex ways to produce the therapeutic effect of the remedy as a whole.

Plants contain hundreds, if not thousands, of different constituent chemicals that interact in complex ways. Frequently, we simply do not know in detail how a particular herb works—even though its medicinal benefit is well established. The pharmacological approach to understanding how whole herbs work is like working on a puzzle where only some of the pieces have been provided. Furthermore, although it is very useful to know that a plant contains certain active constituents, such information can be misleading on its own. For example, Chinese rhubarb (*Rheum palmatum*, p. 130) is a commonly used laxative, containing anthraquinones that irritate the gut wall and stimulate bowel movement. This laxative effect, however, occurs only when large quantities of the herb are used. At lower doses other constituents, notably tannins, which dry and tighten up mucous membranes in the gut, have greater effect. As a result, Chinese rhubarb works in two apparently opposite ways depending on the dosage: as a laxative at moderate to high doses; to treat diarrhea at a lower dose.

This example reveals a couple of fundamental truths about herbal medicine. Firstly, the experience of the herbal practitioner and of the patient often provide the most reliable guide to the medicinal effect of individual herbs. Secondly, the value of a medicinal herb cannot be reduced simply to a list of its active constituents.

Plants as foods & medicines

In general, the human body is much better suited to treatment with herbal remedies than with isolated chemical medicines. We have evolved side-by-side with plants over hundreds of thousands of years, and our digestive system and physiology as a whole are geared to digesting and utilizing plant-based foods, which often have a medicinal value as well as providing sustenance.

The dividing line between "foods" and "medicines" may not always be clear. Are lemons, papayas, onions, and oats foods or medicines? The answer, very simply, is that they are both. Lemon (*Citrus limon*, p. 86) improves resistance to infection; papaya (*Carica papaya*, p. 186) is taken in some parts of the world to expel worms; onion (*Allium cepa*, p. 168) relieves bronchial infections; and oats (*Avena sativa*, p. 179) support convalescence. Indeed, herbal medicine

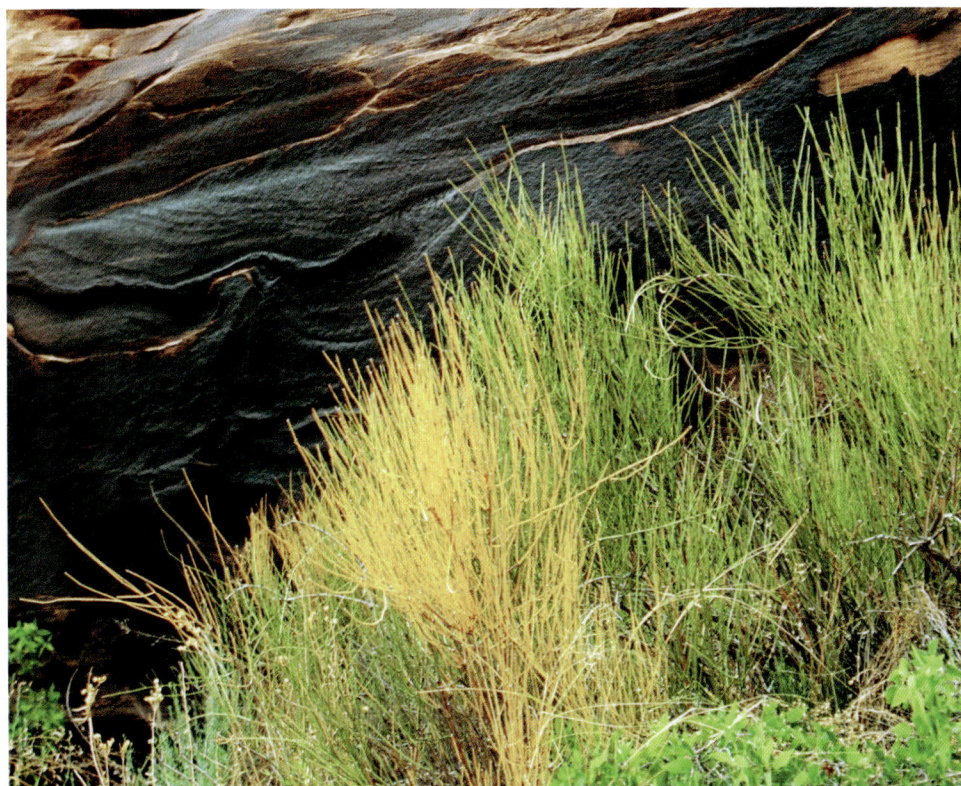

Wild ephedra *growing in Oljeto Canyon in Utah. One of the plant's components, ephedrine, is present in many cold remedies.*

comes into its own when the distinctions between foods and medicines are removed. Though we might eat a bowl of oatmeal oblivious to the medicinal benefits, it will, nonetheless, improve sleep and mental stamina, lower raised blood sugar and cholesterol levels, and maintain regular bowel function. A similar range of benefits is provided by many of the other gentler-acting herbs listed in the *Encyclopedia*.

Herbal treatments

The strategies that herbal practitioners adopt to prevent illness or restore health in their patients are different in the many and varied herbal traditions across the planet, but the effects that herbal medicines have within the body to improve health do not vary. There are many thousands of medicinal plants in use throughout the world, with a tremendous range of actions and degrees of potency. Most have a specific action on particular body systems and are known to be suitable for treating certain types of ailments. See p. 13 for specific actions.

Digestion, respiration, & circulation

Improving the quality of the diet is often an essential starting point in sustaining or regaining good health. The saying "You are what you eat" is by and large true, though herbalists prefer to qualify it, saying "You are what you *absorb* from what you eat." Herbal medicines not only provide nutrients, but when needed they also strengthen and support the action of the digestive system, speeding up the rate of processing food and improving the absorption of nutrients.

The body requires another kind of "nutrient" to function—oxygen. The lungs and respiratory system can be helped with herbs that relax the bronchial muscles and stimulate respiration.

Once taken in by the body, nutrients and medicines are carried to the body's estimated 35 trillion cells. The circulatory system has a remarkable ability to adapt to an endlessly shifting pattern of demand. At rest, the flow of blood is mainly toward the center of the body, while when active, the muscles in the

limbs make huge demands. Herbal medicines work to encourage circulation in particular ways. Some, for example, encourage blood to flow to the surface of the body; others stimulate the heart to pump more efficiently; while others relax the muscles of the arteries, lowering blood pressure. Herbs also work to promote tissue repair, healing, and cell renewal. The body is thought to replace 330 billion cells every day, mainly red blood cells.

Clearing toxicity & soothing skin

After circulation has carried nutrients to the cells, waste matter must be removed. All too often in our polluted world, high levels of toxicity in the body are an underlying cause of ill health, and herbalists use a wide range of cleansing herbs that improve the body's ability to remove toxins. Perhaps the finest example of a detoxifying herb is burdock (*Arctium lappa*, p. 69), which is used extensively in both Western and Chinese medicine. Once herbs such as this reduce the toxic "load," the body is able to invest greater resources in repairing and strengthening damaged tissue and weakened organs.

The skin also plays an important role in good health. Antiseptic plants fight infection, while vulnerary (wound-healing) herbs such as comfrey (*Symphytum officinale*, p. 142) encourage blood clotting and help speed the healing of wounds.

Nervous, endocrine, & immune systems

Good health depends on having a healthy, balanced nervous system. In order to ensure long-term good health of the nervous system, it is important to adapt well to life's daily demands, to avoid excessive anxiety, worry, or depression, and to get sufficient rest and exercise.

Research shows that the nervous system does not work in isolation but is complemented by the endocrine system, which controls the release of a whole symphony of hormones, including the sex hormones, which control fertility and often

affect vitality and mood. The nervous system is also intimately linked with the immune system, which controls the ability to resist infection and to recover from illness and injury.

This incredible complex of systems—part electrical, part chemical, part mechanical—must function harmoniously if good health is to be maintained. In health, the body has a seemingly infinite capacity, via its controlling systems, to adjust and change to external pressures. This ability to adapt to the external world while the body's internal workings remain constant is known as *homeostasis*. Many herbs work with the immune, nervous, and endocrine systems to help the body adapt more effectively to stresses and strains of all kinds: physical, mental, emotional, and even spiritual. They are effective because they work in tune with the body's processes.

Some herbs are *adaptogenic*, meaning that they have an ability to help people to adapt, either by supporting the nervous system and easing nervous and emotional tension, or by working directly with the body's own physiological processes to maintain health. This can make adaptogens hard to understand, as their many different effects on the body can appear exaggerated or contradictory. Ashwagandha (*Withania somnifera* p. 156), native to the Mediterranean and much of Asia, is a prime example of an adaptogen. Its main use is to support stamina and resilience at times of mental or physical stress, but it also has anti-inflammatory activity, relieves anxiety, encourages better sleep, enhances immune resistance, and increases muscle bulk and strength.

Complex natural medicines

As can be seen, an herb is not a "magic bullet" with a single action, but a complex natural medicine composed of many active constituents that work on different body systems. By combining scientific research into active constituents with clinical observation and traditional knowledge of the whole plant, we can develop a rounded picture of each herb's range of actions and medicinal uses.

Herbs & body systems

One of the most common ways of classifying medicinal plants is to identify their actions, for example whether they are sedative, antiseptic, or diuretic, and the degree to which they affect different body systems. Herbs often have a pronounced action on a particular body system, for example a plant that is strongly antiseptic in the digestive tract may be less so in the respiratory tract. Examples of how herbs work on the body are given below.

Skin

Antiseptics, e.g., tea tree (*Melaleuca alternifolia*, p. 116), disinfect the skin. *Emollients,* e.g., marsh mallow (*Althea officinalis*, p. 169), reduce itchiness, redness, and soreness. *Astringents,* e.g., witch hazel (*Hamamelis virginiana*, p. 106), tighten the skin. *Depuratives,* e.g., burdock (*Arctium lappa*, p. 69), encourage removal of waste products. *Healing and vulnerary herbs,* e.g., comfrey (*Symphytum officinale*, p. 142) and calendula (*Calendula officinalis*, p. 77), aid the healing of cuts, wounds, and abrasions.

Immune system

Immune modulators, e.g., echinacea (*Echinacea* spp. p. 96) and pau d'arco (*Tabebuia* spp., p. 143) strengthen the immune system.

Respiratory system

Antiseptics and antibiotics, e.g., garlic (*Allium sativum*, p. 63), help the lungs resist infection. *Expectorants,* e.g., elecampane (*Inula helenium*, p. 111), stimulate the coughing up of mucus. *Demulcents,* e.g., coltsfoot (*Tussilago farfara*, p. 288), soothe irritated membranes.

Endocrine glands

Adaptogens, e.g., ginseng (*Panax ginseng*, p. 123), help the body adjust to external pressures and stress. *Hormonally active herbs,* e.g., chaste tree (*Vitex agnus-castus*, p. 155), stimulate production of sex and other hormones. *Emmenagogues,* e.g., black cohosh (*Cimicifuga racemosa*, p. 61), encourage or regulate menstruation.

Urinary system

Antiseptics, e.g., buchu (*Barosma betulina*, p. 75), disinfect the urinary tubules. *Astringents,* e.g., horsetail (*Equisetum arvense*, p. 210), tighten and protect the urinary tubules. *Diuretics,* e.g. corn silk (*Zea mays*, p. 158), stimulate the flow of urine.

Musculoskeletal system

Analgesics, e.g., yellow jasmine (*Gelsemium sempervirens*, p. 220), relieve joint and nerve pain. *Anti-inflammatories,* e.g., white willow (*Salix alba*, p. 33), reduce swelling and pain in joints. *Antispasmodics,* e.g., cinchona (*Cinchona* spp., p. 84), relax tense and cramped muscles.

Nervous system

Nervines, e.g., rosemary (*Rosmarinus officinalis*, p. 132), support and strengthen the nervous system. *Relaxants,* e.g., lemon balm (*Melissa officinalis*, p. 117), relax the nervous system. *Sedatives,* e.g., mistletoe (*Viscum album*, p. 292), reduce nervous activity.

Circulation & heart

Cardiotonics, e.g., dan shen (*Salvia miltiorrhiza*, p. 134) promote effective heart function. *Circulatory stimulants,* e.g., cayenne (*Capsicum frutescens*, p. 79), improve circulation to the extremities. *Diaphoretics,* e.g., ju hua (*Chrysanthemum × morifolium*, p. 83), stimulate sweating, and lower blood pressure. *Spasmolytics,* e.g., cramp bark (*Viburnum opulus*, p. 154), relax muscle tone and lower blood pressure.

Digestive organs

Antiseptics e.g. ginger (*Zingiber officinale*, p. 159), protect against infection. *Astringents* e.g. bistort (*Polygonum bistorta*, p. 261), tighten up the inner lining of the intestines. *Bitters,* e.g., wormwood (*Artemisia absinthium*, p. 70), stimulate secretion of digestive juices. *Carminatives,* e.g., sweet flag (*Acorus calamus*, p. 163), relieve wind and griping pain. *Cholagogues* and *choleretics* e.g., artichoke (*Cynara scolymus*, p. 203), increase bile flow. *Demulcents,* e.g., psyllium (*Plantago* spp., p. 128), soothe the digestive system and protect against acidity and irritation. *Hepatics,* e.g., bupleurum (*Bupleurum chinense*, p. 76), prevent liver damage. *Laxatives,* e.g., senna (*Cassia senna*, p. 80), stimulate bowel movements. *Stomachics,* e.g., cardamom (*Elettaria cardamomum*, p. 97), protect and support the stomach.

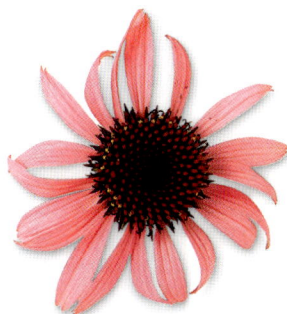

Echinacea
(Echinacea spp.)

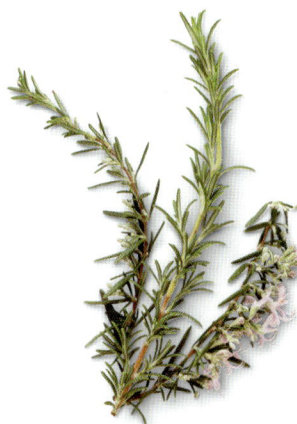

Rosemary
(Rosmarinus officinalis)

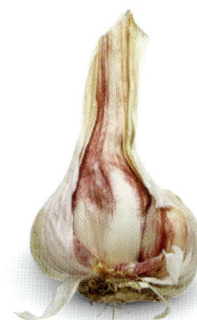

Garlic
(Allium sativum)

Active constituents

The medicinal effects of certain plants are well known. German chamomile, for example, has been taken to soothe digestive problems for thousands of years, and aloe vera was known to Cleopatra as a healing skin remedy. It is only relatively recently, however, that active constituents responsible for the medicinal actions of plants have been isolated and observed. Knowing a little about the chemicals contained in plants helps you understand how they work within the body.

Phenols

Phenols are a very varied group of plant constituents ranging from salicylic acid, a molecule similar to aspirin (acetylsalicylic acid), to complex sugar-containing phenolic glycosides. Phenols are often anti-inflammatory and antiseptic, and are thought to be produced by plants to protect against infection and feeding by insects. Phenolic acids such as caffeic and rosmarinic acids are strongly antioxidant and anti-inflammatory, and can also have antiviral properties. Wintergreen (*Gaultheria procumbens*, p. 220) and white willow (*Salix alba*, p. 133) both contain salicylates. Many mint family members contain phenols—for example, the strongly antiseptic thymol, found in thyme (*Thymus vulgaris*, p. 147).

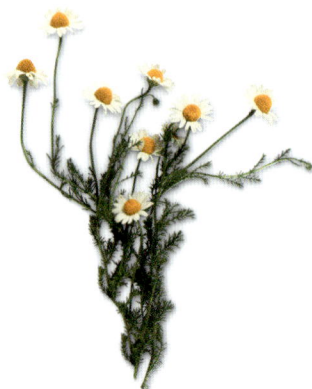

Volatile oils

Volatile oils—which are extracted from plants to produce essential oils—are some of the most important medicinally active plant constituents, and are also used widely in perfumery. They are complex mixtures often of 100 or more compounds, mostly made up of monoterpenes—molecules containing 10 carbon atoms. Essential oils have many uses. Tea tree oil (*Melaleuca alternifolia*, p. 116) is strongly antiseptic, while sweet gale oil (*Myrica gale*, p. 245) is an effective insect repellent. On distillation, some essential oils contain compounds not found in the volatile oil—chamazulene, found in German chamomile (*Chamomilla recutita*, p. 82) essential oil, is anti-inflammatory and anti-allergenic. Resins—sticky oily substances that seep from plants, for example from the bark of Scots pine (*Pinus sylvestris*, p. 257)—are often linked with essential oils (oleoresins) and gums (see Polysaccharides), though they are nonvolatile.

Flavonoids

Found widely throughout the plant world, flavonoids are polyphenolic compounds that act as pigments, imparting color, often yellow or white, to flowers and fruits. They have a wide range of actions and many medicinal uses. They are antioxidant and especially useful in maintaining healthy circulation. Some flavonoids also have anti-inflammatory, antiviral, and liver-protective activity. Flavonoids such as hesperidin and rutin, found in many plants, notably buckwheat (*Fagopyrum esculentum*, p. 215) and lemon (*Citrus limon*, p. 86), strengthen capillaries and prevent leakage into surrounding tissues. Isoflavones, found for example in red clover (*Trifolium pratense*, p. 287), are estrogenic and valuable in treating menopausal symptoms.

Tannins

Tannins are produced to a greater or lesser degree by all plants. The harsh, astringent taste of tannin-laden bark and leaves makes them unpalatable to insects and grazing animals. Tannins are polyphenolic compounds that

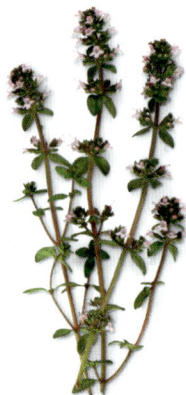

Thyme
(*Thymus vulgaris*)

German Chamomile
(*Chamomilla recutita*)

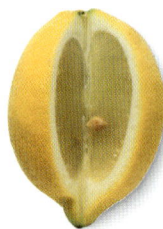

Lemon
(*Citrus limon*)

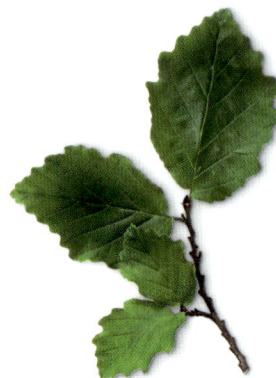

Black Catechu
(*Acacia catechu*)

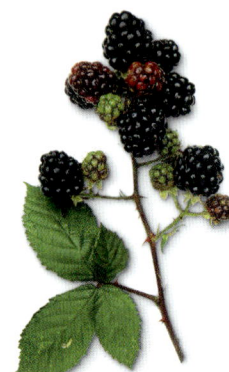

Blackberry
(*Rubus fruticosus*)

contract and astringe tissues of the body by binding with and precipitating proteins—hence their use to "tan" leather. They also help to stop bleeding and to check infection. Tannin-containing herbs are used to tighten up over-relaxed tissues—as in varicose veins—to dry up excessive watery secretions—as in diarrhea—and to protect damaged tissue—such as skin problems resulting from eczema or a burn. Oak bark (*Quercus robur*, p. 268) and black catechu (*Acacia catechu*, p. 278) are both high in tannins.

Proanthocyanidins

Closely related to tannins and flavonoids, these polyphenolic compounds are pigments that give flowers and fruits a blue, purple, or red hue. They are powerfully antioxidant and free-radical scavengers. They protect the circulation from damage, especially the circulation in the heart, hands, feet, and eyes. Blackberry (*Rubus fruticosus*, p. 272), red grapes (*Vitis vinifera*, p. 293), and hawthorn (*Crataegus oxyacantha*, p. 91) all contain appreciable quantities of these proanthocyanins.

Coumarins

Coumarins of different kinds are found in many plant species and have widely divergent actions. The coumarins in melilot (*Melilotus officinalis*, p. 240) and horse chestnut (*Aesculus hippocastanum*, p. 62) help to keep the blood thin, while furanocoumarins such as bergapten, found in celery (*Apium graveolens*, p. 68), stimulate skin tanning, and khellin, found in visnaga (*Ammi visnaga*, p. 65), is a powerful smooth-muscle relaxant.

Saponins

The main active constituents in many key medicinal plants, saponins gained their name because, like soap, they make a lather when placed in water. Saponins occur in two different forms—steroidal and triterpenoid. The chemical structure of steroidal saponins is similar to that of many of the body's hormones, for example estrogen and cortisol, and many plants containing them have a marked hormonal activity. Wild yam (*Dioscorea villosa*, p. 95), from which the contraceptive pill was first developed, contains steroidal saponins. Triterpenoid saponins occur more commonly—for example in licorice (*Glycyrrhiza glabra*, p. 105) and cowslip root (*Primula veris*, p. 264)—but have less hormonal activity. They are often expectorant and aid absorption of nutrients.

Anthraquinones

Anthraquinones are the main active constituents in herbs such as senna (*Cassia senna*, p. 80) and Chinese rhubarb (*Rheum palmatum*, p. 130), both of which are taken to relieve constipation. Anthraquinones have an irritant laxative effect on the large intestine, causing contractions of the intestinal walls and stimulating a bowel movement approximately 10 hours after being taken. They also make the stool more liquid, easing bowel movements.

Cardiac glycosides

Found in various medicinal plants, notably in foxgloves (see common foxglove, *Digitalis purpurea*, p. 207) and in lily of the valley (*Convallaria majalis*, p. 198), cardiac glycosides such as digitoxin, digoxin, and convallatoxin have a strong, direct action on the heart, supporting its strength and rate of contraction when it is failing. Cardiac glycosides are also significantly diuretic. They help to stimulate urine production, thus increasing the removal of fluid from the tissues and circulatory system.

Cyanogenic glycosides

Though these glycosides are based on cyanide, a very potent poison, in small doses they have a helpful sedative and relaxant effect on the heart and muscles. The bark of wild cherry (*Prunus serotina*, p. 265) and the leaves of elder (*Sambucus nigra*, p. 136) both contain cyanogenic glycosides, which contribute to the plant's ability to suppress and soothe irritant dry coughs. Many fruit kernels contain high levels of cyanogenic glycosides, for example those of apricot (*Prunus armeniaca*, p. 264).

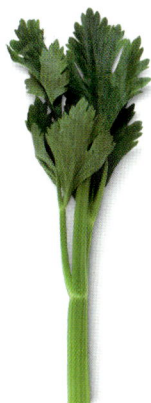

Celery
(*Apium graveolens*)

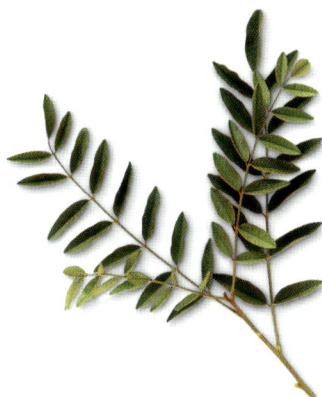

Licorice
(*Glycyrrhiza glabra*)

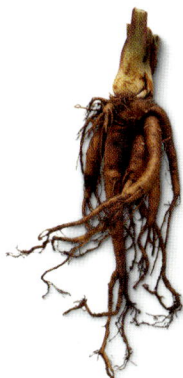

Chinese Rhubarb
(*Rheum palmatum*)

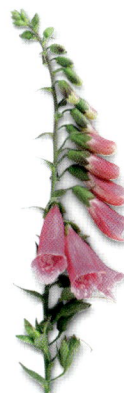

Common Foxglove
(*Digitalis purpurea*)

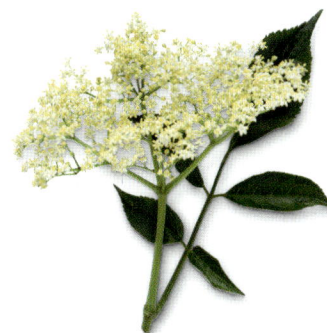

Elderflower
(*Sambucus nigra*)

Polysaccharides

Found in all plants, polysaccharides are multiple units of sugar molecules linked together. From an herbal point of view, the most important polysaccharides are the "sticky" mucilages and gums, which are commonly found in roots, bark, leaves, and seeds. Both mucilage and gum soak up large quantities of water, producing a sticky, jellylike mass that can be used to soothe and protect irritated tissue, for example, dry irritated skin and sore or inflamed mucous membranes in the gut. Mucilaginous herbs, such as slippery elm (*Ulmus rubra*, p. 149) and linseed or flaxseed (*Linum usitatissimum*, p. 113), are best prepared by soaking (macerating) in plenty of cold water. Some polysaccharides stimulate the immune system, for example acemannan, which is found in the leaves of aloe vera (*Aloe vera*, p. 64).

Glucosinolates

Found exclusively in species of the mustard and cabbage family, glucosinolates have an irritant effect on the skin, causing inflammation and blistering. Applied as poultices to painful or aching joints, they increase blood flow to the affected area, helping to remove the buildup of waste products (a contributory factor in many joint problems). On eating, glucosinolates are broken down and produce a strong, pungent taste. Radish (*Raphanus sativus*, p. 269) and watercress (*Nasturtium officinale*, p. 246) are typical glucosinolate-containing plants.

Bitters

Bitters are a varied group of constituents linked only by their pronounced bitter taste. The bitterness itself stimulates secretions by the salivary glands and digestive organs. Such secretions can dramatically improve the appetite and strengthen the overall function of the digestive system. With the improved digestion and absorption of nutrients that follow, the body is nourished and strengthened. Many herbs have bitter constituents, notably wormwood (*Artemisia absinthium*, p. 70), chiretta (*Swertia chirata*, p. 283), and hops (*Humulus lupulus*, p. 108).

Alkaloids

A very mixed group, alkaloids mostly contain a nitrogen-bearing molecule ($-NH_2$) that makes them particularly pharmacologically active. Some are well-known drugs and have a recognized medical use. Vincristine, for example, derived from Madagascar periwinkle (*Vinca rosea*, p. 292), is used to treat some types of cancer. Berberine, from Barberry (*Berberis vulgaris*, p. 181) has antibiotic and anti-inflammatory activity. Other alkaloids, such as atropine, found in deadly nightshade (*Atropa belladonna*, p. 73), have a direct effect on the body, reducing spasms, relieving pain, and drying up bodily secretions.

Vitamins

Though often overlooked, many medicinal plants contain useful levels of vitamins. Some are well known for their vitamin content, for example dog rose (*Rosa canina*, p. 271) has high levels of vitamin C, and carrot (*Daucus carota*, p. 205) is rich in beta-carotene (pro-vitamin A), but many are less well recognized. Watercress (*Nasturtium officinale*, p. 246), for example, contains appreciable levels of vitamins B_1, B_2, C, and E as well as beta-carotene, while sea buckthorn (*Hippophae rhamnoides*, p. 225) can be regarded as a vitamin and mineral supplement in its own right.

Minerals

Like vegetable foods, many medicinal plants provide high levels of minerals. Plants, especially organically grown ones, draw minerals from the soil and convert them into a form that is more easily absorbed and used by the body. Whether plants are eaten as a vegetable, like cabbage (*Brassica oleracea*, p. 183), or taken as a medicine, like bladder wrack (*Fucus vesiculosus*, p. 218), in many cases the mineral content is a key factor in the plant's therapeutic activity within the body. Dandelion leaf (*Taraxacum officinale*, p. 145) is a potent diuretic, balanced by its high potassium content, while the high silica content of horsetail (*Equisetum arvense*, p. 210) supports the repair of connective tissue, making it useful in arthritis.

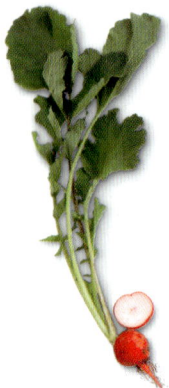

Radish
(Raphanus sativus)

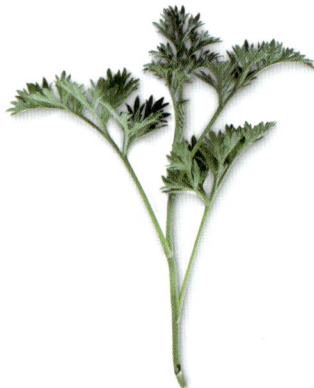

Wormwood
(Artemisia absinthium)

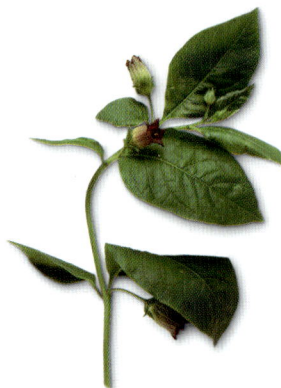

Deadly Nightshade
(Atropa belladonna)

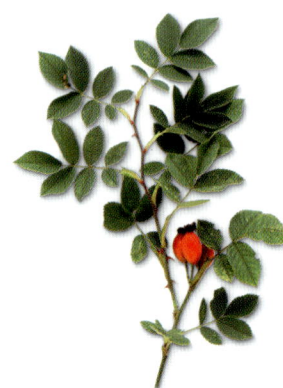

Dog Rose
(Rosa canina)

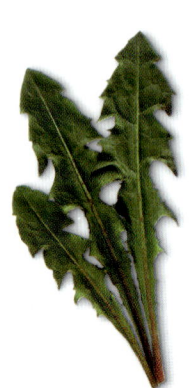

Dandelion
(Taraxacum officinale)

Quality control

Making the most of herbal medicine means ensuring that herbs and herbal products used are of good quality—properly grown, well dried, correctly processed, and within their sell-by date. Using poor-quality herbal produce is all too often a waste of money since there is the strong possibility that you will receive little benefit from it. When it comes to herbal medicine, quality is everything.

Quality is vital for herbal medicine. Without a guarantee that the correct herb of the right quality is being used, it is hard to be confident that the medicine will prove effective. In fact, one reason why the medical profession has generally preferred conventional medicines to herbal ones is the difficulty of guaranteeing quality in herbal remedies. Many herbal products on the market are of high quality but some can be very poor, as Mark Blumenthal, founder and executive director of the American Botanical Council, explains (2018):

The increased popularity of herbs like turmeric attracts producers and suppliers who are often more concerned about making a profit than they are about selling a high-quality botanical ingredient. While there are companies that produce and market high-quality, authentic, reliable turmeric powder and extract supplements, there are also adulterated turmeric ingredients on the market.

Turmeric powder is often diluted with rice flour, but adulterants can include yellow dyes and synthetic curcumin, an artificial version of the main active constituent.

A 2006 US study of black cohosh (*Cimicifuga racemosa*, p. 61) found that only 7 out of 11 over-the-counter products tested contained what was stated on the label. Four contained a cheaper Chinese species instead. The adulteration of herbal products, particularly in Chinese and Indian herbs and powders sold in the West is, regrettably, not unusual, though perhaps counterintuitively, research suggests that herb adulteration occurs more commonly in Europe and the US than in Asia.

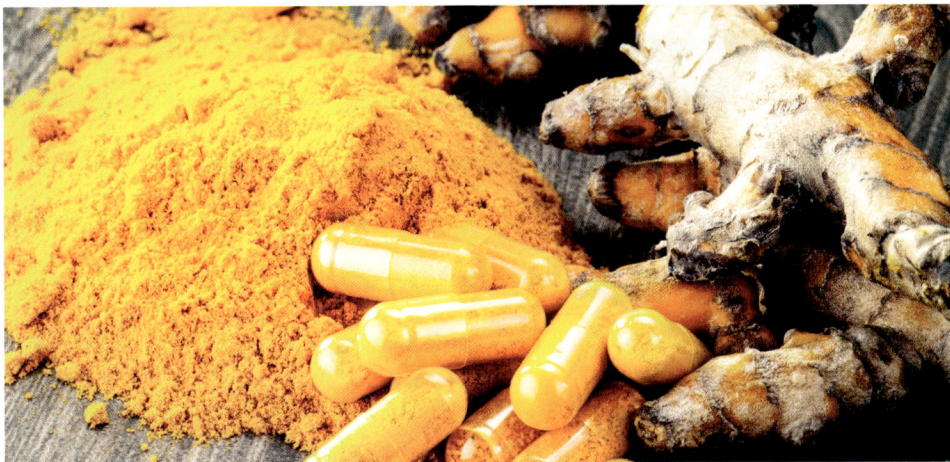

Turmeric powder can be adulterated with yellow dyes and synthetic curcumin. Try to seek out manufacturers that are known to produce high quality, reliable extracts and supplements.

Herb quality may be affected not only by deliberate adulteration, but by the use of wrongly identified or poor-quality material. The herb may have been poorly harvested, dried, or stored, or it may be old or decayed. It may even be that the wrong herb was used. In each case, the lack of attention to quality results in a product with reduced medicinal value—or even none at all.

To try to ensure that only good-quality products are made, manufacturers of genuine herbal medicines use strict quality-control procedures. Usually this involves comparing the dried herb material with listings in an herbal or national pharmacopoeia (a standard reference work that gives the characteristics one would expect to find when analyzing a specific herb). Quality control involves making routine checks to establish that the herbal material is what it claims to be and that it meets a number of minimum requirements. The material is inspected with the naked eye, and assessed microscopically, to see if its botanical profile matches the standard. Other checks are made to see whether it contains appropriate levels of active constituents and to ensure that the material is free from contamination.

More sensitive quality-control methods, however, recognize that the quality of an herb does not depend simply on the presence of one or two key active constituents. Increasingly, people in the world of herbal medicine are focusing on the "fingerprint" of an herb—the unique chemical profile that represents the complex pattern of constituents found when good-quality dried herb material is analyzed by sensitive scientific machinery. By monitoring the sample and comparing it with this unique fingerprint, it is possible to make a much broader assessment of quality than when using only one or two constituents as a standard.

Early origins to the 19th century

In an age of medical specialization in which an expert in neurology will know little about the latest developments in medicine for the ear, nose, and throat, it is difficult to imagine the practices of an earlier time, when healing was holistic in nature and heavily reliant on magic, mysticism, and age-old oral traditions.

From the earliest times, medicinal plants have been crucial in sustaining the health and the well-being of mankind. Flaxseed (*Linum usitatissimum*, p. 113), for example, provided its harvesters with a nutritious food oil, fuel, a cosmetic balm for the skin, and fiber to make fabric. At the same time it was used to treat conditions such as bronchitis, respiratory congestion, boils, and a number of digestive problems. Given the life-enhancing benefits that this and so many other plants conferred, it is hardly surprising that most cultures believed them to have magical as well as medicinal abilities. It is reasonable to assume that for tens of thousands of years herbs were probably used as much for their ritual magical powers as for their medicinal qualities. A 60,000-year-old burial site excavated in Iraq, for instance, was found to contain eight different medicinal plants, including ephedra (*Ephedra sinica*, p. 99). The inclusion of the plants in the tomb suggests they had supernatural significance as well as medicinal value.

In some cultures, plants were considered to have souls. Even Aristotle, the 4th-century BCE Greek philosopher, thought that plants had a "psyche," albeit of a lesser order than the human soul. In Hinduism, which dates back to at least 1500 BCE, many plants are sacred to specific divinities. For example, the bael tree (*Aegle marmelos*, p. 165) is said to shelter Shiva, the god of health, beneath its branches.

In medieval Europe, the Doctrine of Signatures stated there was a connection between how a plant looked—God's "signature"—and how it might be used medicinally. For example, the mottled leaves of lungwort (*Pulmonaria officinalis*, p. 266) were thought to resemble lung tissue, and the plant is still used to treat ailments of the respiratory tract.

Even in Western cultures, beliefs in plant spirits linger. Until the first half of the 20th century, British farm workers would not cut down elder trees (*Sambucus nigra*, p. 136) for fear of arousing the anger of the Elder Mother, the spirit who lived in and protected the tree.

In a similar vein, Indigenous peoples of the Andes in South America believe that the coca plant (*Erythroxylum coca*, p. 211) is protected

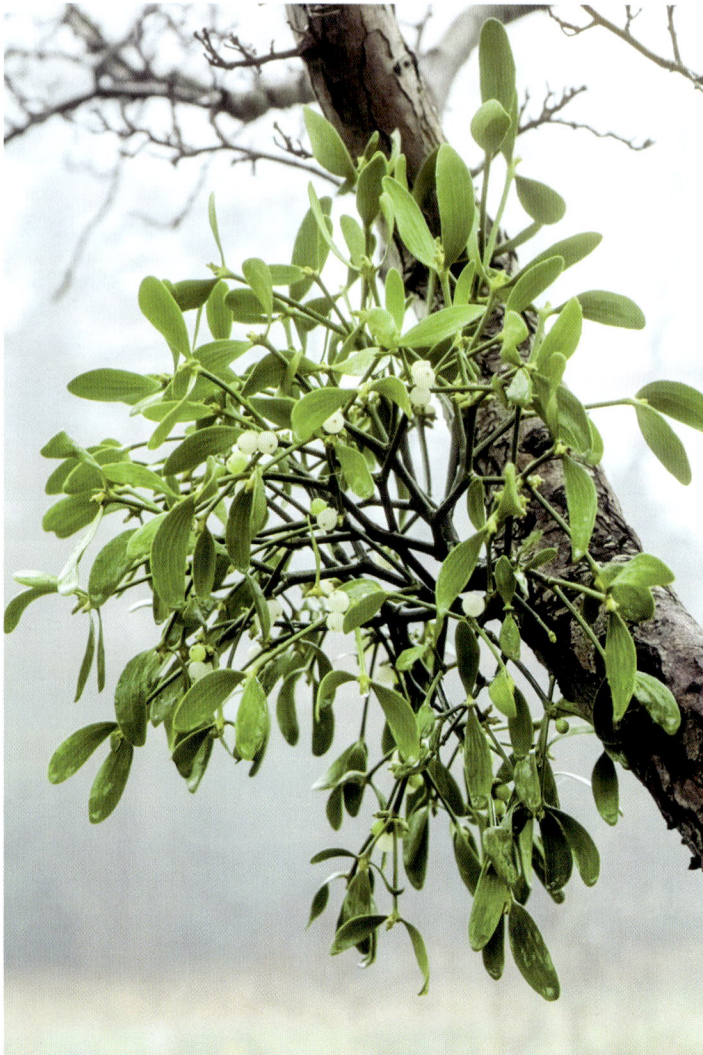

Mistletoe, which the Druids called "golden bough," had a central place in their shamanistic religious and healing ceremonies. The Druids had a well-developed knowledge of medicinal plants.

"It is reasonable to assume that for tens of thousands of years herbs were probably used as much for their ritual magical powers as for their medicinal qualities."

by Mama Coca, a spirit who must be respected and placated if the leaves are to be harvested and used.

Shamanistic medicine

In many traditional societies today, the world is believed to be shaped by good and evil spirits. In these societies, illness is thought to stem from malignant forces or possession by evil spirits. If a member of the tribe falls ill, the shaman (the "medicine" person) is expected to intercede with the spirit world to bring about a cure. Shamans often enter the spiritual realm with the aid of hallucinogenic plants or fungi, such as ayahuasca (*Banisteriopsis caapi*, p. 181), taken by Amazonian shamans, or fly agaric (*Amanita muscaria*), taken by traditional healers of the Siberian steppes.

At the same time, the shaman provides medical treatment for the physical needs of the patient—putting salves and compresses on wounds, boiling up decoctions and barks for internal treatment, stimulating sweating for fevers, and so on. Such treatment is based on a wealth of acutely observed plant lore and knowledge, handed down in an oral tradition from generation to generation.

The development of medicinal lore

It is generally recognized that our ancestors had a wide range of medicinal plants at their disposal, and that they likewise possessed a profound understanding of plants' healing powers. In fact, up until the 20th century, every village and rural community had a wealth of herbal folklore. Tried and tested local plants were picked for a range of

common health problems and taken as teas, applied as lotions, or even mixed with lard and rubbed in as an ointment.

But what were the origins of this herbal expertise? There are no definitive answers. Clearly, acute observation coupled with trial and error has played a predominant role. Human societies have had many thousands of years to observe the effects—both good and bad—of eating a particular root, leaf, or berry. Watching the behavior of animals after they have eaten or rubbed against certain plants has also added to medicinal lore. If one watches sheep or cattle, they almost unerringly steer a path past poisonous plants such as ragwort (*Senecio jacobaea*) or oleander (*Nerium oleander*). Over and above such close observation, some people have speculated that human beings, like grazing animals, have an instinct that recognizes poisonous as opposed to medicinal plants.

Ancient civilizations

As civilizations grew from 3000 BCE onward in Egypt, the Middle East, India, and China, so the use of herbs became more sophisticated, and the first written accounts of medicinal plants were made. The Egyptian Ebers papyrus of c. 1500 BCE is the earliest surviving example. It lists dozens of medicinal plants, their uses, and related spells and incantations. The herbs include myrrh (*Commiphora myrrha*, p. 89), castor oil (*Ricinus communis*, p. 271), and garlic (*Allium sativum*, p. 63).

In India, the *Vedas*, epic poems written c. 1500 BCE, also contain rich material on the herbal lore of that time. The *Vedas* were followed in about 400 BCE by the *Charaka*

Samhita, written by the physician Charaka. This medical treatise includes details of around 350 herbal medicines. Among them are visnaga (*Ammi visnaga*, p. 65), an herb of Middle Eastern origin that has recently proven effective in the treatment of asthma, and gotu kola (*Centella asiatica*, p. 81), which has long been used to treat leprosy.

Medicine breaks from its mystical origins

By about 500 BCE in developed cultures, medicine began to separate from the magical and spiritual world. Hippocrates (460–377 BCE), the Greek "father of medicine," considered illness to be a natural rather than a supernatural phenomenon, and he felt that medicine should be given without ritual ceremonies or magic.

In the earliest Chinese medical text, the *Yellow Emperor's Classic of Internal Medicine* written in the 1st century BCE, the emphasis on rational medicine is equally clear: "In treating illness, it is necessary to examine the entire context, scrutinize the symptoms, observe the emotions and attitudes. If one insists on the presence of ghosts and spirits one cannot speak of therapeutics."

Foundation of major herbal traditions 300 BCE–600 CE

Trade between Europe, the Middle East, India, and Asia was already well under way by the 2nd century BCE, and trade routes became established for many medicinal and culinary herbs. Cloves (*Eugenia caryophyllata*, p. 101), for example, which are native to the Philippines and the Molucca Islands near New

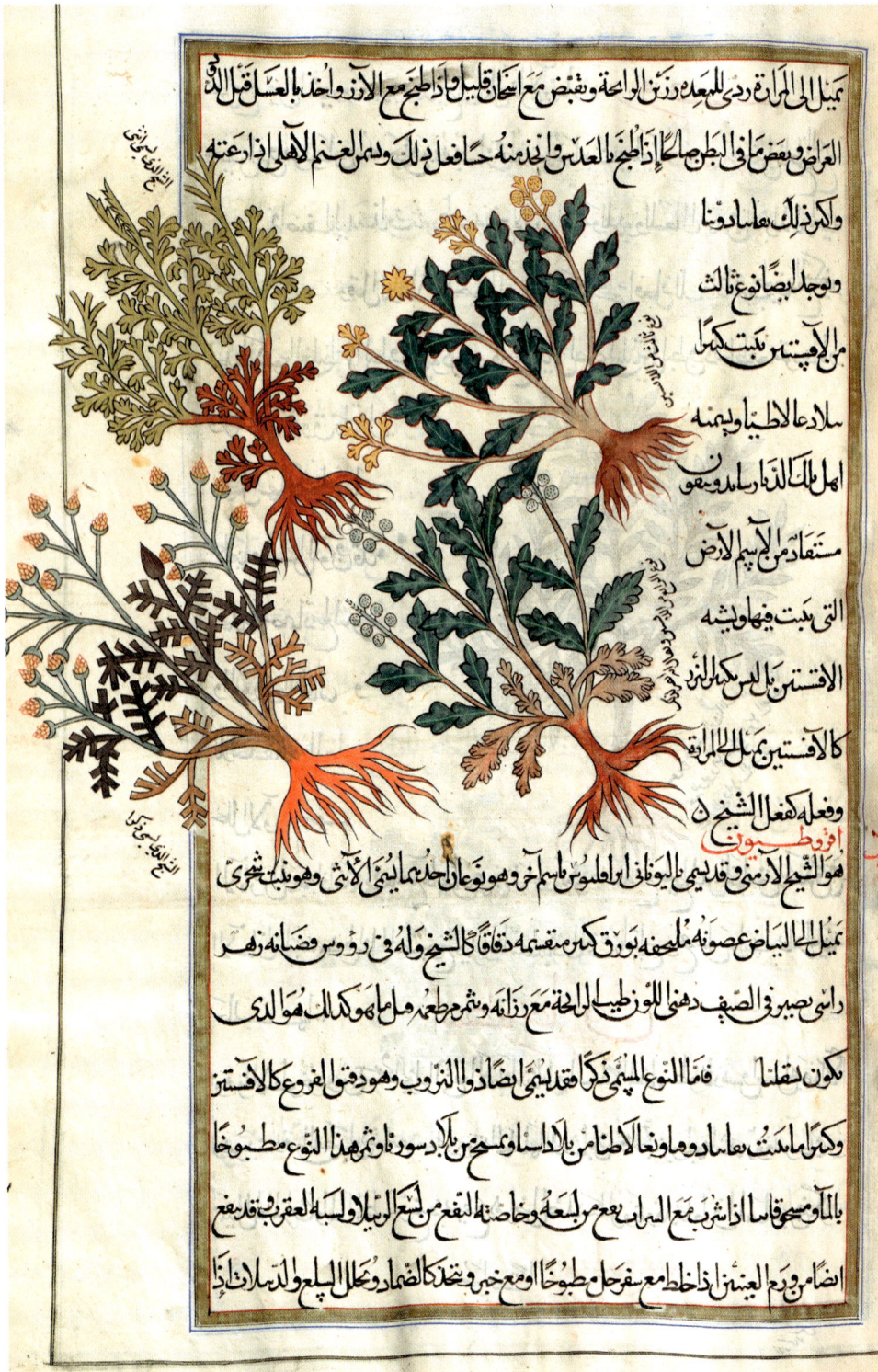

Botanical drawing from a page of the De Materia Medica *by 1st-century CE Greek physician, Dioscorides. His intention was to produce an accurate and authoritative reference work on herbal medicines.*

Guinea, were imported into China in the 3rd century BCE, and first arrived in Egypt around 176 CE. As the centuries passed, the popularity of cloves grew, and by the 8th century CE, their strong aromatic flavor and powerfully antiseptic and analgesic properties were familiar throughout most of Europe.

As trade and interest in herbal medicines and spices flourished, various writers tried to make systematic records of plants with a known medicinal action and record their properties.

In China, the *Divine Husbandman's Classic* (*Shen'nong Bencaojing*), written in the 1st century CE, has 364 entries, of which 252 are herbal medicines, including bupleurum (*Bupleurum chinense*, p. 76), coltsfoot (*Tussilago farfara*, p. 288), and *gan cao* (*Glycyrrhiza uralensis*). This Daoist text laid the foundations for the continuous development and refinement of Chinese herbal medicine up to the present day.

In Europe, a 1st-century CE Greek physician named Dioscorides wrote the first European herbal, *De Materia Medica*. His intention was to produce an accurate and authoritative work on herbal medicines, and in this he was dramatically successful. Among the many plants mentioned are juniper (*Juniperus communis*, p. 229), elm (*Ulmus carpinifolia*), peony (*Paeonia officinalis*, p. 250), and burdock (*Arctium lappa*, p. 69). The text, listing about 600 herbs in all, was to have an astonishing influence on Western medicine, being the principal reference used in Europe until the 17th century. It was translated into languages as varied as Anglo-Saxon, Persian, and Hebrew. In 512 CE, *De Materia Medica* became the first herbal to feature pictures of the plants discussed. Made for Anicia Juliana, the daughter of the Roman emperor Flavius Anicius Olybrius, it contained nearly 400 full-page color illustrations.

Galen (131–200 CE), physician to the Roman emperor Marcus Aurelius, had an equally profound influence on the development of herbal medicine. Galen drew inspiration from Hippocrates and based his theories on the "theory of the four humors" (*see* p. 36). His ideas shaped and, some would say, distorted medical practice for the next 1,400 years.

In India and in China, elaborate medical systems somewhat resembling the theory of the four humors developed (*see* pp. 40–42 and pp. 44–45 respectively) that have endured to the present day.

Though European, Indian, and Chinese systems differ widely, they all consider that imbalance within the constituent elements of the body is the cause of illness, and that the aim of the healer is to restore balance, often with the aid of herbal remedies.

Folk healing in the Middle Ages

The theories of Galenic, Ayurvedic (Indian), and Chinese traditional medicine, however, would have meant practically nothing to most of the world's population. As is still the case today for some Indigenous peoples who have little access to conventional medicines, in the past most villages and communities relied on the services of local "wise" people for medical treatment. These healers were almost certainly ignorant of the conventions of scholastic medicine, yet through apprenticeship and practice in treating illness, attending childbirth, and making use of locally growing herbs as a natural pharmacy, they developed a high level of practical medical knowledge.

We tend to underestimate the medical skills of apparently undeveloped communities—particularly during the so-called Dark Ages in medieval Europe—but it is evident that many people had a surprisingly sophisticated understanding of plant medicine. For example, recent excavations at an 11th-century monastic hospital in Scotland revealed that the monks were using exotic herbs such as opium poppy (*Papaver somniferum*, p. 251) and marijuana (*Cannabis sativa*, p. 78) as painkillers and anesthetics. Likewise, the herbalists in Myddfai, a village in South Wales, obviously knew of Hippocrates' writings in the 6th century CE and used a

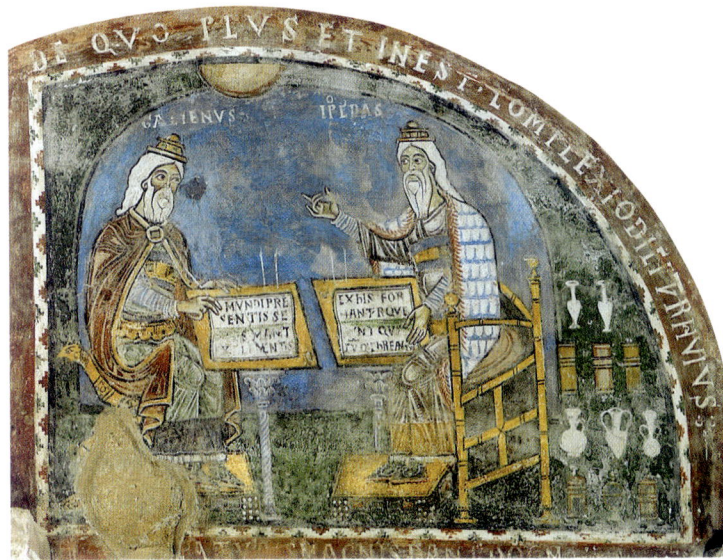

Galen and Hippocrates, *two of the preeminent physicians of the classical era, debate in this imaginary scene depicted in a fresco..*

wide variety of medicinal plants. The texts that have been handed down from that herbal tradition are filled with an engaging blend of superstition and wisdom. Two prescriptions from a 13th-century manuscript illustrate the point. The first recipe could have been written by a modern, scientifically trained herbalist; the second, one must presume, is pure fancy, and would not choose to try it out!:

To strengthen the sight
Take Eyebright and Red Fennel, a handful of each, and half a handful of Rue, distill, and wash your eye daily therewith.

To destroy a worm in the tooth
Take the root of a cat's ear, bruise, and apply to the patient's tooth for three nights, and it will kill the worm.

Islamic & Indian medicine 500–1500 CE

Folk medicine was largely unaffected by sweeping forces of history, but Western scholastic medicine suffered greatly with the decline of the Roman Empire.

It was thanks to the flowering of Arabic culture in 500–1300 CE that the gains of the classical Greek and Roman period were preserved and elaborated. The spread of Islamic culture along North Africa and into present-day Italy, Spain, and Portugal led to the founding of renowned medical schools, notably at Córdoba in Spain. The Arabs were expert pharmacists, blending and mixing herbs to improve their medicinal effect and their taste. Their contacts with both Indian and Chinese medical traditions meant that they had a remarkable range of medical and herbal knowledge to draw on and develop. Ibn Sina (980–1037 CE), author of *Canon of Medicine*, was the most famous physician of the day, but perhaps the most unusual herbal connection was made a century before his time by Ibn Cordoba, an intrepid Arab seafarer, who brought ginseng root (*Panax ginseng*, p. 123) from China to Europe. This valuable tonic herb was to be regularly imported into Europe from the 16th century onward.

Further east, in India, the 7th century saw the arrival of a golden age of medicine. Thousands of students studied Ayurveda at universities across the subcontinent, especially at Nalanda. There, scholars recorded the medical achievements of the time, with advances such as the development of hospitals, maternity homes, and the planting of medicinal herb gardens.

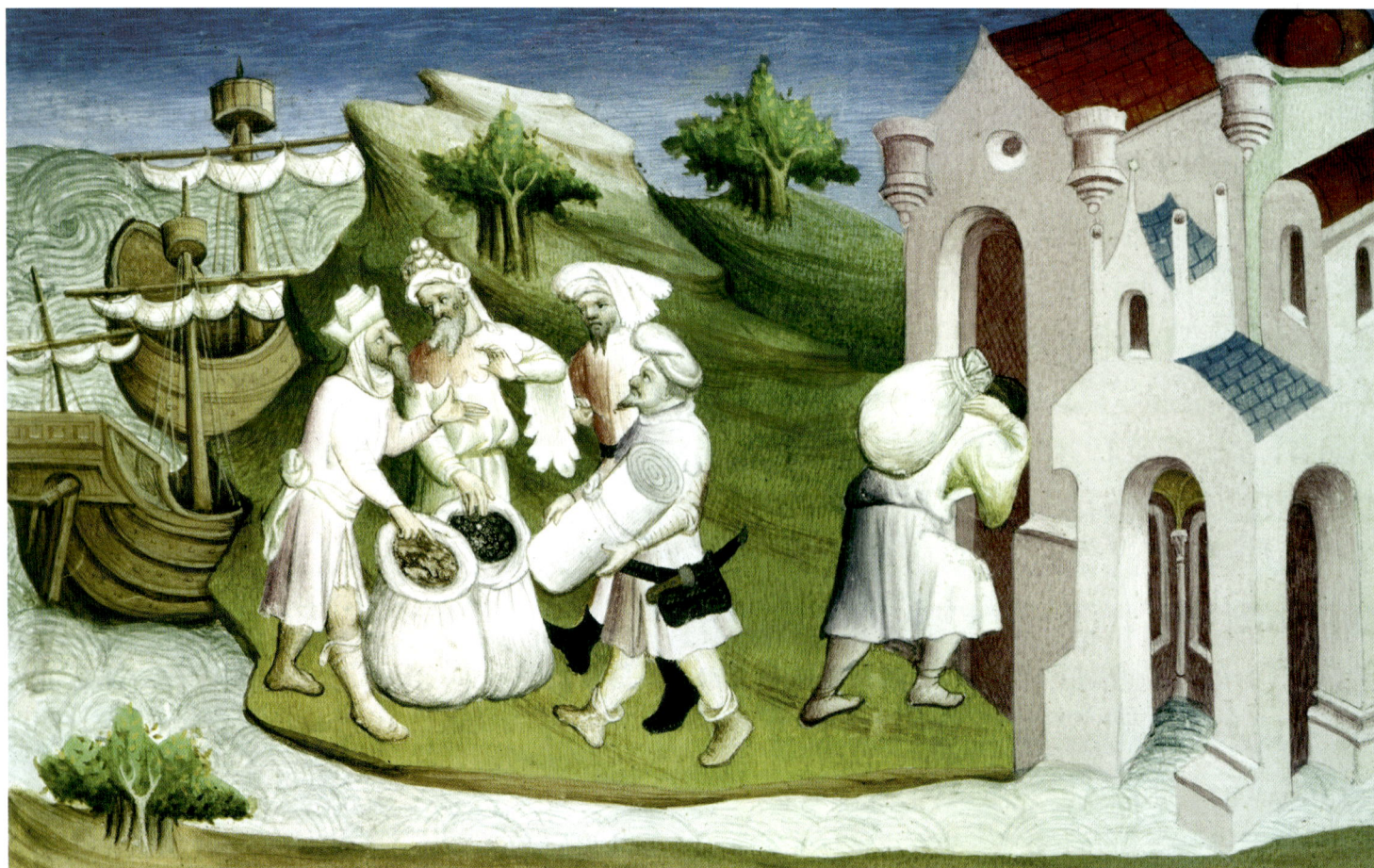

Marco Polo's voyage to China in the 14th century opened the door for a flourishing reciprocal trade in goods, including medicinal herbs, between East and West. Eventually, exotic herbs like ginger, cinnamon, and cloves became widely used in European medicine and cooking.

Central & South American cures

On the other side of the world, the ancient civilizations of Central and South America—Maya, Aztec, and Inca—all had herbal traditions with a profound understanding of local medicinal plants. One account tells of Incas taking local herbalists from what is now Bolivia back to their capital Cuzco in Peru because of the herbalists' great capabilities, which reputedly included growing penicillin on green banana skins.

At the same time, medicine and religion were still closely interwoven in these cultures, possibly even more so than in Europe. One gruesome account tells of Aztec sufferers of skin diseases who sought to appease the god Xipe Totec by wearing the flayed skins of sacrificial victims. Fortunately, a supernatural appeal to the gods was not the sole means to relieve this and other afflictions. Many herbs were available as alternative treatments, including sarsaparilla (*Smilax* spp., p. 279), a tonic and cleansing herb that was used in treatments for a variety of skin complaints including eczema and psoriasis.

Rebirth of European scholarship 1000–1400 CE

As European scholars slowly started to absorb the lessons of Arabic medical learning in the early Middle Ages, classical Greek, Roman, and Egyptian texts preserved in the libraries of Constantinople (later Istanbul) filtered back to Europe, and hospitals, medical schools, and universities were founded. Perhaps the most interesting among them was the medical school at Salerno on the west coast of Italy. It not only allowed students from all faiths—Christian, Muslim, and Jewish—to study medicine, but it also allowed women to train as physicians. Trotula, a woman who wrote a book on obstetrics, practiced and taught there in the 12th century CE. Herbs were, of course, central to the healing process. An adage from the Salerno school on sage (*Salvia officinalis*, p. 135) went as follows: *Salvia salvatrix, natura conciliatrix* (sage, the savior; nature, the conciliator).

By the 12th century, trade with Asia and Africa was expanding and new herbs and spices were being regularly imported into Europe. Hildegard of Bingen (1098–1179), the famous German mystic and herbal

"By the 12th century, trade with Asia and Africa was expanding and new herbs and spices were being regularly imported into Europe."

authority, considered galangal (*Alpinia officinarum*, p. 169)—used in Asia as a warming and nourishing spice for the digestive system— to be the "spice of life," given by God to provide health and to protect against illness.

Asian unification

Marco Polo's travels to China in the 14th century coincided with the unification of the whole of Asia from the Yellow Sea in China to the Black Sea in southeastern Europe by Genghis Khan and his grandson Kublai Khan, whose capital was in China, not far from Beijing. Neither the Chinese nor Ayurvedic medical traditions were directly threatened by this conquest. The Mongol rulers were strict in banning the use of certain toxic plants such as aconite (*Aconitum napellus*, p. 163), but their decree may have held an element of self-preservation, given aconite's alternative use as an arrow poison—one that could have been used against the ruling powers. Moreover, the Mongol unification may have encouraged greater communication between the two medical disciplines.

In other parts of Asia, such as Vietnam and Japan, Chinese culture and medicine exerted the primary influence. While *kampoh*—the traditional herbal medicine of Japan—is distinctive to that country, its roots stem from Chinese practices.

Trade between continents 1400–1700

Trade routes had slowly expanded during the Middle Ages, bringing exotic new herbs in their wake. From the 15th century onward, an explosion in trade led to a cornucopia of new herbs becoming readily available in Europe. They included plants such as ginger (*Zingiber officinale*, p. 159), cardamom (*Elettaria cardamomum*, p. 97), nutmeg (*Myristica fragrans*, p. 119), turmeric (*Curcuma longa*, p. 94), cinnamon (*Cinnamomum* spp., p. 85), and senna (*Cassia senna*, p. 80). The trade in herbs was not entirely one way. The European herb sage, for example, came into use in China, where it was considered to be a valuable *yin* tonic.

The arrival of Columbus's ships in the Caribbean in 1492 was followed by the rapid conquest and colonization of central and south America by the Spanish and Portuguese. Along with their booty of plundered gold, the conquistadors returned to Europe with previously unheard-of medicinal plants. Many of these herbs from the Americas had highly potent medicinal actions, and they soon became available in the apothecaries of the major European cities. Plants such as lignum vitae (*Guaiacum officinale*, p. 223) and cinchona (*Cinchona* spp., p. 84) with strong medicinal actions were used with greater and lesser degrees of success as treatments for fever, malaria, syphilis, smallpox, and other serious illnesses.

For most rural communities, however, the only foreign plants that were used medicinally were those that could also be grown locally as foods. Garlic offers one of the earliest and clearest examples. Originating in central Asia, over time it was cultivated farther and farther west and was grown in Egypt around 4500 BCE. In Homer's 8th-century BCE epic poem *The Odyssey*, the hero is saved from being

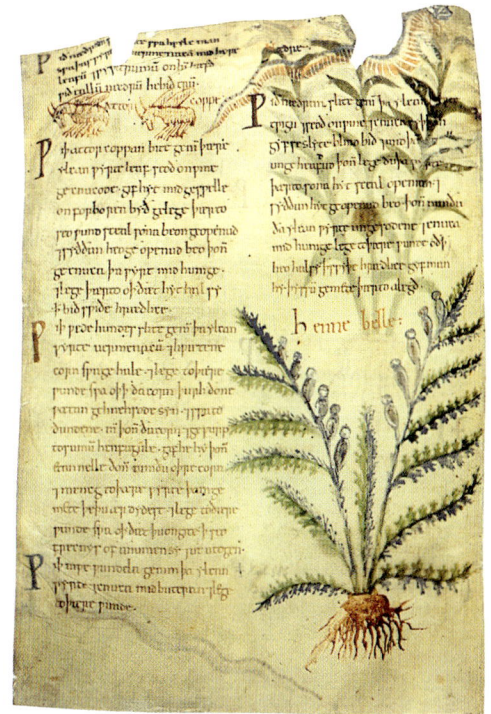

Manuscript page from an Anglo-Saxon herbal of about 1050 CE, illustrating the aerial parts and root system of a medicinal plant.

changed into a pig thanks to garlic. The herb was introduced into Britain after the Roman conquest in the 1st century CE, and by the time it reached the island its remarkable medicinal powers were well understood. In later centuries, potatoes (*Solanum tuberosum*, p. 280) and corn (*Zea mays*, p. 158), both native to South America, would become common foods. These plants have clear medicinal as well as nutritional benefits. Potato juice is a valuable remedy for the treatment of arthritis, while corn silk makes an effective decoction for urinary problems such as cystitis.

Health & hygiene 1400–1700

Between the 12th and 18th centuries, the influx of exotic medicinal plants added to an already large number of useful European herbs. Conceivably, an overall improvement of health in Europe might have resulted. After all, not only were new medicinal plants available,

but Europeans had the opportunity to observe the different medical practices of people in South America, China, Japan, and especially in India, where trade was well established. But, in fact, people living in Europe during this period probably experienced some of the most unhealthy conditions the world has ever seen. In contrast, Indigenous American peoples before the arrival of Columbus lived longer, healthier lives than their counterparts in Europe. This fact is unsurprising given the cities of medieval Europe, with their open sewers, overcrowding,

and ignorance of simple hygiene. Conditions such as these laid fertile ground for the spread of plague-infested rats from the ports of the Mediterranean throughout Western Europe. From the mid-14th century onward, plague killed millions, in some cases close to 50 percent of the population. No medical treatment—herbal or mineral—was able to alter its fatal course. Epidemics continued to decimate the cities of Europe and Asia well into the 18th century. An outbreak in India in 1994 reawakened the terror inspired simply at the mention of the word "plague."

Syphilis was another disease spread by seafarers. It was reputedly brought back from the Caribbean to Naples by Columbus's crew in the 1490s, spreading quickly throughout Europe and to the rest of the world, reaching China in 1550.

European doctors had little success in combating diseases as devastating as plague. The medicine they practiced was based on

the blind acceptance of Galen's humoral principles. Perhaps if, as in Chinese and Indian medicine, European medicine had continued to evolve, revising ancient medical texts and reinterpreting them in the light of new discoveries, it would have had greater success. As it was, European physicians were at least as likely to kill their patients with bloodletting and toxic minerals in misbegotten attempts to balance the humors as they were to cure. Indeed, the increasingly fashionable use of mineral cures such as mercury led to the growth of

chemical formulations, culminating in scientific medicine's ultimate breakaway from herbal practices.

The influence of Paracelsus

One of the key European figures of the 16th century was Paracelsus (1493–1541), a larger-than-life character who rejected the tired repetition of Galen's theories in favor of detailed observation in medicine. "I have not borrowed from Hippocrates, Galen, or anyone else," he wrote, "having acquired my knowledge from the best teacher; that is, by experience and hard work." And again, "What a doctor needs is not eloquence or knowledge of language and of books, but profound knowledge of nature and her works." He also paid great attention to the exact dosage, saying that "it depends only on the dose whether a poison is a poison or not."

As a result, Paracelsus was an influential force in the future development of chemistry, conventional medicine, herbal medicine, and homeopathy. Though he is known as the "father of chemistry," he also explored alchemy, which concerned itself with the transmutation of base materials to gold, and the search for immortal life. Paracelsus also revived interest in the Doctrine of Signatures—the theory that held that medicinal plants contained a sign revealing the ailments it would treat—and affirmed the value of locally grown medicinal herbs over expensive imported specimens.

Culpeper & printed herbals

Paracelsus' advocacy for the use of cheaper local herbs was later fiercely espoused by Nicholas Culpeper (1616–1654). The frontispiece to his *The English Physitian* contains the memorable words: "Containing a Compleat Method of Physick, whereby a Man may preserve his Body in Health, or Cure himself, being Sick, for three pence Charge, with such things only as grow in England, they being most fit for English Bodies."

> "European physicians were at least as likely to kill their patients with bloodletting and toxic minerals in misbegotten attempts to balance the humors as they were to cure."

Wounded during the English Civil War fighting for the Commonwealth, Culpeper championed the needs of the ordinary people who could afford neither the services of a doctor nor the expensive imported herbs and formulations that doctors generally prescribed. Drawing to some degree on Dioscorides, Arabian physicians, and Paracelsus, Culpeper developed a medical system that blended astrology and sound personal experience of the therapeutic uses of local plants. His herbal became an instant "bestseller" and appeared in many subsequent editions. The first herbal published in North America, in 1700, was an edition of his herbal.

While the popularity of *The English Physitian* was notable, other herbals also found a place in households. The development of the printing press in the 15th century brought herbal medicine into homes on a wide scale. Texts such as Dioscorides' *De Materia Medica* were printed for the first time, and throughout Europe herbals were published and ran through many editions.

Deadly cures 1700–1900

By the end of the 16th century, Paracelsus had become the figurehead of the new chemical medicine. However, where he had insisted upon caution in the use of metallic poisons—mercury, antimony, and arsenic—the new medical thinkers were not so inhibited. Larger and larger doses of the purgative known as calomel (mercurous chloride, Hg_2Cl_2) were given to those suffering from syphilis and many other diseases. The treatment was very often worse than the illness, with some patients dying and many more suffering from the long-term consequences of mercury poisoning.

Hippocrates' saying "Desperate cases need the most desperate remedies" was taken very literally, as is evident in the incredible excess of purging and bleeding that developed over the next three

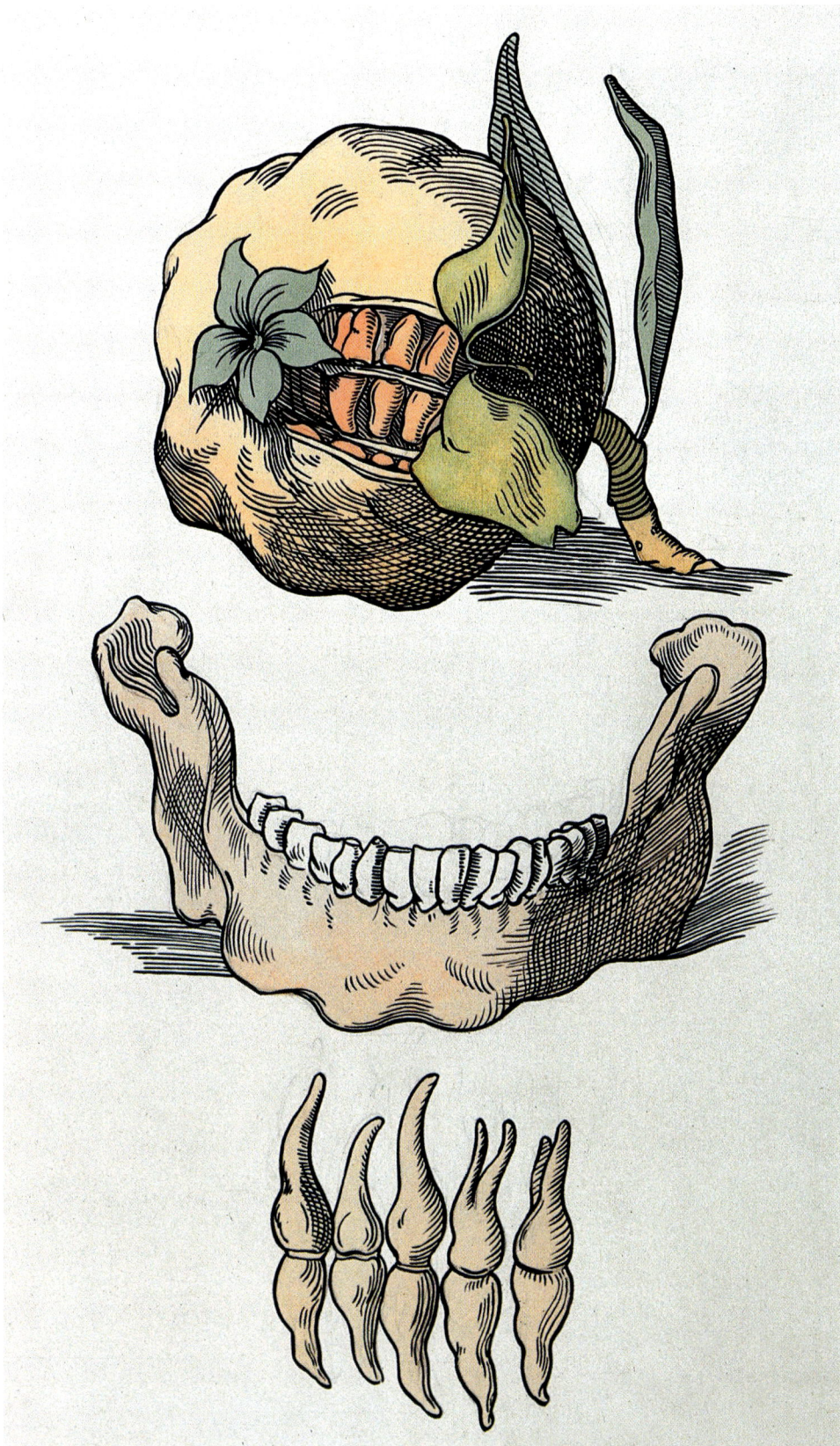

The doctrine of signatures is the ancient theory that held that a plant's appearance indicated the ailments it would treat. A pomegranate was said to resemble the human jaw and teeth.

25

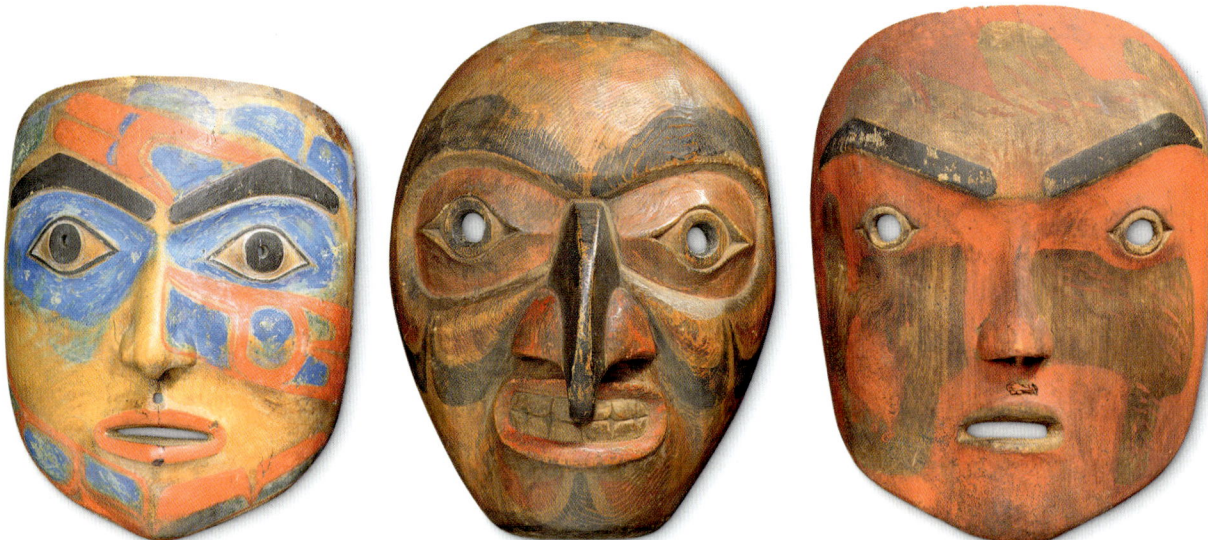

Three shaman masks.
The efficacy of techniques used by Indigenous healers often surpassed that of conventional medical practices of the time.

centuries in Europe and North America. These practices reached a peak in the "heroic" medicine of the early 19th century. Its leading proponent, Dr. Benjamin Rush (1745–1813), maintained that only bloodletting and calomel were required in medical practice. His position was obviously extreme, but it is clear that in this new climate herbal medicines were seen as increasingly irrelevant.

The new rationalism

Along with the new emphasis on chemical cures, modern medicine came to look askance at the notion of the "vital force." Up until the end of the 16th century, nearly all medical traditions had been based on the concept of working with nature, with the body's healing capacities, which could be supported and strengthened with appropriate medicinal herbs. In traditional Chinese medicine, *qi* is the primal energy that maintains life and health. In Ayurveda, it is *prana*, and in the Western tradition, Hippocrates writes about "*vis medicatrix naturae*" or the healing power of nature, while modern Western medical herbalists and homeopaths use the term "vital force."

The importance of the vital force was diminished in the West by the philosophy of René Descartes (1596–1650). This French mathematician divided the world into body and mind, nature and ideas. His philosophy ordained that the intangible vital force that maintains life and governs good health was the province of religion rather than of the newly self-aware "science" of medicine. To the new medical establishment, inching its way forward toward scientifically sound medical practices, "supernatural" concepts such as the vital force were a reminder of the ignorance and superstition that were part and parcel of older healing practices.

Even before Descartes' theories, the rational approach to scientific and medical exploration was beginning to reap rewards. Slowly, medical understanding of bodily functions was gaining ground. William Harvey (1578–1657) made a detailed study of the heart and circulation, proving for the first time that, contrary to Galenic thought, the heart pumped blood around the body. Published in 1628, his study is a classic example of the revolution in medical science.

Since Harvey's time, science has had astounding success in revealing how the body works on a biochemical level and in distinguishing different disease processes. However, despite the revolutionary impact of antibiotic therapy, it has been rather less successful in developing effective medical treatments for the relief and cure of diseases.

The gap in the scientific approach

In hindsight, it seems as if the new science of medicine could only be born in separation from the traditional arts of healing, with which it had always been intertwined. As a result, even though traditional medicine has generally lacked scientific explanation, it has frequently been far ahead of medical science in the way it has been applied therapeutically. In *American Indian Medicine* (University of Oklahoma Press, 1970), Virgil Vogel provides a good example of "ignorant" folk medicine outstripping scientific understanding in therapeutic application:

"During the bitter cold winter of 1535–6, the three ships of Jacques Cartier were frozen fast in the fathom-deep ice of the St Lawrence River near the site of Montreal. Isolated by four feet of snow, the company of 110 men subsisted on the fare stored in the holds of their ships. Soon scurvy was so rampant among them that by mid-March, 25 men had died and the others, 'only three or foure excepted,' were so ill that hope for their recovery was abandoned. As the crisis deepened Cartier had the good fortune to encounter once again the local Indian [sic] chief, Domagaia, who had cured himself of the same disease with 'the juice and sappe of a certain tree.' The Indian women gathered branches of the magical tree, 'boiling the bark and leaves for a decoction, and placing the dregs upon the legs.' All those so treated rapidly recovered their health, and the Frenchmen marveled at the curative skill of the natives."

Naturally, Indigenous North American peoples had not heard of vitamin C deficiency, which causes scurvy, nor would they have been able to explain in rational terms why the treatment worked. Indeed, it was not until 1753 that James Lind (1716–1794), a British naval surgeon, inspired partly by Cartier's account, published *A Treatise of the Scurvy*, which showed conclusively that the disease could be prevented by eating fresh greens, vegetables, and fruit, and was caused by their lack in the diet. James Lind's work is a marvelous example of what can be achieved by combining a systematic and scientific approach with traditional herbal knowledge.

Isolating chemicals

The discovery of the medicinal value of foxglove (*Digitalis purpurea*, p. 207) is another case where traditional herbal knowledge led to a major advance in medicine. Dr. William Withering (1741–1799), a conventionally trained doctor with a long interest in medicinal plants, started to investigate foxglove after encountering a family recipe for curing dropsy (water retention). He found that in some regions of England, foxglove was traditionally used to treat this condition, which is often one of the key indications of a failing heart. In 1785, he published *Account of the Foxglove*, documenting dozens of carefully recorded case histories, and showing how foxglove's powerful (and potentially dangerous) active constituents, now known as cardiac glycosides, made it a valuable plant medicine for dropsy. Cardiac glycosides remain in common use to the present day. Yet despite this clearcut example of the possibilities inherent in a marriage of herbal medicine and scientific method, conventional medicine was to take another path in the 19th century.

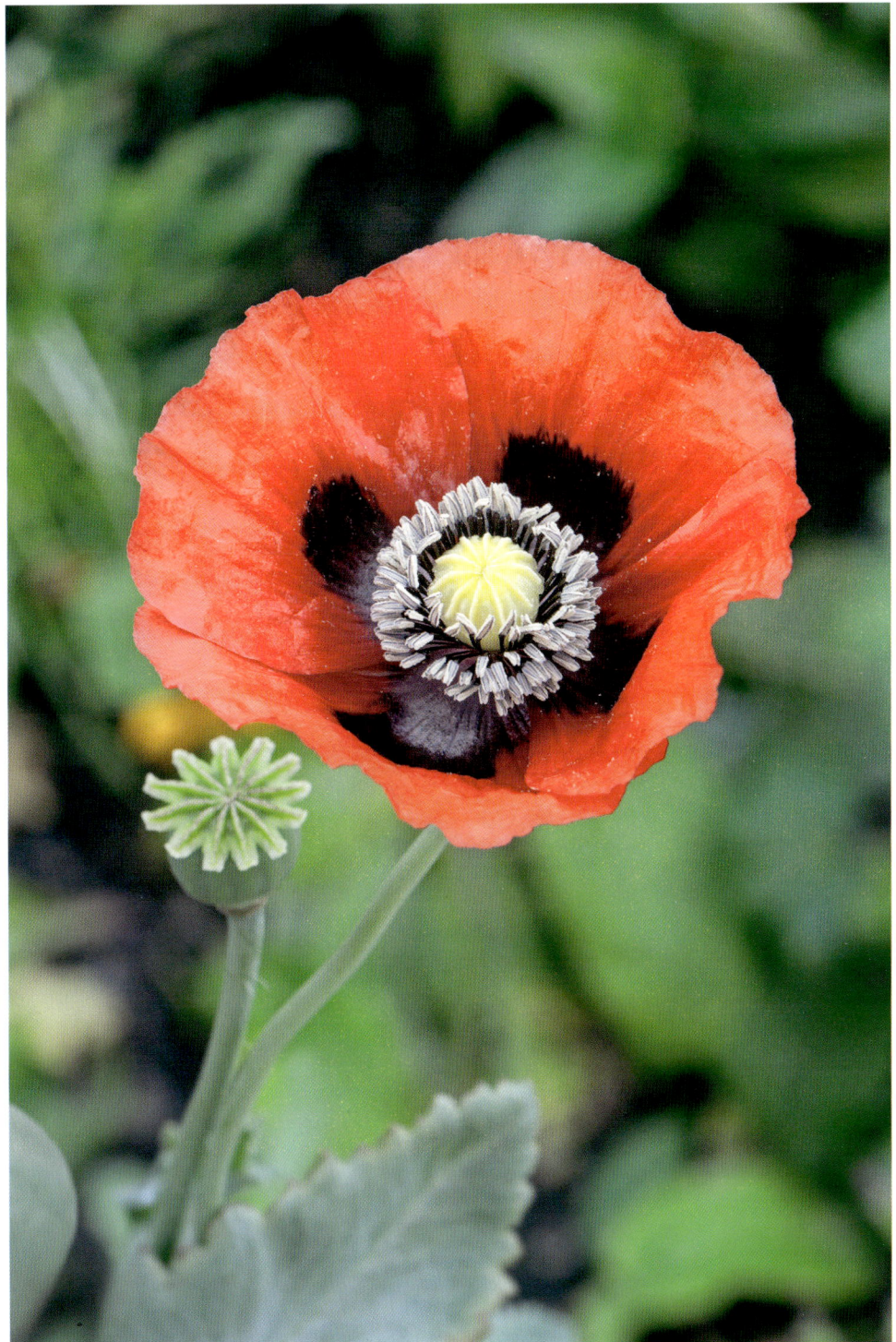

Opium poppy, native to Asia, yields a resin—opium—that has long been smoked for its narcotic effect. The main active constituent, morphine, was first isolated in the laboratory in 1803 and is used to relieve pain.

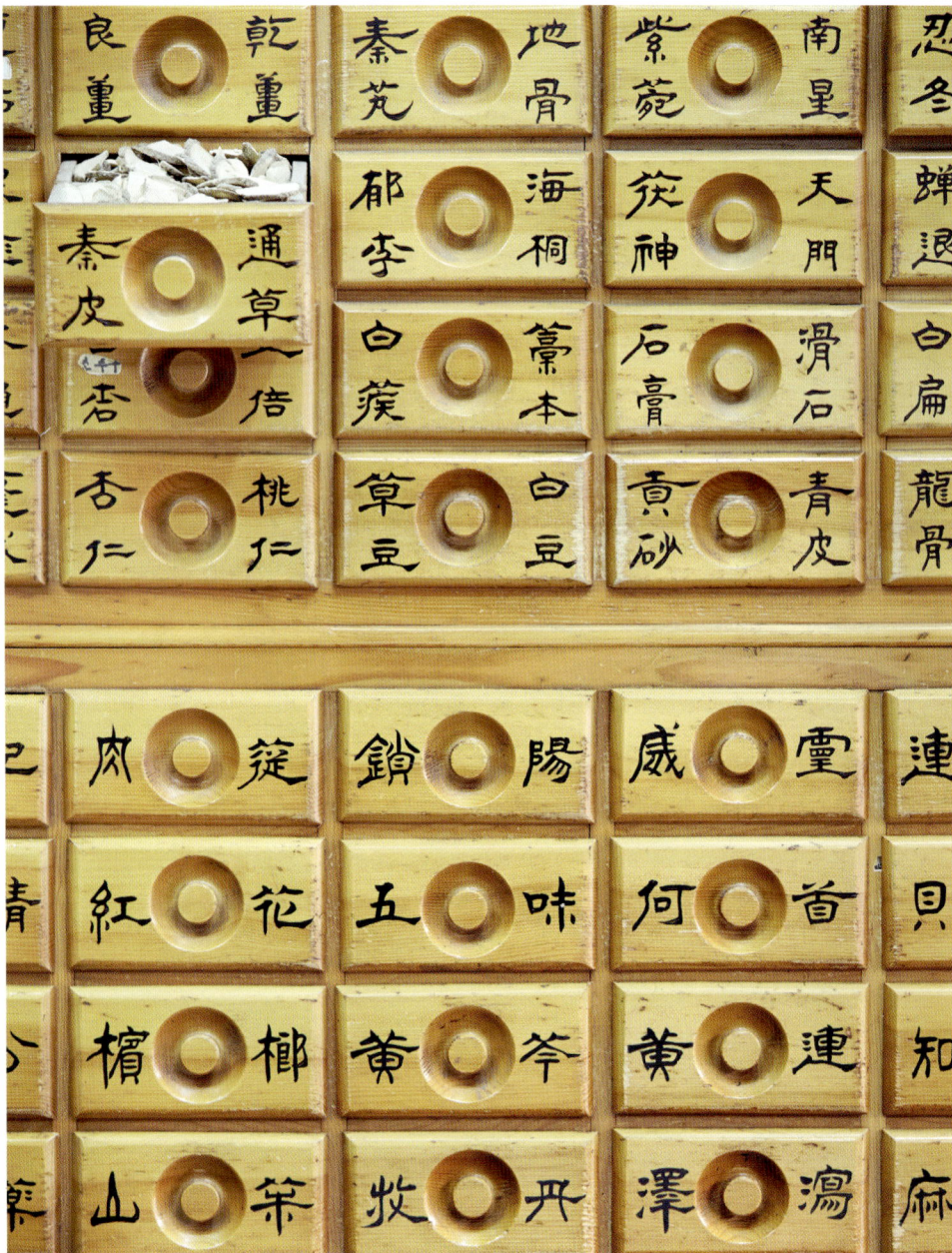

Chinese herbal medicine cabinet. In China the influx of Western biomedicine did not stop the continuing development of traditional herbal practice.

Laboratory versus nature

From the early 19th century, the chemical laboratory began to regularly supplant Mother Nature as the source of medicines. In 1803, narcotic alkaloids were isolated from the opium poppy (*Papaver somniferum*, p. 251). A year later, inulin was extracted from elecampane (*Inula helenium*, p. 111). In 1838, salicylic acid, a chemical forerunner of aspirin, was isolated from white willow bark (*Salix alba*, p. 133), and was first synthesized in the laboratory in 1860. From this point on, herbal medicine and biomedicine were to take separate paths. Aspirin, or acetylsalicylic acid, an entirely new chemical formulation, was first developed in Germany in 1899. But this was still an early step. For the time being, the influence of the universities, medical schools, and laboratories of Europe would remain limited, and herbal medicine would prevail as the predominant form of treatment for most people around the world.

New frontiers, new herbal medicines

Wherever Europeans settled during the great migrations of the 18th and 19th centuries—North America, South America, southern Africa, or Australia—much of the European medicine familiar from home was either unavailable or prohibitively expensive. Settlers came to learn that native peoples were a wellspring of information about the medicinal virtues of indigenous plants. For example, European settlers in southern Africa learned about the diuretic properties of buchu (*Barosma betulina*, p. 75) from Indigenous peoples; and Australian settlers came to understand the remarkable antiseptic properties of tea tree (*Melaleuca alternifolia*, p. 116) from observing the medicinal practices of the Aborigines. Mexican herbal medicine as it exists today isa blend of Indigenous, including Mayan andSpanish, herbs and practices. In North America, Indigenous herbalists were particularly adept at healing external wounds and bites—being superior in many respects to their European counterparts in this area of medicine. This is not surprising, given the range of highly effective medicinal plants Indigenous American peoples had discovered—including well-known herbs such as echinacea (*Echinacea* spp., p. 96), goldenseal (*Hydrastis canadensis*, p. 109), and lobelia (*Lobelia inflata*, p. 114).

European settlers learned much from observing Indigenous practices. Over the course of the 19th and early 20th centuries, as settlers moved west across the frontier territory, new plants were constantly being added to the official record of healing herbs. In addition to the three species mentioned above, about 170 native plants were listed in *The Pharmacopeia of the United States*.

Samuel Thomson & his followers

Lobelia was one of the key herbs, along with cayenne (*Capsicum frutescens*, p. 79), advocated by Samuel Thomson (1769–1843), an unorthodox herbal practitioner who believed that all illness resulted from cold. His simple approach was entirely at odds with the conventional practices of his time (see North America, p. 52). Thomson's methods were often very effective and were well suited to the needs of people living the harsh, restricted lives of frontier territory. His system of medicine—in many ways an early form of naturopathy, in which ill health is treated with naturally grown food, sunlight, fresh air, and natural medicines—became extraordinarily popular, with millions of people across North America following his methods. Thomson's success waned as other more sophisticated herbal approaches were developed, notably the Eclectics and Physiomedicalists, who included medical science in their training and undertook extensive research into plant medicines. The fertile world of 19th century North America also saw the birth of osteopathy (a system of healing based upon the manipulation of bones) and chiropractic (a similar system primarily involving manipulation of the spine).

Western influences on Asian medicine

Across the world in China, Thomson's practices might have been looked on with a measure of surprise, but they would have been familiar. In Chinese medicine, there has always been a debate as to what degree illness arises from cold, and to what degree it arises from heat. *The Shanghanlun (On Cold-Induced Maladies)*, written in the 2nd century CE and revised and reinterpreted in commentaries over the last 1,800 years, recommends the herb cinnamon (*Cinnamomum* spp., p. 85) as a principal remedy when the patient "shivers with fever, breathes heavily, and feels nauseous." In the 14th century, Wang Lu distinguished between cold-induced illness and febrile illness, and treated them in different ways, and this distinction was elaborated in greater and greater detail by different Chinese herbalists right up to the 19th century.

During the early 19th century, the influence of Western biomedicine was beginning to affect traditional practices in both China and India. This was certainly beneficial in many respects. The judicious incorporation of scientific principles and methods into traditional herbal healing offers the possibility of greatly refining the effectiveness of treatment.

But in India under British rule, Western medicine eventually became the only alternative. Ayurveda was seen as inferior to biomedicine (see India & the Middle East, p. 40). Western practice was introduced not as a complement to traditional medicine, but rather as a means to supplant it. According to one authority, "before 1835 Western physicians and their Indian counterparts exchanged knowledge; thereafter only Western medicine was recognized as legitimate and the Eastern systems were actively discouraged" (Robert Svoboda, *Ayurveda, Life, Health and Longevity*, 1992).

In China, the influx of Western ideas was less traumatic. Increasing numbers of Chinese medical students studied Western medicine, but this did not stop the continuing development of traditional herbal practice. By and large, each tradition was recognized as having both advantages and disadvantages.

Herbalism outlawed 1850–1900

In Europe, conventional medicine was seeking to establish a monopoly for its own type of practice. In 1858, the British Parliament was asked to impose legislation banning the practice of medicine by anyone who had not been trained in a conventional medical school. Fortunately, this proposal was rejected, but in countries such as France, Spain, and Italy, and in some states of the US, it became illegal to practice herbal medicine without an orthodox qualification. Herbalists were forced to risk fines or imprisonment simply for providing herbal medicine to patients who had sought their help.

In Britain, concerns such as these, combined with a desire to establish Western herbal medicine as an alternative to conventional practices, particularly in the industrial cities of the North of England, led to the formation in 1864 of what would become the National Institute of Medical Herbalists, the first professional body of herbal practitioners in the world. Its history is an example of how tenacious herbal practitioners have had to be simply to retain their right to give safe, gentle, and effective herbal medicines to their patients.

20th & 21st centuries

For most of us, modern medicine is exemplified by drugs such as antibiotics and highly technical methods of diagnosis and treatment. However, many might be surprised to discover that, for much of the last century, herbal medicines were the primary form of treatment, even in Western countries.

Even as late as the 1930s, around 90 percent of medicines prescribed by doctors or sold over the counter were herbal in origin. It is only during the last 80 years that laboratory-produced medicines have become the norm. During World War I (1914–1918), for example, garlic (*Allium sativum*, p. 63) and sphagnum moss (*Sphagnum* spp.) were used by the ton in the battle trenches to dress wounds and to treat infections. Garlic is an excellent natural antibiotic, and was the most effective antiseptic available at the time, and sphagnum moss, gathered from the moorlands, makes a natural aseptic dressing.

Science & medicine

The development of new medicines in the laboratory—either extracted from medicinal plants or synthesized—stretches back to the early 19th century, when chemists first isolated constituents such as morphine, from opium poppy (*Papaver somniferum*, p. 251), and cocaine, from coca (*Erythroxylum coca*, p. 211). From that time onward, scientists made tremendous progress in understanding how isolated chemicals affect the body, as well as how the body works in health and disease. From the 1860s, scientists—most notably Louis Pasteur (1822–1895)—began to identify the microorganisms that were ultimately responsible for causing infectious diseases, such as tuberculosis and malaria.

Naturally enough, the first aim of those engaged in medical research was to seek out medicines that would act as "magic bullets," directly attacking the microorganisms concerned and ridding the body of the threat. This eventually led to the discovery, or, more accurately, the rediscovery of penicillin by a number of medical researchers, most notably Alexander Fleming (1881–1955) in 1929. However, while 20th-century scientists were the first to scientifically evaluate antibiotics as medicines, they were not the first to employ them in healing. Antibiotic molds had been grown and used to combat infection in ancient Egypt, 14th-century Peru, and in recent European folk medicine.

In the decades following World War II (1939–1945), when antibiotics first came into use, it seemed as though a new era had dawned in which infection could be conquered, and life-threatening diseases such as syphilis, pneumonia, and tuberculosis would cease to be major causes of death in the developed world. Modern medicine also provided other highly effective drugs such as steroid anti-inflammatories, and it seemed as if it was simply a question of time until cures for most illnesses were found.

Ascendancy of biomedicine

As Americans and Europeans became accustomed to medication that led to an almost instant short-term improvement in symptoms (if not in underlying health), herbal medicines came to be seen by the public as outmoded and ineffective. Increasingly, the practice of herbal medicine was outlawed in North America and most of Europe, while the wealthy in developing countries abandoned herbal medicine in favor of the new treatments available.

This was in no small part due to the medical profession itself, which saw herbal medicine as a throwback to the superstitions of the past. From the late 19th century onward, the aim of organizations such as the American Medical Association and the British Medical Association had been to monopolize

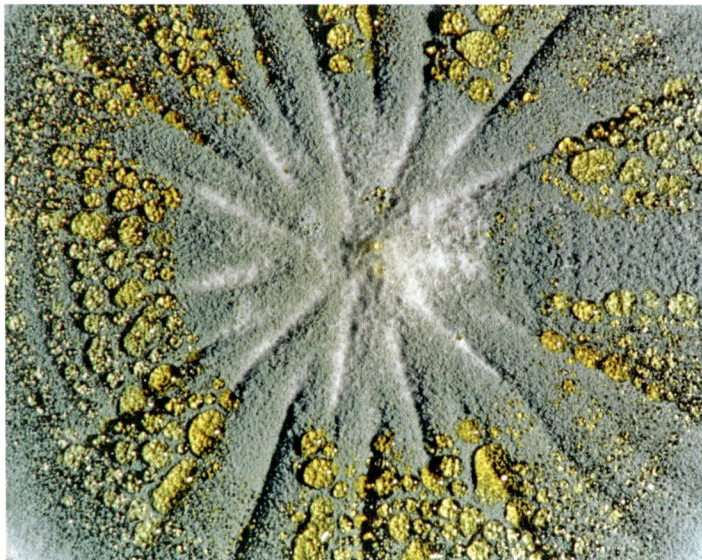

The scientific discovery of penicillin in 1929 revolutionized the treatment of infection, though the earliest identified use of antibiotics was in Egypt and Sudan (350–550 CE).

"Naturally enough, the first aim of those engaged in medical research was to seek out medicines that would act as 'magic bullets,' directly attacking the microorganisms."

conventional medical practice. Herbal medicine thus neared extinction in many countries, especially in the US and Britain. In Britain, for example, from 1941 until 1968 it was illegal to practice herbal medicine without medical qualifications.

The tide turns

Although there were spectacular successes with modern chemical medicines, there were also horrific disasters, most notably the thalidomide tragedy in 1962 in Britain and Germany, when 3,000 deformed babies were born to mothers who had taken the drug for morning sickness during pregnancy. This event marked a turning point in the public's opinion of chemical medicines. People began to realize that a serious cost could accompany the benefits of treatment with modern pharmaceutical drugs. This, and the factors described below, have brought about a sea change in public perceptions of the value of herbal medicine.

The Chinese example

Herbal medicine experienced a major gain in fortune in 1949 in China, when Mao Zedong and the Communist Red Army gained control of the country.

Traditional Western medicine by that time was well established in China, but most of the population had little hope of access to modern hospitals, let alone to new drugs. Out of necessity, traditional Chinese medicine—essentially herbal medicine and acupuncture—once more began to be used alongside Western conventional medicine. The authorities aimed to provide the best of both

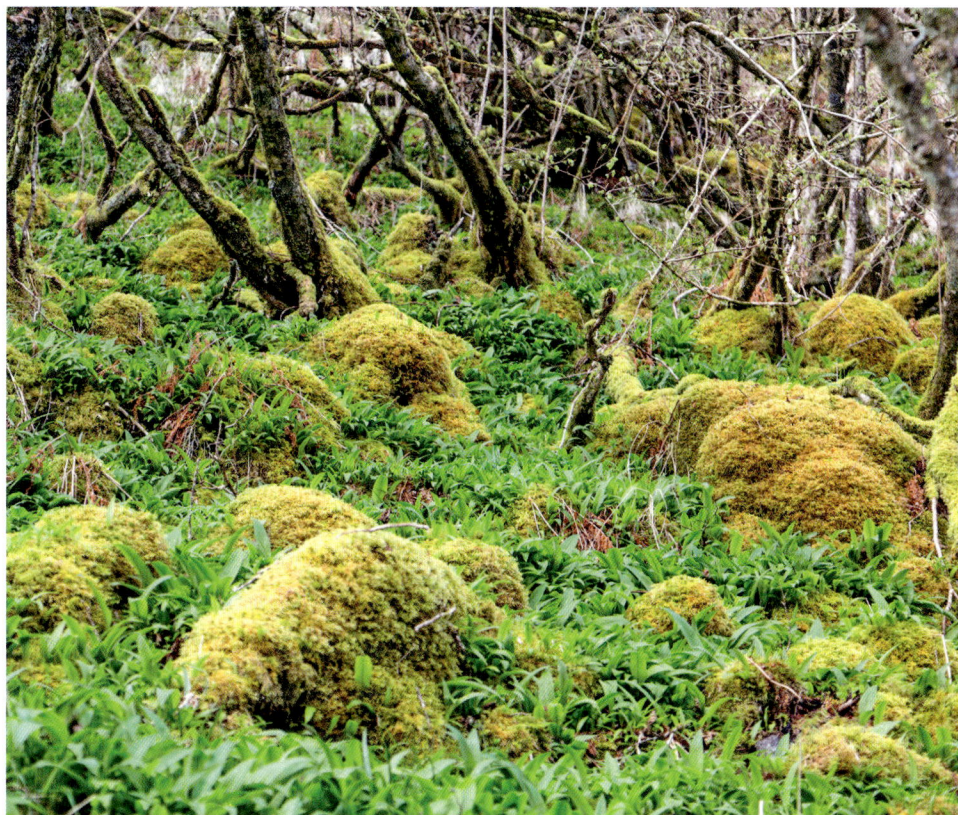

Garlic (Allium sativum) *and sphagnum moss* (Sphagnum spp.), *seen here covering the ground of ancient woodland in Scotland, were used in the battle trenches during World War I to dress wounds and treat infections.*

worlds. Five teaching hospitals for traditional Chinese medicine (TCM) were established, where it was taught on a scientific basis. In addition, great efforts were made to improve the quality of plant medicines.

Contrary to the trend in conventional Western medicine that makes the patient ever more dependent upon the doctor and high-tech machinery, TCM, like other forms of complementary medicine, stresses the

patient's personal responsibility for his or her own cure, encouraging a holistic approach to treatment.

In the 1960s, China also established a system of "barefoot doctors." After a period of basic medical instruction that blended herbal medicine, acupuncture, and Western practices, these practitioners were sent out to provide health care for the millions of rural Chinese too remote from cities to benefit

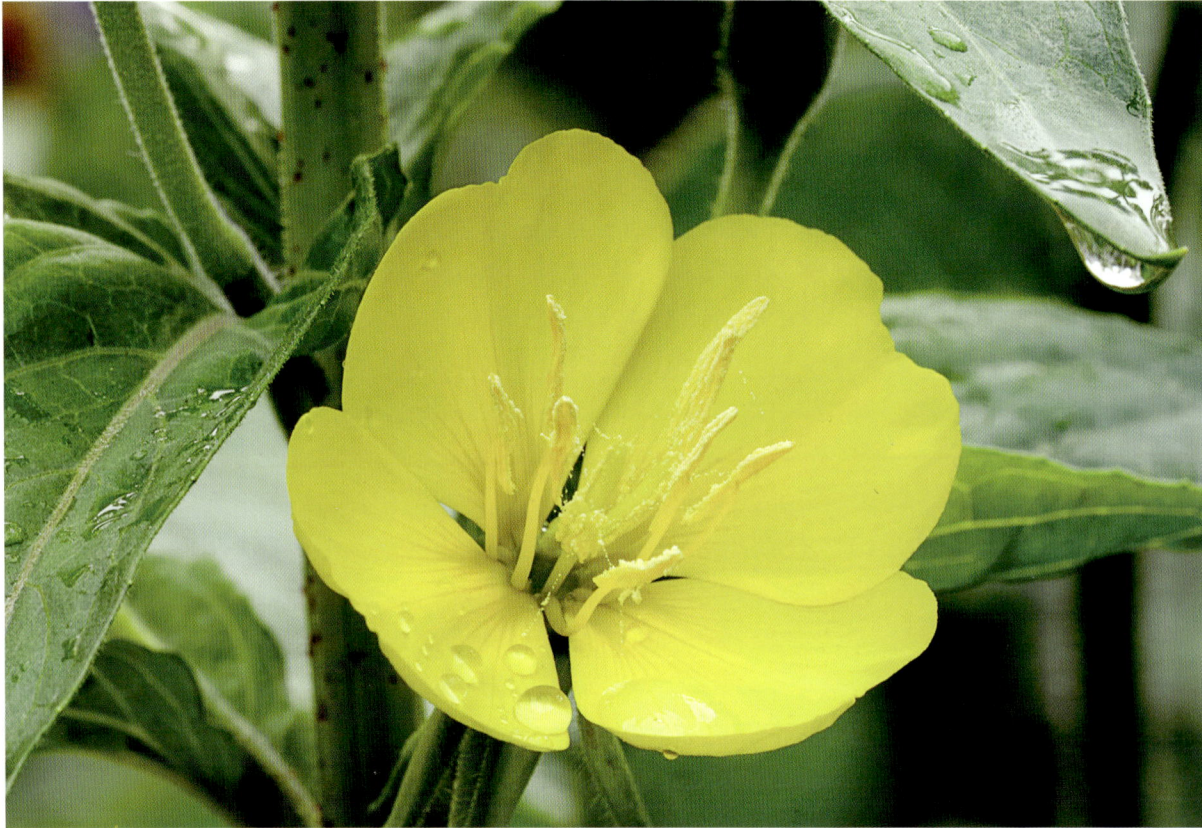

Evening primrose is native to North America and has been used to treat a wide range of conditions, including premenstrual syndrome, asthma, whooping cough, digestive disorders, and eczema.

from the facilities available there. The barefoot doctors in the late 1960s became a model for the World Health Organization, which created a strategy of including traditional herbal practitioners in planning for the health care needs of developing countries.

Western medicine & herbal practices

Further to the initiative by the World Health Organization, experience has shown that traditional (usually herbal) and Western medicine can indeed work well in tandem, although the relationship is often quite complex. J. M. Janzen's *The Quest for Therapy in Lower Zaïre* (University of California Press, 1978) describes one such interaction in Africa:

"The people of Zaïre recognize the advantages of Western medicine and seek its surgery, drugs, and hospital care, but contrary to what might have been expected, native doctors, prophets, and traditional consultations among kinsmen do not disappear with the adoption of Western medicine. Rather a [working relationship] has developed in which different forms of therapy play complementary rather than competitive roles in the thoughts and lives of the people."

The high cost of Western medical treatment is another factor that has encouraged people and governments to reexamine traditional healing. In China, Mexico, Cuba, Egypt, Ghana, India, and Mongolia, to give but a few examples, herbal medicines are being cultivated in greater quantities, and are being used to some degree by conventional as well as traditional practitioners.

Likewise, different types of treatment have evolved to meet the variety of needs within a population. India offers an extraordinary example of the kind of choices available in types of medical care. Alongside physicians who are trained in conventional Western medicine, there are medically trained Ayurvedic practitioners, traditional Ayurvedic practitioners, local healers, and homeopaths.

Changing attitudes

Perhaps the most important factor behind the growing interest in complementary medicine is the poor state of health in Western societies. Conventional medicine has by and large brought serious infectious diseases under control, although there are worrying signs that infectious organisms are becoming resistant to antibiotic treatment, largely as a result of their indiscriminate use. Chronic illness, however, seems to be on the increase. Probably around 50 percent of people in Western countries daily take one or more conventional medicines—for conditions as diverse as high blood pressure, asthma, arthritis, and depression. Many Western countries such as the US and France spend astronomical sums on health care, yet despite this massive investment, much of the population remains demonstrably unhealthy. Even the significant increase in life expectancy in developed countries is showing signs of going into reverse, in part perhaps a result of environmental pollutants and toxic accumulation within the body.

Over the years, changes in public awareness have led to a renewed interest in herbal medicine. In fact, some herbal preparations are now so commonly used that they are accepted as a part of everyday life. One of many possible examples is evening primrose oil, which is used by hundreds of thousands of women in Britain to help relieve premenstrual syndrome. It is extracted from the seeds of *Oenothera biennis* (p. 248), a North American plant. Peppermint oil (*Mentha* x *piperita*, p. 118), prescribed for irritable bowel syndrome and other gut problems, is another example, while senna (*Cassia senna*, p. 80), a simple, effective treatment for short-term constipation, is one of the most frequently used medicines throughout the world.

The growing awareness of how our lives as human beings are interwoven with the fate of our planet also reinforces the value of herbal medicines. As long as care is taken to prevent overharvesting, herbal medicine is ecologically in tune with the environment.

Herbalism & holism

The "germ theory of disease," which holds that illness springs from contact with an infectious organism, remains the dominant view in mainstream medicine. Many people, however, recognize that this is only part of the picture. While illnesses such as cholera and typhoid are highly infectious and are indeed likely to be caught by almost anyone, many infectious diseases are not transmitted automatically from one person to another. The question arises, therefore, what weakness in the patient has allowed the "seed" of infection to find fertile ground? Unlike much conventional medical practice, which focuses on eradicating the "bug" or abnormal condition, herbal medicine also seeks to treat the weakness that gave rise to ill health, and sets this in the context of the patient's life as a whole. A complex web of factors may lie behind the onset of illness. While bodily signs and symptoms are the most obvious indicators, dietary, emotional, and spiritual factors may be of equal importance.

Our bodies contain over 35 trillion cells, which collectively must function in harmony if good health is to be maintained. Used wisely, herbs work in tune with our bodies, stimulating, supporting, or restraining different sets of cells in their allotted tasks within the body, encouraging a return to normal balanced function. Remedies aim to strengthen the patient's own resistance, improve the vitality of weakened tissue, and encourage the body's innate ability to return to good health.

Of course, for people with severe acute illnesses, it may be too late to use an herbal approach to treatment. In these circumstances, strong-acting conventional medicines such as heart drugs, antibiotics, and painkillers, as well as surgery, can all be lifesavers. However, a health-care system that is carefully attuned to the needs of the patient might well provide herbal remedies as a first line of treatment, with conventional medicines held in reserve to be used only when necessary.

Evidence in support of herbal cures

Many medical scientists still find it hard to accept that natural medicines, with their complex chemical makeup and variable constituents, can be as good as chemical cures in treating illness. However, as more and more research reveals that herbal medicines can be as effective as conventional medicines—and are far safer—this thinking is beginning to change.

This is well illustrated by the change in attitude toward St. John's wort (*Hypericum perforatum*, p. 110)—a European plant commonly taken as an antidepressant. Extracts of the herb are now scientifically recognized as having value in mild to moderate depression. By 2022, 267 clinical trials had investigated different aspects of St. John's wort's safety and effectiveness as a medicine. In at least 30 of them, extracts of the herb were found to be as effective as conventional antidepressants, and to produce significantly fewer side effects. In 15 other clinical trials, a St. John's wort extract produced fewer side effects than a placebo (or inert substance) used as a comparison. Other investigations suggest that St. John's wort may have a role in countering viral infections, promoting wound healing, and helping withdrawal from addiction, especially from alcohol.

As is so often the case, research has confirmed traditional views. In the 16th century, Paracelsus (*see* p. 24) had this to say about the herb: "Nothing chases away disease like strength. Therefore, we should seek medicines with power and strength to overcome whatever illnesses they are used against. From this it follows that God has given

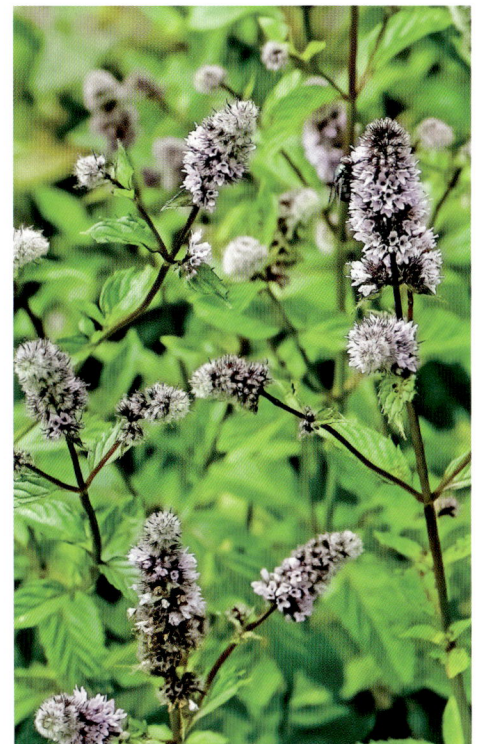

Peppermint essential oil (mentha *x* piperita) *is prescribed for irritable bowel syndrome and other gut problems.*

"Another issue is convincing septics in the medical world that herbal medicine is not just a poor substitute for conventional medicine but a valuable form of treatment in its own right."

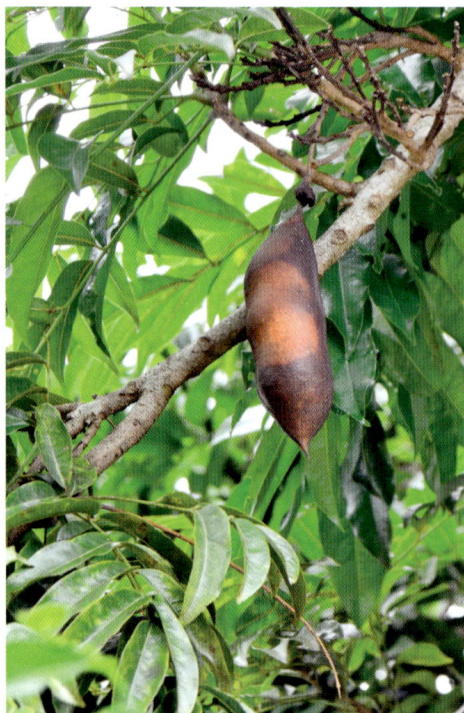

The Moreton Bay chestnut (Castanospermum australe) is being investigated for its anti-HIV activity.

to Perforatum [St. John's wort] the strength to chase [away] the ghosts of nature … and all downheartedness."

As a result of scientific research, today's practitioners have an important advantage—how the plant works in the body is now better understood, so that it is possible to be precise about dosages, aware of side effects, and confident in what form the herb should be taken as a medicine.

All over the world research is now being directed into plants with a traditional use as medicines, in the hope of finding new treatments for all manner of health problems. To give but two examples: the Indian gooseberry (*Emblica officinalis*, p. 209) appears to protect the liver against cancer, lowers blood cholesterol levels, and may prove valuable for acute pancreatitis; while thyme (*Thymus vulgaris*, p. 147), better known as a culinary herb, is a potent antioxidant that may prevent the breakdown of essential fatty acids in the brain and slow the aging process.

Medicinal herbs & big business

The major pharmaceutical companies realized some years ago that rainforests, grasslands, and even along roads and fields are sources of potentially invaluable medicines. As a result, the industry has invested vast resources into screening the active constituents of medicinal plants from all over the world. The drug taxol, first extracted from the Pacific yew (*Taxus brevifolia*), and an effective treatment for breast cancer, was developed in this way.

In this search through the plant world it is probable that other remarkable medicines will be found, though far fewer new drugs

have been successfully developed via this research than was originally anticipated. In fact, there is a key problem to this approach, for it is geared to the production of isolated plant chemicals which can then be synthesized and patented. With a patent, a company can make a profit, recouping the massive investment required to research and develop new medicines. Herbs, however, are whole, naturally occurring remedies. They cannot and should not be patented. Even if the major pharmaceutical companies were able to find an herb such as St. John's wort, which proved to be more effective and safer than conventional medicines, they would prefer to develop synthetic chemical drugs rather than plant medicines.

Herbal synergy

One word more than any other separates herbal from conventional medicine: synergy. When the whole plant is used rather than extracted constituents, the different parts interact, often, it is thought, producing a greater therapeutic effect than the equivalent dosage of isolated active constituents that are generally preferred in conventional medicine.

Increasingly, research shows that herbs such as ephedra (*Ephedra sinica,* p. 99), hawthorn (*Crataegus oxyacantha*, p. 91), ginkgo (*Ginkgo biloba*, p. 104), and lily of the valley (*Convallaria majalis*, p. 198) have a greater-than-expected medicinal benefit thanks to the natural *combination* of constituents within the whole plant. In some cases, the medicinal value of the herb may be due entirely to the combination of substances and cannot be reproduced by one or two "active" constituents alone.

The future of herbal medicine

The main issue for the future of herbal medicine is whether medicinal plants, and the traditional knowledge that informs their use, will be valued for what they are—an immense resource of safe, economical, ecologically balanced medicines—or whether they will be yet another area of life to be exploited for short-term profit.

Another issue is convincing skeptics in the medical world that herbal medicine is not just a poor substitute for conventional medicine, but a valuable form of treatment in its own right. In trials into the effect of certain Chinese herbs on patients with eczema at London's Royal Free Hospital in the 1990s, conventional specialists were astonished when the addition of one extra herb to a Chinese formula containing 10 others resulted in a dramatic improvement in a previously unresponsive patient. This story offers evidence of the skill and art involved in herbal practice. In tailoring the remedy to suit the individual needs of the patient and in treating the underlying cause, major improvements were made. This approach is a far cry from the standard medical view of using a single drug to treat a single disease.

In India and China, there have been university courses in herbal medicine for decades. In the West this process has been slower, with undergraduate courses emerging only in the last 20 years. There are now degree courses in herbal medicine or naturopathy in several Western countries, including Australia, the UK, and the US, while in Germany, medical students have been required to study naturopathy and phytotherapy (herbal medicine) as part of their medical training since 2003. Such developments point toward a future where patients might be able to choose between medical and herbal approaches when considering what medical treatment will suit them best.

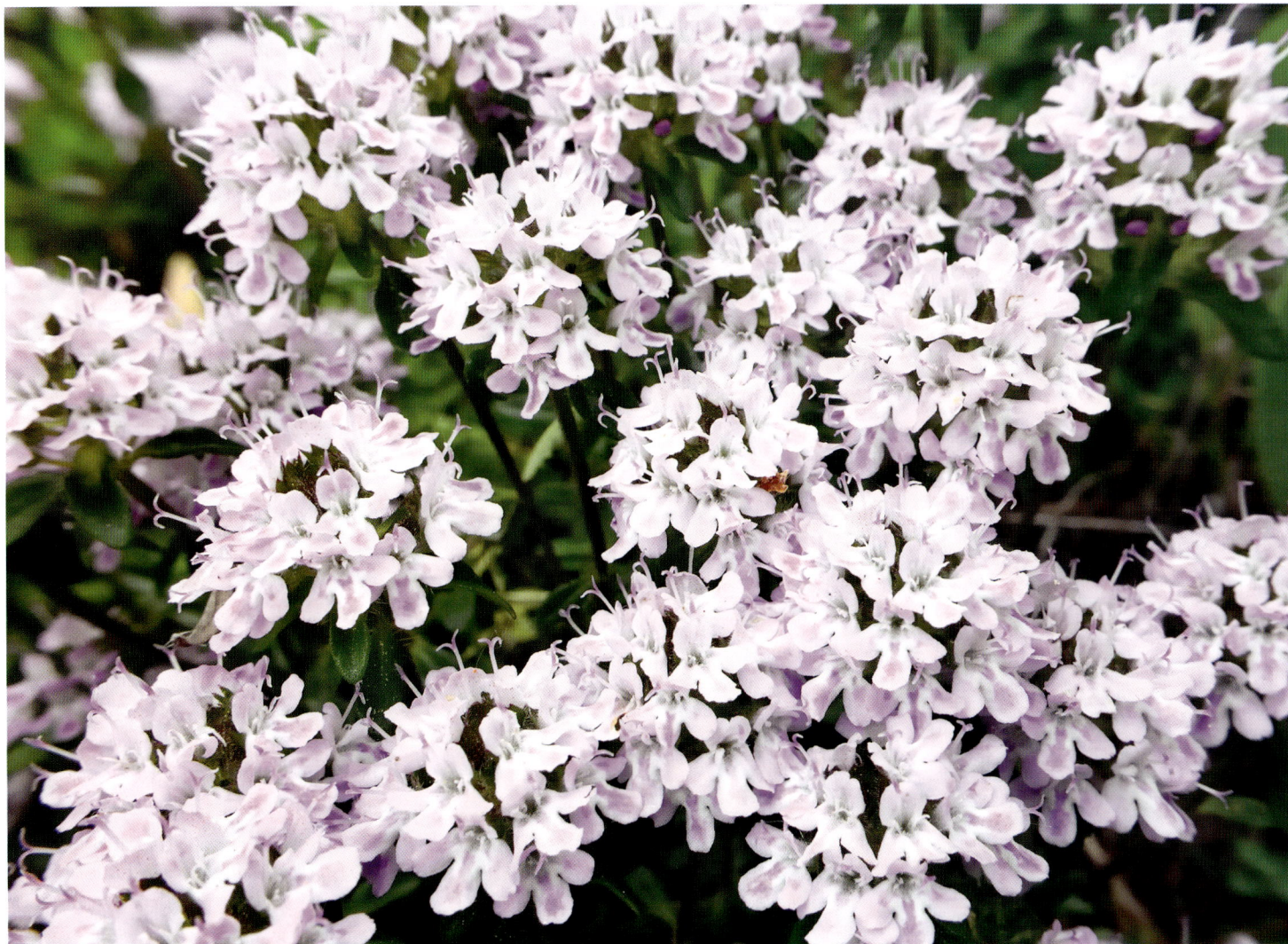

Thyme (**Thymus vulgaris**) *is a potent antioxidant that may prevent the breakdown of essential fatty acids in the brain and slow the aging process.*

Europe

Despite regional variations, European herbal practices largely arose from the common root of the classical tradition. Today, herbalism is increasingly popular in Europe, and in some countries it is widely practiced by orthodox medical practitioners as well as by qualified herbalists.

Each of the world's major herbal traditions developed its own framework for making sense of illness. In Europe, the principal model for understanding and explaining illness was the "theory of the four humors," which persisted well into the 17th century. It was laid down by Galen (131–201 CE), physician to the Roman emperor Marcus Aurelius. Galen was born in Pergamum, and part of his medical practice involved caring for the gladiators of the city, which gave him the opportunity to learn about anatomy and the remedies best suited to healing wounds. He wrote hundreds of books and had a crucial influence on European medicine for over 1,500 years. To this day, plant medicines are sometimes called Galenicals to distinguish them from synthesized drugs.

The theory of the four humors

Galen developed his ideas from the texts of Hippocrates (460–c.377 BCE) and Aristotle (384–322 BCE), who in turn had been influenced by Egyptian and Indian ideas. Hippocrates, expanding on the early belief that the world was made up of the elements fire, air, earth, and water, classified herbs as having hot, dry, cold, and moist properties. Aristotle developed and endorsed the theory of the four humors. According to the theory, four principal fluids—or humors—exist within the body: blood, choler (yellow bile), melancholy (black bile), and phlegm. The "ideal" person bore all four in equal proportion. However, in most people, one or more humors predominate, giving rise to particular temperaments or characters. For instance, excess choler produced a choleric-type person, who was likely to be short-tempered, sallow, ambitious, and vengeful. Galen also believed that *pneuma* (spirit) was taken in with each breath, and processed in the body to form the "vital spirit." Vitality and health depended upon the proper balance between the four humors, the four elements and the correct mix with the inspired *pneuma*.

Influence of classical herbalists

Two other classical writers strongly influenced the European herbal tradition. Dioscorides (40–90 CE), a Greek-born Roman army surgeon, wrote the classical

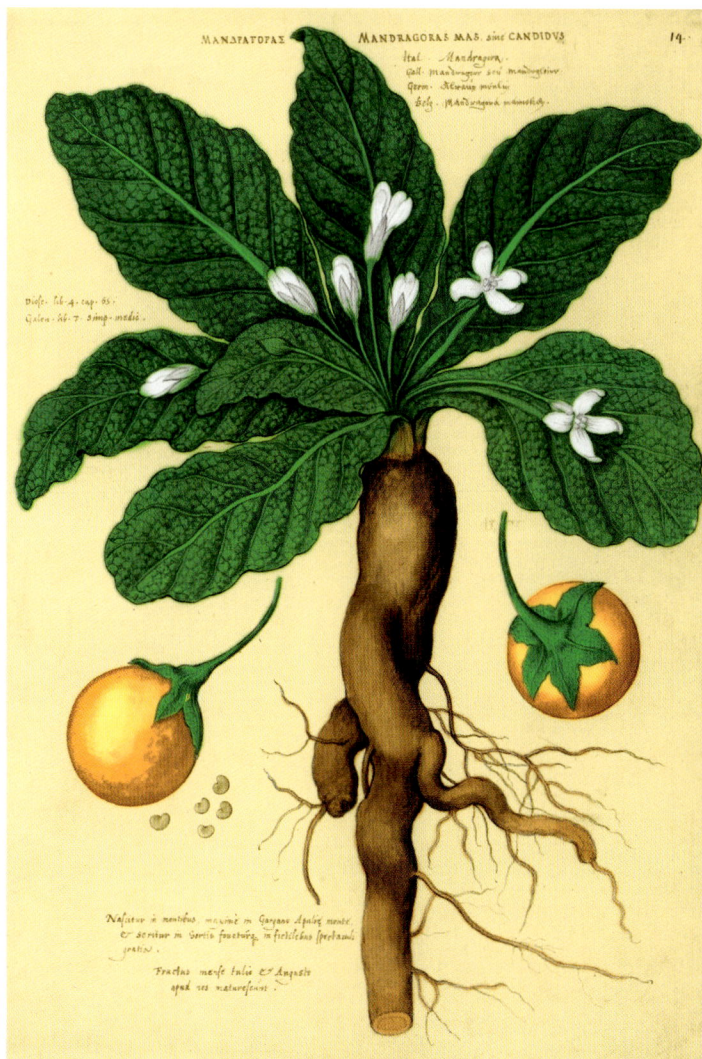

Mandrake (Mandragora officinarum), *with its forked root that appears to resemble the human shape, was credited with great magical and healing powers.*

The ancient theory of the four humors

The ancient theory of the four humors holds that four fluids within the body—black bile, phlegm, yellow bile, and blood—correspond to the four elements (earth, water, air, and fire), the four seasons, and other aspects of the natural world. Until the 17th century, physicians believed that an imbalance of the humoral system caused mental and physical illness.

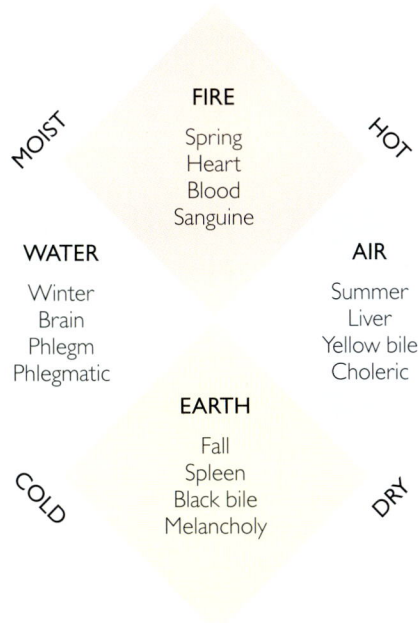

MOIST

FIRE
Spring
Heart
Blood
Sanguine

HOT

WATER
Winter
Brain
Phlegm
Phlegmatic

AIR
Summer
Liver
Yellow bile
Choleric

EARTH
Fall
Spleen
Black bile
Melancholy

COLD

DRY

world's most comprehensive book on herbal medicines, *De Materia Medica*, based on observations of nearly 600 plants. Pliny the Elder (23–79 CE) drew together writings from over 400 authors in his *Natural History*, recording, among other things, herbal lore of the time. Much traditional European knowledge of medicinal herbs comes from Dioscorides and Pliny. One of the most interesting herbs mentioned by both is mandrake (*Mandragora officinarum*, see p. 238). With a forked root that resembles the human shape, mandrake was credited with great magical and healing powers. It was recommended by Dioscorides for many ailments, including sleeplessness and inflammation of the eyes.

With the collapse of the Roman empire in the 5th century CE, the debate about how illness arose and how it should be treated shifted to the East. By the 9th century, Islamic physicians had translated much of Galen's work into Arabic, and his ideas affected the development of Arabic medicine into the Middle Ages, influencing Ibn Sina (980–1037). Later in the Middle Ages, Galen's writings were translated back into Latin from the Arabic and, for 400 years, his ideas held sway and were diligently applied in European medical practice. Even in the 16th and 17th centuries, students in university medical schools were given an academic training in the principles of the humoral system, as established by Galen. They learned how to diagnose an imbalance of the humors, and the methods of restoring equilibrium, primarily bloodletting and purging (see pp. 24–25).

Printing & herbal medicine

The invention of printing in the 15th century changed the face of herbal medicine in Europe. Before that time, European folk medicine had been handed down from

Key herbs from this region

St. John's wort (*Hypericum perforatum*, p. 110)

Valerian (*Valeriana officinalis*, p. 152)

Goldenrod (*Solidago virgaurea*, p. 280)

Marigold (*Calendula officinalis*, p. 77)

Hops (*Humulus lupulus*, p. 108)

Feverfew (*Tanacetum parthenium*, p. 144)

Yarrow (*Achillea millefolium*, p. 60)

Angelica (*Angelica archangelica*, p. 172)

Chaste tree (*Vitex agnus-castus*, p. 155)

Nettle (*Urtica dioica*, p. 150)

Hyssop (*Hyssopus officinalis*, p. 227)

Rosemary (*Rosmarinus officinalis*, p. 132)

Cramp bark (*Viburnum opulus*, p. 154)

Blackberry (*Rubus fruticosus*, p. 272)

Marsh mallow (*Althaea officinalis*, p. 169)

Milk thistle (*Silybum marianum*, p. 141)

Elderflower (*Sambucus nigra*, p. 136)

Sage (*Salvia officinalis*, p. 135)

Hawthorn (*Crataegus oxyacantha*, p. 91)

Cowslip (*Primula veris*, p. 264)

Thyme (*Thymus vulgaris*, p. 147)

Common foxglove (*Digitalis purpurea*, p. 207)

Heartsease (*Viola tricolor*, p. 292)

Lavender (*Lavandula officinalis*, p. 112)

"In several European countries herbal medicines are routinely prescribed by GPs, offering doctors a choice of gentle acting treatments for chronic and more minor health problems."

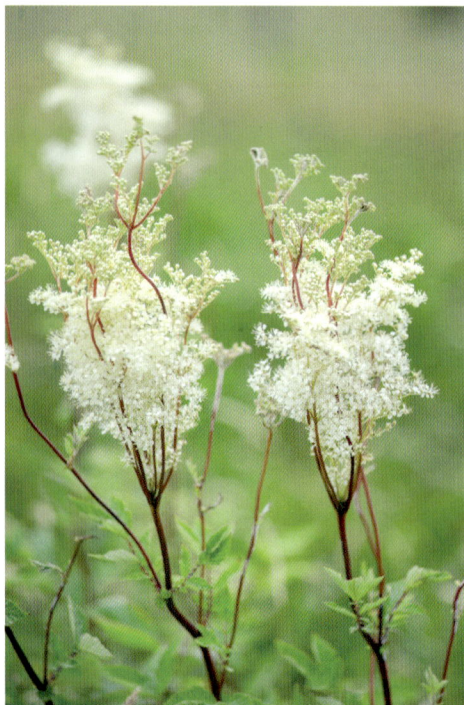

Meadowsweet (**Filipendula ulmaria**) *is often used in combination with other herbs to treat acid indigestion and gastritis.*

generation to generation. While some early herbals were written in Anglo-Saxon, Icelandic, and Welsh, for example, for the most part the tradition was orally based.

During the following centuries, herbals were published throughout Europe in different languages, making standardized catalogs of herbs and their applications accessible to the general public, not just to those who understood Latin. As literacy rates rose, women in particular used the advice in the herbals to treat their families.

In some cases, the printed herbals were written by physicians, and largely reflected the writings of classical authors such as Dioscorides. In other instances they were based directly on first-hand experience—the English herbals of John Gerard (1597) and Nicholas Culpeper (1652) being good examples.

John Gerard's *The Herball* is clearly the work of a horticulturist, rather than of an herbal practitioner, but is nonetheless a mine of information. The book includes many plants that had been recently brought back to Europe by explorers and traders.

Culpeper's *The English Physitian* has been widely used as a practical reference book ever since its publication. It is a rich blend of personal and practical experience, traditional European medicine, and astrological thought. Each herb is assigned a "temperature," a use within the humoral system, and a ruling planet and star sign. Like Dioscorides' *De Materia Medica*, it has the merit of being based on close observation and extensive experience in the use of herbal medicines.

Foreign herbs & synthesized drugs

The growing use of foreign herbs in the 17th century prompted heated debate about the relative value of native European herbs, but for the majority of the population this was irrelevant as the imported herbs were well out of their price range. In the end, it created a rift in herbal medicine. Poor and rural peoples used locally available herbs, while affluent city-dwellers and aristocrats purchased plants of foreign origin, prescribed by university-trained physicians. By the beginning of the 18th century, approximately 70 percent of plant medicines stocked by European apothecaries were imported. Over time, this city-based herbalism evolved into conventional scientific medicine, which in turn rejected its herbal roots and regarded plant medicines as inferior.

Once conventional medicine established its monopoly of practice—in most European countries by the end of the 19th century—it became (and in many cases still remains) illegal to practice herbalism without medical certification. In Greece, traditional herbalists, known as *komboyannites*, were persecuted, and the word itself became an insult meaning "trickster" or "quack." In France and Italy, experienced traditional herbalists were imprisoned for providing treatment to their patients. The renaissance in herbal medicine that has occurred in the last 40 years offers hope that official censure will change.

Modern practitioners

The pattern of herbal medicine across Europe today is remarkably varied, but a common thread runs through the different traditions and practices. Most European herbalists use orthodox methods of diagnosis, looking for signs of infection and inflammation, for example. However, most also try to establish a broad, holistic picture, placing the illness in the context of the patient's life as a whole. Herbalists then choose plant medicines and recommend suitable dietary and lifestyle changes that will allow the body's self-regenerating powers— the modern equivalent of the "vital spirit"— to establish good health once again. Recovery may take longer than it would if treated with conventional medicine, but relief is generally enduring and free from side effects.

A patient with a stomach ulcer, for example, may be treated with a variety of herbs such as meadowsweet (*Filipendula ulmaria*, p. 102), German chamomile (*Chamomilla recutita*, p. 82), marsh mallow (*Althaea officinalis*, p. 169), and deadly nightshade (*Atropa belladonna*, p. 73) to soothe inflammation, astringe, and protect the inner lining of the stomach, and reduce excess acid production. In addition, herbal practitioners also address poor dietary habits, bad posture, and stress—which are all conditions that may have undermined the body's healing ability. Problems such as these are reversed with herbs to relieve stress, a diet rich in non-acidic vegetables and fruits, and exercise.

Popular herbs

In European herbal medicine, native herbs are still highly popular. Alpine plants such as arnica (*Arnica montana*, p. 176) and pulsatilla (*Anemone pulsatilla*, p. 172) are much used in Swiss, German, Italian, and French herbal medicine, while comfrey (*Symphytum officinale*, p. 142) is particularly well liked in Britain. There has also been a surge in demand for exotic herbs. The Chinese ginkgo tree (*Ginkgo biloba*, p. 104), which improves circulation of blood to the head and helps the memory, is now cultivated in vast plantations in France, and has been a best-selling medicine in Germany for over 20 years.

European traditions & the future

Sales of over-the-counter herbal medicines in Europe have continued to increase over the last two decades, though the reasons for this growth vary widely.

It is possibly a reaction to the over-reliance on drug treatment in conventional medicine. Sound advice on a healthy diet and lifestyle, including food herbs, such as turmeric (*Curcuma longa*, p. 94), might well prove more beneficial than conventionally prescribed drugs in helping an aging population to stay healthy for longer.

Nevertheless, in several European countries herbal medicines are routinely prescribed, offering doctors a choice of gentle-acting treatments for chronic and more minor health problems. In Germany and Poland, herbal medicines can be frontline treatments for digestive disorders and chronic problems such as arthritis. This approach leaves conventional drug treatments available for more acute or serious conditions.

In contrast, a barely reported trend is that more and more people are growing medicinal plants. There is a desire to rediscover the magic of cultivating and harvesting plants, and involving them (as food and medicine) in one's daily life.

A 2019 survey conducted by University College, London School of Pharmacy summarizes the situation well:

Herbal medicines are popular, particularly among the 36–55 year old age group. When answers of the group regarding "What, if anything, attracts you to herbal remedies?" were analyzed, 68% indicated that it is because plants are "effective." Other popular reasons for use included that plant medicines are natural and have fewer side effects. Herbal medicines are particularly popular for minor self-limiting conditions like improving sleep or respiratory conditions. Around a third of people grew their own plants for health care, which include mint, lemon balm, and rosemary.

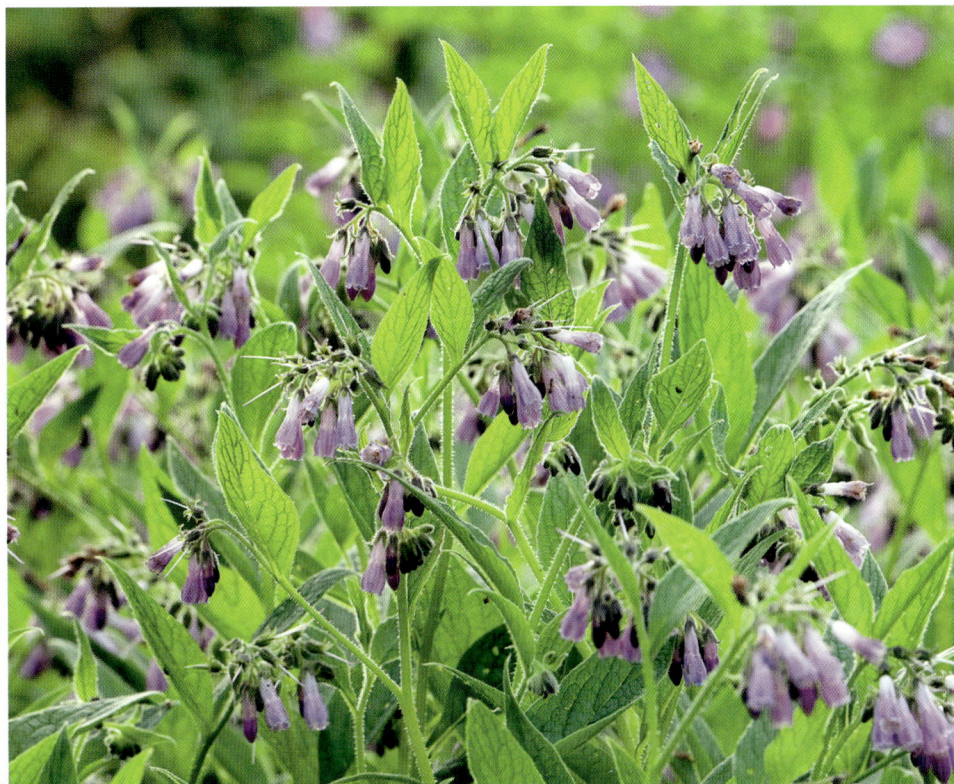

Comfrey (Symphytum officinale), *also known as Knitbone, speeds up tissue healing and has long-standing use as a topical treatment for sprains, fractures, and bruises.*

India and the Middle East

In India and the neighboring regions, a variety of herbal traditions continue to flourish. Ayurveda is the main system of healing in India, but Unani Tibb, traditional Arabic medicine, and Siddha, practiced in Tamil areas of southern India and Sri Lanka, are also major herbal traditions.

The name Ayurveda derives from two Indian words: *ayur* meaning longevity, and *veda* meaning knowledge or science. Ayurveda is as much a way of life as a system of medicine, and encompasses science, religion, and philosophy. Its ultimate aim, drawing on its many different practices—yoga and meditation, for example—is to promote self-realization and a harmonious relationship with the world.

Early origins

Ancient Indian culture developed around 5,000 years ago along the banks of the Indus River in northern India. This is thought of as a time of great spiritual enlightenment, with knowledge and wisdom being transmitted orally from teacher to student over many generations, and eventually set down in Sanskrit poetry known as the *Vedas*. These writings, dating from approximately 1500 BCE, distilled the prevailing historical, religious, philosophical, and medical knowledge, and form the basis of Indian culture. The most important of these texts are the *Rig Veda* and the *Atharva Veda*.

In about 400 BCE, the first Ayurvedic medical school was founded by Punarvasu Atreya. He and his pupils recorded medical knowledge in treatises that would in turn influence Charaka, the scholar who is thought to have written the *Charaka Samhita*. This compendium of writings, in the form that it has come down to us, dates from around 100 CE and describes 341 plant medicines as well as medicines of animal and mineral origin. The second major work was the *Sushruta Samhita*, dating from around the same time; it displays detailed knowledge of surgery, especially plastic surgery, and is still consulted today.

The influence of Ayurveda

Other traditions of medicine share common roots with Ayurveda, and Ayurveda has some claim to being the oldest surviving medical tradition in the world. From the time of the Buddha (563–483 BCE) onward, Ayurvedic medical ideas and practices spread across Asia, accompanying the spread of Buddhism itself. Buddhism, and Ayurvedic approaches to medicine, strongly influenced the development of Tibetan medicine, and these ideas in turn combined fruitfully with traditional Chinese medicine. Ancient civilizations of East and West were linked to one another by trade routes, campaigns, and wars. In each case, this led to the exchange of ideas, medicinal plants, and medical practices, including fertile connections between Ayurveda, Siddha, and traditional Chinese medicine to the east, and ancient Greek and Roman medicine to the west. Later, from

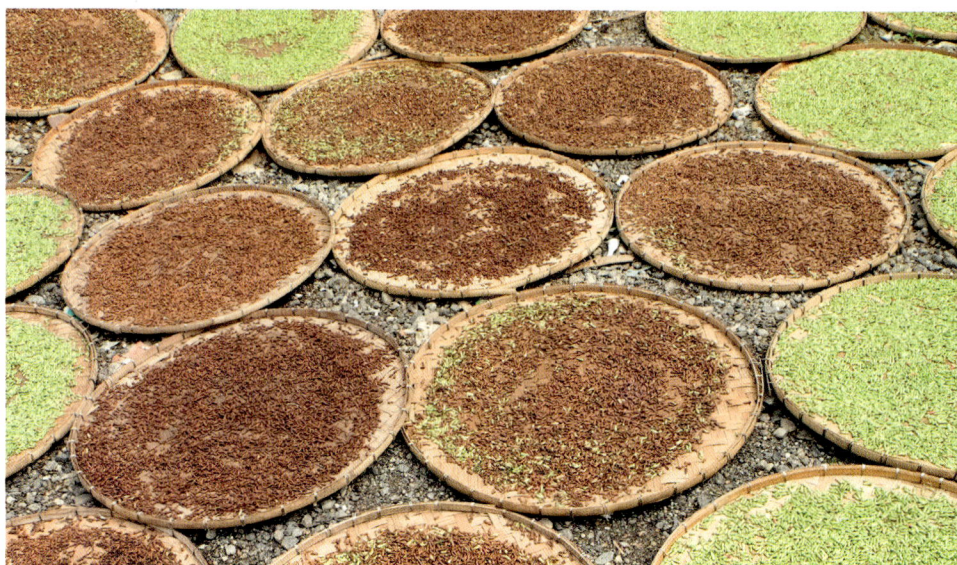

Cloves have been used medicinally for thousands of years in India. The flower buds are dried in the open air.

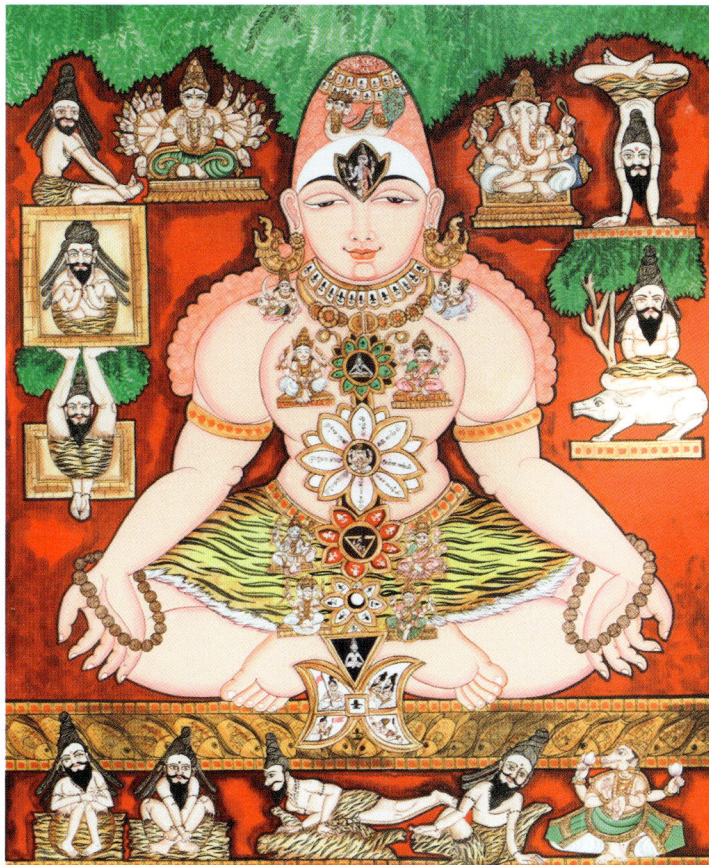

The chakras are represented in this figure. India's medical system, Ayurveda, identifies seven energy centers, chakras, sited along the spinal column from the head to the base of the spine. If they are blocked, illness results. The figures around the edge show some yoga positions.

Key herbs from this region

Myrtle (*Myrtus communis*, p. 246)

Castor oil plant (*Ricinus communis*, p. 271)

Garlic (*Allium sativum*, p. 63)

Cloves (*Eugenia caryophyllata*, p. 101)

Oriental sweetgum (*Liquidambar orientalis*, p. 234)

Licorice (*Glycyrrhiza glabra*, p. 105)

Nutmeg & mace (*Myristica fragrans*, p. 119)

Holy basil (*Ocimum tenuiflorum*, p. 120)

Balloon vine (*Cardiospermum* spp., p. 186)

Turmeric (*Curcuma longa*, p. 94)

Asafoetida (*Ferula assa-foetida*, p. 215)

Lemon (*Citrus limon*, p. 86)

Cardamom (*Elettaria cardamomum*, p. 97)

Cinnamon (*Cinnamomum* spp., p. 85)

Ashwagandha (*Withania somnifera*, p. 156)

Jequirity (*Abrus precatorius*, p. 162)

Soy (*Glycine max*, p. 221)

Sweet flag (*Acorus calamus*, p. 163)

Chiretta (*Swertia chirata*, p. 283)

Pomegranate (*Punica granatum*, p. 261)

Tea (*Camellia sinensis*, p. 185)

Ginger (*Zingiber officinale*, p. 159)

around 700 CE, traditional Greek medicine, based on Hippocratic ideas, developed in the Arabic world as classical Greek texts were translated into Arabic. This tradition, known as Unani Tibb (meaning "Ionian medicine," referring to the island of Iona where Hippocrates lived), at one time spanned from India to Spain, and is still the main form of herbal medicine practiced by hakims in the Middle East.

The five elements

Ayurveda is a unique holistic system, based on the interaction of body, mind, and spirit. In Ayurveda, the origin of all aspects of existence is pure intellect or consciousness. Energy and matter are one. Energy is manifested in five elements—ether, air, fire, water, and earth—which together form the basis of all matter. In the body, ether is present in the cavities of the mouth, abdomen, digestive tract, thorax, and lungs. Air is manifested in the movements of the muscles, pulsations of the heart, expansion and contraction of the lungs, and the workings of the digestive tract and the nervous system. Fire is manifested in the digestive system, metabolism, body temperature, vision, and intelligence. Water is present in the digestive juices, salivary glands, mucous membranes, blood, and cytoplasm. Earth exists in the nails, skin, and hair, as well as in the elements that hold the body together: bones, cartilage, muscles, and tendons.

The five elements manifest in the functioning of the five senses, and they are closely related to our ability to perceive and interact with the environment in which we live. In Ayurveda, ether, air, fire, water and earth correspond to hearing, touch, vision, taste, and smell respectively.

The doshas & health

The five elements combine to form three basic forces, known as the *tridoshas*, which exist in everything in the universe, and influence all mental and physical processes. From ether and air, the air principle *vata* is created; fire and water yield the fire principle *pitta*; and earth and water produce the water principle *kapha*. The principles correspond closely to the three humors of Tibetan medicine and somewhat resemble Galen's theory of the four humors (*see* p. 36).

According to Ayurveda, we are all born with a particular balance of doshas. The proportions are largely determined by the balance of doshas in our parents at the time of our conception. Our body type, temperament, and susceptibility to illnesses are largely governed by the predominant *dosha*. In this way we inherit our basic constitution, called the *prakruti*, which remains unaltered throughout our lives.

The first requirement for health in Ayurveda is a proper balance of the *doshas*. If the balance is upset, illness, *ryadhi*, results. The disruption may be manifested in physical discomfort and pain, or in mental and emotional suffering, including jealousy, anger, fear, and sorrow. While our balance of *doshas* influences vulnerability to certain kinds of illness, the principles do not work in a vacuum.

The effect lifestyle has on our *prakruti*—*vakruti*—has a strong effect on overall health, and may easily disrupt *dosha* balance.

Illness may also result if the flow of energy, *prana*, around the body is interrupted. The flow is relayed via the seven *chakras* (psychic energy centers), which are situated at various points along the spinal column, from the crown of the head to the tailbone. If the energy flowing between these centers is blocked, the likelihood of ill health increases.

Visiting an Ayurvedic practitioner

An Ayurvedic practitioner first carefully assesses *prakruti* and *vakruti*—constitution and lifestyle. This involves taking a detailed case history and carefully examining the body, paying attention to the build, the lines in the face and hands, and skin and hair type—all of which point to more profound aspects of the patient's condition. However, the main foundations on which diagnosis rests are the appearance of the tongue, and the pulse rate. In these respects, Ayurveda has much in common with Chinese and Tibetan medicine, in which these two indicators are also of the greatest importance. A very complex technique for taking the patient's pulse has been developed by Ayurvedic practitioners, requiring many years' experience.

When a *dosha* imbalance has been diagnosed, medical treatment and lifestyle advice are provided. The first step focuses on the elimination of toxins and the main cleansing and rejuvenation program, known as *panchakarma*, includes therapeutic vomiting, purging, enemas, nasal administration of medication, and purification of the blood.

Attributes of remedies

Subsequent treatments fall into three main categories: medicines from natural sources, dietary regimens, and behavioral modifications. Medicines, foods, and lifestyle activities are all classified according to their effect on the three *doshas*. For instance, a health problem associated with an excess of *kapha*, the water principle, is characterized by congestion, excess weight, fluid retention, and lethargy. The practitioner would prescribe the consumption of warm, dry, light foods, because the quality of *kapha* is cool and damp. Avoidance of cold damp foods (such as wheat, sugar, and milk products), which increase *kapha*, would also be advised. Herbal remedies would include warming spices such as ginger (*Zingiber officinale*, p. 159) and cayenne (*Capsicum frutescens,* p. 79), as well as bitters such as turmeric (*Curcuma longa*, p. 94).

The specific choice of herbal remedy depends on its "quality" or "energy," which Ayurveda determines according to twenty attributes (*vimshati guna*) such as hot, cold, wet, dry, heavy, or light. Ayurveda also classifies remedies according to six tastes—sweet, sour, salty, bitter, pungent, and astringent. Sweet, sour, and salty substances increase water (*kapha*) and decrease air (*vata*); bitter, pungent, and astringent remedies increase air and decrease water; and sour, salty, and pungent herbs increase fire (*pitta*).

Preparations & treatments

In addition to plant extracts, Ayurvedic medicines include honey and dairy produce, and sometimes minute doses of minerals such as salt are added. Remedies take the form of pills, powders, balms, and infusions, and most contain several different ingredients, all carefully balanced to individual needs. Treatment might include washes and enemas or the application of poultices as well as massage with warm herbal oil, burning incense, the use of precious stones and metals, and ritual purification for imbalanced mind and emotions. The chanting of mantras (incantations based on sacred texts),

> "In addition to plant extracts, Ayurvedic medicines include honey and dairy produce, and sometimes minute doses of minerals such as salt are added."

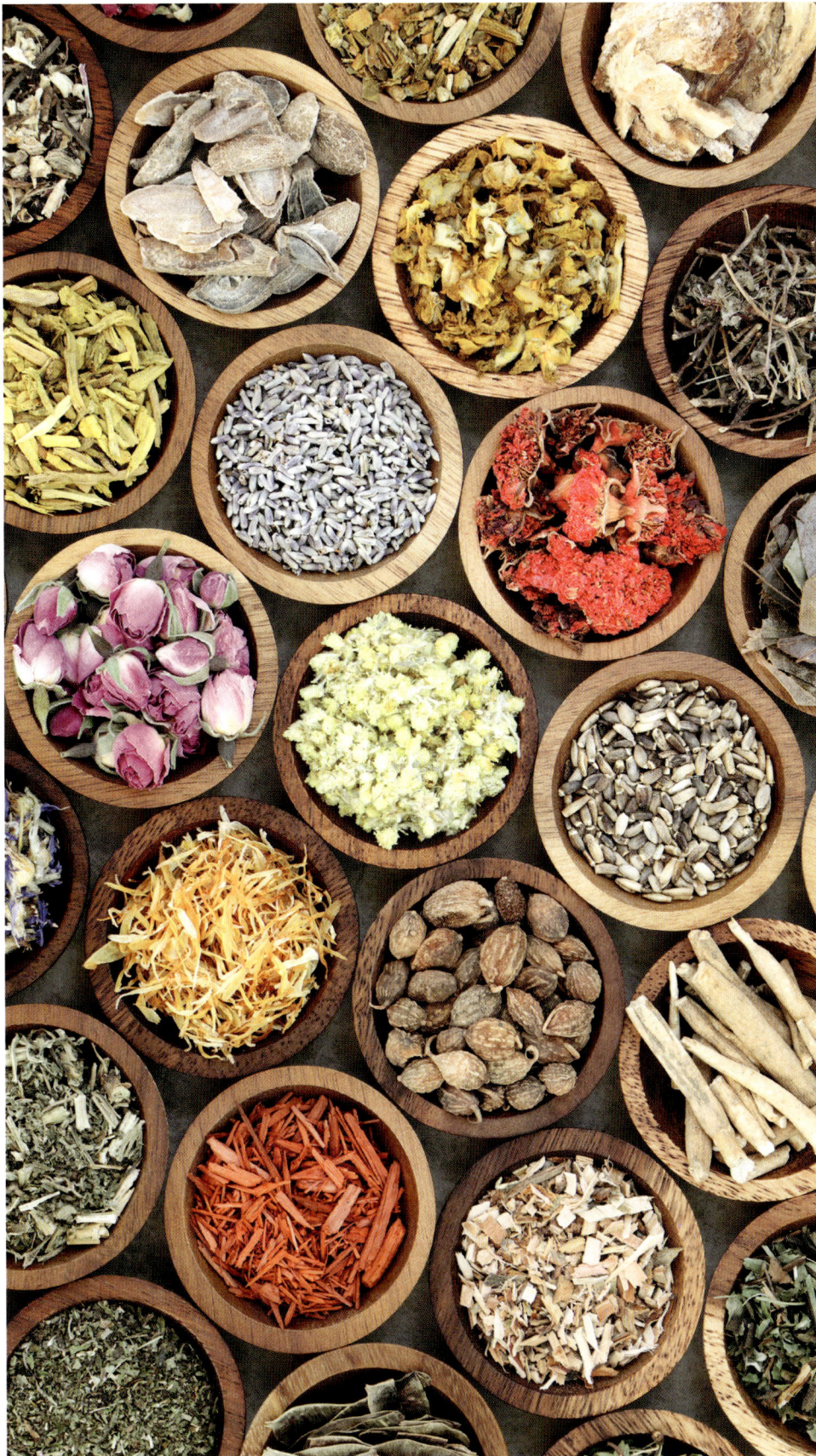

breathing, and meditation exercises may be advised, due to the power of sound and the effect of vibration and meditation on the body, mind, and spirit.

Herbal medicine in India today

In the 19th century, the British dismissed Ayurveda as mere superstition, and in 1833 they closed all Ayurvedic schools and banned the practice. Great centers of Indian learning thus fell apart, and Ayurvedic knowledge retreated into villages and temples. At the turn of the century, however, some Indian physicians and enlightened Englishmen began to reevaluate Ayurveda, and by the time of India's independence in 1947 it had regained its reputation as a valid medical system. Today, Ayurveda flourishes side by side with Unani Tibb and Western conventional medicine and is actively encouraged by the Indian government as an inexpensive alternative to Western drugs. In recent years, Ayurveda has attracted increasing attention from medical scientists in the West and in Japan, and the World Health Organization has resolved to promote its practice in developing countries.

Ayurveda's value lies in the fact that it is not a medical science dealing solely with treatment of disease. Instead, it offers practical guidelines that apply to every facet of daily existence. It also seeks to reconcile health and lifestyle with universal aspects of existence, and to enhance well-being and promote longevity.

The specific choice of herbal remedy depends on its "quality" or "energy," which Ayurveda determines according to twenty attributes (vimshati guna).

China, Japan, and Southeast Asia

China's ancient herbal tradition has survived intact into the 21st century, and in China it is now accorded equal status with Western conventional medicine. Today, many Chinese universities teach and research herbal medicine, a factor of crucial importance in the reemergence of herbalism worldwide.

Traditional Chinese medicine (TCM) and the herbal tradition that is part of it developed separately from Chinese folk medicine. It arose from ideas recorded between 200 BCE and 100 CE in the *Yellow Emperor's Classic of Internal Medicine (Huang Di Nei Jing)*. This text is based on detailed observations of nature and a deep understanding of the way that all life is subject to natural laws. It contains concepts that are fundamental to TCM, including *yin* and *yang*; the five elements (*wu xing*); and the theory of the effect of nature upon health.

In TCM, living in harmony with these principles is the key to good health and longevity. According to the *Yellow Emperor's Classic*, members of previous generations lived for a hundred years, and had constitutions so strong that illness was cured by incantations alone. Only later, as human vitality, or *qi*, declined and people became "overactive … going against the joy of life," did herbal medicine, acupuncture, and other branches of TCM become necessary.

Key theories

Unlike other herbal traditions that have a unified theory for making sense of illness and disease (for example, the European theory of the four humors), TCM has two quite different systems—the *yin* and *yang* theory and the five elements. They developed quite separately in China, and the five elements system was only accepted and fully incorporated into Chinese medicine during the Song dynasty (960–1279 CE). To this day, differences between these theories are reflected in practitioners' approaches to diagnosis and treatment.

In Chinese thought, everything in the universe is composed of *yin* and *yang*—words that were first used to denote the dark and light side of a valley. Everything has *yin* and *yang* aspects, or complementary opposites—such as day and night, up and down, wet and dry. Every yin or yang category can itself also be subdivided—so that while the front of the body is *yin* relative to the back, which is *yang*, the abdomen is *yin* relative to the chest, which is *yang*.

The five elements theory associates constituents of the natural world—wood, fire, earth, metal, and water—with other fundamentals such as seasons, emotions, and

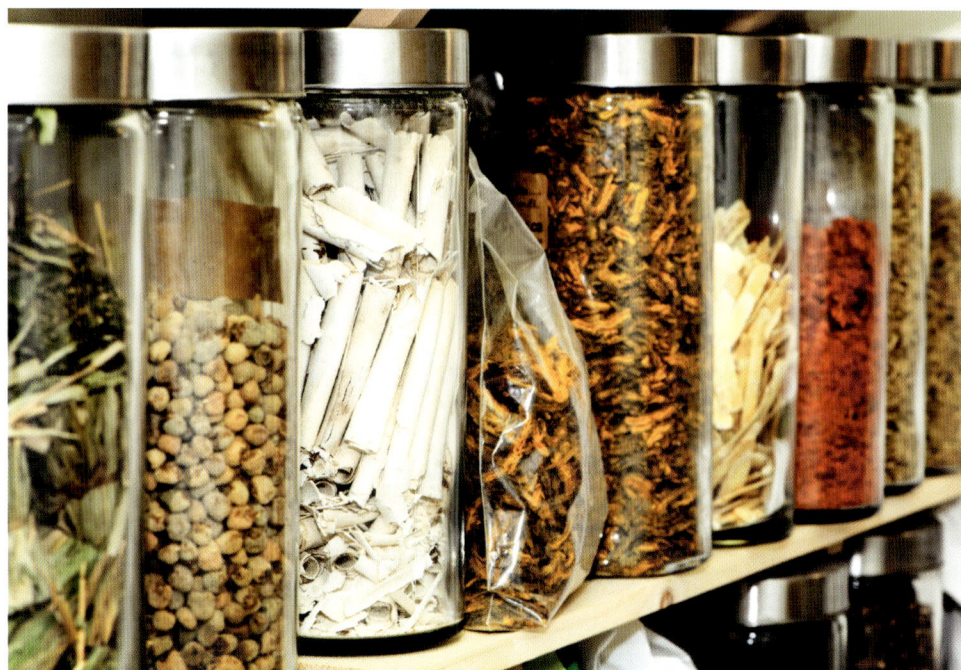

On the streets of Hong Kong herbal pharmacists are a familiar sight. Prescriptions are formulated during a consultation with an herbalist, and the patient then obtains the appropriate herbs.

The ancient five elements theory

The ancient five elements theory is used by the Chinese when writing prescriptions. It associates herbs with the natural world, including elements, seasons, and parts of the body. In the circular movement, each element gives rise to the next (for example, winter gives rise to spring). The five-angled movement is a controlling one, in which each element restrains another.

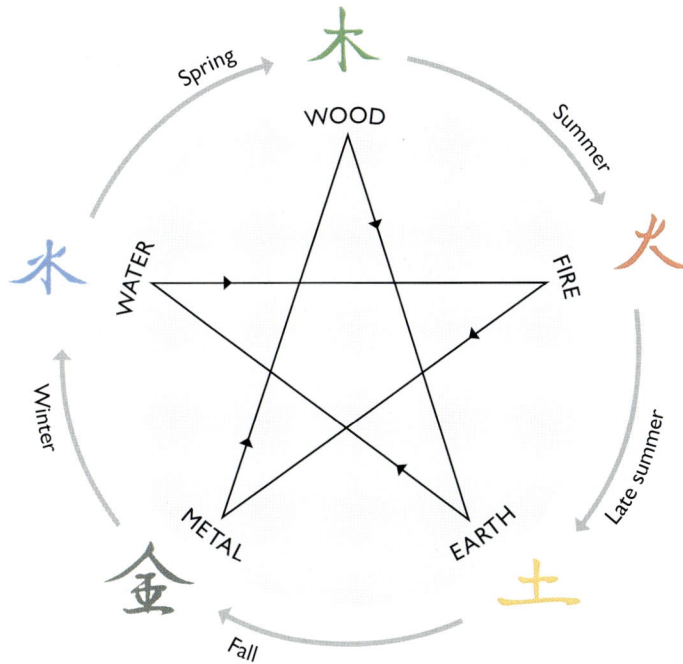

	WOOD	FIRE	EARTH	METAL	WATER
Season	Spring	Summer	Late summer	Fall	Winter
Climate	Windy	Hot	Damp	Dry	Cold
Emotion	Anger	Joy	Reflection	Grief	Fear
Taste	Sour	Bitter	Sweet	Pungent	Salty
Herb	Schisandra	Chinese rhubarb	Jujube	Ginger	Chinese figwort
Actions	Astringent	Cooling	Tonic, Restorative	Stimulant, Warming	Drains fluids
Parts of the body	Liver Gallbladder Eyes Tendons	Heart Small intestine Tongue Blood vessels	Spleen Stomach Mouth Flesh	Lungs Large intestine Nose Skin	Kidneys Bladder Ears Hair

Key herbs from this region

Magnolia (*Magnolia officinalis*, p. 237)

Baikal skullcap (*Scutellaria baicalensis*, p. 138)

Fu ling (*Poria cocos*)

Chou wu tong (*Clerodendrum trichotomum*, p. 195)

Ginseng (*Panax ginseng*, p. 123)

Schisandra (*Schisandra chinensis*, p. 137)

Sang ye (*Morus alba*, p. 244)

Codonopsis (*Codonopsis pilosula*, p. 87)

Jing jie (*Schizonepeta tenuifolia*, p. 276)

Fo ti (*Polygonum multiflorum*, p. 129)

Chinese angelica (*Angelica sinensis*, p. 67)

Galangal (*Alpinia officinarum*, p. 169)

Cinnamon (*Cinnamomum cassia*, p. 85)

Notopterygium root (*Notopterygium incisum*, p. 247)

Ginkgo (*Ginkgo biloba*, p. 104)

Su xian hua (*Jasminum officinale*, see *J. grandiflorum*, p. 228)

Goji berry (*Lycium chinense*, p. 115)

Hong hua (*Carthamus tinctorius*, p. 187)

White peony (*Paeonia lactiflora*, p. 122)

Huo xiang (*Agastache rugosa*, p. 165)

Ephedra (*Ephedra sinica*, p. 99)

Chinese rhubarb (*Rheum palmatum*, p. 130)

Ju hua (*Chrysanthemum* x *morifolium*, p. 83)

Corydalis (*Corydalis yanhusuo*, p. 90)

Zhe bei mu (*Fritillaria thunbergii*)

Huang lian (*Coptis chinensis*, p. 199)

Shan yao (*Dioscorea opposita*)

Suan zhoa ren (*Ziziphus spinosa*, see *Z. jujuba*, p. 293)

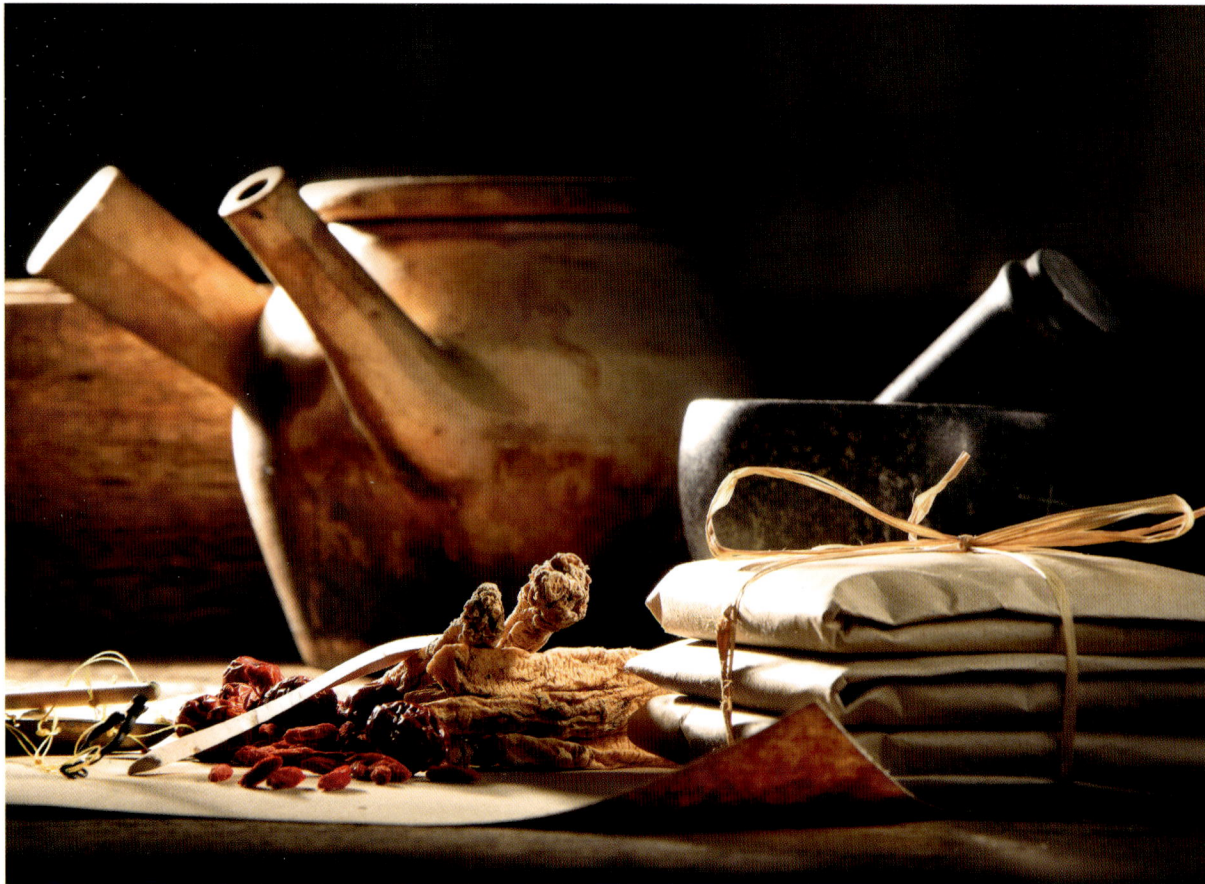

Many herbal preparations are available to Chinese practitioners.

parts of the body. Each element gives rise to the next in a perpetual fashion (see diagram above). For this reason, the system might be more accurately described as the five phases, representing the process of continual movement in life. The five elements have a central role in Chinese herbal medicine, especially in the grouping of tastes of herbs and parts of the body.

Diagnosis & treatment

Instead of looking for causes of illness, Chinese practitioners seek patterns of disharmony, which are expressions of imbalance between *yin* and *yang*. Particular attention is given to reading the pulse and tongue, both of which are very important for an accurate diagnosis. Ill health results from a deficiency or excess of either *yin* or *yang*. A cold, for example, is not just the result of a virus (though this clearly is a cause), but a sign

that the body is not adapting to external factors such as "wind-heat," "wind-cold," or "summer-heat." A high temperature denotes too much *yang* and shivering is the result of an excess of *yin*. The art of the Chinese herbal practitioner is to restore harmony between *yin* and *yang* both within the patient's body and between the patient and the world at large.

Chinese herbs

Over the centuries, the number of medicinal herbs has grown, and the 1977 Encyclopedia of *Traditional Chinese Medicinal Substances* has 5,757 entries, the majority of which are herbs. The Communist Revolution in 1949 helped swell the number of plants used in TCM, because herbs that had previously only been employed in folk medicine were incorporated into the tradition.

As the herbal tradition developed within

TCM, the taste and other characteristics of herbs became closely linked with their therapeutic uses. *The Divine Husbandman's Classic* (*Shen'nong Bencaojing*, 1st century CE) lists 252 herbal medicines specifying their tastes and "temperatures," and today, Chinese herbalists still relate the taste and temperature of an herb directly to its therapeutic use. Sweet-tasting herbs such as ginseng (*Panax ginseng*, p. 123) are prescribed to tone, harmonize, and moisten, while bitter-tasting herbs such as *dan shen* (*Salvia miltiorrhiza*, p. 134) are employed to drain and dry excess "dampness." Hot-tasting herbs are used for treating "cold" conditions and vice versa. Together, an herb's taste and temperature link it to specific types of illness. For example, Baikal skullcap (*Scutellaria baicalensis*, p. 138), which is bitter-tasting and "cold," is a drying, cooling herb for conditions such as fever and irritability, brought on by patterns of excess heat.

"The Chinese tradition relies heavily on formulas, which are set mixtures of herbs that have proven effectiveness as tonics or remedies for specific illnesses."

Taking medicines

The Chinese tradition relies heavily on formulas, which are set mixtures of herbs that have proven effectiveness as tonics or remedies for specific illnesses. Many are available over the counter and are used by millions of people every day in China and around the world. Chinese herbalists often take a formula as a starting point and then add other herbs to the mixture. There are hundreds of formulas, one of the most famous being "Four Things Soup," a tonic given to regulate the menstrual cycle and tone the reproductive system. It consists of *dong quai* (*Angelica sinensis*, p. 67), rehmannia (*Rehmannia glutinosa*, p. 270), *chuang xiong* (*Ligusticum wallachii*), and white peony (*Paeonia lactiflora*, p. 122).

Chinese herbal medicine uses tinctures or alcoholic extracts of herbs, but only infrequently. Generally, patients are given mixtures of roots and bark to take as decoctions two or three times a day.

The Chinese influence in Japan & Korea

Japan and Korea have been strongly influenced by Chinese medical ideas and practices. *Kampoh*, traditional Japanese medicine, traces its origins back to the 5th century CE, when Buddhist monks from Korea introduced their healing arts, largely derived from Chinese medicine, into Japan. In the following century, the Empress Suiko (592–628 CE) sent envoys to China to study that country's culture and medicine. Direct Chinese influence on Japanese medicine, which was practiced for the most part by the monks, continued for 1,000 years. In the 16th century, Japan started to assert its cultural identity, and kampoh developed its own characteristic traits, emphasizing the Japanese ideals of simplicity and naturalness. However, certain Chinese concepts, such as *yin* and *yang* and *ki* (*qi*), continued to have a central role.

In 1868, the Japanese embraced Western conventional medicine. Formal training in *kampoh* officially ceased in 1885, but a few committed practitioners passed their knowledge on to younger generations, keeping the tradition alive. In the last 40 years the number of medical practitioners who use *kampoh* within their practice has greatly increased. Many Japanese medical schools now include training in *kampoh* as part of the curriculum.

Korean herbal medicine is very similar to mainstream Chinese herbal medicine, and almost all the Chinese herbs are used in Korea. Ginseng (*Panax ginseng*, p. 123) has been cultivated in Korea for home use and export since 1300.

Importance of Chinese herbal medicine

Since 1949 when the Chinese Communist Party gained control, the herbal tradition has flourished in China (*see* p. 31) and today it is recognized as a valid medical system, available to the Chinese on an equal footing with conventional Western medicine. As is often the case elsewhere, herbs seem to be used mainly for chronic conditions, while Western medicine is more frequently employed for serious acute illness.

Chinese herbal medicine, however, is not just of significance in China and the surrounding regions, but is practiced by trained practitioners in every continent and, in some countries, now has official government recognition. For example, there has been a traditional Chinese medicine hospital in Paris since 1996, and in 2013 the French government agreed to open three new traditional Chinese medicine hospital centers. Herbal medicine is now taught in 34 Chinese universities. This development (and the massive input of resources involved) has helped revitalize herbal medicine around the world over the past 30 to 40 years.

The impact of these developments has not been confined solely to those taking herbal medicines—whether in China or elsewhere. In 2015 Dr. Tu Youyou, a researcher trained in traditional Chinese medicine and conventional medicine, was awarded the Nobel Prize for medicine for her lifelong study of sweet Annie (*Artemisia annua*, p. 71) and its key active constituent artemisinin. From her base at the Academy of Traditional Chinese Medicine in Beijing, she proved that the herb (and its active constituent) had unusually potent antimalarial activity. Artemisinin has now become the standard treatment for acute malaria.

Africa

In Africa there is a greater variety of herbal traditions than on any other continent. During the colonial period, indigenous herbal practices were largely suppressed, but today, in a marked turnaround, practitioners of conventional medicine often work closely with traditional healers.

The therapeutic use of medicinal plants in Africa dates back to the earliest times. Ancient Egyptian writings confirm that herbal medicines have been valued in North Africa for millennia. The Ebers papyrus (c.1500 BCE), one of the oldest surviving medical texts, includes over 870 prescriptions and formulas, 700 medicinal herbs—including gentian (*Gentiana lutea*, p. 103), aloe (*Aloe vera*, p. 64), and opium poppy (*Papaver somniferum*, p. 251)—and covers conditions ranging from chest complaints to crocodile bite. The medicinal arts put forward in this and other Egyptian texts formed the intellectual foundation of classical medical practice in Greece, Rome, and the Arabic world.

Trade & the Arabian influence

Herbal medicines have been traded between the Middle East, India, and northeastern Africa for at least 3,000 years. Herbs widely used in the Middle East, such as myrrh (*Commiphora myrrha*, p. 89), originally came from Somalia and the Horn of Africa. From the 5th century CE to the 13th century, Arab physicians were at the forefront of medical advancement, and in the 8th century, the spread of Arabic culture across northern Africa had an influence on North African medicine that lasts to this day. In the mid-13th century, the botanist Ibn El Beitar published a *Materia Medica* that considerably increased the range of North African plant medicines in common use.

Ancient beliefs & indigenous herbs

In the more remote areas of Africa, nomadic peoples, such as the Berber of Morocco and the Topnaar of Namibia, have herbal traditions that until recently have remained largely unaffected by changes in medicine in the world at large. For these people, traditional healing linked to a magical world in which spirits influence illness and death. In Berber culture, possession by a *djinn* (spirit) is a major cause of sickness, and herbs with "magical" properties are given to restore health. If the patient fails to recover, their condition is likely to be attributed to a curse or to the "evil eye."

The Topnaar formerly depended completely on their environment for medicines, using the few medicinal plants that grow in such harsh and arid conditions. Although they are now heavily influenced by the Western way of life and have lost much of their plant lore, they continue to employ many indigenous plants medicinally. The stem of the seaweed *Ecklonia maxima*, for example, is roasted, mixed with petroleum jelly, and

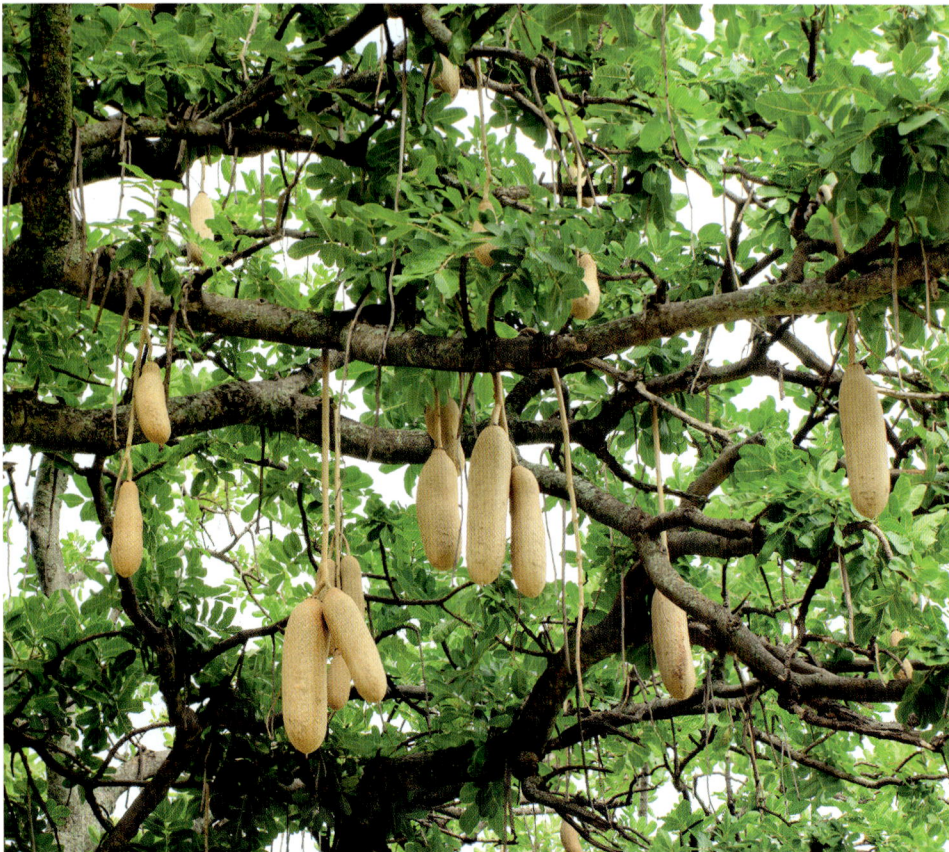

Kigelia (**Kigelia pinnata**)—*an African tree from the region south of the Sahara—has been shown to have a marked ability to prevent and treat inflammatory skin conditions such as psoriasis.*

rubbed into wounds and burns, while *Hoodia currori*, a low-lying cactus, is stripped of its thorns and outer skin and eaten raw to treat coughs and colds.

Throughout Africa, thousands of different wild and locally grown medicinal plants are sold in the markets. Some are prescribed as medicines for home use. Others, such as kanna (*Mesembryanthemum* spp.) and iboga (*Tabernanthe iboga*), are chewed to combat fatigue, and are taken as intoxicants in religious ceremonies. According to local accounts in the Congo and Gabon, iboga's stimulant effect was discovered when observers saw wild boars and gorillas dig up and eat the roots, and subsequently become frenzied.

Traditional & conventional care

Conventional Western medicine is well established throughout Africa, but in rural areas, far from medical and hospital services, traditional medicine remains the only form of health care available. Even in urban areas conventional health care services can be limited, and in this situation traditional providers of care such as traditional healers, herbalists, and midwives are the main source of treatment available for the majority of the population. The World Health Organization aims to achieve a level of health care that will permit all people to lead socially and economically productive lives. In an attempt to meet this, African countries have pioneered the training of traditional medicine practitioners in simple medical techniques and basic hygiene procedures. In one center in Mampong, Ghana, conventionally trained medical staff work hand in hand with traditional herbal practitioners, encouraging the safer use of herbal medicines and researching them in detail. In nearby Kumasi, the university now offers a BS degree in herbal medicine. This represents a remarkable change in attitude. In the 19th and much of the 20th centuries, colonial governments and Christian missionaries viewed traditional herbalists as witch doctors, whose practices were best suppressed.

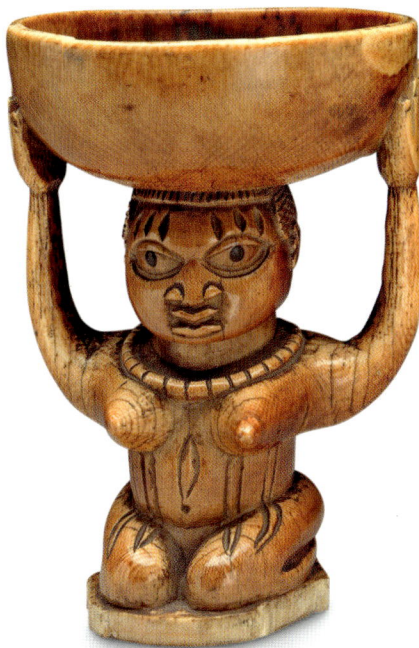

This Nigerian divination bowl was used by traditional healers to guide their understanding in diagnosing and treating illness. Sixteen palm nuts were placed in the bowl and their positioning interpreted.

The discovery of new herbal cures

Along with encouraging the safer use of herbal medicines, medical centers are researching their use in detail. The benefits of pygeum (*Pygeum africanum*, p. 268) have been conclusively established. This tree is traditionally used in central and southern Africa to treat urinary problems. Today, it is regularly prescribed in conventional French and Italian medicine for prostate problems. Of the plants under investigation in Africa, Kigelia (*Kigelia pinnata*, p. 230)—a tree from the region south of the Sahara, and Sutherlandia (*Sutherlandia frutescens*)—a small South African shrub, are of particular interest. Kigelia has a marked ability to prevent and heal skin lesions, including psoriasis, while Sutherlandia is an adaptogen with anticancer activity.

The reevaluation of traditional herbal medicine in Africa may result in the acceptance of additional plant-based medicines. Today, the opportunity exists to combine the best of traditional practice with conventional medical knowledge, for mutual gain.

Key herbs from this region

Calumba (*Jateorhiza palmata*, p. 229)
Buchu (*Barosma betulina*, p. 75)
Coffee (*Coffea arabica*, p. 196)
Visnaga (*Ammi visnaga*, p. 65)
Myrrh (*Commiphora myrrha*, p. 89)
Devil's claw (*Harpagophytum procumbens*, p. 107)
Kola nut (*Cola acuminata*, p. 197)
Grains of paradise (*Aframomum melegueta*)
Pellitory (*Anacyclus pyrethrum*, p. 171)
Senna (*Cassia senna*, p. 80)
Aloe vera (*Aloe vera*, p. 64)

Australia and New Zealand

Regrettably, much of the herbal knowledge of the Australian Aborigines was lost after the arrival of the Europeans. The predominant strains of Australian herbalism today derive from the West, China, and, increasingly, from other countries on the Pacific Rim.

The cradle of the oldest continuous culture on earth, Australia is also the home of an ancient herbal tradition. The Aboriginal people, believed to have settled in Australia over 60,000 years ago, developed a sophisticated empirical understanding of native plants, many of which, such as eucalyptus (*Eucalyptus globulus*, p. 100), are unique to Australia. While much of this knowledge has vanished with its keepers, there is currently a high level of interest in Indigenous herbal traditions.

Aboriginal herbal medicine

The Aboriginal people probably had a more robust health than the early European colonizers who displaced them. They had very different ideas of health, disease, and illness, in which the influence of the spirit world played a major role. In common with other indigenous societies, the Aboriginal people devoted much time to ritual, which reinforced the sense of place and purpose in the lives of each individual. They used healing plants and the laying on of hands in a complex weave of culture and medicine. Contrary to current perceptions, Aboriginal peoples had complex, permanent settlements that included ecologically balanced forms of agriculture and land management.

The influx of Europeans in the 18th century was disastrous for the Aboriginal people. They were exploited and driven off the land, and their population was decimated by killings and infectious Western diseases. Not only did the Europeans fail to discern any value in Indigenous customs, but much of the orally based herbal tradition was lost through death of the elders and the dispersal of tribal groupings.

Nevertheless, a little is known of Aboriginal medicine. Aromatic herbs, such as eucalyptus, were crushed and inhaled to treat many common illnesses, including respiratory diseases such as flu. Without metal technology, water could not be boiled, but decoctions were made by heating water with hot stones. These were drunk or applied externally. Skin eruptions, such as boils and scabies, were common and were treated with acacia (*Acacia* spp., p. 290), while acute diarrhea was treated with eucalyptus or kino (*Pterocarpus marsupium*, p. 266). In Queensland, fever bark (*Alstonia* spp., p. 169) was used to treat fevers.

Native & foreign herbs

Over the past 200 years, many native Australian plants have become popular around the world. Research into fever bark resulted in the discovery of the alkaloid reserpine, which markedly lowers blood pressure. The substance is now prescribed by herbalists and conventional practitioners alike. Eucalyptus and tea tree (*Melaleuca alternifolia*, p. 116) yield essential oils that are employed worldwide as antiseptics. Other native Australian plants are now used in Australian herbalism because of their medicinal use elsewhere, for example gotu kola (*Centella asiatica*, p. 81) and visnaga (*Ammi visnaga*, p. 65), which have a long history of medicinal use in India and the Middle East. Early British colonizers imported European medicinal plants, such as vervain (*Verbena officinalis*, p. 153), hawthorn (*Crataegus oxyacantha*, p. 91), mullein (*Verbascum thapsus*, p. 291), and dandelion (*Taraxacum officinale*,

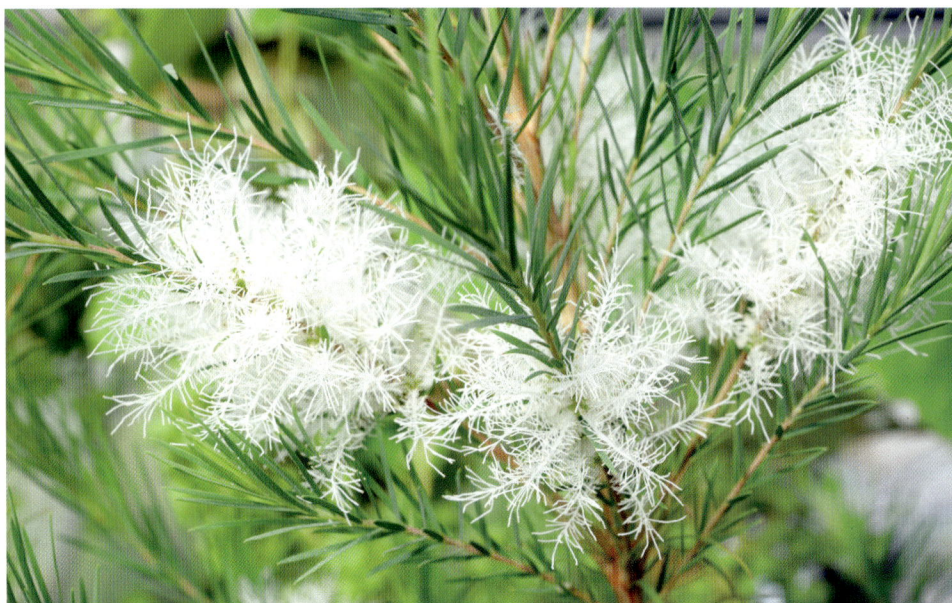

The commercial cultivation of Australian medicinal plants is on the increase, notably the key essential-oil-bearing plants such as tea tree (Melaleuca alternifolia).

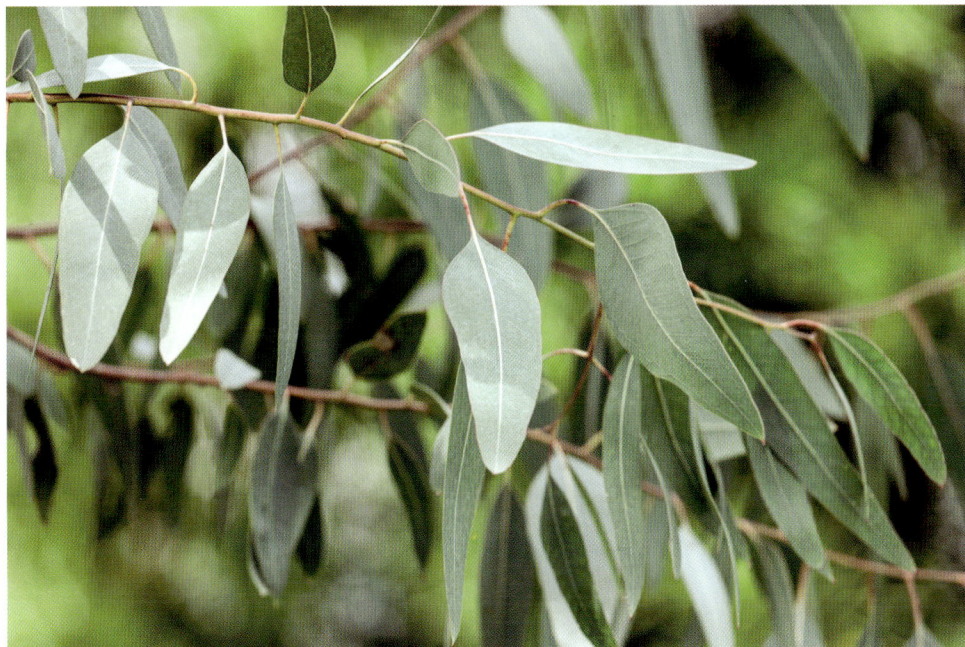

Red river gum (Eucalyptus camaldulensis) has aromatic, astringent leaves. When taken internally, typically to treat diarrhea, it turns the saliva red.

p. 145), which have now all become naturalized. Native American plants have also found their way to Australia, including prickly pear (*Opuntia ficus-indica*, p. 248) and Canadian fleabane (*Conyza canadensis*, p. 199). As Australian herbalists generally follow the Anglo-American herbal tradition, these plants are often employed in local practice.

Chinese influence

Traditional Chinese medicine has substantially influenced herbalism in Australia. Following the arrival of Chinese immigrants in the 19th century, herbal formulas gained a reputation for effectiveness, and Chinese medicine maintained a small but loyal following in all the major cities. During the 1980s, a renaissance in all branches of herbal medicine began, and today Australia has seven colleges of traditional Chinese medicine. In 2012, traditional Chinese medicine became a nationally regulated form of medicine, with practitioners required to register with the Chinese Medicine Board of Australia. Naturopathy and Western herbal medicine are yet to achieve this status.

The future

With the passing of enlightened legislation—the Therapeutic Goods Act—in 1989, herbal medicine became a dynamic growth industry in Australia. Quality standards for over-the-counter herbal medicines have been raised, many new herbal products have been developed, and university training and herbal research has expanded. The commercial cultivation of medicinal plants is on the increase, notably the key essential-oil-bearing plants, tea tree (*Melaleuca alternifolia* p. 116) and sandalwood (*Santalum album* p. 275), though many other native essential-oil-bearing plants, such as lemon myrtle (*Backhousia citriodora*) and manuka (*Leptospermum scoparium*), are now also in cultivation. In this environment, Australians are becoming increasingly sophisticated in their use of natural medicines and are regularly incorporating them into their daily lives.

With its ancient culture, ties to Western herbalism, and location on the Pacific Rim, Australia is host to many herbal traditions. The next 20 years will doubtless see further exciting developments.

North America

Many ancient herbal traditions in North and Central America not only withstood the influx of European settlers but helped to reinvigorate Western herbalism. In parts of Central America herbal medicine is widely practiced, and in the US and Canada it is again enormously popular.

Stretching from the Arctic wilds of Canada and Alaska to the tropical regions of Panama, North and Central America cover diverse geographical regions and harbor an immense variety of medicinal plants. Most of them are native, but others—such as nutmeg, ginger, and tamarind—were introduced from Europe, Asia, and Africa from the 16th century onward. Likewise, native American medicinal plants—such as corn, cocoa, cayenne, and sunflower—were introduced to Europe, Asia, and Africa. This trade of species was an important part of the interplay between the herbal traditions around the globe.

Herbal traditions in Central America

Herbal medicine is commonly practiced in rural areas of Central America, especially in Guatemala and Mexico. In the Mexican tradition, loss of "balance" between hot and cold elements within the body is thought to be the underlying cause of illness, and the healer's art is to restore balance and vitality.

Mexican herbal medicine is not a static tradition, but has evolved from a shifting blend of Indigenous pre-Hispanic and Spanish influences. Long before Hernán Cortéz and his conquistadors came ashore in 1519, Indigenous Mexican peoples, such as the Maya and Zapotec, had a profound understanding of plant medicines. The *Badianus Manuscript*, the first American herbal (written by an Aztec, Martin de la Cruz, in 1552), lists the medicinal uses of 251 Mexican species. They include damiana (*Turnera diffusa*, p. 148), taken by the Maya as an aphrodisiac, and mesquite (*Prosopis juliflora*), used by the Aztecs as an eye lotion. Both species are still used medicinally, alongside European herbs such as pennyroyal (*Mentha pulegium*, p. 241) and thyme (*Thymus vulgaris*, p. 147). It is thought that approximately 65 percent of the plants used today by traditional Mexican herbalists originated in Europe.

In other Central American countries efforts are being made to encourage people to use herbal medicine as the first line of treatment for illness. Projects in the Dominican Republic and Nicaragua, for example, are teaching women how to use local herbs within their communities, while in Cuba doctors routinely prescribe medicinal herbs to make up for the scarcity of conventional medicines.

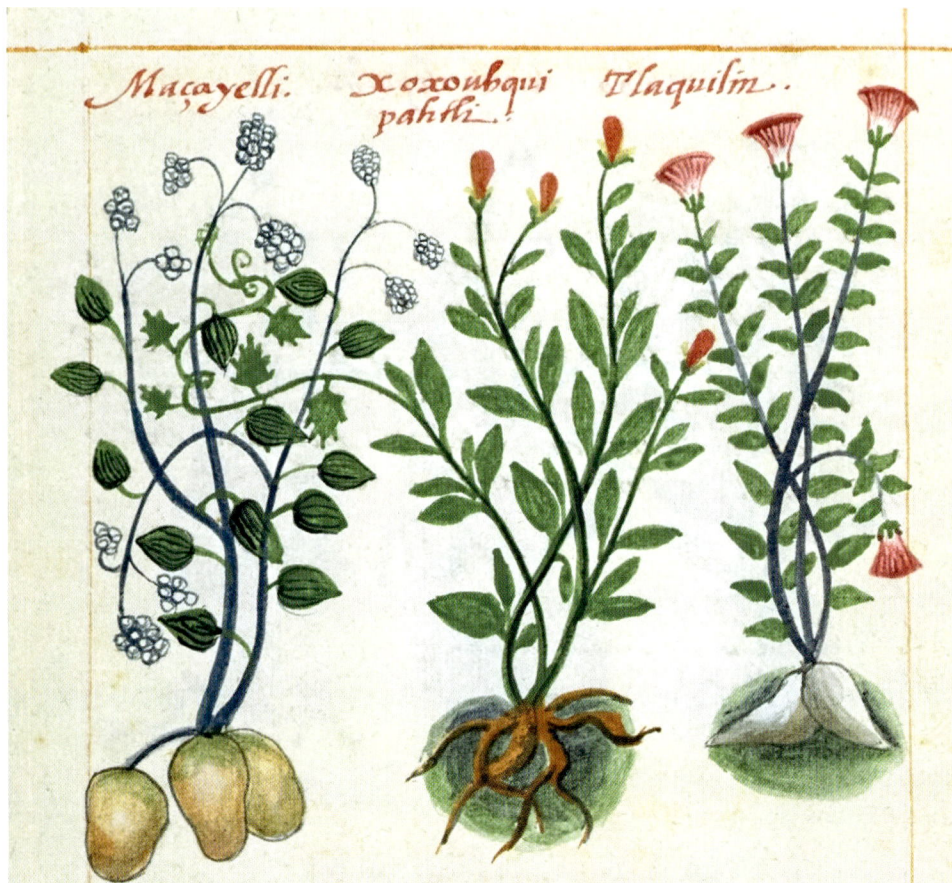

The Badianus Manuscript—the first American herbal, written by an Aztec, Martin de la Cruz, in 1552—lists the medicinal uses of 251 Mexican species.

Caribbean herbal medicine

Throughout the Caribbean, domestic herbal medicine remains popular. Some of the widely used herbs include fever grass or lemongrass (*Cymbopogon citratus*, p. 203), which, as its name suggests, is used to treat fevers, and kerala (*Momordica charantia*, p. 242), a creeping vine that is prized as a "cure-all" on many of the islands. Kerala has been shown to have an ability to lower blood-sugar levels and may help to slow down the onset of diabetes, a relatively common illness among Afro-Caribbeans. The medical and religious customs on each Caribbean island vary, but on many they reflect the African traditions of transported slaves, especially of the Yoruba people shipped from West Africa, who carried on the practices of their homelands. In some of these traditions, herbs are valued for their magical power as well as for their medicinal properties. Tobacco (*Nicotiana tabacum*, p. 247) for example, is used for divination in many American cultures, including in Santeria and Voodoo religious rituals, as are other herbs, including garlic (*Allium sativum*, p. 63) and cayenne (*Capsicum frutescens*, p. 79).

Shamanism

Moving north, Indigenous herbal medicine in what is now the United States was and is primarily shamanistic in nature, involving herbal lore, ritual, and magic. Shamanistic societies from Siberia to the Amazon believe that, in serious illness, the soul of the sick person has been taken over by malign forces. The shaman's role is to heal both the physical *and* the spiritual dimension of the illness. The patient cannot be truly cured until his or her soul has been freed from evil spirits. Shamanistic ceremonies and rites to heal the sick person's spirit include dancing, chanting, drumming, playing games, and the stirring of ashes or sprinkling of water. By taking hallucinogens such as peyote (*Lophophora williamsii*, p. 235), a Mexican cactus, the shaman is able to reach out to the spirit world and heal both the individual and the community as a whole.

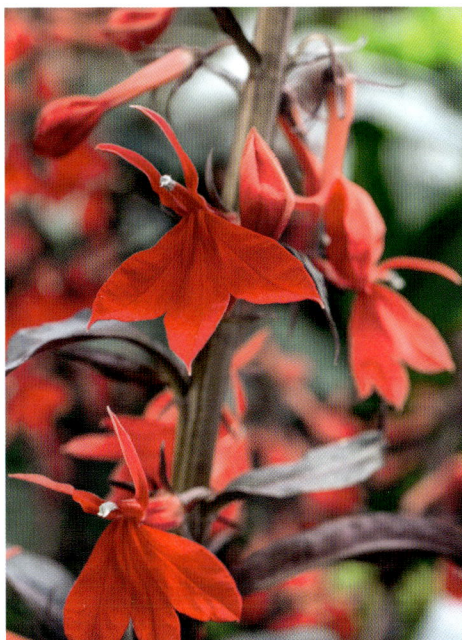

Cardinal lobelia (Lobelia cardinalis) *has the ability to heal or harm, according to the Iroquois, and should be picked with respect, and stored and used with great care.*

Power of herbs

In all Indigenous American cultures from Canada to Chile, herbs are thought to have spiritual energy, and many of them are invested with great magical power. The Iroquois believe that cardinal lobelia (*Lobelia cardinalis*, see *L. inflata*, p. 114) and morning glory (*Ipomoea pandurata*) have the ability to heal or harm, and should be picked, stored, and used with great care. Morning glory is considered so powerful that even touching it could cause harm. The Iroquois use the plant as a remedy for coughs, tuberculosis, and other ailments, and also take it as a decoction with sunflower seeds (*Helianthus annuus*) as a sacrament in spring and fall rituals.

Tobacco, now considered an addictive drug, was a sacred shamanistic herb for most Indigenous American peoples. It was smoked in pipes and "thrown into fires as an offering, cast into the wind and water to abate storms, scattered about a fish weir to improve the catch, and offered to the air in thanksgiving for escape from danger," according to Virgil Vogel's *American Indian Medicine* (1970).

Key herbs from this region

Corn silk (*Zea mays*, p. 158)
Slippery elm (*Ulmus rubra*, p. 149)
Saw palmetto (*Serenoa repens*, p. 140)
Gravel root (*Eupatorium purpureum*, p. 214)
Prickly ash (*Zanthoxylum americanum*, p. 157)
Wild yam (*Dioscorea villosa*, p. 95)
Lobelia (*Lobelia inflata*, p. 114)
Goldenseal (*Hydrastis canadensis*, p. 109)
Pokeweed (*Phytolacca americana*, p. 255)
Skullcap (*Scutellaria lateriflora*, p. 138)
Cramp bark (*Viburnum opulus*, p. 154)
Pleurisy root (*Asclepias tuberosa*, p. 177)
Witch hazel (*Hamamelis virginiana*, p. 106)
Avocado (*Persea americana*, p. 126)
California poppy (*Eschscholzia californica*, p. 212)
Blue cohosh (*Caulophyllum thalictroides*, p. 188)
Damiana (*Turnera diffusa*, p. 148)
Cayenne (*Capsicum frutescens*, p. 79)
Evening primrose (*Oenothera biennis*, p. 248)
Black cohosh (*Cimicifuga racemosa*, p. 61)
Helonias (*Chamaelirium luteum*, p. 190)

European colonizers

The first European colonizers in North America, arriving in the early 17th century, tended to dismiss Indigenous American medical practices as nothing more than primitive savagery. The colonizers relied largely on imported herbal medicines, or on European plants hardy enough to grow in eastern North America.

As time went by, however, increased contact with indigenous peoples in frontier regions fostered a healthy respect for their medicinal and healing skills. Sometimes Europeans adopted not just the plants but the harvesting and therapeutic methods as well. Joseph Doddridge, in *Notes on the Settlement and Indian Wars* (1876), relates that butternut bark (*Juglans cinerea*, p. 229) was peeled downward if it was to be used as a purgative (acting "downward" by purging the bowels), and upward for use as an emetic (acting "upward" by provoking vomiting).

The types of healing regimens practiced by Indigenous American peoples eventually gained widespread popularity. Toward the end of the 18th century, Samuel Thomson (1769–1843) developed a simple therapeutic regimen based on Indigenous American herbal practice. Thomson never acknowledged the debt, but it is clearly evident—from the use of emetics, purgatives, and stimulants, to the central role of sweating and vapor baths (based in part on Indigenous American sweat lodges), to the deep knowledge of American medicinal plants. Thomson considered that "all disease is caused by cold" and his system worked well for those with a robust health struck down by infection or injury. The two main herbs in his system—cayenne, a stimulating herb, and lobelia, an emetic, relaxant, and stimulant— act to raise body temperature and dilate the blood vessels. Taking these plants helps to increase resistance to infection and speeds the healing of wounds.

Eclecticism & its influence

The fertile marriage between Indigenous American and Western herbal medicine led to the establishment of more sophisticated herbal systems, such as Eclecticism, founded by Dr. Wooster Beech (1794–1868) in the 1830s. Beech studied both herbal and conventional medicine and tried to combine the new scientific knowledge of physiology and pathology with the best of the herbal tradition. Beech rejected Thomson's theories as being overly simplistic, and aimed to use the lowest dosages possible to achieve good results. His approach was so successful that at Eclecticism's height in 1909, over 8,000 members were in practice, all with recognized medical qualifications. Another significant medical movement, inspired by Thomson's regimen and influenced by the Eclectics, was Physiomedicalism. Using many herbs, these practitioners sought to harmonize "the organic tissues with the vital force," with the aim of restoring equilibrium within the body. Believing the stomach was the source of disease, Physiomedicalists used herbs that induced vomiting, such as pokeweed (*Phytolacca americana,* p. 255), to cleanse the organ. Other herbs, such as echinacea (*Echinacea* spp., p. 96), now recognized as an effective immune modulator, and goldenseal (*Hydrastis canadensis*, p. 109), a tonic and anti-inflammatory, were then prescribed to aid recovery.

The second half of the 19th century was an extraordinary time for American natural medicine. In addition to engendering osteopathy and chiropractic at the turn of the century, it also reinvigorated herbal medicine in Britain to such a degree that Physiomedicalism became an Anglo-American herbal tradition. To this day, British herbalists use a far wider variety of American medicinal herbs than other European herbalists.

North American herbal medicine today

In the US, herbal medicine went into steep decline after 1907 because of the government's decision to limit financial support for herbal medical training at conventional medical schools. Since that time, herbal medicine in both the US and Canada

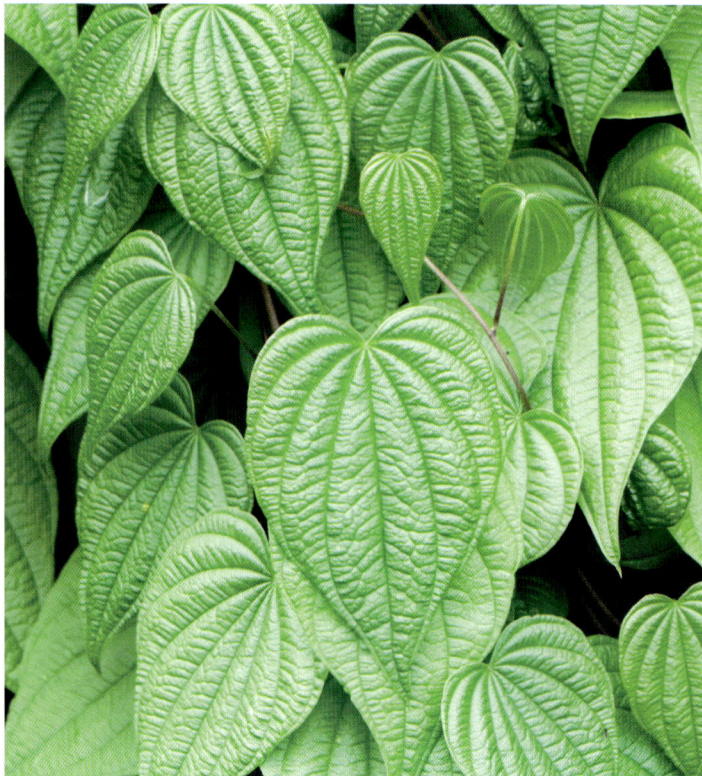

Wild yam is found growing in Mexico. Its rhizome relaxes smooth muscle and it is used as an antispasmodic.

has existed mostly on the fringes of conventional health care. In some US states, it is illegal to practice herbal medicine without medical qualifications, but courses in herbalism are not offered at medical schools.

With the passing of liberal legislation in 1994, use of herbal medicine in the US exploded and sales of St. John's wort (*Hypericum perforatum*, p. 110)—the most extreme example—are thought to have increased by 3,900 percent between 1995 and 1997. Such growth could not be sustained, and led to lower-quality herbal products being sold over the counter. The American Botanical Council has been at the forefront of the campaign to raise quality standards of herbal medicines, and many bona fide herbal manufacturers have signed up to their Botanical Adulterants program. At the same time, greater resources are being put into researching herbal medicines, for example through the US National Center for Complementary and Integrative Health, which has so far funded over 15 clinical trials into herbs such as garlic (*Allium sativum*, p. 63) and saw palmetto (*Serenoa repens*, p. 140).

Over the past 20 years, North Americans have become increasingly savvy about herbal medicines and their role in maintaining well-being and treating ill health. Best-selling herbs include turmeric (*Curcuma longa*, p. 94) and elderberry (*Sambucus nigra*, p. 136), and their use fits well with the American tradition of self-reliance.

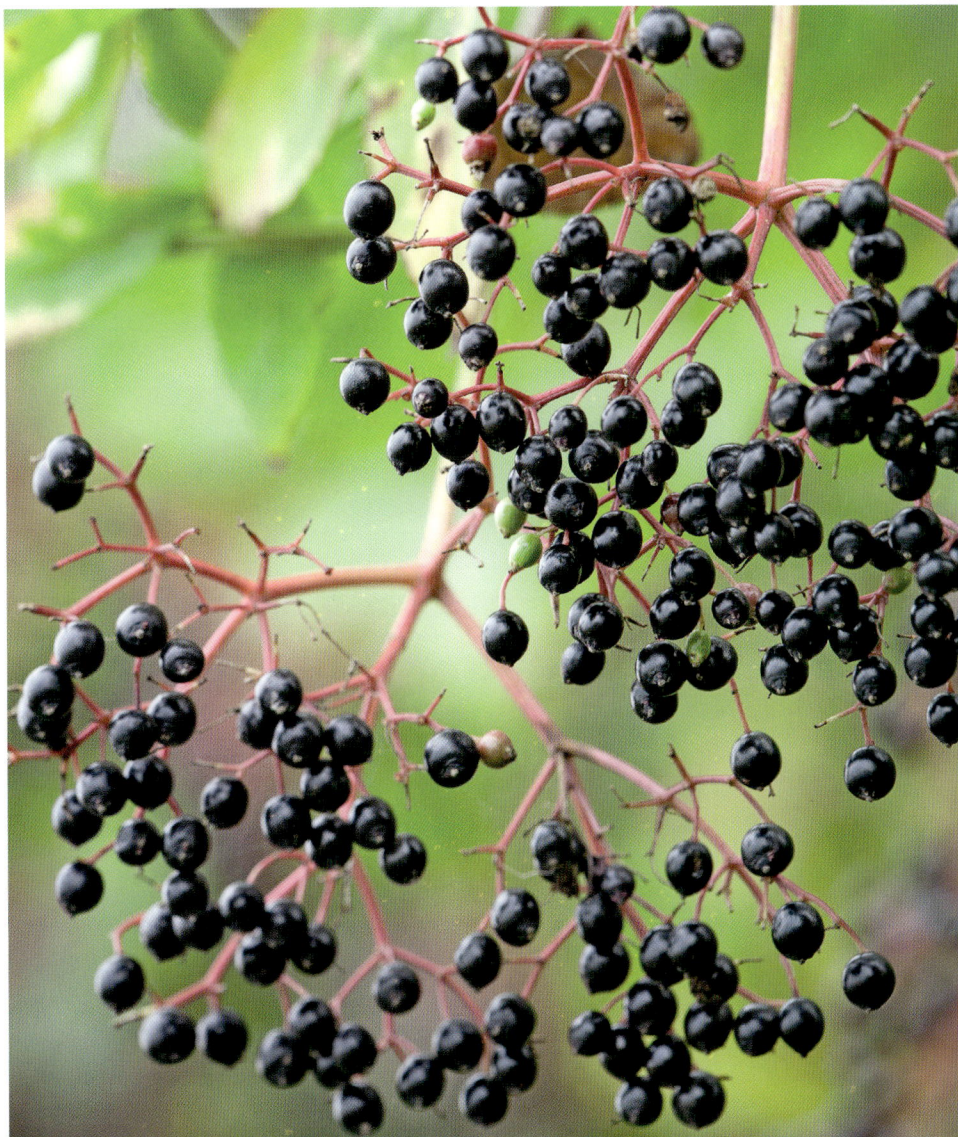

*Elderberry (**Sambucus nigra**) is one of the best-selling medicinal herbs in North America. Both fresh and dried berries have antiviral activity and support improved immune function.*

"The fertile marriage between Indigenous American and Western herbal medicine led to the establishment of more sophisticated herbal systems, such as Eclecticism."

South America

Herbal medicine is a part of the struggle for survival for the Indigenous peoples of South America, as they seek to protect their culture and natural habitats. As the great rainforests disappear we are losing thousands of plant species, some of which may have had great medicinal value.

Herbal medicine in South America conjures up images of shamanistic rituals and a collection of thousands of as yet unclassified plants under the thick canopy of the rainforest. But these are only two facets of the continent's herbal tradition—those of the Amazon and Orinoco regions. Distinctly different plants and practices are found in other areas, for example on the Bolivian Andes plateau, on the humid plains of Paraguay, and in cities such as Rio de Janeiro.

Wealth of native plants

Ever since the Spanish conquest in the early 16th century, European writers have remarked on the huge variety of plant medicines used by Indigenous peoples. The most important of these was cinchona (*Cinchona* spp., p. 84), a traditional Andean fever remedy, which the Spaniards first discovered around 1630. Quinine, produced from this plant, became the most effective treatment for malaria for nearly 300 years

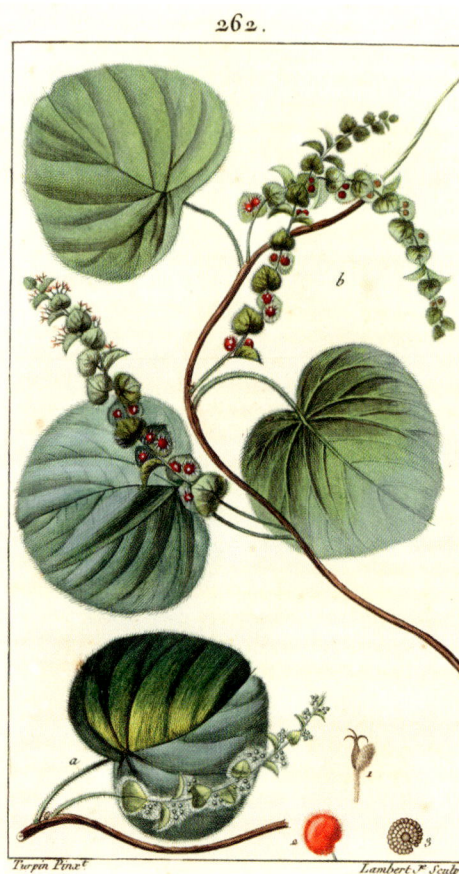

262.

Pareira (Chondrodendron tomentosum) is a climbing vine of the Amazon rainforest that yields the poison curare, used in hunting. It is also taken medicinally to treat water retention and bruising.

Turpin Pinx.ᵗ   Lambert.F.ᶜ Sculpᵗ

PAREIRA - BRAVA.

and is still widely used as a tonic, bitter, and muscle relaxant. Other important plants originating in South America include the potato (*Solanum tuberosum*, p. 280), which was cultivated in over 60 different varieties by the Inca. Its uses are wide-ranging, but it is particularly effective as a poultice for skin conditions. Ipecac (*Cephaelis ipecacuanha*, p. 189)—now commonly found in over-the-counter cough preparations—was taken by Brazilian peoples to treat amebic dysentery. Maté (*Ilex paraguariensis*, p. 227), which grows in southern regions of the continent, makes a stimulating beverage that is prepared and drunk like tea. Maté has become so popular it is now cultivated in Spain and Portugal as well as in South America.

Since the 1950s, specialized ethnobotanists have lived within Indigenous communities, particularly in the Amazon region, where most peoples have a highly developed herbal lore. Their work has resulted in a wealth of knowledge about Amazonian species. Pareira (*Chondrodendron tomentosum*, p. 193), a climbing vine of the rainforest, for example, yields the poison curare used in hunting, and is taken medicinally to treat water retention, bruising, and insanity. Sadly, however, the herbal medicine of many Indigenous groups is now under threat as the rainforests, and their culture, disappear.

Mind-altering remedies

Notorious in the West as the source of cocaine, coca (*Erythroxylum coca*, p. 211) is an important medicine in South America for nausea and vomiting, toothache, and asthma. It is also completely interwoven into the

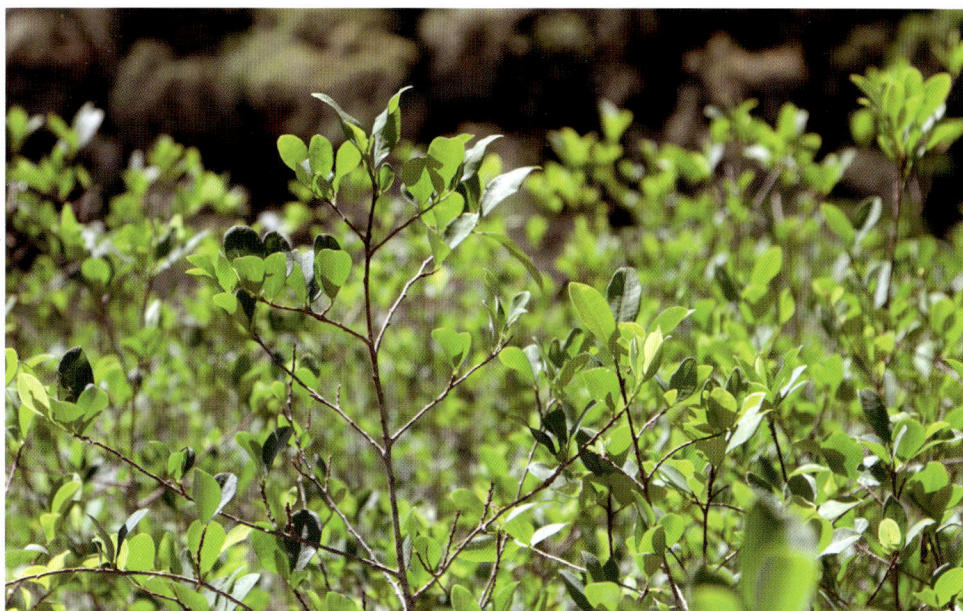

Coca harvest in Bolivia. *The leaves are picked when they begin to curl. They have been used as a stimulant for centuries by the Indigenous peoples of the Andes.*

culture of Indigenous Amazonian and Andean peoples and serves as a precise example of the unique relationship that traditional peoples have with the plant world. Many different myths confirm coca's sacred and ancient origins in South America, and great ritual and significance is attached to the leaves, which, when mixed with lime and chewed, reduce appetite and increase endurance.

Many hallucinogenic plants are used within South American shamanistic societies, notably ayahuasca (*Banisteriopsis caapi*, p. 180). This powerful "medicine" enables the shaman (priest) to communicate with the spirit world and cure the patient's ill health.

The European influence

In more westernized areas of South America, herbal medicine is often a blend of both Spanish and local traditions (as is also the case in Central America, see p. 52). Large herb markets exist in some cities, such as La Paz and Quito, which provide an astonishing variety of indigenous and European herbs. In Ecuadorian markets, for example, anise (*Pimpinella anisum*, p. 256), a digestive remedy for colic and cramps that originally came from the Mediterranean, is sold alongside unusual native medicines such as arquitecta (*Culcitium reflexum*), a diuretic and detoxifying herb traditionally used to treat toxicity and infections, including syphilis.

Research & new hopes

Research into native herbs has led to the use of certain plants in conventional medicine. Brazilian investigation into pau d'arco (*Tabebuia impetiginosa*, p. 143) indicates significant therapeutic potential for fungal infections, inflammation of the cervix, HIV, and cancer. While pau d'arco's effectiveness in treating cancer is controversial, it is currently prescribed both by local doctors and in hospitals.

Research into herbal medicine is expanding, with hospital-based studies taking place in centers such as Belem in northeastern Brazil and Bogotá in Colombia. These locally based researchers, unlike most multinational drug companies, are willing to develop medicines based on simple extracts, which may ultimately prove more effective than the isolated constituents often used in conventional drugs.

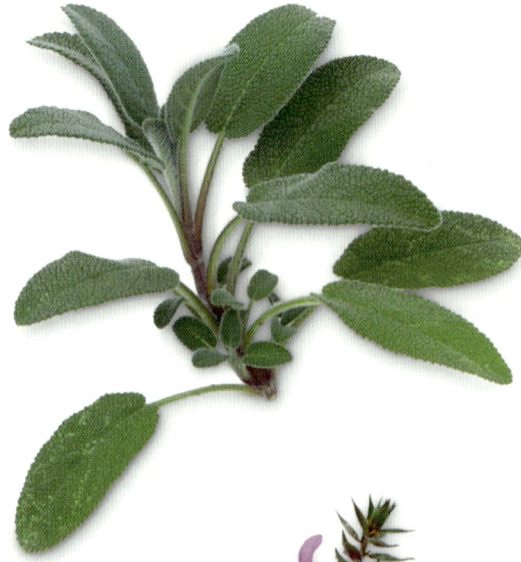

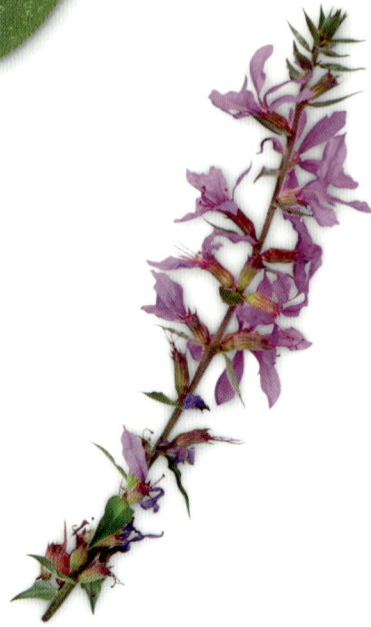

Key medicinal plants

Of the estimated 500,000 plants on our planet, it is thought that around 10,000 are used regularly for medicinal purposes. The index of Key Medicinal Plants features 100 of the best-known medicinal plants in Latin name order. Many are commonly available and widely used in different herbal traditions around the world, for example German chamomile (*Chamomilla recutita*, p. 82) and ginger (*Zingiber officinale*, p. 159). Others such as neem (*Azadirachta indica*, p. 74), from Asia, are key herbs within their native region. A significant proportion of these herbs have been well researched and most are excellent for home use.

Achillea millefolium (Asteraceae)

Yarrow, Milfoil

Yarrow is a native European plant, with a long history as a wound healer. In classical times, it was known as *herba militaris*, and used to staunch war wounds. It has long been taken as a strengthening bitter tonic, and all kinds of bitter drinks have been made from it. Yarrow helps recovery from colds and flu and is beneficial for hay fever. It is also helpful for menstrual problems and circulatory disorders.

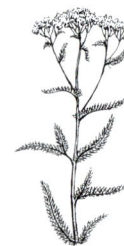

A creeping perennial, growing to 3 ft (1 m), with white flower heads and finely divided leaves.

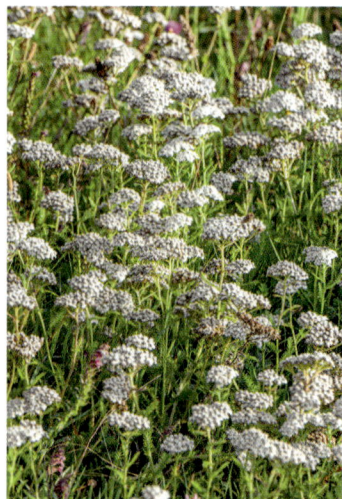

Yarrow was once known as "nosebleed" because its leaves were used to staunch blood.

Habitat & cultivation

Native to Europe and western Asia, yarrow can be found growing wild in temperate regions throughout the world, in meadows and along roadsides. The herb spreads via its roots, and the aerial parts are picked in summer when in flower.

Key constituents

• Volatile oil with variable content (linalool, camphor, sabinene, azulene)
• Sesquiterpene lactones
• Flavonoids • Alkaloids (achilleine)
• Triterpenes • Phytosterols
• Tannins

Key actions

• Antispasmodic • Astringent • Bitter tonic • Increases sweating • Lowers blood pressure • Reduces fever
• Mild diuretic and urinary antiseptic
• Stops internal bleeding • Promotes menstruation • Anti-inflammatory

Research

Despite its many uses and similarity to German chamomile (*Chamomilla recutita*, p. 82), yarrow has been poorly researched. The herb and its volatile oil have been shown to be anti-inflammatory; the azulenes are also anti-allergenic. The sesquiterpene lactones are bitter and have antitumor activity. Achilleine and the flavonoids help arrest internal and external bleeding; the flavonoids may be responsible for yarrow's antispasmodic action. Laboratory studies indicate that yarrow dilates blood vessels, thereby lowering blood pressure. It works, in part, like conventional medicines known as ACE inhibitors, which are commonly prescribed for high blood pressure.

Traditional & current uses

Healing wounds Achilles reputedly used yarrow to heal wounds, hence its botanical name. It has been used for this purpose for centuries, and in Scotland a traditional wound ointment was made from yarrow.

Gynecological herb Yarrow helps regulate the menstrual cycle, reduces heavy menstrual bleeding, and eases period pain.

Other uses Combined with other herbs, yarrow helps colds and flu. Its bitter tonic properties make it useful for weak digestion and colic. It also helps hay fever, lowers high blood pressure, improves venous circulation, and tones varicose veins.

Self-help uses

• Cleansing wounds, p. 314.
• Colds & flu, p. 321. • Digestive infections, p. 315. • Fever, p. 321.
• Varicose veins, p. 312.

Parts used

Aerial parts contain flavonoids, which are thought to give yarrow its antispasmodic properties.

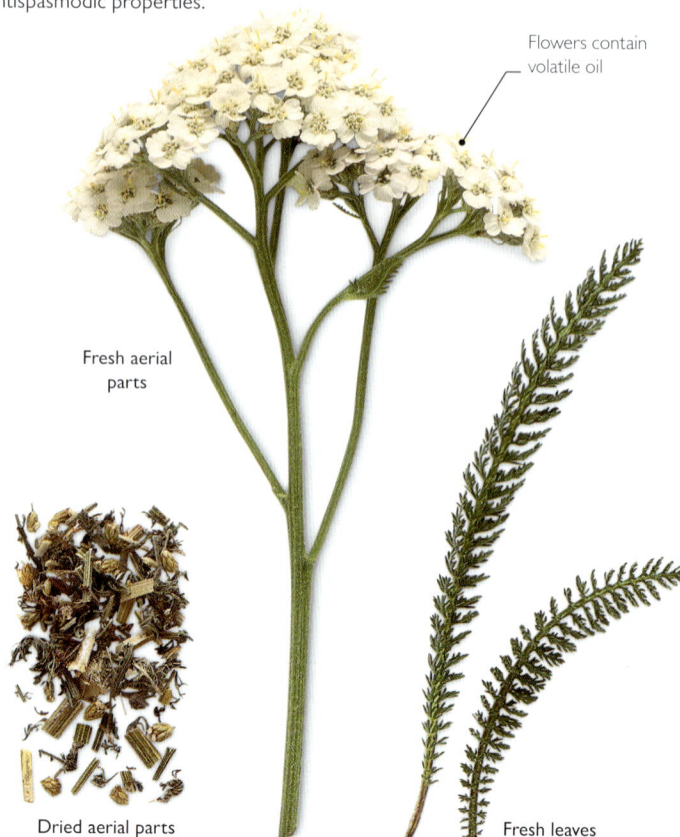

Flowers contain volatile oil

Fresh aerial parts

Dried aerial parts

Fresh leaves

Key preparations & their uses

Remedy For colds, mix equal parts of yarrow, peppermint, and elderflower. Infuse 1 tsp with ¾ cup (150 ml) water for 10 minutes (*see* p. 301). Take 3 times a day.

Tincture (to make, p. 302). For indigestion, take 20 drops 3 times a day.

Essential oil extracted from the flowers is used by herbalists to treat congestion.

Poultice (to make, p. 305). Apply to grazes, cuts, and bruises.

Cautions May cause allergic reaction in rare cases. Use the essential oil only under professional supervision. Do not take during pregnancy.

Actaea racemosa syn. Cimicifuga racemosa

Black cohosh

Black Cohosh root has a long history of use in North America and has become well known as a key remedy for women's health issues, especially painful menstruation and problems associated with the menopause. It benefits rheumatic problems, including rheumatoid arthritis, and nerve conditions such as tinnitus, and was used by Penobscot peoples for kidney troubles. The root has a bitter, acrid taste and a disagreeable odor.

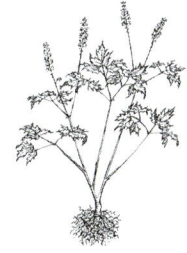

An herbaceous perennial growing to about 8 ft (2.5 m), with creamy-white flower spikes.

Habitat & cultivation

Black cohosh is native to Canada and eastern parts of the US, growing as far south as Florida. It prefers shady positions in woods and hedgerows. The herb is now grown in Europe and can be found in the wild, having self-seeded from cultivated plants. It is propagated from seed and the root is harvested in the fall.

Related species

A number of *Cimicifuga* species are used in traditional Chinese medicine, including *sheng ma* (*C. dahurica*) and *C. foetida*. They are thought to "clear heat" and relieve toxicity, and are used to treat asthma, headaches, and measles, among other conditions.

Key constituents

• Triterpene glycosides (actein, cimicifugoside) • Isoflavones (formononetin) • Isoferulic acid

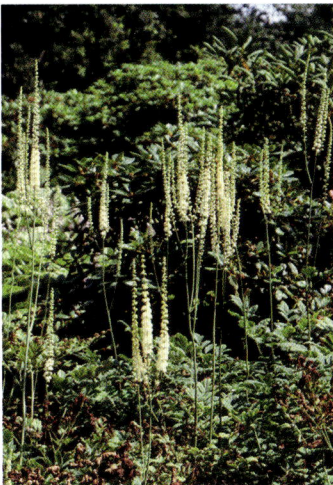

Black cohosh was used by Indigenous peoples in North America to treat gynecological problems and complaints such as rheumatism and headaches.

Key actions

• Anti-inflammatory • Sedative
• Antirheumatic • Estrogenic
• Expectorant

Research

Menopause At least 10 clinical trials have found that black cohosh helps relieve menopausal symptoms. A 1995 German study using black cohosh and St. John's wort found that the combination was 78% effective in such cases.

Estrogenic properties It seems black cohosh does not contain estrogen but has an estrogenic action within the body due to specific hormonal effects within the brain. It is suggested that black cohosh may slow or prevent the development of osteoporosis, and it has potential in treating polycystic ovary syndrome.

Safety concerns Research strongly suggests that black cohosh is a safe and valuable medicine. Concerns have been raised that it might cause liver damage or be unsuitable for women at risk of developing breast cancer. No effect on liver function was found during the clinical trials, and it is thought that it has some preventative activity against breast cancer.

Traditional & current uses

Gynecological uses Also known as "squaw vine", indigenous American people saw black cohosh as a valuable remedy for many women's health problems. It is used today for period pain; menstrual problems where estrogen levels are too low; and for menopausal symptoms, especially hot flashes and night sweats.

Inflammation Black cohosh is useful for inflammatory arthritis, especially when it is associated with menopause, and it also finds use as a remedy for rheumatic problems, including rheumatoid arthritis.

Sedative properties Black cohosh's sedative action makes it valuable for treating many conditions, including high blood pressure, tinnitus (ringing in the ears), whooping cough, and asthma.

Self-help uses

• Arthritis, p. 323. • Decreased estrogen & progesterone levels, p. 326.

Parts used

Root is unearthed in the fall. Dried root is most commonly used in herbal medicine.

The active constituents are strongest in mature roots

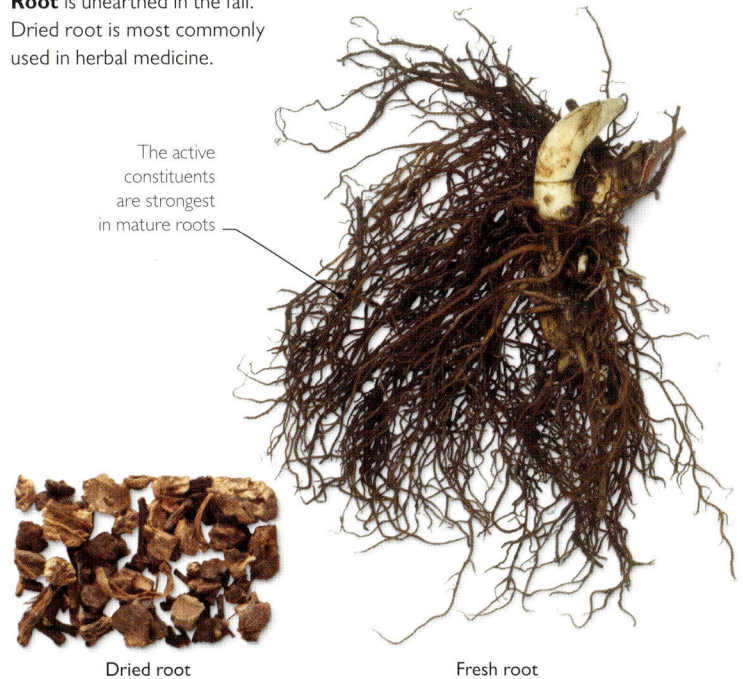

Dried root

Fresh root

Key preparations & their uses

Decoction (to make, p. 301). For rheumatism, take ⅓ cup (75 ml) twice a day.

Tablets are made from powdered herb. Take for menopausal symptoms, such as mood swings and hot flashes.

Tincture (to make, p. 302). To relieve period pain, add 40 drops to ½ cup (100 ml) water and take 3 times a day.

Cautions Do not take in pregnancy or if breastfeeding. Larger doses can cause stomach upsets and headache.

Aesculus hippocastanum (Sapindaceae)

Horse chestnut

Extracts of horse chestnut seed—the shiny brown "conkers" collected by British children in the fall—have a scientifically established ability to relieve the symptoms of varicose veins, and promote their repair. Taken by mouth, or applied as a lotion, horse chestnut will help tighten up the tissues and reduce the pain and swelling of varicose veins. It is also useful in helping to reduce fluid retention.

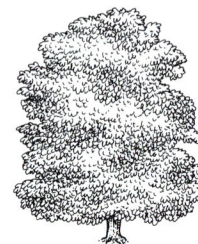

A deciduous tree with divided leaves, white and pink flowers, and spiny green fruit. It grows to 80 ft (25 m).

Habitat & cultivation

Native to mountain woods from the Balkans through western Asia to the Himalayas, horse chestnut is now cultivated as an ornamental and shade tree in temperate regions around the world, especially in northern and western Europe. It is propagated from seed in the fall or spring. Leaves are harvested in summer, the bark and seeds in the fall.

Related species

Do not use Ohio Buckeye (A. glabra), as it is toxic if taken internally.

Key constituents

• Triterpenoid saponins, including about 5% aescin, a complex mixture of glycosides • Polysaccharides (about 50%) • Coumarins, including aesculin • Flavonoids • Tannins, including proanthocyanidins • Fixed oil (2–3%)

Key actions

• Venous tonic • Astringent
• Anti-inflammatory • Antioxidant
• Reduces fluid retention

Research

Clinical trials Numerous trials have confirmed horse chestnut's value as a

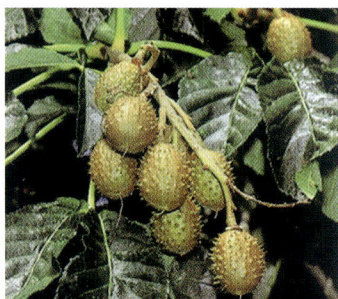

Horse chestnut seeds are the main herbal medicine for venous disorders.

medicine in venous problems such as varicose veins, venous ulcers, hemorrhoids, and frostbite. In one London-based study, published in 1996, horse chestnut extract was shown to be as effective in treating varicose veins as compression stockings. In Germany, horse chestnut extracts and aescin are now routinely used to treat varicose veins.

Venous insufficiency A 2006 review of clinical trials by the Cochrane Database assessed the use of horse chestnut extract for chronic venous insufficiency—a condition that includes leg swelling and spider and varicose veins. The review concluded that horse chestnut extract was a safe and effective short-term treatment for this problem.

Traditional & current uses

Circulatory system Although horse chestnut has a beneficial effect on the heart and arteries, it is primarily a remedy for the veins. It helps improve the tone of the vein walls, which when slack or distended result in varicose veins, piles, and similar problems. It also reduces edema (fluid retention) caused by fluid leaking from distended veins. Horse chestnut is taken internally for leg ulcers, varicose veins, piles, and frostbite, and applied locally as a lotion, gel, or ointment. A decoction of the bark or leaf can be used as an astringent lotion for varicose veins.

Rheumatism In France, an oil extracted from the seeds has been used as a topical application for rheumatism.

Chest remedy Horse chestnut makes a serviceable chest remedy, and in Turkey has been used to treat chest complaints in horses. In the US, a decoction of the leaves has been considered useful for whooping cough.

Parts used

Leaves can be used to make a lotion for varicose veins and hemorrhoids.

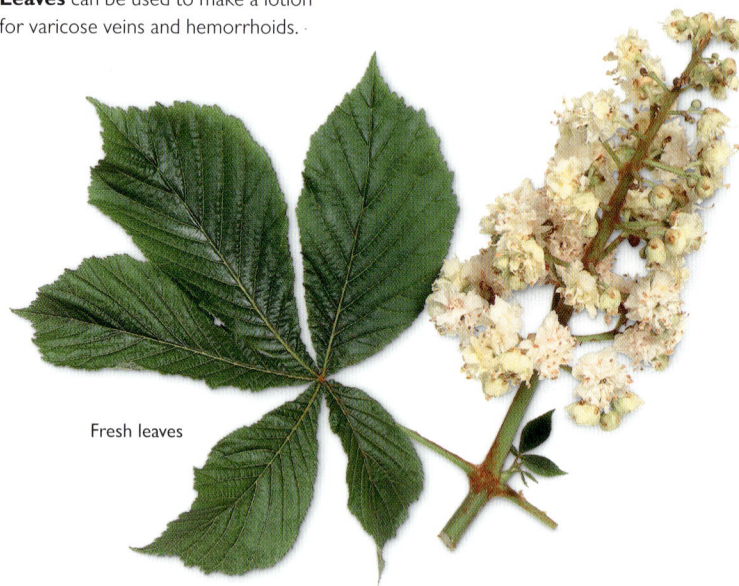

Fresh leaves

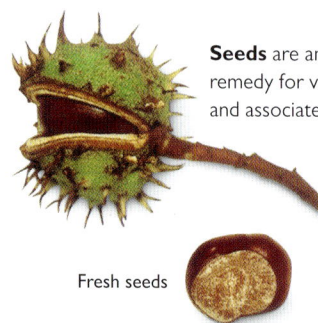

Fresh seeds

Seeds are an excellent remedy for varicose veins and associated fluid retention.

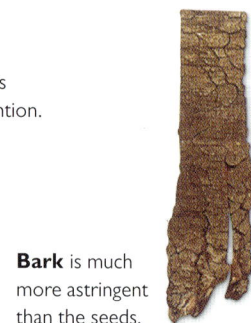

Bark is much more astringent than the seeds.

Key preparations & their uses

Tablets may have a higher aescin content than other preparations.

Lotion (to make, p. 306). Apply twice daily to varicose veins.

Capsules are convenient for long-term use.

Cautions Best taken with professional advice. Horse chestnut can cause gastrointestinal upset at normal dosage (discontinue if symptoms develop) and is toxic at excess dosage. Not suitable for children. Do not apply to broken or ulcerated skin. May interact with blood-thinning drugs.

Allium sativum (Liliaceae)

Garlic

Known for its pungent odor and taste, garlic is an ideal herbal medicine, being completely safe for home use and a powerful treatment for a host of health problems. It counters many infections, including those of the nose, throat, and chest. It also reduces cholesterol; helps circulatory disorders, such as high blood pressure; and lowers blood-sugar levels, making it a useful dietary addition in type 2 diabetes.

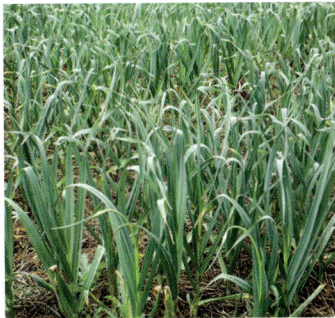

A bulbous perennial growing to 1–3 ft (30 cm–1 m), with pale pink or green-white flowers.

Garlic is widely cultivated commercially for use in cooking.

Habitat & cultivation

Originally from central Asia, garlic is now grown worldwide. It is grown by dividing the bulb and is harvested late the following summer.

Related species

Onion and ramsons (*A. cepa* and *A. ursinum*, p. 168) are both important medicinal herbs.

Key constituents

• Volatile oil (alliin, alliinase, allicin)
• Scordinins • Selenium • Vitamins A, B, C, and E

Key actions

• Antibiotic • Expectorant
• Increases sweating • Lowers blood pressure • Reduces blood clotting
• Antidiabetic • Expels worms

Research

Invaluable remedy Over 1,000 research papers have been published on the medicinal effects of garlic. They show that it helps normalize blood fat levels, to keep the blood thin and protect against blood clots, to lower raised blood pressure, to lower blood sugar levels and has antibiotic properties.

• **Unknown action** While it is understood that when the fresh clove is crushed, alliin is broken down by alliinase into allicin (which has strong antiseptic activity), authorities still disagree on precisely how garlic achieves its medicinal effects. Nevertheless, research indicates that it is best to crush garlic cloves, and then to wait 10 minutes before using it in food or as medicine. This allows sufficient time for allicin to form.

Traditional & current uses

Traditional remedy Garlic has always been esteemed for its healing powers, and before the development of antibiotics it was a treatment for all manner of infections, from tuberculosis to typhoid. It was also used to dress wounds in World War I.

Bronchial infections Garlic is an excellent remedy for all types of chest infections. It is good for colds, flu, and ear infections, and it helps reduce mucus.

Digestive tract Digestive infections respond well to garlic. The herb can also rid the body of intestinal parasites.

Circulatory remedy Garlic prevents circulatory problems and strokes by keeping the blood thin. It lowers cholesterol levels and blood pressure.

Other uses Garlic has been used to treat diverse health problems, from hay fever and asthma to an enlarged prostate and osteoarthritis. It is useful when taken alongside conventional antibiotics to help prevent side-effects such as diarrhea. Strongly antifungal, garlic can be an effective treatment in fungal skin conditions, taken internally and applied to the skin. It has anticancer activity and helps protect against stomach and colon cancer.

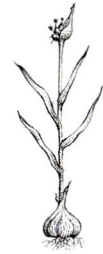

Parts used

Garlic whole, chopped, or crushed, has been used as a medicine and as a tonic food for thousands of years.

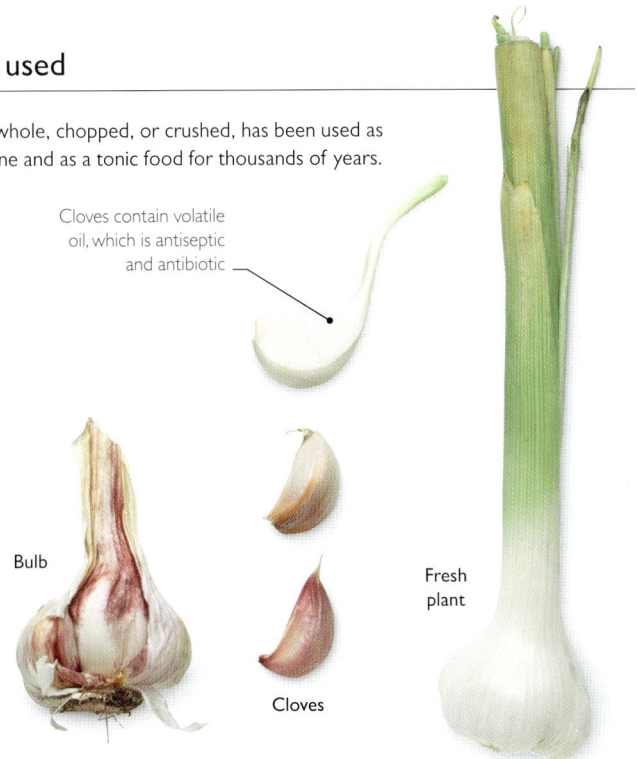

Cloves contain volatile oil, which is antiseptic and antibiotic

Bulb

Cloves

Fresh plant

Key preparations & their uses

Pearls contain garlic oil. Take to increase resistance to infections.

Chopped cloves Use regularly in cooking to help reduce cholesterol levels and boost the immune system.

Garlic syrup (to make, p. 303). For coughs, take 1 tsp every 3 hours.

Capsules (to make, p. 302). For bronchitis, take 2 x 100 mg capsules 3 times a day.

Tablets Take for high blood pressure and bronchitis.

Caution Consult a professional practitioner before giving garlic as a medicine to children under 12. Ask professional advice if taking blood-thinning medication.

Self-help uses

• Acne & boils, p. 315. • Athlete's foot, p. 314. • Colds & flu, p. 321. • Cold sores, p. 314. • Coughs & bronchitis, p. 320. • Digestive infections, p. 315. • Earache, p. 322. • Fungal infections, p. 324. • High blood pressure, p. 311. • Old age tonic, p. 329. • Tonsillitis, p. 321. • Urinary infections, p. 324.

Aloe vera syn. *A. barbadensis* (Xanthorrhoeaceae)

Aloe vera, Aloes

Native to Africa, aloe vera is commonly cultivated as a potted plant and has two distinct types of medicinal use. The clear gel contained in the leaf is a remarkably effective healer of wounds and burns, speeding up the rate of healing and reducing the risk of infection. The yellow sap from the base of the leaf when dried is known as "bitter aloes." It is a strong laxative, useful for short-term constipation.

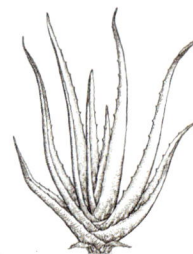

A perennial with succulent leaves 2 ft (60 cm) long and a spike of yellow or orange flowers.

Habitat & cultivation

Native to eastern and southern Africa, aloe vera grows wild in the tropics and is cultivated extensively worldwide. (Aloe vera plants grown as potted plants have a low anthraquinone content.) Aloe vera is propagated by breaking off small rooted plantlets. To collect the gel and bitter liquid, the leaves are cut and drained.

Related species

Cape aloes (*A. ferox*) is used in herbal medicine as an irritant laxative. Many other *Aloe* species are also useful medicinally.

Key constituents

- Anthraquinones (aloin, aloe-emodin) • Resins • Tannins
- Polysaccharides • Aloectin B

Key actions

- Heals wounds • Emollient •
Stimulates secretions of bile • Laxative

Research

Healing properties Extensive research since the 1930s in the US and Russia has shown that the clear gel has a dramatic ability to heal wounds, ulcers, and burns, putting a protective coat on the affected area and speeding up the rate of healing. This action is in part due to the presence of aloectin B, which stimulates the immune system.

Traditional & current uses

Beauty treatment Aloe vera has a long history as a skin lotion—Cleopatra is said to have attributed her beauty to it.

Western remedy In the West, aloe vera first became popular in the 1950s when its ability to heal burns, in particular radiation burns, was discovered.

First aid Aloe vera is an excellent first aid remedy for burns, scrapes, scalds, and sunburn. A leaf, broken off, releases soothing gel, which may be applied to the affected part.

Skin conditions The gel is useful for almost any skin condition that needs soothing and astringing, and will help varicose veins to some degree.

Ulcers The protective and healing effect of aloe vera also works internally, and the gel can be used for mouth ulcers, sore tongue, peptic ulcers, and irritable bowel syndrome.

Laxative The bitter yellow liquid in the leaves (bitter aloes) contains anthraquinones, which are strongly laxative. They cause the colon to contract, generally producing a bowel movement 8–12 hours after consumption. At higher doses, bitter aloes are laxative and purgative.

Self-help uses

- Minor burns & sunburn, p. 313.
- Stretch marks, p. 327. • Warts, p. 314. • Weeping skin, p. 313.
- Wounds, p. 314.

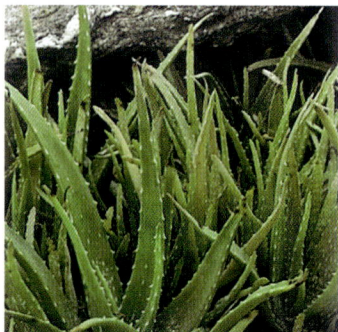

Aloe vera has prickly, gray-green, succulent leaves that yield effective medicinal substances.

Parts used

Leaves exude a bitter liquid, which is dried and known as "bitter aloes." They also contain a clear gel, which is a soothing skin remedy.

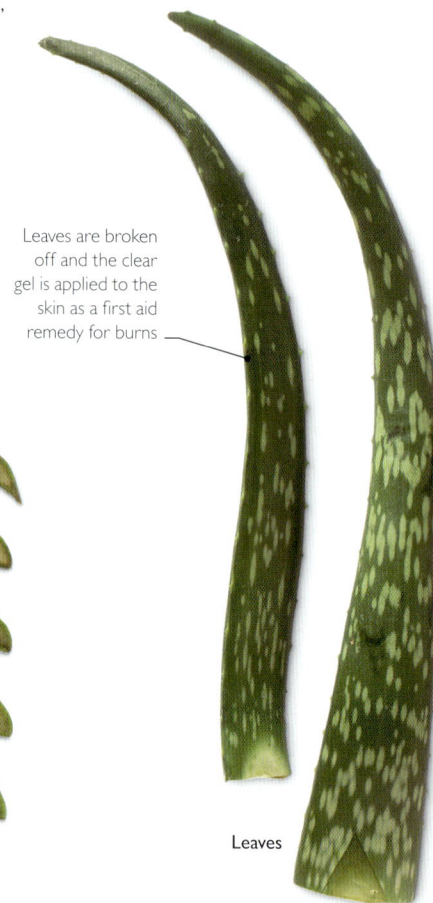

Leaves are broken off and the clear gel is applied to the skin as a first aid remedy for burns

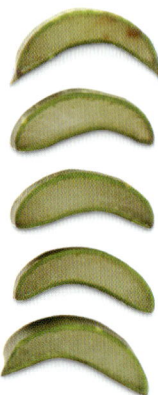

Chopped leaves

Leaves

Key preparations & their uses

Bitter aloes are used by herbalists to treat constipation.

Juice is made commercially from the gel. For peptic ulcers, take 2½ tbsp 3 times a day.

Leaves Break off a leaf and split open to collect the gel. For burns and eczema, apply liberally twice a day.

Tincture made from bitter aloes (see p. 302). To stimulate the appetite, take 3 drops with water before meals.

Cautions Do not use the bitter yellow juice from the base of the leaves (bitter aloes) on the skin. Its use is restricted in some countries. Do not take internally during pregnancy or while breast-feeding. Do not take if suffering from hemorrhoids or kidney disease.

Visnaga daucoides (Apiaceae)

Visnaga, Khella

Visnaga, with its aromatic, bitter scent and flavor, has greater medicinal than culinary value. It is an effective muscle relaxant and has been used for many centuries to alleviate the excruciating pain of kidney stones. Scientific research has confirmed the validity of this traditional use. Visnaga contains khellin, from which particularly safe pharmaceutical drugs for the treatment of asthma have been derived.

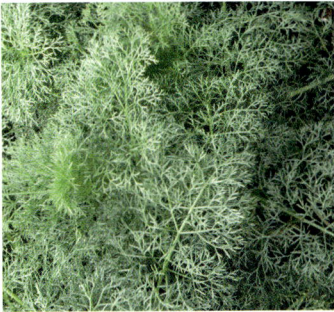

An erect annual growing to 3 ft (1 m), with leaves divided into wisps and clusters of small white flowers.

Visnaga is a member of the carrot family and has the characteristic delicate, wispy leaves.

Habitat & cultivation
Native to North Africa, visnaga grows wild in the Middle East and around the Mediterranean. It is naturalized in Australia and South America. Grown from seed, visnaga is widely cultivated. The tiny fruits containing the seeds are picked in late summer before they have fully ripened.

Related species
Bishop's weed (*A. majus*, p. 170) is a close relative. This plant has been used to treat asthma but is mainly taken as a diuretic and to treat psoriasis.

Key constituents
• Furochromones including khellin (1%) and visnagin • Coumarins
• Flavonoids • Volatile oil
• Phytosterols

Key actions
• Antispasmodic • Anti-asthmatic
• Relaxant

Research
Strong antispasmodic Research by a pharmacologist working in Egypt in 1946 revealed that visnaga (in particular its constituents khellin and visnagin) has a powerful antispasmodic action on the smaller bronchial muscles, the coronary arteries that supply blood to the heart, and on the urinary tubules. Visnaga's ability to relax the small bronchi lasts for up to 6 hours, and the plant has practically no side effects.
Khellin Intal, an asthma drug formerly much used in conventional medicine, is derived chemically from khellin.

Traditional & current uses
Kidney stones Visnaga is a traditional Egyptian remedy for kidney stones. It was mentioned in the Ebers papyrus of Egypt (c. 1500 BCE) and is still used there to relieve kidney stones. By relaxing the muscles of the ureter, visnaga reduces the pain caused by the trapped stone and helps ease the stone down into the bladder.
Asthma remedy Following research into its antispasmodic properties, visnaga is now given for asthma, and is safe even for children to take. Although it does not always relieve acute asthma attacks, it does help prevent their recurrence.
Other respiratory conditions Visnaga is an effective remedy for various respiratory problems, including bronchitis, emphysema, and whooping cough.
Circulatory herb By relaxing the coronary arteries, visnaga helps improve blood supply to the heart muscle and thereby ease angina and reduce blood pressure.
Dental hygiene In Andalusia in Spain, the largest and best-quality visnaga seeds were employed to clean the teeth. The high value given to the herb in general was reflected in the saying: "Oro, plata, visnaga, o nada!" (Gold, silver, visnaga, or nothing!).

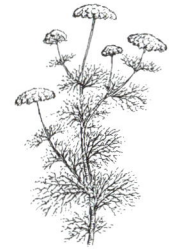

Parts used

Seeds from the fruit of the fresh plant are collected in late summer and dried for use in infusions and powders.

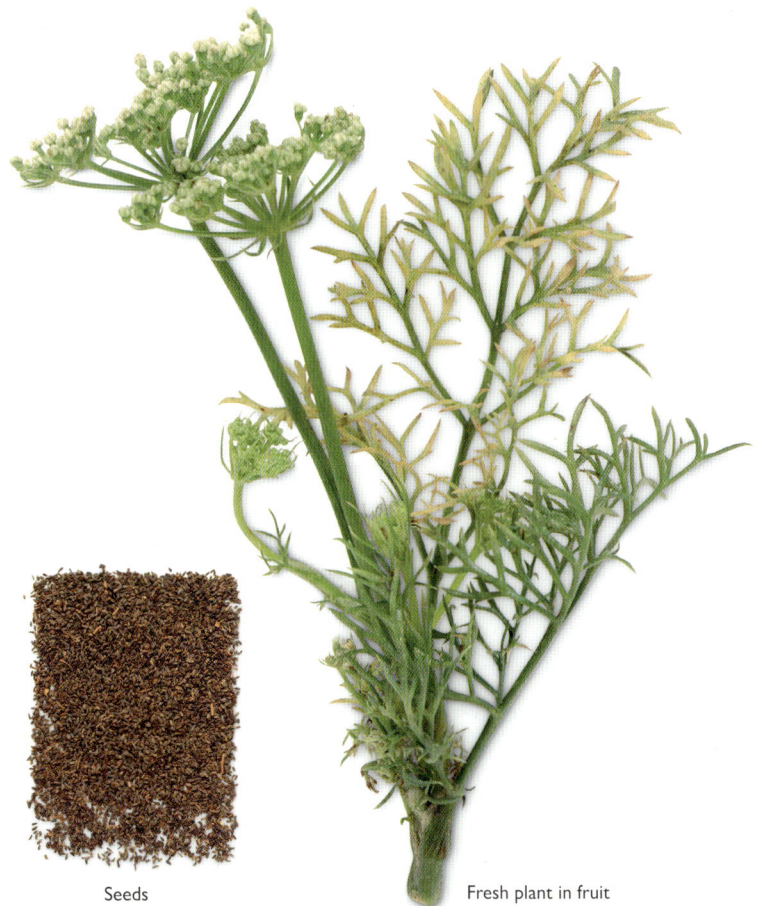

Seeds

Fresh plant in fruit

Key preparations & their uses

Infusion alleviates asthma, bronchitis, and kidney stones.

Powder is prescribed by doctors and medical herbalists to relieve angina.

Cautions Take only under professional supervision. Long-term use produces symptoms such as nausea, headaches, and insomnia. Subject to legal restrictions in some countries.

Andrographis paniculata (Acanthaceae)

Andrographis, Green chiretta

Known as the "King of Bitters" in India, due to its profoundly bitter taste, Andrographis has been used in traditional Indian and Chinese medicine for several thousand years. Prized for its ability to ease cold, flu, and cough symptoms, as well as more serious illnesses such as malaria and tuberculosis, current research suggests that the herb has a potent ability to treat upper respiratory tract infections. Andrographis may also have significant nerve protective activity.

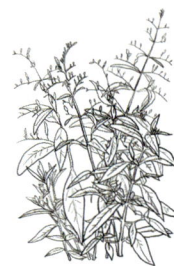

An upright annual growing to 3 ft (1 m) with lanceolate leaves and clusters of small pink flowers.

Habitat and cultivation

Andrographis grows throughout much of the Indian subcontinent and southeast Asia, on plains and as undergrowth in forests. Readily grown from seed, it is cultivated in tropical and subtropical regions throughout the world.

Key constituents

- Diterpenoids (andrographolides)
- Flavonoids • Polyphenols
- Phytosterols

Key actions

- Immune modulating • Liver protective • Anti-inflammatory
- Lowers blood sugar levels
- Antibacterial/antiviral
- Neuroprotective

Research

Acute respiratory infections After reviewing 33 clinical trials, researchers (2017) concluded that andrographis had a significant effect in improving and shortening the duration of symptoms of acute respiratory tract infection, such as sore throat, catarrh and cough.

Liver protection Andrographolide and extracts of the herb have demonstrated an effect similar to, or better than, silymarin (from *Silybum marianum p.*) in supporting healthy liver function.

Nerve protection Ongoing research into the nerve protective effects of andrographolide, which is able to cross the blood-brain barrier, point to multiple positive effects on the central nervous system. It counters inflammatory processes; protects against clot formation and reduced oxygen levels, as in stroke; and may have protective activity in conditions such as dementia, Parkinson's disease and multiple sclerosis. A clinical trial in Chile is currently underway, that is investigating the effects of an andrographis extract in people with multiple sclerosis.

Traditional & current uses

Immune support A classically bitter and tonic herb, Andrographis exerts a wide range of protective effects on the body—mostly through its ability to strengthen the immune system and protect the liver from damage, whether by infection or poisoning.

Fever, colds and flu Like most bitters, it will help counter fever and is a traditional remedy for colds, coughs, and influenza.

Covid-19 In several African and Asian countries, notably Nigeria and Thailand, andrographis has been used as a frontline treatment for Covid-19 infection.

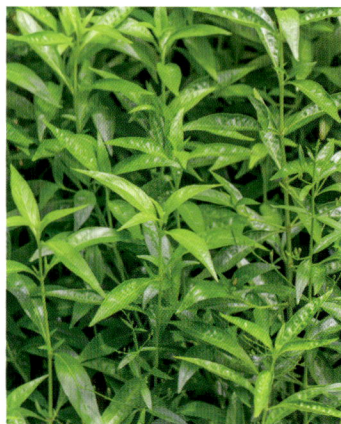

*An **annual** growing to about 3 ft (1 m), Andrographis has a strongly bitter taste and is a valued medicine in India and China.*

Parts used

Aerial parts—all parts of the plant are profoundly bitter and have major liver protective activity.

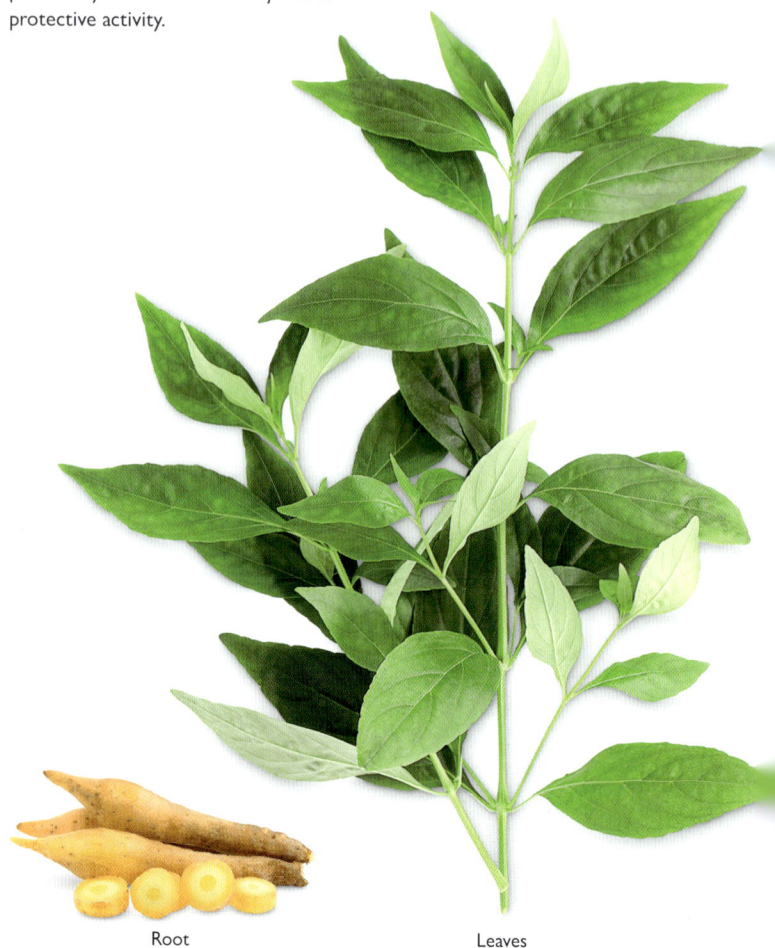

Root

Leaves

Key preparations & their uses

Infusion (to make, p. 301) Use ½ cup (100 ml) as a gargle for sore throat, then swallow.

Tincture (to make, p. 302) For upper respiratory tract infection, take ½ tsp in water 1–3 times a day

Capsule (to make, p. 302) Take 1–2 capsules a day to aid liver health.

Cautions Do not take during pregnancy or if trying to conceive. High doses may cause nausea and vomiting.

Angelica sinensis syn. *A. polymorpha* (Apiaceae)

Dong quai, Chinese angelica, *Dang gui* (Chinese)

In China, *dong quai* is the main tonic herb for conditions suffered by women. It is taken on a daily basis by millions of women as an invigorating tonic, helping to regulate menstruation and tonify the blood. It also improves the circulation. *Dong quai* has a sweet, pungent aroma that is very distinctive, and in China it is often used in cooking, which is the best way to take it as a blood tonic.

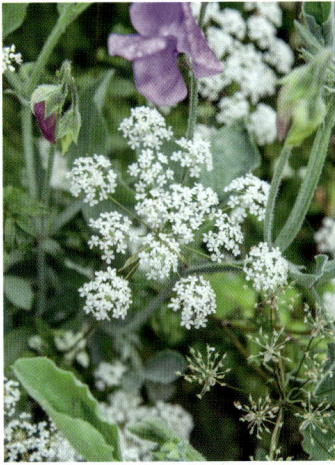

A stout, erect perennial growing to 6½ ft (2 m), with large, bright green leaves and hollow stems.

Dong quai has attractive clusters of white flowers in summer.

Habitat & cultivation

Dong quai is native to China and Japan, where it is now cultivated. The best rhizomes are in Gansu province in China. Seed is sown in spring and the rhizomes are lifted in the fall.

Related species

American angelica (*A. atropurpurea*) has similar properties, though it is less aromatic. European angelica (*A. archangelica*, p. 172) is a warming tonic herb for digestion and circulation, but does not have the same tonic action as *dong quai*.

Key constituents

- Volatile oil (ligustilide, sesquiterpenes, carvacrol)
- Coumarins • Phytosterols
- Polyacetylenes • Ferulic acid

Key actions

- Tonic • Anti-inflammatory
- Antispasmodic • Thins blood
- Promotes menstrual flow

Research

Gynecology Research in China from the 1970s on has shown that the herb helps to regulate uterine contractions, which may explain its benefit for period pain.

Circulation The root can help normalize heart function and has been shown to thin the blood. It may therefore interact with anticoagulant medicines.

Traditional & current uses

Blood tonic Famous in China as a tonic, *dong quai* is taken for "deficient blood" conditions, anemia, and for the symptoms of anemia due to blood loss—a pale complexion, palpitations, and lowered vitality.

Women's health *Dong quai* regulates the menstrual cycle, relieves period pain and cramps, and is an ideal tonic for women with heavy menstruation who risk becoming anemic. However, as it stimulates menstrual bleeding, other tonic herbs such as nettle (*Urtica dioica*, p. 150) are best taken during menstruation if the flow is heavy. It is also a uterine tonic, and helps infertility.

Circulation *Dong quai* is a "warming" herb, improving the circulation to the abdomen and to the hands and feet. It strengthens the digestion and is also useful in the treatment of abscesses and boils.

Self-help uses

- Aiding conception, p. 326.
- Menstrual problems, p. 325.

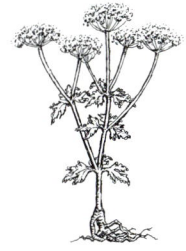

Parts used

Rhizome is valued for its medicinal properties and is often used in cooking.

Rhizome is large and brownish on the outside and white inside

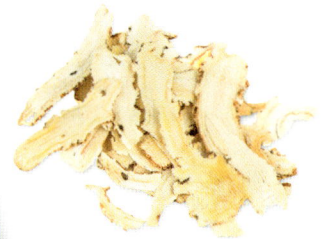

Slices from the rhizome interior

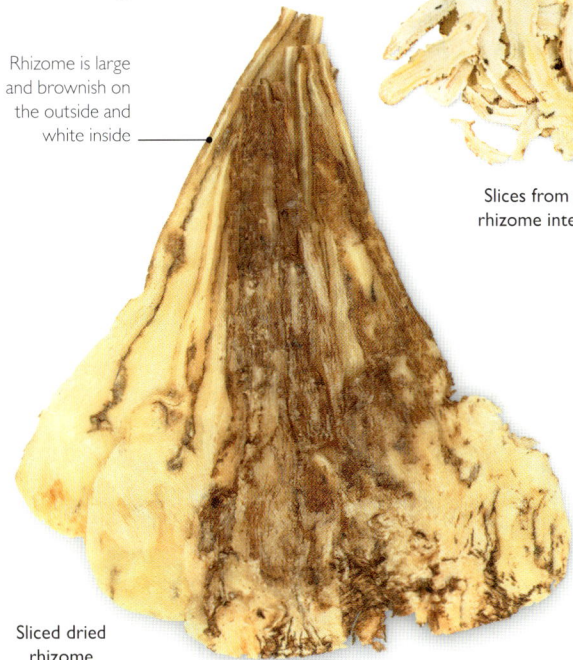

Sliced dried rhizome

Key preparations & their uses

Tonic wine Make with *dong quai* and other tonic or bitter herbs (see p. 303). To improve vitality, drink a ¾ cup (150 ml) daily.

Chopped rhizome is commonly added to soups in China.

Tincture (to make, p. 302). For period pain, take ½ tsp with water up to 4 times a day.

Infusion For poor circulation, infuse 1 tsp with ¾ cup (150 ml) water (see p. 301). Drink this mixture 1–2 times a day.

Decoction (to make, p. 301). For anemia, take ¾ cup (150 ml) 2–3 times a day.

Tablets Take as a general female tonic.

Cautions Do not take during pregnancy or while breastfeeding. Should not be used for heavy menstrual bleeding, bleeding disorders, and diarrhea. May interact with prescribed blood-thinning medication.

Apium graveolens (Apiaceae)

Celery

More familiar as a vegetable than as a medicine, celery stems and seeds have long been taken for urinary, rheumatic, and arthritic problems. Celery is a good cleansing, diuretic herb, and the seeds are used specifically for arthritic complaints where there is an accumulation of waste products in the joints. The seeds also have a reputation as a carminative with a mild tranquilizing effect. The stems are less significant medicinally.

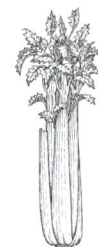

A biennial with a ridged, shiny stem; glossy leaves; and small flowers, growing to about 20 in (50 cm).

Habitat & cultivation

Native to Britain and other European countries, celery is found growing wild along the English and Welsh coasts, and in marshlands. Widely grown as a vegetable, cultivated celery is less fragrant than the wild variety. It is propagated from seed in spring and harvested from midsummer to fall.

Related species

Celeriac (*A. graveolens* var. *rapaceum*) is a "turnip-rooted" variety of celery. A medicinal food, it has some of the same qualities as celery.

Key constituents

- Volatile oil (1.5–3%) containing limonene (60–70%), phthalides, and beta-selinene • Coumarins
- Furanocoumarins (bergapten)
- Flavonoids (apiin)

Key actions

- Antirheumatic • Carminative
- Antispasmodic • Diuretic • Lowers blood pressure • Urinary antiseptic
- Anti-inflammatory

Research

Volatile oil Research in the 1970s and 1980s showed that the volatile oil

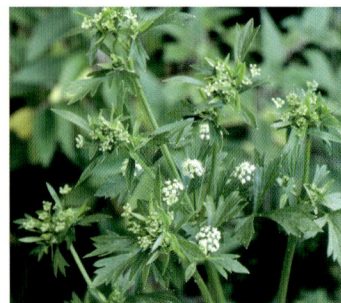

Celery is an important medicinal herb as well as a vegetable.

has a calming effect on the central nervous system.

Other research A 1995 study in India found the seeds to have marked liver-protective activity. Extracts of the seeds may also lower blood fat levels. Iranian laboratory research from 2013 found that celery seed had a marked effect in lowering high blood pressure.

Traditional & current uses

Ancient herb Records show that celery has been cultivated for at least 3,000 years, notably in pharaonic Egypt, and it was known in China in the 5th century BCE. Throughout history, celery has been used as a food, and at various times both the whole plant and the seeds have been taken medicinally.

Cleansing properties Today, the seeds are used for treating rheumatic conditions and gout. They help the kidneys dispose of urates and other waste products, and work to reduce acidity in the body as a whole. The seeds are useful in arthritis, helping to detoxify the body and improve the circulation of blood to the muscles and joints.

Diuretic Celery seeds have a mildly diuretic and significantly antiseptic action. They can be an effective treatment for cystitis, disinfecting the bladder and urinary tubules.

Nutritious drink Celery and organic carrot juice make a nutritious, cleansing drink that is good for many chronic illnesses.

Other uses Celery seeds are beneficial for chest problems such as asthma and bronchitis, and, in combination with other herbs, can help reduce blood pressure.

Self-help uses

- Arthritis, p. 323. • Gout, p. 323.

Parts used

Stems are eaten as a nourishing vegetable and made into juice.

Seeds contain volatile oil and are the main part used medicinally.

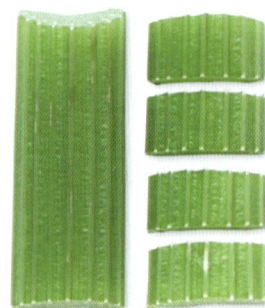

Chopped stem

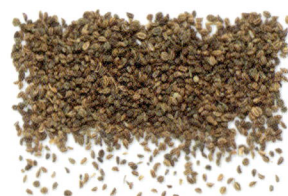

Seeds

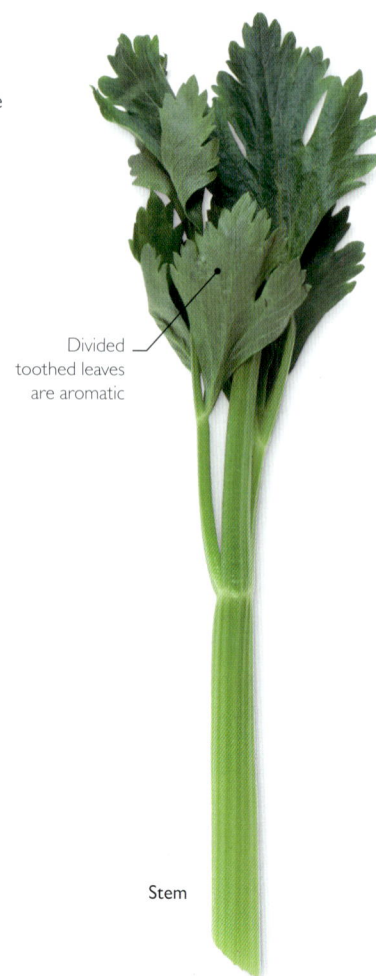

Divided toothed leaves are aromatic

Stem

Key preparations & their uses

Remedy As a cleansing drink, take ¾ cup (150 ml) of organic carrot and celery juice a day.

Infusion of seeds (to make, p. 301). For gout and arthritis, take ¾ cup (150 ml) daily.

Tincture of seeds (to make, p. 302). For rheumatism, take 30 drops 3 times a day.

Powder of seeds. For arthritis, mix 1 tsp with food each day.

Cautions Do not take celery seed during pregnancy or if suffering from kidney disease. Do not use seeds sold for cultivation in medicinal preparations. Do not take the essential oil internally except under professional supervision.

Arctium lappa (Asteraceae)

Burdock, *Niu bang zi* (Chinese), *Gobo* (Japanese)

Burdock is one of the foremost detoxifying herbs in both Western and Chinese herbal medicine. It is used to treat conditions caused by an "overload" of toxins, such as throat and other infections, boils and rashes, and chronic skin problems. The root and the seeds help cleanse the body of waste products, and the root is thought to be particularly good at helping to eliminate heavy metals.

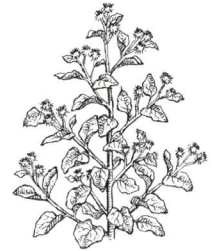

A biennial, with stems that grow to 5 ft (1.5 m), reddish-purple flower heads, and hooked bracts.

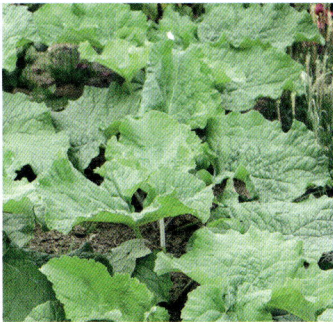

Burdock in its first year produces a rosette of large leaves.

Habitat & cultivation
Native to Europe and Asia, burdock now grows in temperate regions throughout the world, including the US. Burdock is also cultivated in Europe and China and is propagated from seed in spring. The seeds are harvested in summer and the whole plant is unearthed in high summer.

Related species
A. minus and *A. tomentosum* are related species with a similar use to burdock.

Key constituents
• Bitter glycosides (arctiopicrin)
• Flavonoids (arctiin) • Tannins
• Polyacetylenes • Volatile oil • Inulin (up to 45%) • Lignans

Key actions
• Detoxifying • Mild diuretic
• Antibiotic • Antiseptic
• Anti-inflammatory

Research
Antibiotic Studies in Germany (1967) and Japan (1986) showed that the polyacetylenes, especially within the fresh root, have an antibiotic effect.

Other research Burdock has antibacterial and antifungal properties, and diuretic and hypoglycemic (lowering blood-sugar levels) effects. It also seems to have an antitumor action. Recent studies suggest the seeds are anti-inflammatory, antioxidant, and hepatoprotective.

Traditional & current uses
History Burdock was a traditional remedy for gout, fevers, and kidney stones. In the 17th century, Culpeper wrote, "The seed is much commended to break the stone and cause it to be expelled by urine."

Cleansing herb Burdock is used in both Western and Chinese herbal medicine as a detoxifying herb. The seeds are used to remove toxins in fevers and infections such as mumps and measles, and the root helps the body eliminate waste products in chronic skin and arthritic conditions.

Skin problems Burdock's diuretic, antibiotic, and mildly bitter actions make it helpful for skin disorders, especially where toxicity is a key factor, such as in acne, abscesses, local skin infections, eczema, and psoriasis.

Combination remedies Burdock is rarely used on its own in remedies. It is generally mixed with herbs such as dandelion (*Taraxacum officinale*, p. 145) or yellow dock (*Rumex crispus*, p. 273). These help the body remove accumulated waste products drawn out of tissues by burdock's detoxifying action. Use of burdock alone can cause a flare-up of skin conditions such as eczema.

Self-help uses
• Acne & boils, p. 315. • Skin rashes, p. 313.

Parts used

Leaves and fruit (containing seeds) are harvested in late summer.

Dried root is most used to aid detoxification.

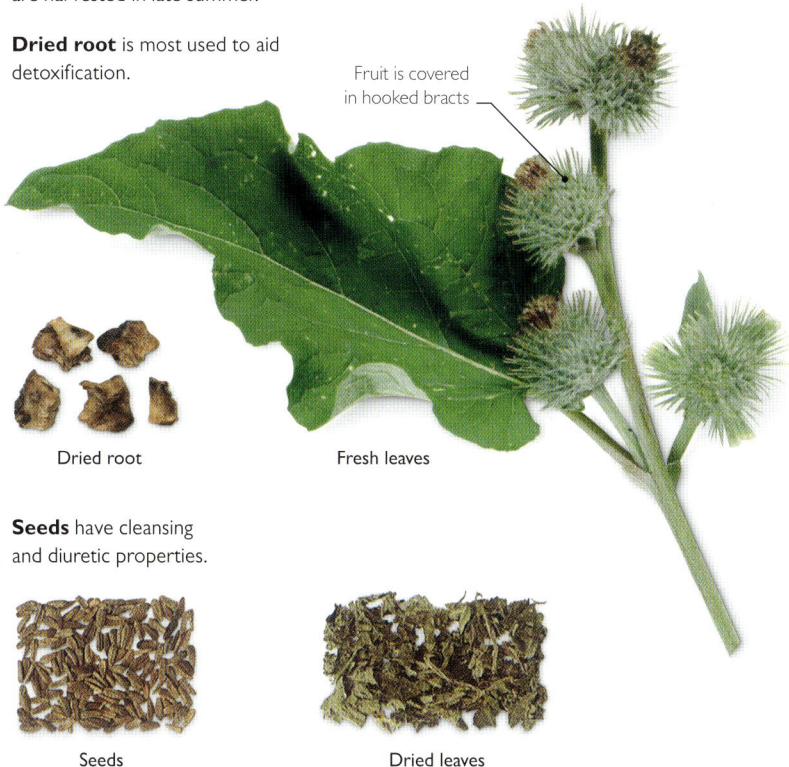

Fruit is covered in hooked bracts

Dried root

Fresh leaves

Seeds have cleansing and diuretic properties.

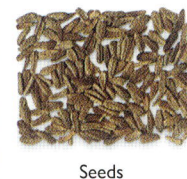

Seeds

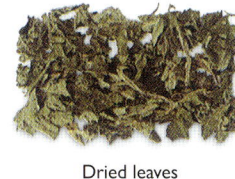

Dried leaves

Key preparations & their uses

Remedy For acne, make a decoction (see p. 301) with 2 tsp burdock root and 5 tsp dandelion root. Drink ¾ cup (150 ml) twice a day.

Tincture of root (to make, p. 302). For arthritis and skin disorders, take 20 drops diluted with water 2–3 times a day for up to 4 weeks.

Decoction of root (to make, p. 301) is an alternative to tincture for arthritis and skin disorders. Drink 7 tsp once a day for up to 4 weeks.

Infusion of seeds (to make, p. 301). Use as a wash for acne and boils.

Poultice of leaves (to make, p. 305). Apply to abscesses and boils.

Cautions Very rarely can cause contact dermatitis.

Artemisia absinthium (Asteraceae)

Wormwood

One of the truly bitter plants—*absinthium* means "without sweetness"—wormwood has a strong tonic effect on the digestive system, especially on the stomach and gallbladder. It is taken in small doses and sipped, the intensely bitter taste playing an important part in its therapeutic effect. In the past, wormwood was one of the main flavorings of vermouth (whose name derives from the German for wormwood).

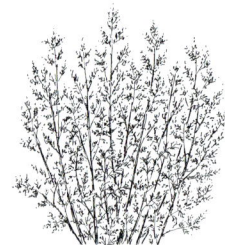

A perennial reaching 3 ft (1 m), with gray-green stems and feathery leaves, both covered in fine hairs.

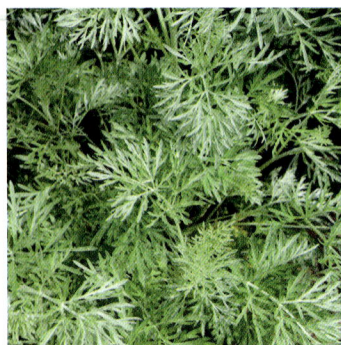

Wormwood is strongly aromatic and was used to flavor many alcoholic drinks.

Habitat & cultivation

Wormwood is a wayside plant, native to Europe. It now grows wild in central Asia and in eastern parts of the US. It is also cultivated in temperate regions worldwide. Wormwood is propagated from seed in spring or by dividing the roots in the fall. The aerial parts are harvested in late summer.

Related species

Artemisia species with a medicinal use include *A. abrotanum* (p. 176); *A. annua* (p. 71); *A. anomala*; *A. capillaris* and *A. cina* (p. 176); *A. vulgaris* and *A. dracunculus* (p. 177).

Key constituents

• Volatile oil containing sesquiterpene lactones (artabsin, anabsinthin); thujone; azulenes • Flavonoids
• Polyphenols • Lignans

Key actions

• Aromatic bitter • Stimulates secretion of bile • Anti-inflammatory
• Eases stomach pain • Mild antidepressant • Antimicrobial
• Antiparasitic

Research

Bitter herb Research into wormwood, mostly during the 1970s, has established that a range of the constituents within the plant contributes to its medicinal activity. Many are very bitter, affecting the bitter taste receptors on the tongue which sets off a reflex action, stimulating stomach and other digestive secretions.

Gut inflammation A German clinical trial in 2007 found that wormwood helped in treating Crohn's disease (an inflammatory bowel disorder). Wormwood prevented the return of symptoms in 90% of those taking it, and reduced required dosage of powerful steroid drugs taken to control inflammation. Patients also experienced lower levels of depression.

Other research Constituents within wormwood, notably the essential oil, are thought to have wide-ranging therapeutic effects, including neuroprotective, antidepressant, antibacterial, antifungal, and antimalarial activity.

Traditional & current uses

Absinthe Wormwood is the source of *absinthe*, an addictive drink favored in 19th-century France. Flavored with wormwood essential oil, *absinthe* was toxic due to its high level of thujone. This is a nerve stimulant that is safe at low dosage but is toxic in excess.

Digestive stimulant Wormwood is an extremely useful medicine for those with weak and underactive digestion. It increases stomach acid and bile production and therefore improves digestion and the absorption of nutrients, making it helpful for many conditions, including anemia. Wormwood also eases gas and

Parts used

Aerial parts contain bitter substances and have a wide range of medicinal uses.

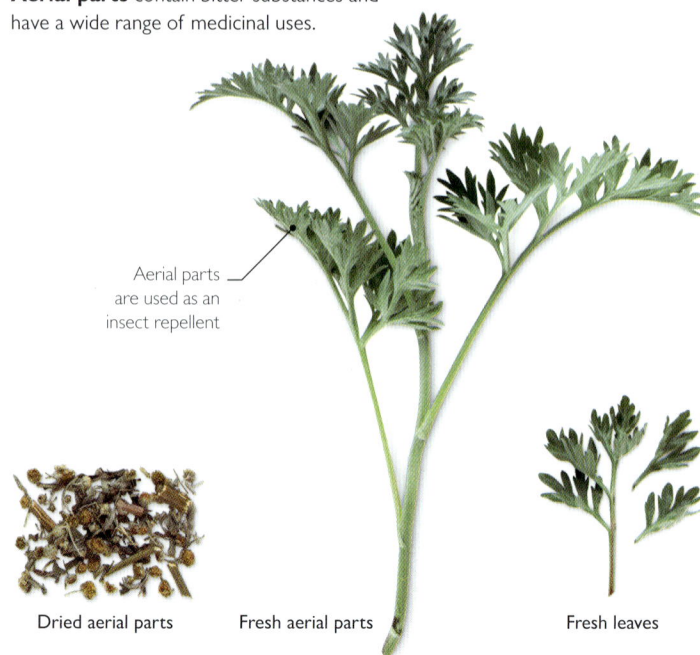

Aerial parts are used as an insect repellent

Dried aerial parts

Fresh aerial parts

Fresh leaves

Key preparations & their uses

Infusion made from wormwood can be taken in small doses to stimulate appetite.

Tincture is used to treat chronic digestive infections.

Cautions Take only under professional supervision. Take only in small doses, generally for no more than 4–5 weeks at a time. Do not take during pregnancy.

bloating and, if the tincture is taken regularly, it slowly strengthens digestion and helps the body return to full vitality and wellness after a prolonged illness.

Worms Wormwood is commonly used by herbalists and naturopaths to treat parasitic infections of the gut, such as worm infestation, amebic dysentery, and *Shigella* infection.

Traditional insect repellent Wormwood is a good insecticide and insect repellent.

Other uses The anti-inflammatory action of wormwood makes it useful for infections, and it has occasionally been given as an antidepressant.

Self-help uses

• Anemia, p. 311. • High fever, p. 321.

Artemisia annua (Asteraceae)

Sweet Annie, *Qing hao*

Until the 1970s, sweet Annie was regarded as just another *Artemisia*, though one used in traditional Chinese medicine for treating malaria. After extensive research, sweet Annie and its key constituent artemisinin were shown to have powerful antimalarial activity and few side effects. Artemisinin rapidly became the key treatment for severe malaria worldwide, and is still the treatment of choice in many acute cases of the illness.

A perennial growing to about 3 ft (1 m), with green feathery leaves covered in fine hairs.

Habitat & cultivation

Sweet Annie grows in grasslands and in open areas in Vietnam, Japan, China, Russia, and North America. It is cultivated in eastern China. The herb is propagated from seed in spring or by dividing the rootstock in the fall. It is harvested in summer before flowering.

Related species

The related *A. apiacea* is used interchangeably with sweet Annie in China and is employed as a general tonic in Vietnam. Many other *Artemisia* species are used medicinally: *A. abrotanum* (p. 176); *A. absinthium* (p. 70); *A. capillaris* and *A. cina* (p. 176); *A. dracunculus* and *A. vulgaris* (p. 177).

Key constituents

- Artemisinin (sesquiterpene lactone) • Essential oil (abrotamine, beta-bourbonene) • Flavonoids
- Polyphenols

Key actions

- Bitter • Reduces fever
- Antimalarial • Antiparasitic
- Anticancer

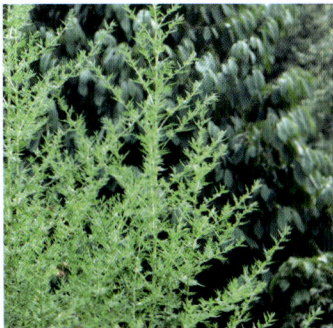

Sweet Annie has bright green, saw-toothed leaves. It is used widely around the world as an effective antimalarial.

Research

Chinese research Sweet Annie was extensively researched in China in the 1980s, and studies have demonstrated that its key active constituent is an effective antimalarial, having a powerful action against the malaria parasite *Plasmodium*, a protozoan introduced into the body by the mosquito.

Artemisinin Clinical trials, notably in Thailand, show that it can provide vital treatment in the acute stages of malaria, proving up to 90% effective in countering the infection. Artemisinin has a lesser role to play in chronic malaria and prevention of the disease.

Anticancer potential Laboratory studies suggest that sweet Annie has marked anticancer activity, promoting programmed cell death and inhibiting blood vessel growth. No clinical trials have so far been undertaken, but sweet Annie is claimed to be useful particularly in breast cancer and leukemia. Synthetic molecules modeled on artemisinin are also being researched as potential anticancer drugs.

Traditional & current uses

History The first mention of sweet Annie was in a Chinese text of 168 BCE. Traditionally, it was seen as an herb that helped "to clear and relieve summer heat."

Cooling properties Sweet Annie has a cool, bitter taste and is used for conditions brought on by heat, especially with symptoms such as fever, headaches, dizziness, and a tight-chested sensation. It is used to treat chronic fevers, night fevers, and morning chills and is a traditional remedy for nosebleeds associated with heat.

Antimalarial Sweet Annie has been used to treat the fevers and chills of malaria for thousands of years, and artemisinin is now used in many countries as an antimalarial. Artemisinin reduces the risk of developing malaria and aids a quick recovery, though drug resistance to it is now being seen. The whole plant may also be used to treat malaria and act as a preventative, though large doses are required.

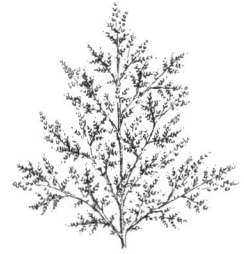

Parts used

Leaves contain artemisinin, which is a powerful antimalarial.

Leaves are harvested in summer

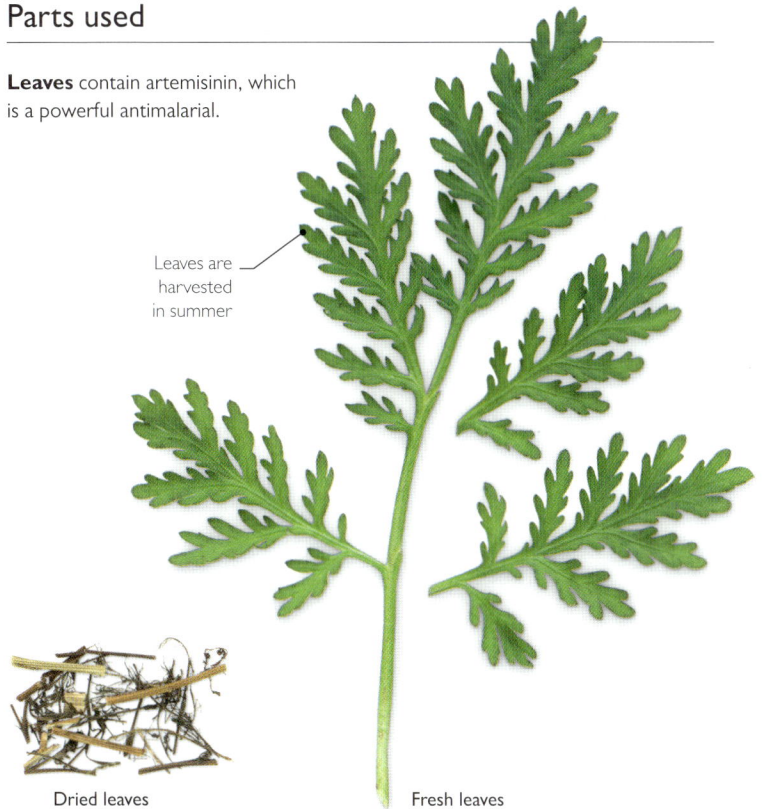

Dried leaves

Fresh leaves

Key preparations & their uses

Tincture is prescribed to prevent malaria. It is also used to treat the illness itself.

Infusion is strongly bitter. Herbalists use it to treat headaches and fever.

Tablets containing artemisinin, which is extracted from the herb, are taken for malaria throughout the tropics.

Cautions Only take sweet Annie under professional supervision. Do not take during pregnancy.

Astragalus membranaceus (Fabaceae)

Astragalus, *Milk vetch, Huang qi* (Chinese)

Despite the fact that astragalus is one of the most popular tonic herbs in China, it is not that well known in the West. In China, the root, known as *huang qi*, has been used for thousands of years. It has a sweet taste and is a warming tonic particularly suited to young, active people, increasing stamina and endurance, and improving resistance to the cold. It is often combined with other herbs as a blood tonic.

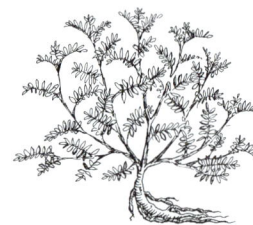

A perennial growing to 16 in (40 cm) with hairy stems and leaves divided into 12–18 pairs of leaflets.

Habitat & cultivation

Astragalus is native to Mongolia and northern and eastern China. It is grown from seed in spring or fall and thrives in sandy, well-drained soil, with plenty of sun. The roots of 4-year-old plants are harvested in the fall.

Key constituents

• Triterpene saponins (astragolosides)
• Isoflavonoids (formonentin)
• Polysaccharides • Phytosterols

Key actions

• Adaptogenic • Immune stimulant
• Diuretic • Vasodilator • Antiviral

Research

Chinese investigations

Investigations in China indicate that astragalus is diuretic and that it lowers blood pressure and increases endurance. A 2012 clinical trial found that 5 grams of astragalus root a day helped stabilize kidney function in patients with chronic kidney disease, delaying the need for dialysis.

Western research Recent American research has focused on the ability of astragalus to restore normal immune function in cancer patients. Clinical evidence suggests that, as with a number of other herbs, cancer patients undergoing chemotherapy or radiotherapy recover faster and live longer if given astragalus concurrently.

Traditional & current uses

Tonic & endurance remedy

Astragalus is a classic energy tonic, perhaps even superior to ginseng (*Panax ginseng*, p. 118) for young people. In China, it is believed to warm and tone the *wei qi* (a protective energy that circulates just beneath the skin), helping the body adapt to external influences, especially to the cold. Astragalus raises immune resistance and manifestly improves physical endurance.

Control of fluids Though a vasodilator (encouraging blood to flow to the surface), astragalus is used for excessive sweating, including night sweats. It is also helpful in both relieving fluid retention and reducing thirstiness. It supports normal kidney function and is thought to protect the kidneys from damage.

Immune stimulant Not an herb for acute illness, astragalus is nonetheless a very useful medicine for viral infections such as the common cold.

Other uses Astragalus is used to treat prolapsed organs, especially the uterus, and it is beneficial for uterine bleeding. Astragalus is often used in combination with dong quai (*Angelica sinensis*, p. 67) in order to act as a blood tonic for treating anemia.

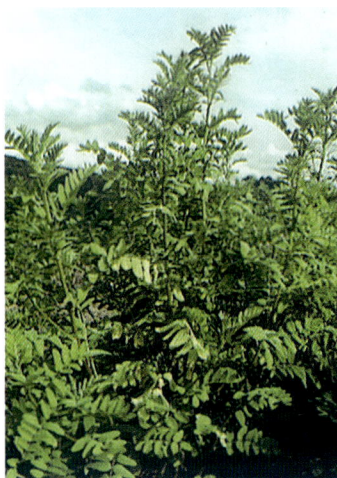

Astragalus is a typical member of the pea family and is closely related to licorice.

Parts used

Root is a traditional tonic remedy in China, improving energy levels and helping the body to resist cold.

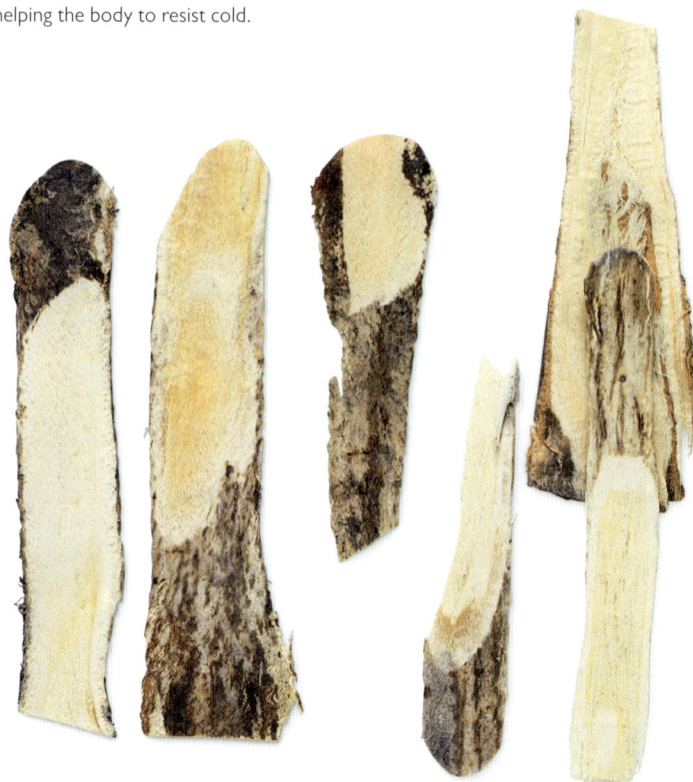

Dried root

Key preparations & their uses

Decoction For anemia, decoct (*see* p. 301) with 12 g root and 12 g Chinese angelica. Take 1¼ cups (300 ml) daily.

Dry-fried root As a stimulant tonic, each day fry 5–10 g root by itself or with 1 tsp of honey and eat with meals.

Remedy For cold and numbness, make a decoction (*see* p. 301) with 20 g root and 5 g cinnamon. Drink ¾ cup (150 ml) twice a day.

Tincture (to make, p. 302). For night sweats, take 1 tsp with water 1–2 times daily.

Cautions Do not take astragalus if suffering from skin disorders, or during acute illness.

Atropa belladonna (Solanaceae)

Deadly nightshade, Belladonna

Although deadly nightshade conjures up images of poison and death, like many plants it is an important and beneficial remedy when used correctly. Some of its constituents are employed in conventional medicine, for example to dilate the pupils for eye examinations and as an anesthetic. In herbal medicine, deadly nightshade is mainly prescribed to relieve intestinal colic and to treat peptic ulcers.

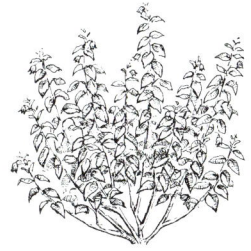

A perennial with large leaves and black berries, growing to 5 ft (1.5 m).

Habitat & cultivation

Deadly nightshade is native to Europe, western Asia, and northern Africa, and is now cultivated worldwide. It thrives in chalky soils, in woods, and in open areas. The leaves are harvested in summer, and the root is collected from the first year onward in the fall.

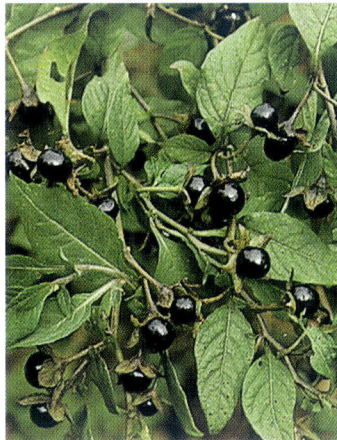

Related species

Many of the Solanaceae family are powerful medicines, including Thorn Apple (*Datura stramonium*, p. 205), tobacco (*Nicotiana tabacum*, p. 247), and henbane (*Hyoscyamus niger*, p. 226).

Key constituents

• Tropane alkaloids (up to 0.6%), including hyoscyamine and atropine
• Flavonoids • Coumarins • Volatile bases (nicotine)

Key actions

• Smooth muscle antispasmodic
• Narcotic • Reduces sweating
• Sedative

Research

Tropane alkaloids The action of the tropane alkaloids is well understood. They inhibit the parasympathetic nervous system, which controls involuntary bodily activities. This reduces saliva; gastric, intestinal, and bronchial secretions; as well as the activity of the urinary tubules, bladder, and intestines. Tropane alkaloids also increase heart rate and dilate the pupils.

Traditional & current uses

Folklore Deadly nightshade was believed to help witches fly. Its other name "belladonna" (beautiful woman) is thought to refer to its use by Italian women to dilate the pupils of their

Deadly nightshade produces unmistakable cherry-size, glossy black berries in the fall.

eyes, making them more attractive.
Relaxant Deadly nightshade has been used in the same way throughout history. It is prescribed to relax distended organs, especially the stomach and intestines, relieving intestinal colic and pain. It helps peptic ulcers by reducing gastric acid production, and it relaxes spasms of the urinary tubules.
Parkinson's disease The herb can be used to treat the symptoms of Parkinson's disease, reducing tremors and rigidity, and improving speech and mobility.
Anesthetic Muscle relaxant properties of deadly nightshade have for many centuries made it a valued anesthetic in operations, particularly when digestive or bronchial secretions need to be kept to a minimum.

Parts used

Leaves are harvested in early summer. They have a weaker action than the root, and are more commonly used.

Root is collected in the fall.

Leaves, like the root, have relaxant properties.

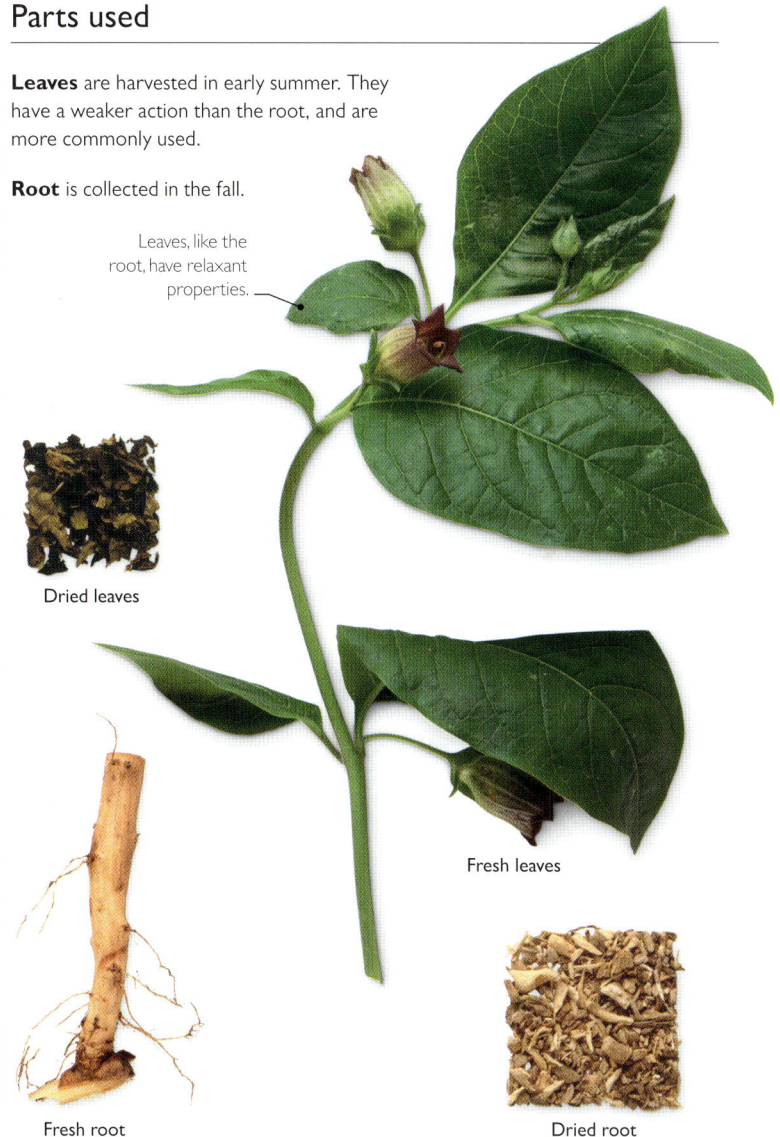

Dried leaves

Fresh leaves

Fresh root

Dried root

Key preparations & their uses

Tincture made from the leaves or the root, is a strong relaxant. It is prescribed by herbal practitioners to relieve colic and to treat Parkinson's disease.

Cautions Take only if prescribed by a medical herbalist or doctor. Deadly nightshade can be fatal if taken at the wrong dosage.

Azadirachta indica (Meliaceae)

Neem

Neem is one of the most valued herbs in Indian and Ayurvedic medicine. Extracts of the leaves are used to treat conditions such as asthma, eczema, diabetes, and rheumatism, while neem oil has been applied as a hair lotion to treat head lice, and to calm angry skin rashes. Research indicates that neem may prove useful as an insecticide and a contraceptive. The tree itself is said to purify the air and is widely planted in India.

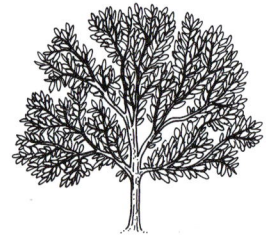

An evergreen tree, growing to 52 ft (16 m), with compound leaves and white flowers.

Habitat & cultivation

Native to Iran, Pakistan, India, and Sri Lanka, neem is found throughout the subcontinent in forests and woods, often being planted on roads to provide shade. It is now naturalized in other tropical regions, including Malaysia, Indonesia, Australia, and West Africa. It is grown from seed. Leaves and seed are harvested throughout the year.

Related species

Melia azedarach, also an Indian plant, is a very close relative with particular value in treating intestinal worms. It is often used as a substitute for neem.

Key constituents

- Meliacins • Liminoids
- Triterpenoid bitters • Sterols
- Tannins • Flavonoids

Key actions

- Anti-inflammatory • Lowers fever
- Antimicrobial • Promotes wound healing • Antiparasitic • Antimalarial

Research

Recent research This indicates that neem oil is both anti-inflammatory and antibacterial, and to some degree

reduces fever and lowers blood-sugar levels.

Insecticide Extensive research shows that liminoid azadirachtins are insecticidal and inhibit feeding and growth—making neem an inexpensive and ecologically sound insecticidal agent. The azadirachtins are also linked to the tree's antimalarial activity.

Diabetes Research indicates that neem leaf and oil act to stabilize blood-sugar levels and may be helpful in treating or delaying type 2 diabetes.

Traditional & current uses

Medicine chest Thought of in India as almost a pharmacy in its own right, all parts of the neem tree may be used medicinally. The bark is bitter and astringent and a decoction is used for hemorrhoids. The leaves are taken as an infusion for malaria, peptic ulcers, and intestinal worms, and may be applied locally as a juice, infusion, or ointment to skin problems including ulcers, wounds, boils, and eczema. The juice of the leaves is also applied to the eyes to treat night blindness and conjunctivitis. The twigs are used as a tooth cleanser, firming up the gums and preventing gum disease.

Neem oil and sap Neem oil, expressed from the seeds, is commonly used as a hair dressing and is strongly antifungal and antiviral, preventing scabies and ringworm, among other things. It can be made into a useful and easily applied treatment for head lice. The oil is also used to treat skin conditions such as eczema, psoriasis, and even leprosy, and as a vehicle for other active ingredients. Neem oil should be avoided when attempting to conceive a child as it can reduce fertility in both women and men.

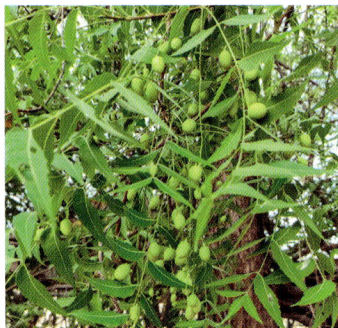

Neem has so many medicinal uses that the tree is considered a "natural pharmacy."

Parts used

Leaves can be infused and applied as a lotion to many skin rashes, including acne, eczema, and psoriasis.

Twigs are used as toothpicks to improve oral hygiene.

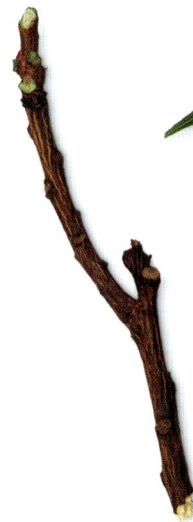

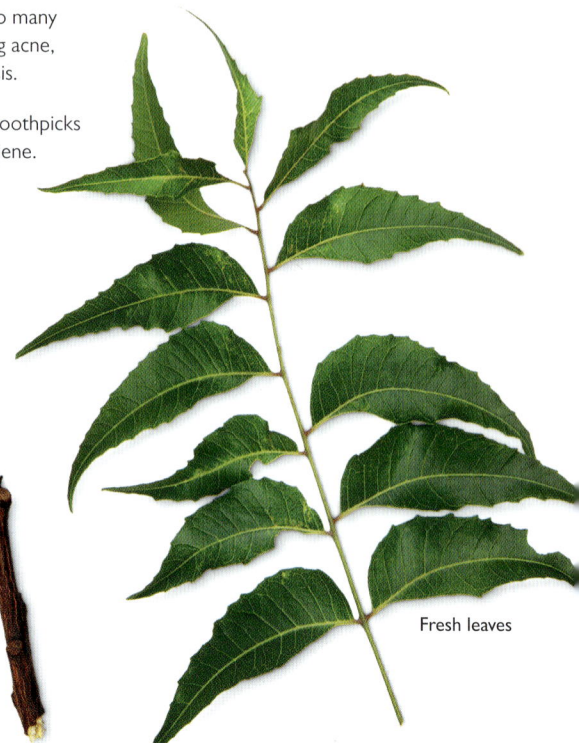

Fresh leaves

Twig

Seeds contain neem oil, which can be expressed and used to treat head lice in adults and children.

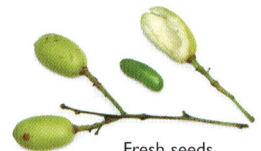

Fresh seeds

Key preparations & their uses

Oil from the seeds is used to prevent and treat infestations of head lice. Apply daily to the scalp.

Cream (to make, p. 306) is used to treat many skin disorders, including eczema. Apply as required.

Tincture (to make, p. 302) is bitter and can be used to treat fevers.

Infusion of the leaves (to make, p. 301) can be used for conjunctivitis.

Decoction of the bark (to make, p. 301) is strongly bitter and astringent.

Cautions Do not take during pregnancy, while breastfeeding, or during fertility treatment. In children, use topically only. Long term high-dose treatment is not advisable.

Barosma betulina syn. *Agathosma betulina* (Rutaceae)

Buchu

A traditional South African remedy, buchu is taken as a stimulant, a diuretic, and to relieve digestive complaints. In Western herbal medicine, it is valued as a urinary antiseptic and diuretic, and is used specifically to treat cystitis and other infections of the urinary tract. Buchu has a strongly distinctive aroma and taste, reminiscent of black currant but described by some as a mixture between rosemary and peppermint.

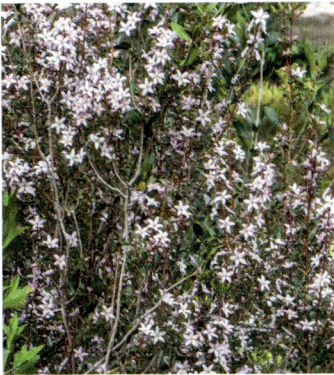

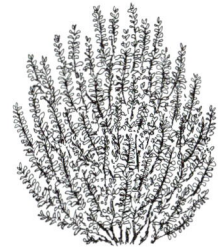

A bushy shrub growing to 6½ ft (2 m), with stemless, slightly leathery leaves dotted with oil glands.

Buchu is grown commercially and used to enhance the black-currant flavor of cassis.

Habitat & cultivation

Buchu is native to South Africa, where is it widely cultivated on hillsides. It is also grown in parts of South America. The herb is grown from cuttings in late summer and requires well-drained soil and plenty of sun. The leaves are harvested when the plant is flowering or fruiting in summer.

Related species

Two closely related species, *B. crenulata* and *B. serratifolia*, are used in a similar way to buchu, but contain less volatile oil and are not so effective.

Key constituents

• Volatile oil (1.5–2.5%), including pulegone, menthone, diosphenol
• Sulfur compounds • Flavonoids (diosmin, rutin) • Mucilage

Key actions

• Urinary antiseptic • Diuretic
• Stimulant • Uterine stimulant

Traditional & current uses

Traditional remedy Buchu is a traditional remedy of the Khoisan people of South Africa. It is used as a general stimulant and a diuretic. Strongly aromatic, it is taken as a carminative, helping to relieve gas and bloating.

Early Western uses The herb was first exported to Britain in 1790 and became an official medicine in 1821, being listed in the *British Pharmacopoeia* as an effective remedy for "cystitis, urethritis, nephritis, and catarrh of the bladder."

Modern urinary treatment Broadly speaking, buchu is used today in Western herbal medicine for the same type of urinary complaints as in the 19th century. It is commonly prescribed for urinary tract infections, often proving effective in curing acute cystitis when combined with other herbs such as corn silk (*Zea mays*, p. 158) and juniper (*Juniperus communis*, p. 229). Taken regularly, it can help prevent recurrent attacks of chronic cystitis or urethritis. It is also taken for prostatitis and irritable bladder, often in combination with herbs such as uva-ursi (*Arctostaphylos uva-ursi*, p. 174) and corn silk. The key active constituent diosphenol has a diuretic action, and may partly account for the herb's antiseptic effect on the urinary system.

Gynecological uses Buchu infusion or tincture is useful in treatments for cystitis and urethritis, especially when they are related to a preexisting *Candida* problem, such as yeast infections. The infusion is generally preferable to the tincture, particularly when onset of infection is sudden. The infusion is also used as a douche for leukorrhea (white vaginal discharge), and occasionally for yeast infections. The herb is a uterine stimulant and contains pulegone, which is also present in large quantities in pennyroyal (*Mentha pulegium*, p. 241). Pulegone is an abortifacient and a powerful emmenagogue (stimulates menstrual flow). Buchu should not, therefore, be taken during pregnancy.

Parts used

Leaves are harvested in summer and used in preparations for urinary infections.

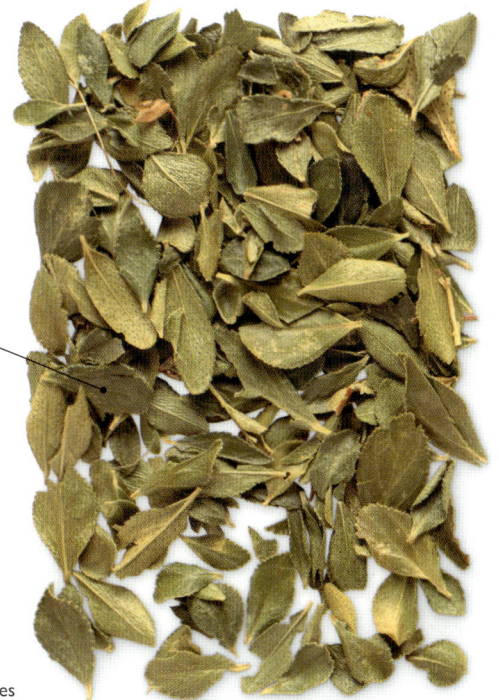

Leaves contain volatile oil, which is antiseptic

Dried leaves

Key preparations & their uses

Infusion (to make, p. 301). For prostatitis, drink ¾ cup (150 ml) twice a day.

Tincture (to make, p. 302). For chronic urinary infections, take 40 drops with water 3 times a day.

Capsules (to make, p. 302). For cystitis, take a 500 mg capsule twice daily.

Cautions During pregnancy take only on advice of your health care practitioner. Potentially toxic at excessive dosage.

Self-help use

• Urinary infections, p. 324.

Bupleurum chinense syn. *B. scorzonerifolium* (Apiaceae)

Bupleurum, Hare's ear root, *Chai hu* (Chinese)

First mentioned in texts from the 1st century BCE, bupleurum is one of China's "harmony" herbs, balancing different organs and energies within the body. It is used as a tonic, strengthening the action of the digestive tract, improving liver function, and helping to push blood to the surface of the body. Recent research in Japan has endorsed traditional use, showing that bupleurum protects the liver.

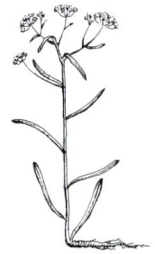

A perennial growing to 3 ft (1 m) high, with sickle-shaped leaves and clusters of small yellow flowers.

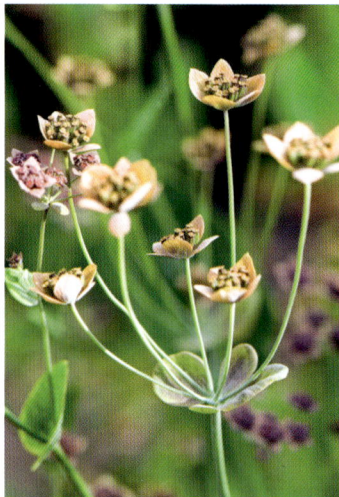

Bupleurum is commonly on sale in medicinal herb shops in China. It is widely taken as a liver tonic.

Habitat & cultivation

Bupleurum grows in China and is cultivated throughout the central and eastern parts of that country. It is also found in other parts of Asia and in Europe. Bupleurum is propagated from seed in spring or by root division in the fall and requires well-drained soil and plenty of sun. The root is unearthed in spring and fall.

Key constituents

• Triterpenoid saponins—saikosides (saikosaponins) • Flavonoids
• Polysaccharides

Key actions

• Protects liver • Anti-inflammatory
• Tonic • Induces sweating

Research

Saikosides Research in Japan from the 1960s onward into the *Bupleurum* genus has revealed that the saikosides are potent medicines. They appear to protect the liver from toxicity, and strengthen liver function, even in people with immune system disorders. Following this discovery, clinical trials during the 1980s in Japan showed that the root is effective in the treatment of hepatitis and other chronic liver problems. Saikosides also have antitumor activity.

Anti-inflammatory The saikosides stimulate the body's production of corticosteroids as well as increasing their anti-inflammatory effect.

Traditional & current uses

Ancient Chinese remedy
Bupleurum has been taken in China for over 2,000 years as a liver tonic. It is traditionally believed to strengthen liver *qi* and to have a tonic action on the spleen and stomach. In Chinese medicine, bupleurum is used to treat "disharmony" between the liver and the spleen, a condition that manifests itself in problems of the digestive system such as abdominal pain, bloating, nausea, and indigestion.

Liver problems In common with milk thistle (*Carduus marianus*, p. 141) and members of the *Glycyrrhiza* genus, for example licorice (*G. glabra*, p. 105), bupleurum is an excellent remedy for a poorly functioning or compromised liver. Its anti-inflammatory action may contribute to its overall use in the treatment of liver disease.

Fever In China, bupleurum is taken to treat fevers, flu, and colds, especially where accompanied by a bitter taste in the mouth, irritability, and either vomiting and abdominal pain, or dizziness and vertigo.

Modern Japanese remedy
The traditional uses of bupleurum and scientific research accord so well that many Japanese doctors practicing conventional Western medicine now use extracts of bupleurum root to treat patients with liver problems.

Other uses Bupleurum is sometimes useful in the treatment of hemorrhoids, and of prolapsed tissue in the pelvis, such as a prolapse of the uterus.

Parts used

Root is harvested in spring and fall, when it contains the most nutrients. It is used to make a valuable liver tonic.

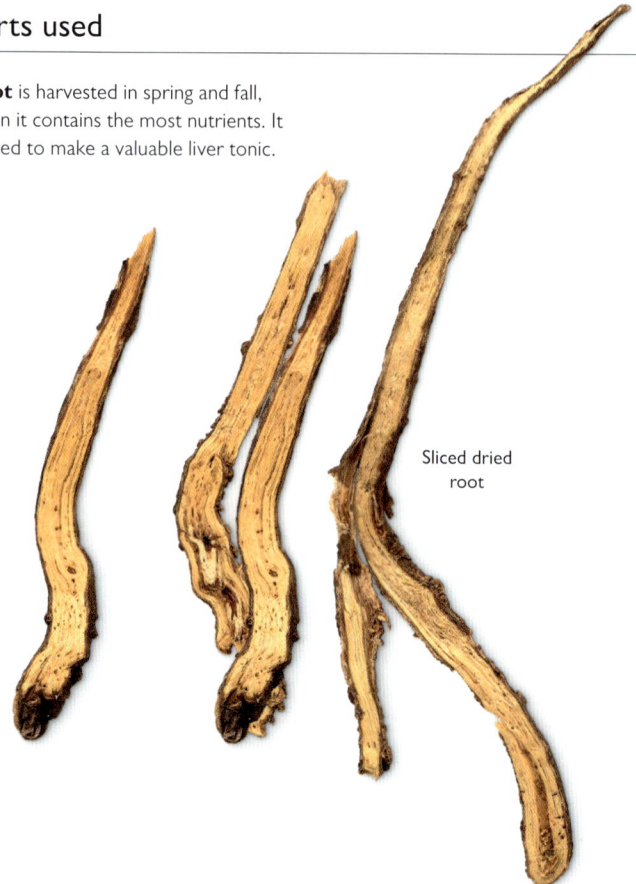

Sliced dried root

Key preparations & their uses

Decoction (to make, p. 301). To stimulate sweating and so reduce fever, drink ¾ cup (150 ml) 3 times a day.

Remedy To improve liver function, decoct 15 g bupleurum, 5 g licorice, and 3 cups (750 ml) water (*see* p. 301). Take in 3 doses during a 24-hour period.

Cautions Do not exceed the dose. Can occasionally cause nausea or vomiting.

Calendula officinalis (Asteraceae)

Calendula, Pot marigold, English marigold

Calendula is one of the most well-known and versatile herbs in Western herbal medicine. The bright orange petals are an excellent remedy for inflamed and angry skin; their antiseptic and healing properties help prevent the spread of infection and speed up the rate of repair. Calendula is also a cleansing and detoxifying herb, and the infusion and tincture are used to treat chronic infections.

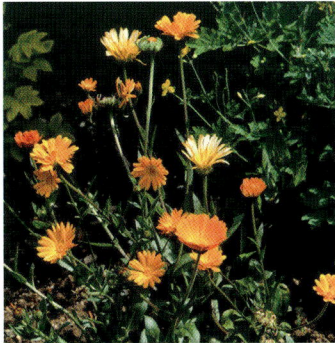

An annual growing to 2 ft (60 cm), with vivid orange flower heads similar in structure to daisies.

Calendula's colorful flowers were thought to lift the spirits and encourage cheerfulness.

Habitat & cultivation

Calendula, native to southern Europe, is cultivated in temperate regions around the world. Easily propagated from seed, it flourishes in almost all soils. The flowers are harvested as they open in early summer, and are dried in the shade.

Related species

C. arvensis, a wild species, seems to have similar therapeutic properties to calendula.

Key constituents

• Triterpenes • Resins • Bitter glycosides • Volatile oil • Phytosterols • Flavonoids • Mucilage • Carotenes

Key actions

• Anti-inflammatory • Relieves muscle spasms • Astringent • Prevents hemorrhaging • Heals wounds • Antimicrobial • Detoxifying • Mildly estrogenic

Traditional & current uses

Therapeutic properties Calendula is antiseptic. Some constituents are antifungal (particularly the resins), antibacterial, and antiviral, and have shown significant activity against *Candida albicans*. The herb also astringes the capillaries, an action that explains its effectiveness for cuts, wounds, varicose veins, and various inflammatory conditions.

Skin remedy Calendula is above all a remedy for the skin, providing effective treatment for most minor skin problems. It is used for cuts, scrapes, and wounds; for red and inflamed skin, including minor burns and sunburn; for acne and many rashes; and for fungal conditions such as ringworm, athlete's foot, and thrush. It is very helpful for diaper rash and cradle cap, and soothes nipples that are sore from breastfeeding.

Digestive disorders Taken internally, calendula infusion or tincture helps inflammatory problems of the digestive system such as gastritis, peptic ulcers, regional ileitis, and colitis.

Detoxifying Calendula has long been known as an anti-inflammatory and detoxifying herb, helping to cleanse the toxicity that underlies many chronic health conditions. Laboratory studies suggest that the herb's traditional use as a background treatment in cancer, notably breast cancer, is likely to be justified. Other conditions such as inflammatory bowel disease and psoriasis may also benefit from the herb.

Gynecological uses Calendula has a mild estrogenic action and is often used to help reduce pain during menstruation and to regulate menstrual bleeding. The infusion makes an effective douche for yeast infections.

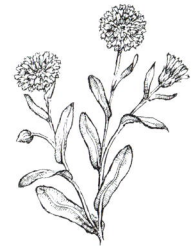

Parts used

Flowers are harvested in summer. Flower heads and petals are removed for use in a wide range of preparations.

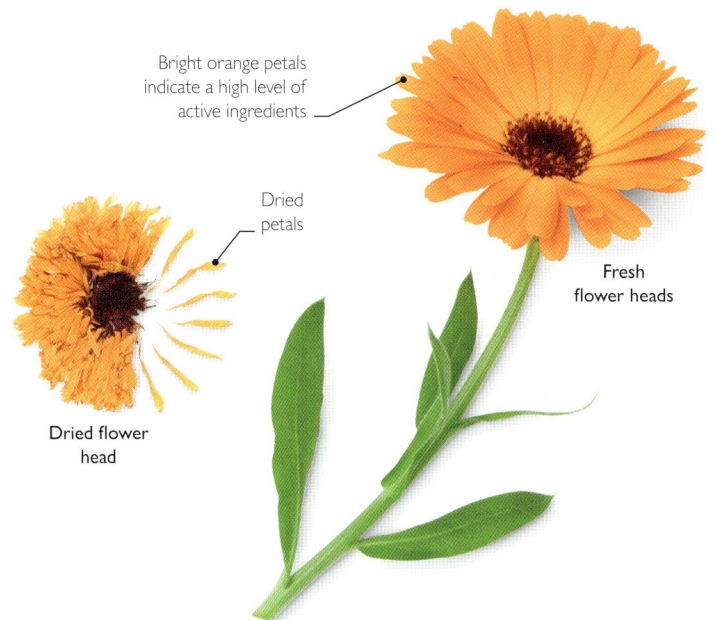

Bright orange petals indicate a high level of active ingredients

Dried petals

Dried flower head

Fresh flower heads

Key preparations & their uses

Infusion (to make, p. 301). For chronic fungal infections, such as ringworm or thrush, drink ¾ cup (150 ml) 3 times a day.

Cream is easy to make (see p. 306). Apply to cuts and grazes.

Ointment (to make, p. 305). For minor burns, apply up to 3 times a day.

Infused oil (to make, p. 304). For inflamed dry skin, rub into the area 2–3 times a day.

Tincture (to make, p. 302). For eczema, take 30 drops with water 3 times a day.

Caution May cause allergic reaction in rare cases.

Self-help uses

• Acne & boils, p. 315. • Athlete's foot, p. 314. • Bites & stings, p. 313. • Breast tenderness & sore nipples, p. 325.
• Digestive infections, p. 315.
• Inflamed skin rashes, p. 313.
• Diaper rash, p. 328. • Hives, p. 313.
• Varicose veins, p. 312. • Wounds & bruises, p. 314.

Cannabis sativa (Cannabaceae)

Marijuana

First records of marijuana use date back to 800 BCE in India, where it was used to clear catarrh. Famously, Queen Victoria took marijuana as an analgesic—it was the standard remedy in the 19th century for menstrual pain and cramps. With ever-increasing research confirming marijuana's medicinal benefits, the herb is now a legal drug in some countries, and cannabidiol (CBD) extracts, which help relieve pain and anxiety and promote better sleep, are commonly available over the counter.

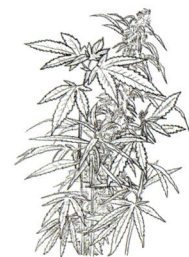

A rough, slightly hairy, upright annual with distinctive palmate leaves, growing to 13 ft (4 m).

Habitat and cultivation

Native to the Caucasus, China, northern India, and Iran, marijuana is cultivated the world over for fiber and seeds, as a pain-relieving medicine, and as a recreational drug. It can be readily grown from seed.

Key constituents

- Phytocannabinoids (over 100)
- tetrahydrocannabinol (THC), cannabidiol (CBD) • Flavonoids
- Alkaloids • Volatile oil

Key actions

- Analgesic • Sedative
- Anti-inflammatory • Antiemetic

Research

Pain relief Marijuana's ability to relieve pain is not in doubt. A 2015 article in the Journal of the American Medical Association found a "30% or greater improvement in pain with cannabinoid compared to placebo."

Substance abuse The availability of medical grade marijuana appears to be correlated with a reduction in substance abuse. One study found a 15–35% reduction in substance abuse admissions to hospital after legalization of marijuana. In particular, this suggests that addiction to other painkillers, such as the opioids codeine and morphine, might be reduced by marijuana.

Cancer research Several laboratory studies indicate that a combined THC and CBD extract might reduce brain tumor cell growth. A small 2021 UK clinical study found that a THC/CBD extract extended the survival time of patients with brain cancer receiving chemotherapy. At the time of writing, a larger trial is underway at 15 hospitals across the UK.

Traditional & current uses

Pain relief With its long history of use, marijuana has, at one time or another, been recommended for almost every illness. As an analgesic, the flowering tops (and CBD extracts) relieve pain with minimal side-effects, proving potentially helpful in pain of all types, from asthma and menstrual cramps to pain associated with cancer and chemotherapy.

Muscle & nerve relaxant Its relaxant properties make it a valuable medicine in multiple sclerosis and cerebral palsy. Marijuana lowers raised blood pressure and can provide effective treatment for glaucoma.

Constipation Marijuana seeds are used in Chinese medicine as a strong but safe laxative, particularly for constipation in the elderly.

Marijuana is a graceful, upright, annual growing to 13 ft (4 m), with fine, serrated, segmented leaves, and flowers on both male and female plants.

Parts used

Flowering tops—extracts are taken to relieve pain and to treat some cancers.

CBD oil is extracted from the flowers and whole plant.

Seeds are used in traditional Chinese medicine as a laxative.

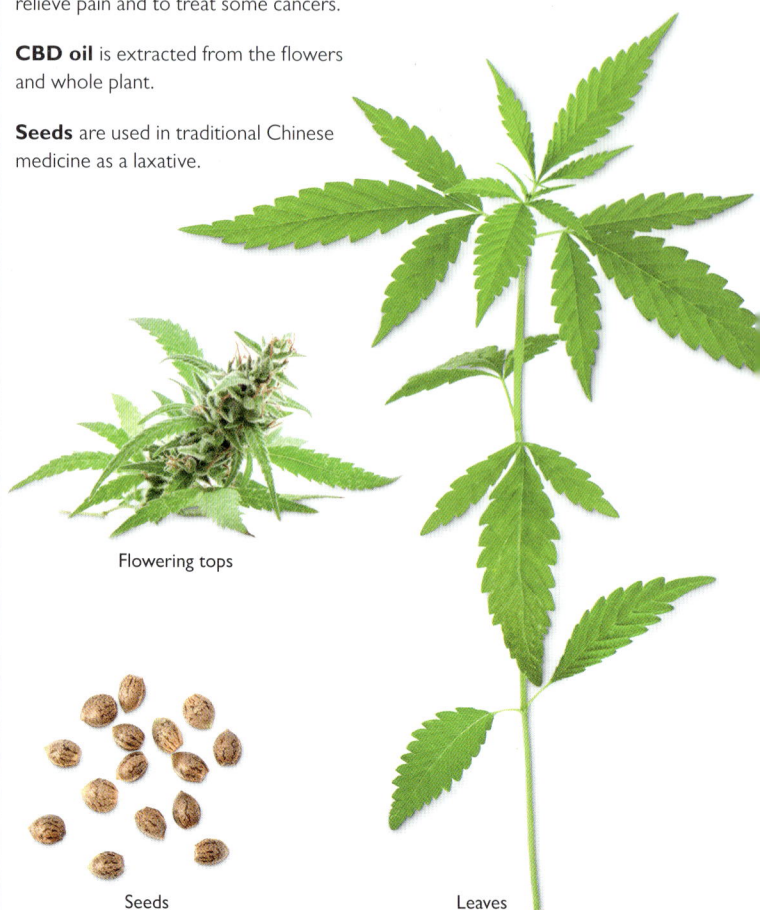

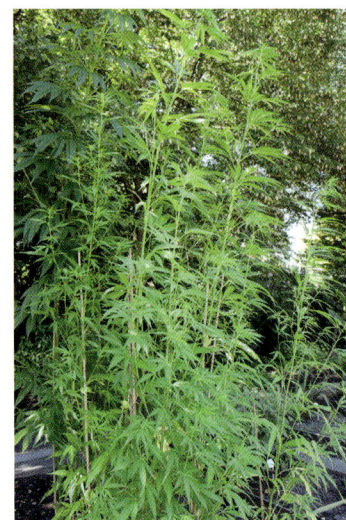

Flowering tops

Seeds

Leaves

Key preparations & their uses

Leaf extracts Take as recommended for health problems such as asthma and multiple sclerosis.

CBD oil Take as recommended for pain relief and to aid sleep.

Seeds Take 1–3 tsp with food or water to aid constipation.

Cautions It is illegal to grow or possess cannabis in any form under federal law in the US. However, individual states permit various uses, including medical, industrial, and recreational. The long-term effects of THC are unknown, but have been associated with impaired mental health.

Capsicum annuum & C. frutescens (Solanaceae)

Cayenne, Cayenne pepper, Chile, Chili

Originally from the tropical regions of the Americas, cayenne was first introduced to Europe in the 16th century. In cooking, it is renowned for its hot, burning taste, and it is not surprising to learn that, medicinally, it is a powerful warming stimulant. It acts on the circulation and digestion and is used to treat a wide range of complaints from arthritis and chilblains to colic and diarrhea.

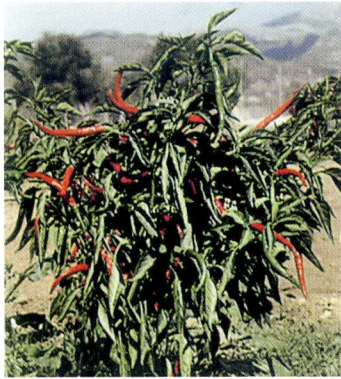

A perennial, spiky shrub growing to 3 ft (1 m), with scarlet-red conical fruits filled with white seeds.

Cayenne is so popular in Mexico where it originates that it is even used to flavor ice cream.

Habitat & cultivation

Chile is native to the tropical Americas, and is now cultivated throughout the tropics, especially in Africa and India. It is grown from seed in early spring and flourishes in hot, moist conditions. The fruit is harvested when ripe in summer and is dried in the shade.

Related species

Many closely related species and varieties of *C. frutescens* exist, all with different grades of pungency. Paprika, or Hungarian pepper (one of the mildest peppers), and the large green and red peppers that are eaten as vegetables are both varieties of *C. annuum* and are important medicinal foods.

Key constituents

- Capsaicin (0.1–1.5%) • Carotenoids
- Flavonoids • Volatile oil • Steroidal saponins (capsicidins—in seeds only)

Key actions

- Stimulant • Tonic • Carminative
- Relieves muscle spasms • Antiseptic

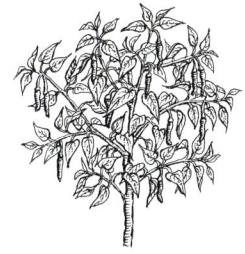

- Increases sweating • Increases blood flow to the skin • Analgesic

Research

Capsaicin Extensive clinical research shows that capsaicin, the compound in cayenne mostly responsible for its hot, pungent taste, has strong, local analgesic activity in certain types of nerve pain. Applied to the skin, capsaicin desensitizes nerve endings and acts as a counterirritant. It is standardly prescribed for relief of neuralgic pain. It may also provide effective pain relief in conditions such as arthritis and headache.

Traditional & current uses

Warming stimulant The herb's heating qualities make it a valuable remedy for poor circulation. It improves blood flow to the hands and feet and to the central organs.

Antimicrobial In Mayan herbal medicine, cayenne was used to counter microbial infections— different *Capsicum* species including cayenne are now known to have significant antimicrobial activity. Adding cayenne to food reduces the chances of developing gastric or intestinal infection, and the herb is frequently used by herbalists to treat gastroenteritis and dysentery.

External uses Applied locally to the skin, chile is mildly analgesic. It is also rubefacient, increasing blood flow to the affected part, and this helps to stimulate the circulation in "cold" rheumatic and arthritic conditions, aiding the removal of waste products and increasing the flow of nutrients to the tissues. Chile may also be applied to unbroken chilblains.

Internal uses Chile is taken to relieve gas and colic and to stimulate

Parts used

Fruit improves digestion and circulation.

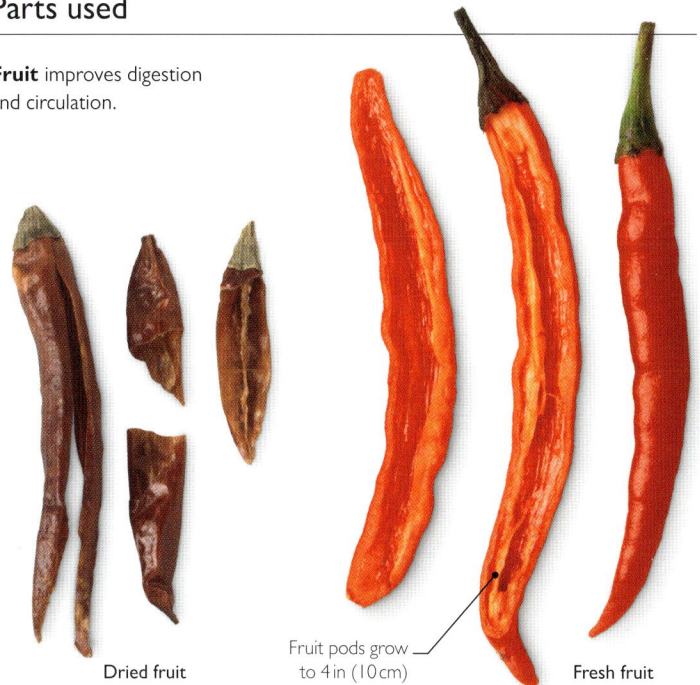

Fruit pods grow to 4 in (10 cm)

Dried fruit

Fresh fruit

Key preparations & their uses

Powder For sore throats, add a pinch to 5 tsp lemon juice. Dilute with hot water, add honey, and use as a gargle.

Infused oil Add 100 g chopped cayenne to 2 cups (500 ml) oil and simmer (*see* p. 304). Gently massage into rheumatic limbs.

Tincture (to make, p. 302). For arthritis, combine 20 drops with ½ cup (100 ml) willow bark tincture. Take 1 tsp with

water twice a day.

Tablets are convenient for long-term use. Take for poor circulation.

Ointment (to make, p. 305). Apply to chilblains (only if the skin is unbroken).

Cautions Nontoxic at normal doses, although caution is required when eating or handling cayenne. Can cause intense pain and burning, and contact dermatitis.

digestive juices. It may be taken in frequent, small doses for a weak heart. A pinch of chile can be used in gargles for sore throats. Chile is also helpful in relieving acute diarrhea.

Self-help uses

- High fever, p. 321.
- Poor circulation, p. 312.

Cassia senna syn. *Senna alexandrina* (Fabaceae)

Senna, Alexandrian senna

Almost everyone will have taken a preparation containing senna at some time in their lives. Senna is probably one of the best known herbal medicines, not least because it is still widely used in conventional medicine. It is a very efficient laxative and is a particularly useful remedy for the occasional bout of constipation. It has a slightly bitter, nauseating taste, and is therefore generally mixed with other herbs.

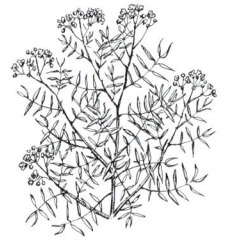

A small perennial shrub growing to 3 ft (1 m), with a straight, woody stem and yellow flowers.

Habitat & cultivation

Senna is native to tropical Africa and is now cultivated throughout that continent. It is grown from seed in spring or from cuttings in early summer and requires plenty of sun. The leaves may be picked before or while the plant is in flower, and the pods are collected when they are ripe in the fall.

Related species

There are over 400 species of *Cassia*. Tinnevelly senna (*C. angustifolia*) is grown in the Indian subcontinent and has the same therapeutic properties as *C. senna*. In Ayurvedic medicine, it is used for skin problems, jaundice, bronchitis, and anemia, as well as for constipation. *Jue ming zi* (*C. obtusifolia*) is used in traditional Chinese medicine for "liver fire" patterns, constipation, and atherosclerosis.

Key constituents

• Anthraquinone glycosides (sennosides) • Naphthalene glycosides • Mucilage • Flavonoids • Volatile oil

Key actions

• Stimulant • Laxative • Cathartic

Research

Sennosides Extensive research during the last 50 years has led to a clear understanding of senna's action. The sennosides irritate the lining of the large intestine, causing the muscles to contract strongly, resulting in a bowel movement about 10 hours after the dose is taken. The sennosides also stop fluid being absorbed from the large intestine, helping to keep the stool soft.

Traditional & current uses

Early records The herb was first used medicinally by Arabian physicians in the 9th century CE.

Constipation Senna has always been specifically used for constipation. It is particularly appropriate when a soft stool is required, for example in cases of anal fissure. Senna is a good short-term laxative but should not be taken for more than 10 days as this leads to weakening of the large intestine muscles.

Cathartic As a cathartic (very strong laxative), senna can cause cramping and colic, and is therefore normally taken with aromatic, carminative herbs that relax the intestinal muscles.

Self-help use

• Constipation, p. 317.

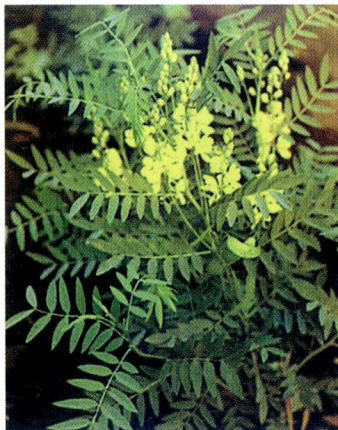

Senna shrubs have pairs of lance-shaped leaflets arranged either side of a central stem.

Parts used

Leaves are stronger in action than the pods and are not as commonly used.

Pods are milder in effect than the leaves. They are made into tablets and other preparations.

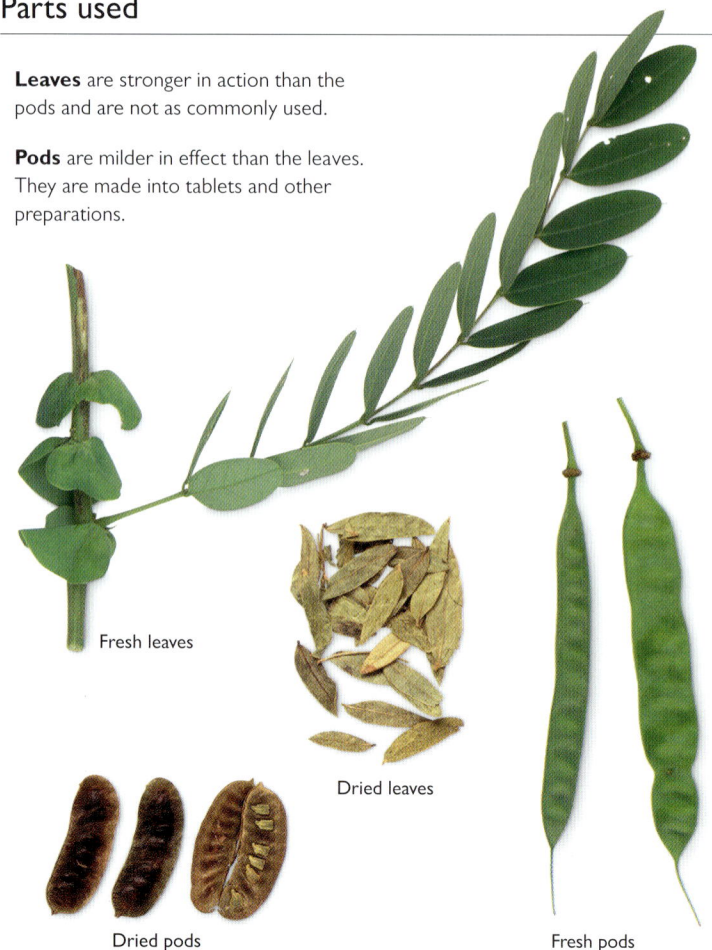

Fresh leaves

Dried leaves

Dried pods

Fresh pods

Key preparations & their uses

Tablets are the standard senna preparation and are convenient. Take for occasional constipation.

Decoction For constipation, steep 3–6 senna pods and 1 g fresh ginger in ¾ cup (150 ml) freshly boiled water for 6–12 hours. Strain and drink.

Infusion For mild constipation, infuse 1–2 senna pods, 1 g fresh ginger, and 1–2 cloves in ¾ cup (150 ml) freshly boiled water for 15 minutes. Strain.

Tincture is prescribed by herbalists to treat short-term constipation.

Cautions Do not give to children under 12. Do not take for more than 10 days at a time. Do not take if suffering from colitis. During pregnancy, take on advice of your health care practitioner.

Centella asiatica syn. *Hydrocotyle asiatica* (Apiaceae)

Gotu kola (Hindi), Indian pennywort

Gotu kola is an ancient Ayurvedic remedy that is now used extensively in the West. It is a useful tonic and cleansing herb for skin problems and digestive disorders. In India, it is used to treat a variety of conditions, including leprosy, but it is valued chiefly as a revitalizing herb that strengthens nervous function and memory. It has a bittersweet, acrid taste, and in India it is sometimes used in salads and as a vegetable.

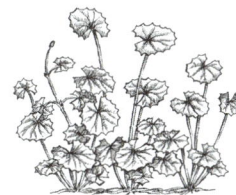

A perennial, herbaceous creeper, growing to 20 in (50 cm), with fan-shaped leaves.

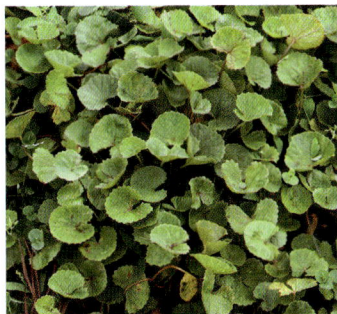

Gotu kola is found growing wild throughout India.

Habitat & cultivation

Gotu kola is native to India and the southern US. It also grows in tropical and subtropical parts of Australia, southern Africa, and South America. It prefers marshy areas and riverbanks. Though usually gathered wild, *gotu kola* can be cultivated from seed in spring. The aerial parts are harvested throughout the year.

Related species

Marsh pennywort (*Hydrocotyle vulgaris*) is a related European species, but, unlike *gotu kola*, has no known therapeutic uses.

Key constituents

• Triterpenoid saponins (asiaticoside, brahmoside, thankuniside) • Alkaloids (hydrocotyline) • Bitter principles (vellarin)

Key actions

• Wound healer • Tonic
• Anti-inflammatory • Sedative
• Peripheral vasodilator

Research

Wound healing *Gotu kola* has an established ability to promote wound healing and tissue repair, making it useful as a cosmetic agent, in skin disorders such as psoriasis, and in arthritis. Asiaticoside, in particular, has been shown to speed up collagen formation and the laying down of new blood vessels. This healing effect extends to the blood vessels, so that *gotu kola* extracts aid venous repair, notably in chronic venous insufficiency, a condition that includes symptoms such as leg swelling and varicose veins. Recent US research has investigated the effectiveness of high-strength extracts to help in diabetic neuropathy (nerve pain due to poor circulation) with signs of positive benefit.

Brain function Over the last 15 years, research has focused on gotu kola's ability to relieve anxiety and act as a brain tonic, enhancing memory and central nervous system brain function. A Thai clinical trial in 2008 found that *gotu kola* extract improved attention, working memory, alertness, and mood in 28 healthy volunteers with an average age of 65.

Traditional & current uses

Wound healing *Gotu kola's* main traditional use lies in treating wounds and skin problems. In Ayurveda, it is used specifically to promote healing in skin ulcers and serious skin problems, as well as to prevent scarring. The herb may be applied directly to the skin, or taken internally, where it appears to promote tissue repair throughout the body. It supports peripheral circulation and can be taken to strengthen blood vessels, e.g. varicose veins. Many people swear by *gotu kola's* ability to prevent and relieve arthritis and rheumatic problems.

Tonic The herb has a longstanding reputation in India and southern Asia as a "rejuvenator," aiding concentration and memory, particularly in the elderly. In Western herbal medicine, it is understood to be an adaptogen and can be taken long-term to help support healthy brain function, slow aging, and calm anxiety. It is also thought to have a tonic effect on digestion.

Parts used

Aerial parts have valuable tonic and cleansing properties.

In India, fresh leaves are eaten as a tonic herb in salads

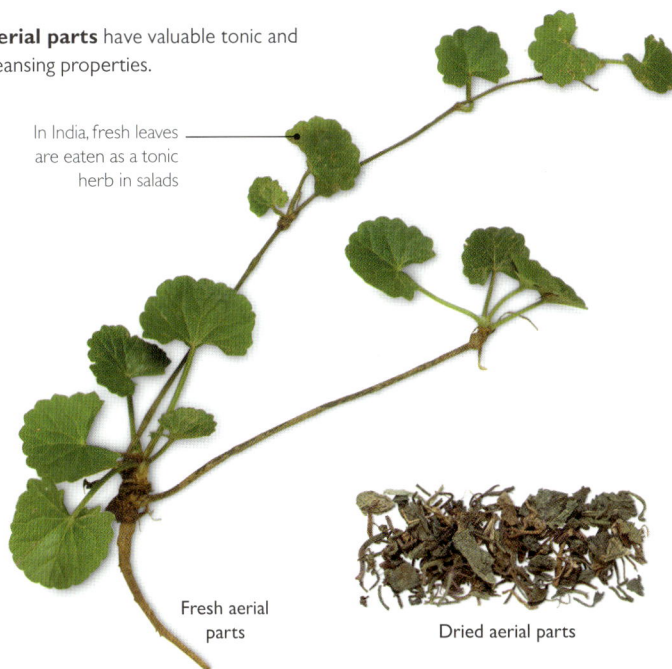

Fresh aerial parts

Dried aerial parts

Key preparations & their uses

Powder is an important Ayurvedic remedy. Take 1–2 g a day with water as a general tonic.

Paste made from powder. Mix 2 tsp powder with 5 tsp (25 ml) water and apply to patches of eczema.

Infusion (to make, p. 301). For rheumatism, take 7 tsp twice a day.

Tincture (to make, p. 302). For poor memory and concentration, take 40 drops with water 3 times a day.

Cautions Can occasionally cause sensitivity to sunlight. Restricted herb in some countries. May cause allergic reactions in rare cases.

Self-help uses

• Eczema, p. 310.
• Maintaining vitality, p. 319.

Chamomilla recutita syn. *Matricaria recutita* (Asteraceae)

German chamomile

German chamomile's aromatic, slightly bitter taste, reminiscent of apples, is familiar to herbal tea drinkers. The herb's varied medicinal uses, however, are not as well known. It is an excellent herb for many digestive disorders and for nervous tension and irritability. Externally, it is used for sore skin and eczema. Roman chamomile (*Chamaemelum nobile*, p. 190) is a close relation, used in a similar way.

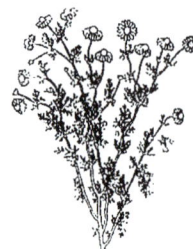

A sweetly aromatic annual growing to 2 ft (60 cm), with finely cut leaves and white flower heads.

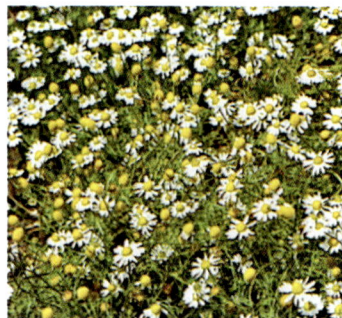

German chamomile is a useful herb to cultivate for home use.

Habitat & cultivation

German chamomile grows in much of Europe and other temperate regions. The seeds are sown in spring or fall and the flower heads are picked in full bloom, in summer.

Key constituents

• Volatile oil (proazulenes, farnesine, alpha-bisabolol, spiroether)
• Flavonoids • Bitter glycosides (anthemic acid) • Coumarins

Key actions

• Anti-inflammatory • Anti-allergenic
• Antispasmodic • Relaxant
• Carminative

Research

Candidiasis A 2021 clinical trial investigating the use of chamomile cream in vaginal candidiasis found that in 89% of cases, women using the chamomile cream recovered after 2 weeks treatment.

Premenstrual syndrome An Iranian clinical trial compared chamomile with mefenamic acid for relief of premenstrual syndrome symptoms. Both were found effective in relieving the physical symptoms of premenstrual syndrome, but chamomile proved better in relieving emotional symptoms.

Other research Clinical studies have shown that chamomile cream strongly promotes wound healing and tissue repair. A 1993 trial using chamomile and four other herbs showed them to be highly effective in easing infantile colic.

Traditional & current uses

Digestive problems Chamomile has been taken for digestive problems since at least the 1st century CE. Gentle and efficacious, it is suitable for children. The herb is valuable for pain, indigestion, acidity, gastritis, gas, bloating, and colic. It is also used for hiatal hernia, peptic ulcer, Crohn's disease, and irritable bowel syndrome.

Relaxation Chamomile, which contains spiroether, a strong antispasmodic, eases tense muscles and period pain. Women in ancient Rome commonly took chamomile to relieve menstrual cramps. The flowers also reduce irritability and promote sleep—especially helpful for children.

Irritation The herb is useful for hay fever and asthma. On steam distillation, the proazulenes produce chamazulene, which is anti-allergenic. Externally, it can be applied to sore, itchy skin, sore nipples, and eczema. It also relieves eyestrain. A poultice can be applied to sore breasts.

Self-help uses

• Bites & stings, p. 313. • Congestion & hay fever, p. 322. • Colic, p. 328.
• Eczema, p. 310. • Indigestion, p. 317.
• Insomnia, p. 319. • Mild asthma, p. 311. • Morning sickness, p. 327. • Sore & tired eyes, p. 320. • Sore nipples, p. 325. • Stomach spasm, p. 315.

Parts used

Flower heads may be used fresh or dried. They should be picked on the day they open, when the active constituents are at their strongest.

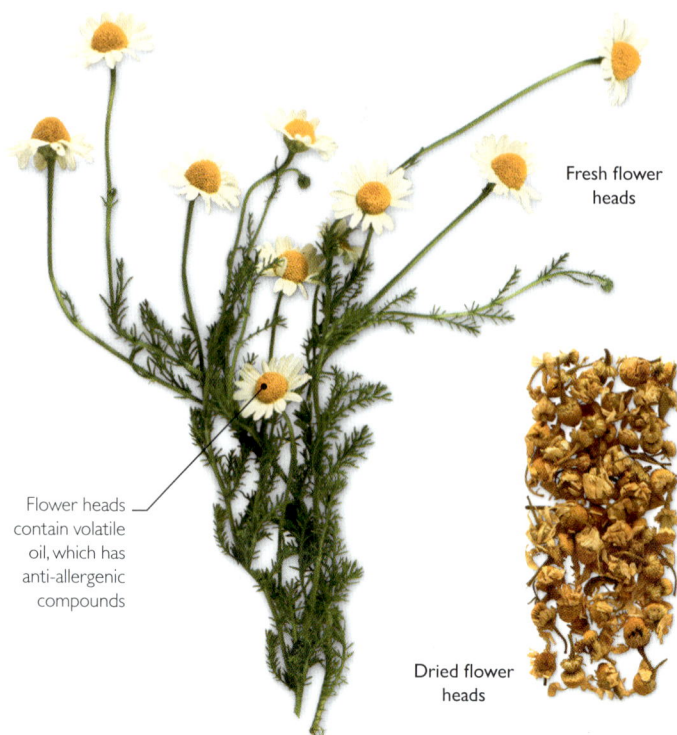

Fresh flower heads

Flower heads contain volatile oil, which has anti-allergenic compounds

Dried flower heads

Key preparations & their uses

Cream (to make, p. 306). Rub onto sore or itchy skin.

Essential oil For diaper rash, combine 5 drops with 1 tbsp carrier oil and apply.

Making infusion with flower heads (see p. 301). For a good night's sleep, drink ¾ cup (150 ml) before bed.

Infusion To relax irritable and overtired children, infuse 4 tsp dried herb in 2 cups (500 ml) water (see p. 301) and strain into a bath.

Ointment (to make, p. 305). Rub onto sore or inflamed skin.

Tincture (to make, p. 302). For irritable bowel syndrome, take 1 tsp diluted with ½ cup (100 ml) water 3 times a day.

Cautions The fresh plant can cause dermatitis. Do not take the essential oil internally except under professional supervision. Take only on professional advice if using blood-thinning medication. Do not use the oil externally during pregnancy.

Chrysanthemum × morifolium (Asteraceae)

Ju hua (Chinese), Florists' chrysanthemum

Ju hua is known in the West as florists' chrysanthemum and is valued for its ornamental qualities. In China, however, it is a popular medicinal herb and it is also commonly drunk as a refreshing tisane. *Ju hua* is used to improve vision and soothe sore eyes, to relieve headaches, and to counter infections such as colds and flu. Furthermore, research has demonstrated that it is a valuable remedy for high blood pressure.

A perennial growing to about 5 ft (1.5 m), with flower heads composed of yellow ray florets.

Habitat & cultivation

Ju hua is native to China. Today, it is mostly cultivated, and is propagated from cuttings in spring or early summer. The flower heads are gathered in the fall when fully open. They are usually dried in the sun, which can take a long time.

Related species

Wild chrysanthemum, *ye hu hua* (*C. indicum*), has a similar use in Chinese herbal medicine. Many other closely related species have an established therapeutic value, for example tansy (*Tanacetum vulgare*, p. 284) and feverfew (*T. parthenium*, p. 144).

Key constituents

• Alkaloids, including stachydrine
• Volatile oil • Sesquiterpene lactones
• Flavonoids, including apigenin
• Betaine & choline • Vitamin B$_1$

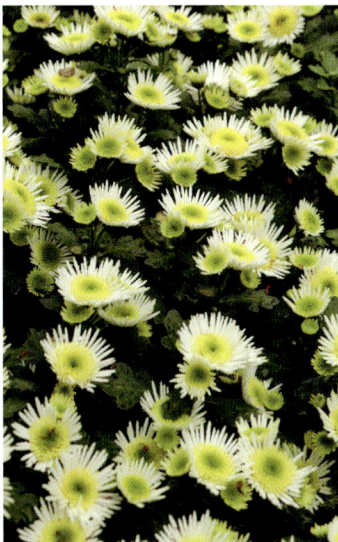

Key actions

• Increases sweating • Antiseptic
• Lowers blood pressure • Cooling
• Reduces fever

Research

Blood pressure A number of Chinese and Japanese clinical trials during the 1970s showed that *ju hua* is most effective at lowering blood pressure and relieving associated symptoms such as headaches, dizziness, and insomnia. In these trials, *ju hua* was mixed with *jin yin hua* (*Lonicera* spp., p. 235).

Other research *Ju hua* has proven to be helpful in the treatment of angina, and to have an antibiotic effect against a range of pathogens. In laboratory studies, some of the flavonoids were found to have anti-HIV activity. Extracts of the flowers reduce inflammation.

Traditional & current uses

Long-standing remedy *Ju hua* has been taken in China as a medicine and as a beverage for thousands of years. It was first categorized in the *Divine Husbandman's Classic (Shen'nong Bencaojing)*, written in the 1st century CE.

Eye problems In China, the infused flower heads are popular as a remedy for red, sore eyes, especially after long periods of close work, such as reading or working at a computer. The warm flower heads are placed on closed eyes and then replaced when cool. *Ju hua* infusion is taken in China as a remedy to improve eyesight.

Cooling & antiseptic *Ju hua* infusion is used to reduce fever, to counter infection, and to detoxify the body. It relieves mild fevers and tension headaches, soothes a dry mouth or throat, and treats bad breath.

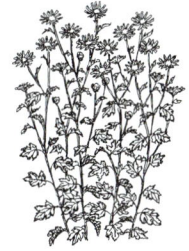

Skin complaints The fresh leaves make an antiseptic poultice for acne, pimples, boils, and sores.

High blood pressure Symptoms often associated with high blood pressure, such as dizziness, headaches, and tinnitus, are treated with *ju hua*.

Ju hua flowers are colorful and have been used medicinally in China since the 1st century CE.

Parts used

Flower heads are gathered in late fall. In China, they are steamed before drying to reduce bitterness.

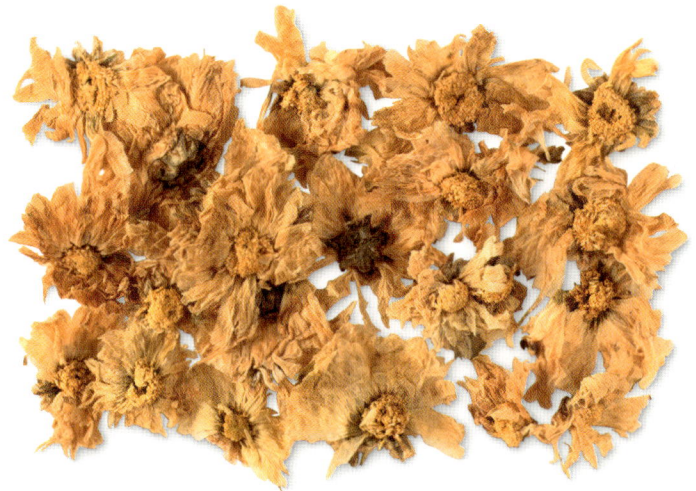

Dried flower heads

Key preparations & their uses

Infusion of flower heads (p. 301). For tension headaches, drink ¾ cup (150 ml) at hourly intervals.

Poultice (to make, p. 305). For eyestrain, steep flower heads in hot water for 10 minutes and place them on closed eyes.

Powdered leaves For acne, mix 1 tsp with 2–3 tsp water and apply to pimples.

Poultice of fresh leaves (to make, p. 305). For boils and pimples, apply directly to the skin.

Caution May cause allergic reactions in rare cases.

Self-help use

• Sore & tired eyes, p. 320.

Cinchona spp. (Rubiaceae)

Cinchona, Peruvian bark, Jesuit bark

Cinchona is best known as the source of quinine, which for centuries was the most widely taken antimalarial remedy in the world. It was first documented in Peru by a Jesuit missionary in 1633. As well as being a remedy for malaria, the herb is also used for fevers and digestive problems. Various *Cinchona* species are used medicinally, including *C. calisaya*, *C. ledgeriana*, and *C. officinalis*.

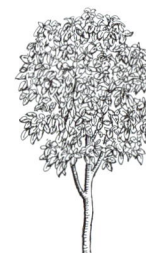

An evergreen tree reaching 80 ft (25 m), with reddish bark and leaves that grow to 20 in (50 cm).

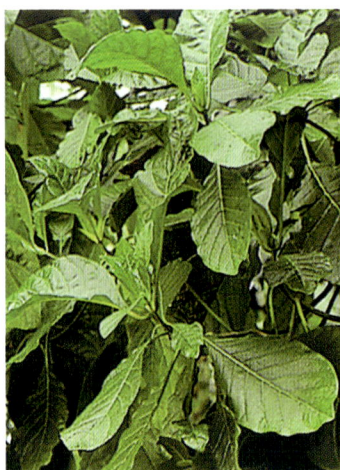

Cinchona bark has a bitter taste, and it, or its constituent quinine, is used to flavor tonic water.

Habitat & cultivation

Native to mountainous tropical regions of South America, especially Peru, cinchona is now also grown in India, Java, and parts of Africa and is cultivated intensively in plantations. The trees are propagated from cuttings in late spring, and the bark of the trunk, branches, and root are removed from 6- to 8-year-old trees, and then dried in the sun. The annual production of cinchona bark has been estimated at about 8,000 tons (8,200 metric tons) a year.

Key constituents

• Alkaloids (up to 15%), mainly quinoline alkaloids (quinine, quinidine) and indole alkaloids (cinchonamine)
• Bitter triterpenic glycosides (quinovin) • Tannins • Quinic acid

Key actions

• Bitter • Reduces fever
• Antimalarial • Tonic • Stimulates

the appetite • Antispasmodic • Astringent • Antibacterial

Research

Pharmacology Cinchona has been thoroughly researched and its pharmacological actions are well established.

Quinine Quinine is both strongly antimalarial and antibacterial. Like the other alkaloids, it is antispasmodic.

Bitter Cinchona contains bitter constituents including alkaloids and quinovin, which produce a reflex stimulation of the digestion as a whole, increasing stomach secretions.

Quinidine Quinidine is a cardiac depressant and is known to reduce heart rate and improve irregularity of heartbeat.

Traditional & current uses

Traditional remedy The Indigenous peoples of Peru have taken cinchona for many centuries, and it is still a well-used remedy for fevers, digestive problems, and infections.

Homeopathic proving Samuel Hahnemann, the founder of homeopathy, prepared the first homeopathic medicine, or proving, from cinchona in about 1790.

Antimalarial Cinchona, and in particular quinine, were the principal remedies for malaria until World War I. From the 1960s, resistance of the malarial parasite to the synthetic drug chloroquine led to quinine's use once again in preventing and treating malaria. Quinine is also used to treat other acute feverish conditions.

Digestive stimulant As a bitter tonic, cinchona stimulates saliva, digestive secretions, and appetite, and improves weak digestive function.

Parts used

Bark of the trunk, branches, and root contains alkaloids, especially quinine. The bark of the trunk is most commonly used medicinally.

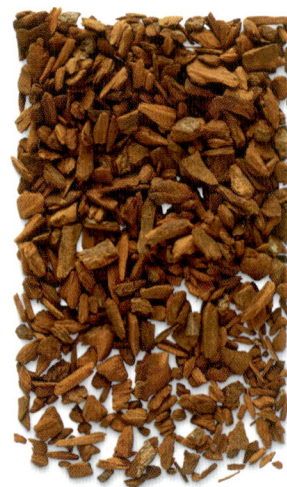

Dried bark

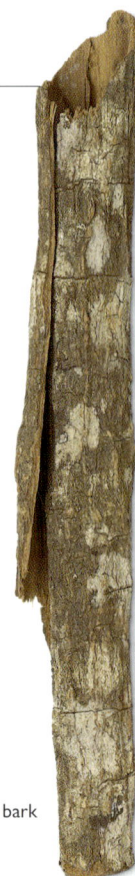

Fresh bark

Key preparations & their uses

Powder is used to treat malaria.

Decoction is a well-known remedy for fevers. It is also used as a gargle for sore throats.

Tincture is strongly bitter and is prescribed to improve digestion.

Cautions Take only under professional supervision. Do not take during pregnancy. Excessive use causes "cinchonism," which in extreme cases leads to coma and death. Restricted in some countries.

Gargle Cinchona is useful as a gargle for sore, infected throats.

Muscle spasms The herb is used in herbal medicine for cramps, especially night cramps. It also relieves arthritis.

Indian remedy In India, cinchona is used for various conditions, including sciatica, dysentery, and problems with *kapha* (see p. 42).

Cinnamomum spp. (Lauraceae)

Cinnamon, *Dalcini* (Hindi), *Rou gui* (Chinese)

One of the world's most important spices, cinnamon is an ancient medicine, first mentioned in the Jewish religious text, the Torah. The bark has a long history of use in India and Southeast Asia, and is thought to have arrived in Egypt around 2000 BCE, reaching Europe around 500 BCE. Traditionally used to treat colds, flu, and digestive problems, cinnamon is now commonly taken to help stabilize blood-sugar levels.

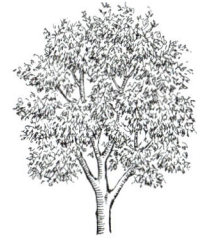

An evergreen tree growing to 26–59 ft (8–18 m), with soft, reddish-brown bark and yellow flowers.

Habitat & cultivation

Cinnamon (*C. zeylanicum*) is native to India and Sri Lanka, growing in tropical forests to an altitude of 1,600 ft (500 m). It is widely cultivated throughout tropical regions, especially in the Philippines and the Caribbean. The tree is propagated from cuttings and every second year, the young trees are cut back to just above ground level. The bark is stripped from the shoots that emerge the following year, and the inner layer is set out to dry in the sun, forming the characteristic quills.

Related species

Several species are used besides "true" cinnamon (*C. zeylanicum* and *C. verum*). Cassia (*C. cassia*), native to China and Japan, is used as a *yang* tonic (see p. 44) in Chinese herbal medicine. Cassia is the most commonly used species in commerce.

Key constituents

• Volatile oil up to 4% (cinnamaldehyde 65–80%, eugenol 5–10%) • Phenolics (procyanidins) • Coumarins (*C. cassia*) • Mucilage

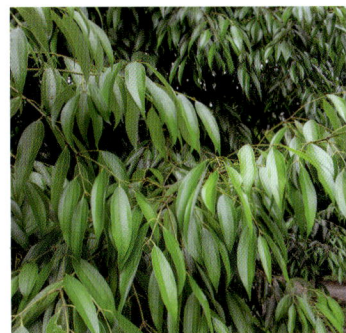

Cinnamon is now widely cultivated as a spice and a medicine, but, traditionally, only bark from wild trees was used medicinally.

Key actions

• Warming stimulant • Carminative
• Antidiabetic • Antimicrobial
• Antifungal

Research

Metabolic syndrome Research suggests the bark helps prevent and treat type 2 (late-onset) diabetes, increasing cells' ability to respond to insulin and aiding the stabilization of blood-sugar levels. It also aids weight loss, reduces high blood pressure, and may slightly lower cholesterol, so could help treat metabolic syndrome.
Other uses Similarities of the phenolic procyanidins to grape seed (*Vitis vinifera*, p. 293) and green tea (*Camellia sinensis*, p. 185) indicates cinnamon is strongly antioxidant and aids healthy circulation. The essential oil is sedative, analgesic, and has marked antimicrobial and antifungal activity. There are hints that cinnamon helps brain health.

Traditional & current uses

Ancient warming remedy
Cinnamon has always been used as a warming herb for "cold" conditions, often in combination with ginger (*Zingiber officinale*, p. 159). The bark stimulates circulation and blood flow to the extremities. It has long been used for flu symptoms, and makes an excellent mouthwash for conditions such as oral thrush.
Convalescence Cinnamon is a gentle acting herb that helps to support both digestion and circulation. It is used specifically in the treatment of debility and in convalescence.
Gynecological remedy It can help relieve period cramps and might have a normalizing effect on menstrual

Parts used

Inner bark is used in preparations and is distilled for essential oil.

Twigs of closely related *C. cassia* are widely used in Chinese medicine to relieve "cold" conditions.

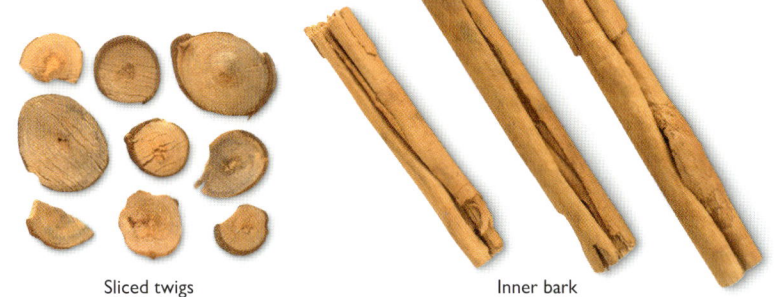

Sliced twigs

Inner bark

Key preparations & their uses

Infusion (to make, p. 301). For colds and flu, drink ½ cup (100 ml) 2–3 times a day.

Essential oil For wasp stings, dab on oil as often as required.

Tincture To make, infuse the herb in alcohol (see p. 302). For flatulence, take

20 drops with water up to 4 times a day.

Powder take up to 3 tsp a day to support stable blood-sugar levels.

Cautions Occasionally causes allergic reaction; excessive doses may cause low blood sugar; do not take essential oil internally.

bleeding—controlling heavy bleeding but stimulating flow where it is light. It is valuable in the treatment of PCOS (polycystic ovary syndrome) as it helps to reduce insulin levels and stabilize estrogen levels.
Insulin resistance It has a distinct role to play in promoting better blood glucose levels and in preventing insulin resistance—the impaired uptake of sugar by cells that is a warning sign of diabetes. One suggestion, as part of a wider regimen for diabetes and

metabolic syndrome, is to take 3 tsp of cinnamon powder a day for 4 months.
Gastrointestinal problems It has always been used as a warming and soothing remedy for digestion, aiding in nausea, indigestion, and flatulence, as well as colic and diarrhea. Its antifungal activity means that it can be of value in gut dysbiosis (disordered gut bacteria).

Self-help use

• Colds, p. 321.

Citrus limon (Rutaceae)

Lemon, *Ning Meng* (Chinese), *Neemboo* (Hindi)

Lemon is one of the most important and versatile natural medicines for home use. A familiar food as well as a remedy, it has a high vitamin C content that helps improve resistance to infection, making it valuable for colds and flu. It is taken as a preventative for many conditions, including stomach infections, circulatory problems, and arteriosclerosis (thickening of the arterial walls).

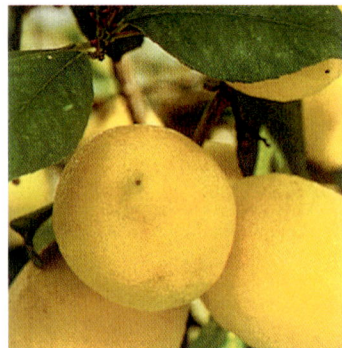

A small, evergreen tree growing to about 23 ft (7 m), with light green, toothed leaves.

Lemons were a remedy for scurvy (caused by lack of vitamin C) long before vitamin C was identified.

Habitat & cultivation

Thought to be native to India, lemon trees were first grown in Europe in the 2nd century CE and are now cultivated in Mediterranean and subtropical climates worldwide. Propagated from seed in spring, they prefer well-drained soil and plenty of sun. The fruit is harvested in winter when the vitamin C content is at its highest.

Key constituents

• Volatile oil (about 2.5% of the peel), limonene (up to 70%), alpha-terpinene, alpha-pinene, beta-pinene, citral • Coumarins
• Flavonoids • Phenolic acids
• Vitamins A, B_1, B_2, B_3, and C (40–50 mg per 100 g of fruit)

Key actions

• Antiseptic • Antirheumatic • Antibacterial • Antioxidant • Reduces fever

Traditional & current uses

Valuable medicine Spanish popular medicine ascribes so many medicinal uses to lemon that whole books have been written about it.

Established properties Despite its acid content, once digested, lemon has an alkaline effect within the body, making it useful in rheumatic conditions where acidity is a contributory factor. The volatile oil is antiseptic and antibacterial. The bioflavonoids are antioxidant and strengthen the inner lining of blood vessels, especially veins and capillaries, and help counter varicose veins and easy bruising.

Preventative Lemon is a valuable preventative medicine. Its antiseptic and cleansing actions make it useful for those prone to arteriosclerosis, and to infections and fevers (especially of the stomach, liver, and intestines). Its ability to strengthen blood vessel walls helps prevent circulatory disorders and bleeding gums. Lemon is also useful as a general tonic for many chronic illnesses. Above all, it is a food that helps maintain general good health.

Strengthening vein walls The whole fruit, especially the pith, treats arteriosclerosis, weak capillaries, and varicose veins.

Juice Lemon juice is good for colds, flu, and chest infections. It stimulates liver detoxification, improves the appetite, and helps ease stomach acidity, ulcers, arthritis, gout, and rheumatism. As a gargle, lemon juice is helpful for sore throats, gingivitis, and mouth ulcers. Externally, lemon juice can be applied directly to acne, athlete's foot, chilblains, insect stings, ringworm, sunburn, and warts.

Self-help uses

• Acne & boils, p. 315. • Arthritis, p. 323. • Bites & stings, p. 313.
• Chilblains, p. 312. • Colds & flu, p. 321. • Cold sores, p. 314. • Sore throats, p. 321. • Weak digestion, p. 316.

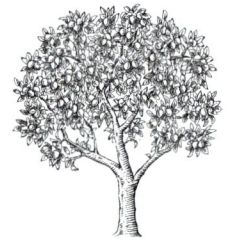

Parts used

Fruit and peel improve the circulation and increase resistance to infection.

Pith and peel contain volatile oil and most of the bioflavonoids.

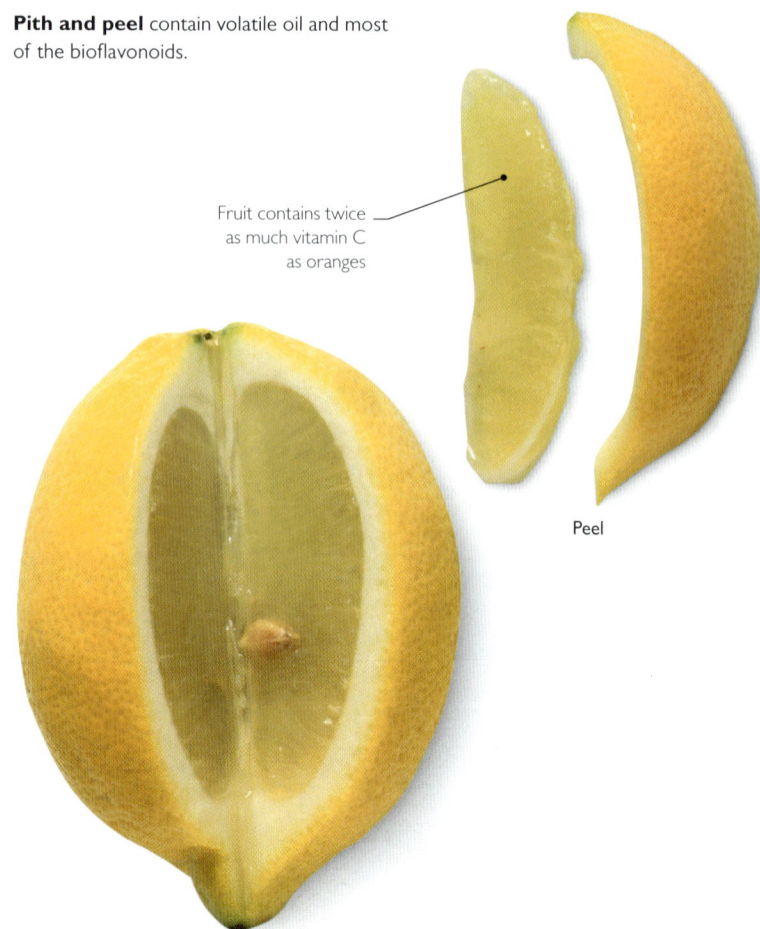

Fruit contains twice as much vitamin C as oranges

Peel

Key preparations & their uses

Remedy For colds, combine 1 tbsp lemon juice with 2½ tbsp hot water, a crushed garlic clove, and a pinch of cinnamon. Drink up to 3 times a day.

Essential oil Dilute 5 drops with 1 tsp carrier oil. Dab onto mouth ulcers.

Juice For sore throats, dilute 1 tbsp lemon juice with 1 tbsp hot water and use as a gargle.

Caution Do not take essential oil internally except under professional supervision.

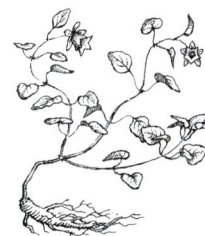

Codonopsis pilosula (Campanulaceae)

Codonopsis, *Dang shen* (Chinese)

Codonopsis has a central place in Chinese herbal medicine as a gentle tonic that increases energy levels, improves physical and mental well-being, and helps the body adapt to stress. Codonopsis is an adaptogen similar in action to ginseng (*Panax ginseng*, p. 123) but with a milder and shorter-lasting effect. It is given to those who find ginseng too strong a tonic, and is used interchangeably with ginseng in Chinese herbal formulas.

A twining perennial growing to 5 ft (1.5 m), with oval leaves and pendulous green and purple flowers.

Habitat & cultivation

Codonopsis is native to northeastern China and grows throughout much of the region, especially in the Shanxi and Szechuan provinces. It is propagated from seed in spring or fall. The root is harvested in the fall once the aerial parts have died down.

Key constituents

• Sterols • Alkaloids • Terpenes
• Polysaccharides • Alkanes

Key actions

• Adaptogen • Tonic • Antianemic

Research

Blood remedy Laboratory experiments have demonstrated that codonopsis increases hemoglobin and red blood cell levels, and lowers blood pressure.
Stamina Other research has confirmed the ability of codonopsis to help increase endurance to stress and to maintain alertness.

Traditional & current uses

Tonic herb In Chinese herbal medicine, codonopsis is considered to tone the *qi* (vital force—see pp. 26–27), lungs, and spleen. It improves vitality and helps balance metabolic function. It is a gentle tonic remedy that helps revive the system as a whole.
Primary uses Codonopsis is taken in particular for tired limbs, general fatigue, and for digestive problems such as appetite loss, vomiting, and diarrhea. It is thought to nourish the *yin* (see pp. 44–45) of the stomach without making it too "wet," and at the same time to tone the spleen without making it too "dry." It is beneficial in any chronic illness

where "spleen *qi* deficiency" is a contributory factor.
False fire Perhaps most interestingly, codonopsis is given as a tonic to people who are stressed and have "false fire" symptoms, including tense neck muscles, headaches, irritability, and high blood pressure. Such symptoms can be aggravated by stronger adaptogens such as ginseng (*Panax ginseng*, p. 123), while codonopsis is also more effective in helping reduce adrenaline levels and associated stress.
Breastfeeding tonic The herb is taken regularly by nursing mothers in China to increase milk production and as a tonic to "build strong blood."
Respiratory problems Codonopsis clears excessive mucus from the lungs, and is useful for respiratory problems including shortness of breath and asthma.

Self-help uses

• Loss of appetite & vomiting, p. 316.
• Nervous exhaustion, muscle tension, & headaches, p. 318. • Stress or convalescence, p. 329.

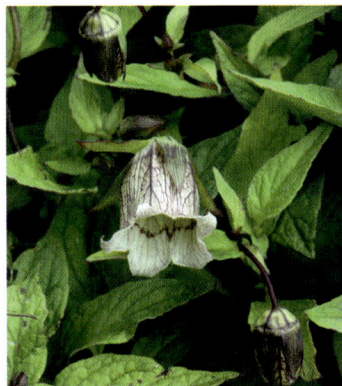

Codonopsis *bears solitary, bell-shaped flowers with purple markings in summer.*

Parts used

Root is used in cooking or dried for use in tinctures and decoctions.

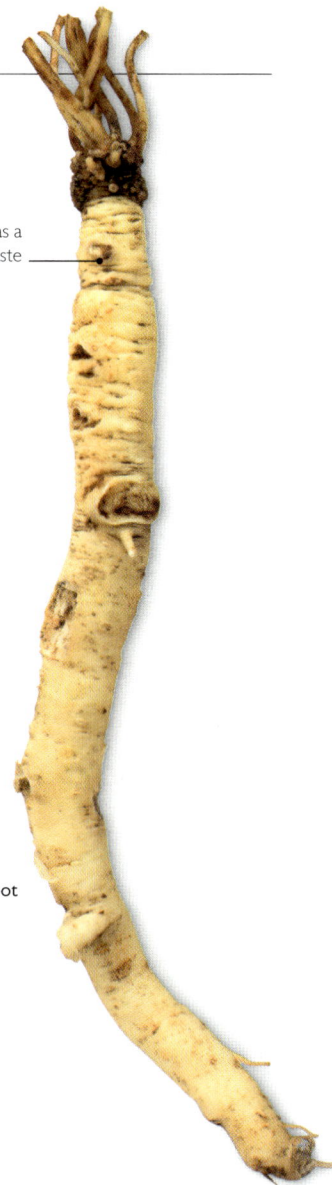

Root has a sweet taste

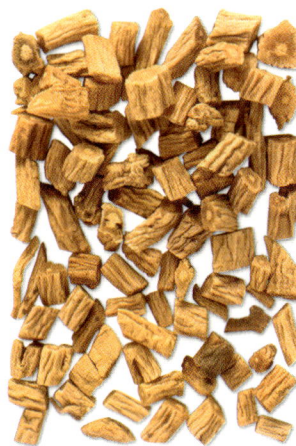

Dried root

Fresh root

Key preparations & their uses

Remedy Simmer 4 tsp codonopsis, 4 tsp astragalus, and 2 tsp lycium berries with 3 cups (750 ml) water for 40 minutes. Drink regularly as a tonic.

Decoction (to make, p. 301). For fatigue, drink ⅓ cup (75 ml) twice a day.

Tincture (to make, p. 302) is used in the West, but not in Chinese herbal medicine. As a tonic, take ½ tsp with water 3 times a day.

Coleus forskohlii syn. *Plectranthus barbatus* (Lamiaceae)

Coleus

Native to India, coleus is used in Indian folk medicine rather than within the Ayurvedic tradition, and is a traditional digestive remedy. It shot to fame in Western medical circles when one of its constituents, forskolin, was first isolated in the 1970s. Research by an Indian/German company showed that forskolin was a powerful medicine for various conditions, including heart failure, glaucoma, and bronchial asthma.

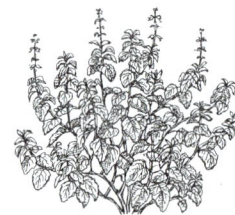

An aromatic perennial, with tuber-like roots and an erect stem, reaching 2 ft (60 cm).

Habitat & cultivation

Native to India, coleus grows on the dry slopes of the Indian plains and in the foothills of the Himalayas. It is also found in subtropical or warm temperate areas, including Nepal, Sri Lanka, Myanmar, and parts of eastern Africa. Coleus was popular as an ornamental in the 19th century. Today it is cultivated on a large scale in Gujarat, India, for use in pickles—around 980 tons (1,000 metric tons) are harvested each year. The plant is propagated by stem cuttings or root division in spring or summer and flourishes in well-drained soil in sun or partial shade. Both root and leaves are harvested in the fall.

Related species

Six other species of *Coleus* have been investigated but only *C. forskohlii* contains forskolin. Indian borage (*C. amboinicus*) is used traditionally within Ayurvedic and Unani Tibb herbal medicine to help reduce inflammation and is prescribed for bronchitis and asthma.

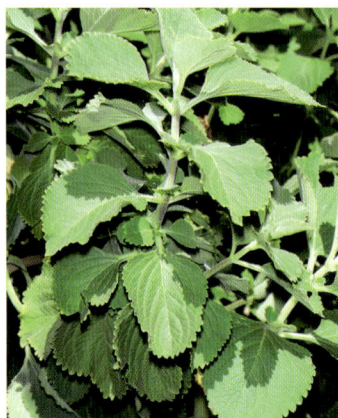

Coleus is strongly aromatic and the leaves have a distinctive camphor-like scent.

Key constituents

• Volatile oil • Diterpenes (forskolin)

Key actions

• Lowers blood pressure
• Antispasmodic • Dilates the bronchioles (small airways of the lungs) • Dilates the blood vessels
• Heart tonic

Research

Forskolin The active constituent forskolin was first isolated in the 1970s. It has important therapeutic benefits, which include lowering high blood pressure, relaxing smooth muscle, increasing the release of hormones from the thyroid gland, stimulating digestive secretions, and reducing pressure within the eye.

Whole herb A 2016 Japanese review of 7 clinical studies investigating the anti-obesity effects of Coleus extracts found that the herb had a significant positive benefit in aiding weight loss in overweight and obese people.

Traditional & current uses

Traditional uses Coleus is a traditional herb in India for a wide range of digestive problems. It is given to relieve gas, bloating, and abdominal discomfort.

Circulatory remedy An important heart and circulatory tonic, coleus is used to treat congestive heart failure and poor coronary blood flow. It also improves circulation of blood to the brain.

Respiratory problems Its antispasmodic action makes coleus valuable for respiratory complaints, including asthma and bronchitis.

Glaucoma Coleus is used topically in treatments to relieve glaucoma (excess pressure within

Parts used

Leaves have valuable medicinal properties and are also eaten in pickles.

Root is unearthed in the fall when the active constituents are most concentrated.

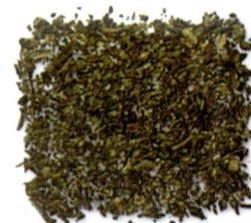

Dried leaves

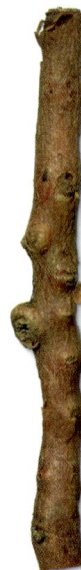

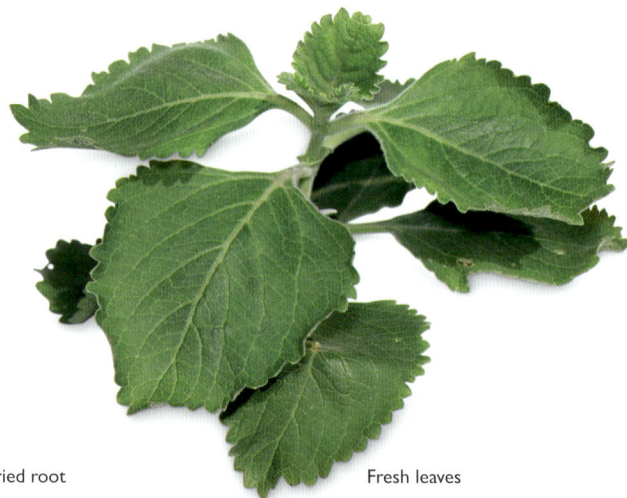

Dried root · Fresh leaves

Key preparations & their uses

Decoction of the root. For bronchial asthma, make a decoction with 15 g root and 2 cups (500 ml) water (*see* p. 301). Drink in small doses over 2 days.

Infusion of the leaves (to make, p. 301). To relieve gas and bloating, drink ¾ cup (150 ml) twice a day.

Cautions Do not take for circulatory problems or glaucoma without professional advice.

the eye, which, if untreated, can result in loss of vision).

Weight loss Recently, coleus has been marketed as a weight-loss aid. It is argued that because coleus

stimulates cellular metabolism, it will help promote weight loss. There is no evidence to support this, though it may be of use if weight gain is due to poor thyroid function.

Commiphora myrrha (Burseraceae)

Myrrh

Myrrh has been used in perfumes, incense, and embalming, and, as a symbol of suffering, was one of the three gifts offered to the infant Jesus by the Three Wise Men. Myrrh is also one of the oldest known medicines and was extensively used by the ancient Egyptians. It is an excellent remedy for mouth and throat problems, with a drying, slightly bitter taste, and it is also useful for skin problems.

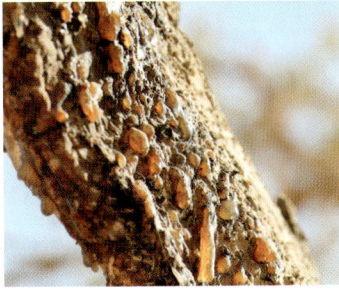

A spiny, deciduous tree growing to 16 ft (5 m), with yellow-red flowers and pointed fruit.

Myrrh trees yield a thick, yellow resin that has a distinct, aromatic odor. It is used in mouthwashes.

Habitat & cultivation

Native to northeast Africa, especially Somalia, myrrh is now also found in Ethiopia, Saudi Arabia, India, Iran, and Thailand. It grows in thickets and likes well-drained soil and sun. Myrrh is propagated from seed in spring or from cuttings at the end of the growing season. The resin is collected from cut branches and is dried for use.

Related species

A number of closely related *Commiphora* species are used interchangeably with myrrh. See guggul (*C. mukul*, p. 198).

Key constituents

• Gum (30–60%), acidic polysaccharides • Resin (25–40%)
• Volatile oil (3–8%), including heerabolene, eugenol, and many furanosesquiterpenes

Key actions

• Antiseptic • Astringent
• Antiparasitic • Anti-inflammatory
• Anti-ulcer • Wound healer

Research

Antibiotic Egyptian research confirms that myrrh is a key treatment for certain parasitic infections, notably liver flukes and schistosomiasis (both common and serious waterborne diseases). In one clinical study, myrrh extract cleared all signs of liver fluke infection within 6 days, with patients remaining clear 3 months later. Others have been similarly successful. It is also being studied as a gastric ulcer remedy and for anticancer properties. The gum resin has thyroid-stimulating activity.

Traditional & current uses

Mouth & throat remedy Being astringent and strongly antiseptic, myrrh is a favored remedy for sore throats, canker sores, and gingivitis (gum disease). As myrrh is not soluble in water, tincture or essential oil is used and diluted. The resulting mouthwash or gargle is often swiftly effective (though tastes very bitter). Myrrh's key actions also make it valuable in countering infection throughout the digestive tract, while at the same time it promotes healing in inflamed areas, notably gastric ulcers.

Ayurvedic remedy In Ayurvedic medicine, myrrh is considered a tonic and aphrodisiac, and to cleanse the blood. It has a reputation for improving intellect. Myrrh is also taken for irregular or painful menstruation.

External uses Myrrh is an underused treatment for skin problems such as acne, boils, and inflammatory conditions. The herb's drying and slightly anesthetizing effect has led to its use in Germany as a treatment for pressure sores caused by prosthetic limbs.

Self-help uses

• Acne & boils, p. 315. • Mouth & tongue ulcers, p. 316. • Canker sores & gum problems, p. 316. • Oral thrush, p. 324. • Sore throats, p. 321.

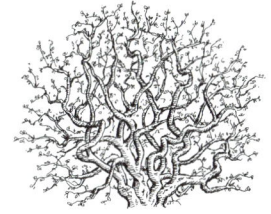

Parts used

Gum resin oozes from fissures or cuts in the bark of the tree and dries into yellow-red solid pieces.

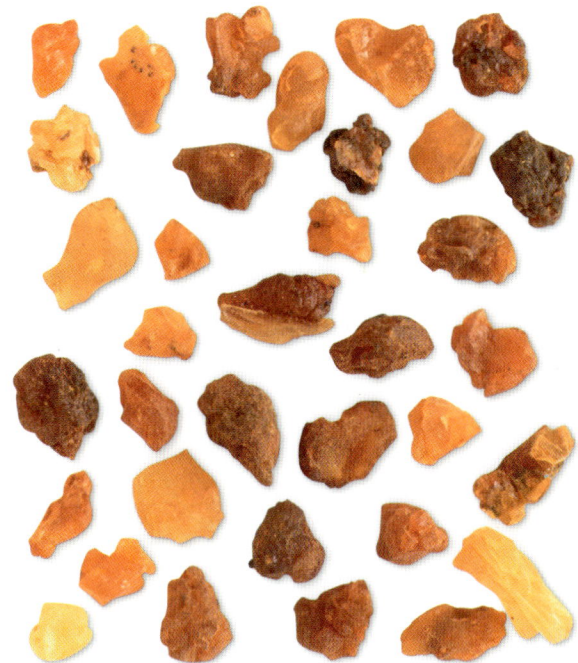

Dried gum resin

Key preparations & their uses

Mouthwash Dilute 1 tsp tincture (to make, p. 302) with ½ cup (100 ml) water and use as a mouthwash or for sore throats.

Tincture (to make, p. 302). For mouth ulcers, carefully dab on a little every hour.

Essential oil For congested sinuses, dilute 3 drops in 1 tsp carrier oil and massage gently (see p. 307).

Powder Rub a little onto sore gums 3 times daily.

Capsules (to make, p. 302). For bronchial congestion, take a 300 mg capsule twice a day.

Cautions Do not use in pregnancy. Do not take the essential oil internally.

Corydalis yanhusuo (Papaveraceae)

Corydalis, *Yan hu suo* (Chinese)

Corydalis is an important Chinese remedy that has been used at least since the 8th century to help "invigorate the blood" and relieve almost any painful condition. It is used particularly for menstrual cramps and for chest and abdominal pain. Research in China has confirmed the validity of corydalis' traditional use, revealing that it contains powerful alkaloids that are responsible for its analgesic effect.

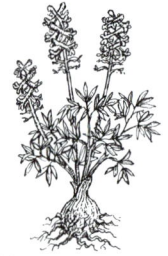

A small, herbaceous plant growing to 8 in (20 cm) with narrow leaves and pink flowers.

Habitat & cultivation

Native to Siberia, northern China, and Japan, corydalis is commonly cultivated in eastern and northeastern parts of China. It is propagated from seed in early spring or fall, and the rhizome is harvested in late spring and early summer when the top growth has died back.

Related species

C. cava, a related species from southern Europe, has been shown to provide relief from involuntary tremors and ataxia (shaky movements). *C. gariana*, native to the Himalayas, is used in India as a detoxifying and tonic herb for skin problems and genito-urinary infections. Fumitory (*Fumaria officinalis*, p. 218), used to treat skin problems, is also closely related.

Key constituents

• Alkaloids (including corydalis L, corydaline, tetrahydropalmatine [THP], protopine) • Protoberberine-type alkaloid (leonticine)

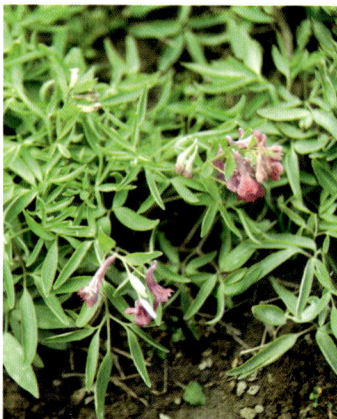

Corydalis is commonly prescribed by the Chinese in formulations for period pain.

Key actions

• Analgesic • Antispasmodic
• Sedative

Research

Analgesic properties Research in China from the 1950s onward has shown that corydalis has useful pain-relieving properties. The powdered rhizome has up to one-tenth of the analgesic potency of morphine—an alkaloid derived from the opium poppy (*Papaver somniferum*, p. 251). Morphine is highly concentrated and the strongest nonsynthetic analgesic in medical use. Although this research shows corydalis to be much weaker in its effect than morphine, it nonetheless indicates the value of corydalis in pain relief.

Alkaloids The strongest analgesic alkaloid in corydalis is corydaline. Tetrahydropalmatine (THP), another alkaloid, is analgesic and sedative and has been shown to work, at least in part, by blocking the dopamine receptors in the central nervous system. This constituent is also known to stimulate secretion of the adrenocorticotropic hormone (ACTH) by the anterior pituitary gland, which controls aspects of stress.

Menstrual pain Several clinical trials in China have shown corydalis to be very effective in relieving menstrual pain.

Traditional & current uses

Pain relief Corydalis is specifically taken to treat pain, and is used in Chinese herbal medicine to relieve pain resulting from almost any cause. It is rarely taken on its own, being combined with various other herbs as appropriate.

Period pain Corydalis is well worth

Parts used

Rhizome contains powerful alkaloids that research shows help alleviate pain. It is unearthed in the fall and dried and chopped.

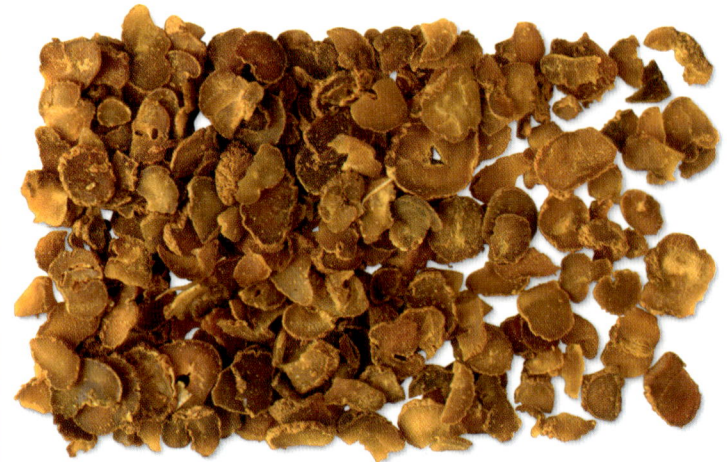

Dried rhizome

Key preparations & their uses

Decoction Make a decoction with 10 g corydalis, 3 g cinnamon, and 2 cups (500 ml) water (see p. 301). For period pain, take ½ cup (100 ml) twice a day.

Powder To ease pain, take 2 g of powder with food twice a day.

Tincture (to make, p. 302). For abdominal pain, take up to 1 tsp with water twice a day.

Caution Do not take during pregnancy.

trying as a natural treatment for period pain, and combines well with cramp bark (*Viburnum opulus*, p. 154).

Abdominal conditions Many types of abdominal pain, whether in the lower abdomen as in appendicitis, or in the upper abdomen as in peptic ulcer, are treated with corydalis.

Injuries In Chinese medical theory, and in other herbal traditions, pain is often thought to stem from obstruction of normal blood flow. As corydalis is thought to "invigorate the blood," it is considered to be especially useful as a treatment for the pain that results from a traumatic injury.

Crataegus oxyacantha & C. monogyna (Rosaceae)

Hawthorn

Hawthorn is an extremely valuable medicinal herb. It was known in the Middle Ages as a symbol of hope and taken for many ailments. Today it is used mainly for heart and circulatory disorders, in particular for angina. Western herbalists consider it literally to be a "food for the heart," increasing blood flow to the heart muscles and restoring normal heartbeat. Recent research has confirmed the validity of these uses.

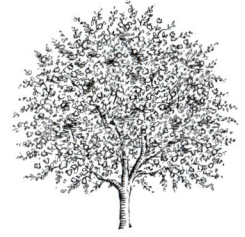

A deciduous, thorny tree with small leaves, white flowers, and red berries, growing to 26 ft (8 m).

Habitat & cultivation

The hawthorn tree grows along roadsides, and in thickets and fields throughout the British Isles and in all temperate regions of the northern hemisphere. It can be propagated from seed, but it takes 18 months to germinate, so the trees are usually cultivated from cuttings. The flowering tops are harvested in late spring and the berries in late summer to early fall.

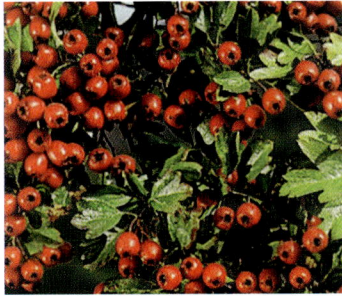

Key constituents

- Polyphenols • Proanthocyanins
- Bioflavonoids • Triterpenoids
- Coumarins • Amines
(trimethylamine—in flowers only)

Key actions

- Cardiotonic • Circulatory tonic
- Lowers blood pressure
- Antioxidant

Research

Bioflavonoids Hawthorn has been fairly well researched. Its main medicinal benefit is due to its high bioflavonoid and proanthocyanin content. These constituents relax and dilate the arteries, especially the coronary arteries. This increases the flow of blood to the heart muscles and reduces the symptoms of angina. Both the bioflavonoids and the proanthocyanins are also strongly antioxidant, helping to prevent or reduce degeneration of the blood vessels.

Cardiac herb Several clinical trials have explored hawthorn's ability to lower blood pressure and support heart function, with substantially positive findings and strong evidence of the herb's safety.

Traditional & current uses

Historical uses Hawthorn was

Hawthorn has bright red berries in the fall. They are used in remedies to treat a variety of circulatory disorders.

traditionally used in Europe for kidney and bladder stones, and as a diuretic. The 16th- and 18th-century herbals of Gerard, Culpeper, and K'Eogh all list these uses. Its current use for circulatory and cardiac problems stems from an Irish physician who started using it successfully for such conditions toward the end of the 19th century.

Heart remedy Hawthorn is used today to treat angina and coronary artery disease. It specifically improves heart function and is useful for mild congestive heart failure and irregular heartbeat. Like many herbs, hawthorn works in tune with the body's own physiological processes and it takes time for change to occur.

Blood pressure Hawthorn is best thought of as a remedy that normalizes blood pressure. It clearly works to lower high blood pressure, but also appears to support blood pressure levels where these tend to be low.

Poor memory Combined with ginkgo (*Ginkgo biloba*, p. 104), hawthorn is used to enhance poor memory. It works by improving the circulation of blood within the head, thereby increasing the amount of oxygen to the brain.

Parts used

Flowering tops contain trimethylamine, which stimulates circulation.

Berries help the heart function normally.

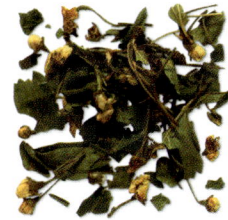

Dried flowering tops

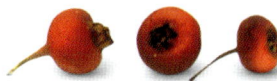

Fresh berries

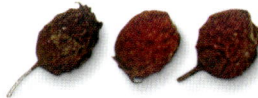

Dried berries

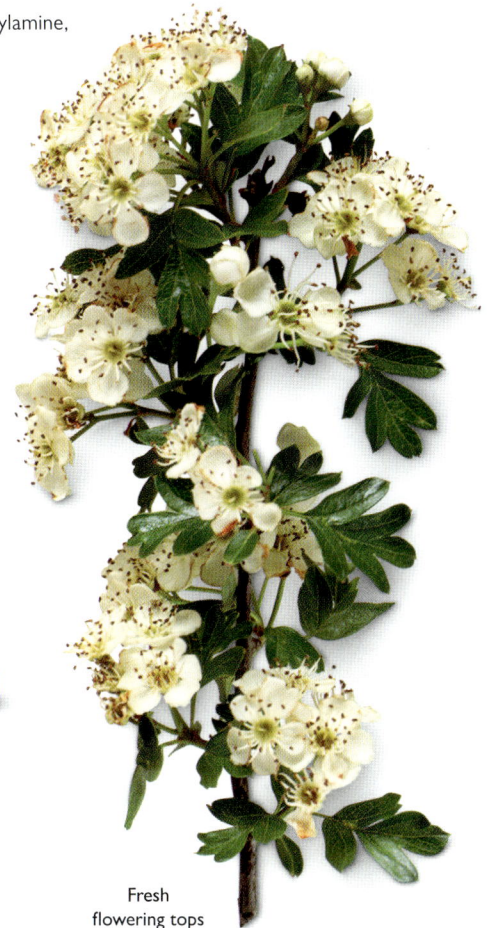

Fresh flowering tops

Key preparations & their uses

Tincture of flowering tops or berries is the most commonly used preparation.

Decoction of flowering tops is valuable for circulatory disorders.

Tablets containing powdered flowering tops are convenient for long-term use.

Infusion, made from the flowers or leaves, helps restore blood pressure levels to normal.

Cautions Interactions with prescribed medicines can occur. Seek advice from an herbal or medical practitioner if taking prescribed medicines, especially for high blood pressure and heart disorders.

Crataeva nurvala (Capparaceae)

Varuna, *Barun* (Hindi), Three-leafed caper

The bark of the varuna tree is an important herb for problems affecting the kidneys and bladder, especially kidney and bladder stones. In Ayurvedic medicine, it has been used for around 3,000 years to treat these problems, and, as is the case with so many herbs, recent scientific research is confirming the appropriateness of its traditional usage, demonstrating that it prevents the formation of kidney stones.

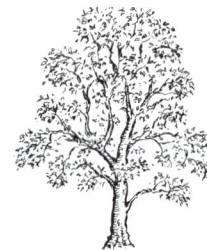

A large deciduous tree growing to 33 ft (10 m), with smooth bark and pale yellow flowers.

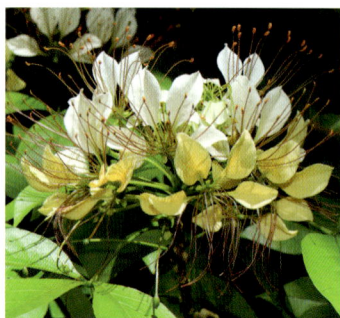

***Varuna** is frequently cultivated in the vicinity of temples in central India and Bangladesh.*

Habitat & cultivation

Varuna grows throughout India and is often found along riverbanks. Grown from seed in spring, the leaves are harvested in spring and the bark is collected throughout the year.

Key constituents

- Triterpenes • Saponins • Flavonoids
- Sterols • Alkaloids • Glucosilinates

Key actions

- Diuretic • Inhibits the formation of stones

Research

Bladder & kidney stones Clinical research in India from the 1980s onward indicates that varuna increases bladder tone and inhibits the formation of bladder stones. It reduces the production within the body of oxalates, substances that can precipitate in the kidneys and bladder to form stones. The herb also seems to reduce the rate at which stone-forming constituents within the urine are deposited in the kidneys.
Urinary system Indian research in the 1980s and 1990s points to varuna being valuable in the treatment of urinary

tract infections and bladder problems caused by an enlarged prostate gland. In one clinical trial, 85% of patients with chronic urinary tract infections were symptom-free after undergoing 4 weeks' treatment with varuna.

Traditional & current uses

Ancient urinary remedy Texts dating back to the 8th century BCE document varuna's use in Ayurvedic medicine for kidney and bladder problems. From around 1100 CE, varuna became the main Indian herbal medicine for kidney stones.
Other traditional uses Traditionally, varuna bark is considered useful in Ayurveda (see p. 40–44) for weakened conditions of *vata* (air) and *kapha* (earth), and is used to treat many conditions, including asthma, bronchitis, and skin diseases. The bark is also used to treat fevers, gastritis, and vomiting, as well as snake bite. The fresh leaves, bruised and mixed with vinegar, relieve sore and inflamed joints.
Kidney stones Today, varuna is beginning to be used in the West, as well as in India, in the prevention and treatment of kidney stones. It is given to people who are prone to develop kidney stones, reducing the tendency to stone formation. It is also prescribed for people who already have small stones. Varuna improves smooth muscle tone and encourages the removal of stones in the urine.
Urinary tract remedy Combined with antiseptic and immune-stimulating herbs, varuna is very useful for urinary tract infections, including cystitis. It is also sometimes effective for bladder conditions involving poor muscle tone, some cases of incontinence, and urinary problems associated with prostate enlargement.

Parts used

Bark contains constituents that inhibit the formation of kidney stones.

Leaves are harvested in spring and are used in infusions.

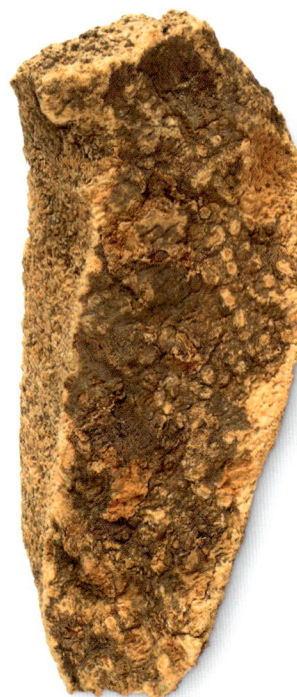
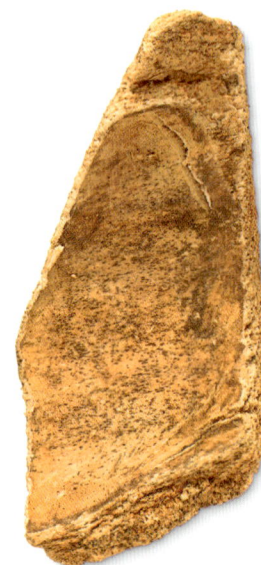

Dried bark

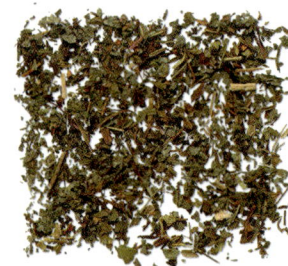

Dried leaves

Key preparations & their uses

Infusion of leaves (to make, p. 301). For painful joints, apply as a lotion 3 times a day (see p. 306).

Powdered bark is used in Ayurveda. For urinary infections, take 15 g with water daily.

Decoction of bark (to make, p. 301) is the most common preparation. To prevent kidney stone formation, take ¾ cup (150 ml) once a day.

Caution Best taken under professional supervision.

Crocus sativus (Iridaceae)

Saffron, Saffron crocus

Perhaps most familiar as an ingredient in the Spanish dish paella, saffron is a prized herbal medicine that by weight is more valuable than gold. The thin, deep-orange filaments picked from the saffron flower have longstanding traditional use as a remedy for lowered mood, menstrual disorders, and as a sexual tonic. Current research is endorsing some of these findings, and saffron clearly offers significant health benefits.

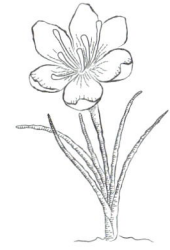

A perennial growing to 1 ft (30 cm), saffron has slender leaves and multiple lilac to mauve flowers.

Habitat & cultivation

Saffron prefers a sunny, well-drained site. It is cultivated in Iran, which grows roughly 90% of world production. The stigma are collected in the fall when the plant is in flower. The flowers are first cut, the stigma then being plucked from within. The corms (bulbs) naturally reproduce themselves—one corm producing five after 3 years.

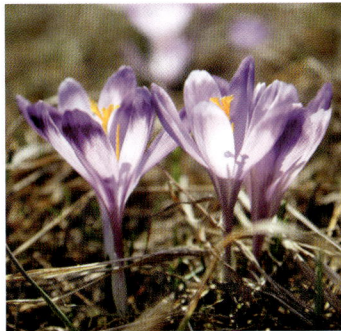

Related species

Saffron should not be confused with meadow saffron (*Colchicum autumnale*, p. 197), an important (but toxic) medicinal plant that is only distantly related to saffron.

Key constituents

- Crocins (carotenoid glucosides)
- Volatile oil (including safranal)
- Bitter substances

Key actions

- Neuroprotective • Antidepressant
- Antispasmodic • Aphrodisiac
- Stomach tonic

Research

Depression Several clinical trials have found saffron to be beneficial in depression. In 2005, Iranian researchers found that saffron was as effective as fluoxetine (Prozac) for mild to moderate depression. In a different clinical trial, saffron was shown to help relieve the symptoms of sexual dysfunction (in both men and women) that can sometimes present themselves as a side effect of taking fluoxetine.

Eye health Research from a combined Italian-Australian study suggests that saffron has a useful role to play in helping to support eye health in the early stages of macular degeneration. The study found that

Saffron's golden-red threads may help support eyesight and prevent macular degeneration.

retinal function improved in those taking saffron. Other research suggests that saffron might prove useful in treating glaucoma.

Cognitive function Saffron appears to have marked neuroprotective activity (*see Depression and Eye health*). Iranian clinical research has examined saffron's therapeutic potential in people with moderate Alzheimer's disease. Though still at a very early stage, two small studies indicate that saffron, and particularly the crocins within it, act on the brain to improve memory and cognitive function, including in those with dementia.

Adulteration Due to its high cost, saffron is frequently adulterated. For medicinal purposes, good-quality material is essential.

Traditional & current uses

Traditional uses Ibn Sina (Avicenna), a 10th-century physician famous for his *Canon of Medicine*, described saffron in detail, noting that it was an "exhilarant and cardiac tonic [that] strengthens eyesight, reduces appetite, [and is] a stimulant of sexual desire." A rereading of the *Canon* paved the way

Parts used

Stigma are the three deep orange-red threads at the center of the flower.

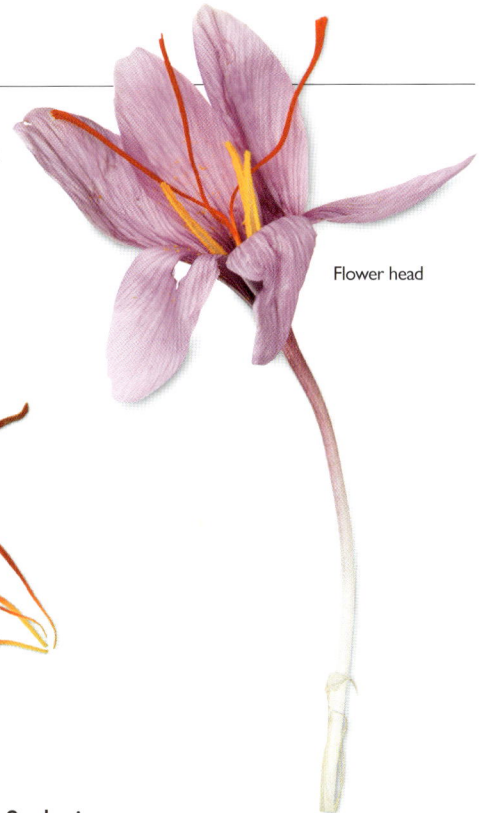

Flower head

Stigma

Key preparations & their uses

Dried stigma For low mood, take 5 threads 1–2 times a day.

Capsules (to make, p. 302). For menstrual cramps, take a 300 mg capsule up to five times a day.

Cautions Do not take as a medicine during pregnancy. Excessive doses can be toxic.

for much of the Iranian research over recent years. The herbalist Christopher Catton, following the English view of saffron as a "cordial" or heart tonic, wrote in 1862 that "Saffron hath power to quicken the spirits, and the virtue thereof pierceth by and by to the heart, provoking laughter and merriness." It is said that rubbed into the palm, saffron has an immediate action on the heart.

Chinese herbal medicine In Chinese medicine, saffron is used for depression and shock. It also has long use as a remedy for menstrual difficulties such as period cramps and premenstrual syndrome (PMS). Saffron is also used to treat skin disorders, stomach weakness, and to reduce appetite.

Curcuma longa syn. *C. domestica* (Zingiberaceae)

Turmeric, *Haldi* (Hindi), *Jiang huang* (Chinese)

Although best known for its bright yellow color and spicy taste in Indian food, turmeric is now recognized as a medicinal food that offers major health benefits. Its significant anti-inflammatory activity makes it potentially useful in many chronic health conditions, including allergies, arthritis, diabetes, and psoriasis, where long-term inflammation is usually a key underlying factor.

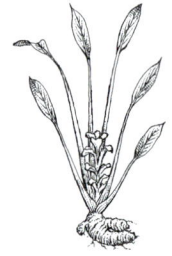

A perennial reaching 3 ft (90 cm), with a short stem, lance-shaped leaves, and a knobbly rhizome.

Habitat & cultivation

Turmeric is native to India and southern Asia and is now cultivated throughout the tropics. It is propagated by cuttings from the root, and needs well-drained soil and a humid climate. The rhizome is unearthed in winter.

Key constituents

• Curcumin • Volatile oil (3–5%), including zingiberen and turmerone • Bitter principles • Resin

Key actions

• Anti-inflammatory • Lowers cholesterol levels • Antimicrobial • Antiplatelet (blood-thinning)

Research

Combining with black pepper or piperine Curcumin is poorly absorbed across the gut wall. Scientific studies endorse the Ayurvedic tradition of eating black pepper with turmeric root and have shown that the combination can increase the bioavailability of curcumin by up to 2,000%.

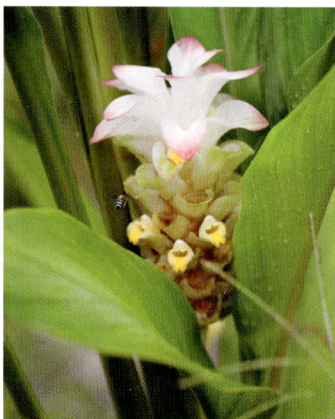

Turmeric is a valuable remedy for arthritic and skin conditions.

Covid-19 Many of the symptoms associated with Covid-19 infection result from acute and chronic inflammation. Curcumin has been suggested as an adjuvant treatment for Covid-19 infection. A small clinical study in India (2021) found that patients who "received curcumin/piperine treatment showed early symptomatic recovery (fever, cough, sore throat, and breathlessness), less deterioration, fewer red flag signs, better ability to maintain oxygen saturation above 94% on room air, and better clinical outcomes than the control group".

Potent anti-inflammatory Research into turmeric, and more specifically curcumin, took off in the early 2000s as the herb's potent anti-inflammatory activity was conclusively established. Turmeric works by blocking several different inflammatory pathways within the body, making it a key remedy to counter chronic inflammation. Conditions such as arthritis, metabolic syndrome, raised cholesterol levels, and post-exercise inflammation can all benefit from turmeric supplementation.

Curcumin When applied to the skin and exposed to sunlight, turmeric is strongly antibacterial. Curcumin is the constituent responsible for this action. Curcumin is also more strongly antioxidant than vitamin E.

Cholesterol Chinese clinical trials in 1987 indicate that turmeric lowers cholesterol levels.

Cancer Research suggests that turmeric and curcumin are useful supplements for people at risk of developing cancer.

Other actions Research has shown that turmeric has an anticoagulant action, keeping the blood thin. It also increases bile production and flow, and has a protective action on the stomach and liver.

Parts used

Rhizome is carefully unearthed and broken into sections. It is boiled or steamed before drying.

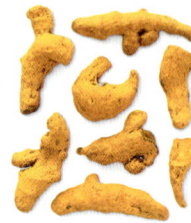

Fresh rhizome is bright orange inside

Dried rhizome

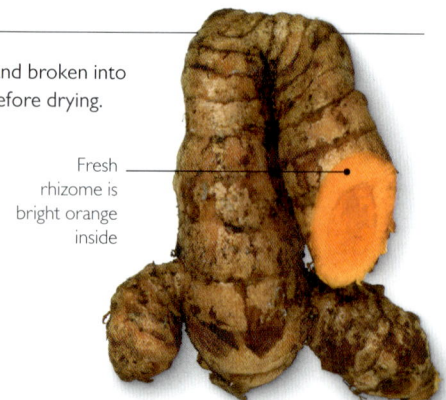

Fresh rhizome

Key preparations & their uses

Decoction (to make, p. 301). For gastritis, take ⅓ cup (75 ml) 3 times a day.

Poultice using a paste made with powder. For psoriasis, mix 1 tsp with a little water and apply 3 times a day.

Powder is the most common preparation in Ayurvedic medicine. For gastritis, take 1 tsp with water 3 times a day.

Tincture (to make, p. 302). For eczema, take 1 tsp diluted with ½ cup (100 ml) of water 3 times a day.

Cautions If taking blood-thinning medication, or if gallstones are present, take only with professional advice. Turmeric occasionally causes skin rashes.

Traditional & current uses

Traditional remedy Turmeric improves the action of the liver and is a traditional remedy for jaundice in both Ayurvedic and Chinese herbal medicine. It is also an ancient herb for digestive problems such as gastritis and acidity, helping to increase mucus production and protect the stomach. The herb also alleviates nausea.

Arthritis & allergies Even though turmeric does not relieve pain, its anti-inflammatory action makes it useful for arthritis and other inflammatory conditions such as asthma and eczema.

Circulatory disorders Due to its anti-inflammatory, blood-thinning, and cholesterol-lowering properties, turmeric is now used to reduce the risk of strokes and heart attacks.

Skin conditions Applied to the skin, turmeric is useful in treating a number of conditions, including psoriasis, and fungal infections such as athlete's foot.

Self-help uses

• Athlete's foot, p. 314. • Nausea & motion sickness, p. 316.

Dioscorea villosa (Dioscoreaceae)

Wild yam, Colic root

Wild yam is the plant source of a steroid-like substance, diosgenin, which was the starting point in the creation of the first contraceptive pill. There is no suggestion that the plant was used as a contraceptive in the past, though it has traditionally been taken in Central America to relieve menstrual, ovarian, and labor pains. The herb is also valuable for digestive problems, arthritis, and muscle cramps.

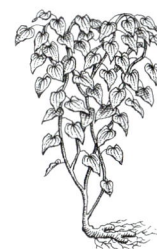

A deciduous perennial vine climbing to 20 ft (6 m) with heart-shaped leaves and tiny green flowers.

Habitat & cultivation

Wild yam is native to North and Central America, and has now become naturalized in tropical, semitropical, and temperate climates around the world. The plant is propagated from seed in spring, or from sections of tubers or by root division in spring or fall. It thrives in sunny conditions and rich soil. The root and tuber of wild yam are harvested in the fall.

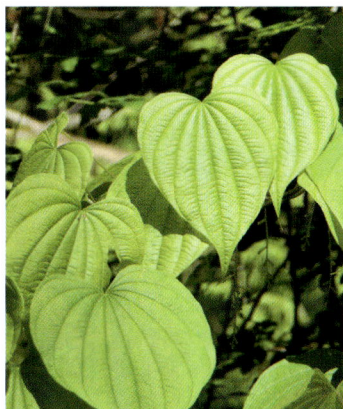

Related species

Many yam species have a hormonal action. Shan yao (*Dioscorea opposita*) is an important tonic for the stomach and digestion in traditional Chinese medicine, and is taken for appetite loss and wheezing.

Key constituents

• Steroidal saponins (mainly dioscin)
• Phytosterols (beta-sitosterol)
• Alkaloids • Tannins • Starch

Key actions

• Antispasmodic • Anti-inflammatory
• Antirheumatic • Increases sweating
• Diuretic

Research

Synthesis of hormones Diosgenin, a breakdown product of dioscin, was first identified by Japanese scientists in 1936. This discovery paved the way for the synthesis of progesterone (one of the main female sex hormones) and of corticosteroid hormones such as cortisone. Wild yam does not contain estrogen or progesterone, and wild yam "natural progesterone" products are derived from chemically processed diosgenin, and have little or no relationship with naturally occurring wild yam.

Wild yam can be found growing wild in damp woodlands in North America.

Anticholesterol activity Research indicates that diosgenin reduces the absorption of cholesterol from the gut and increases its elimination from the body.

Traditional & current uses

Traditional uses Both the Maya and the Aztec peoples used wild yam medicinally—possibly to relieve pain. The plant is also known as colic root and rheumatism root in North America, indicating its use by European colonizers for these conditions.

Gynecological problems A traditional remedy for painful periods and ovarian pain, wild yam has estrogen-modulating activity and is used to treat menopausal symptoms.

Arthritis & rheumatism The herb's combination of anti-inflammatory and antispasmodic actions makes it extremely useful in treatments for arthritis and rheumatism. It reduces inflammation and pain, and relaxes stiff muscles in the affected area.

Parts used

Root and tuber have valuable antispasmodic properties. They are used to treat colic and menstrual cramps.

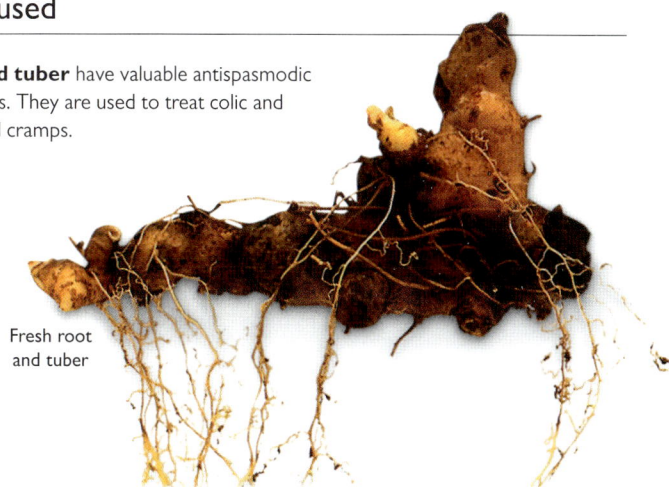

Fresh root and tuber

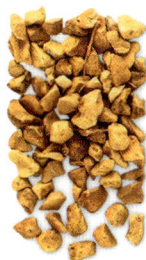

Chopped dried root and tuber

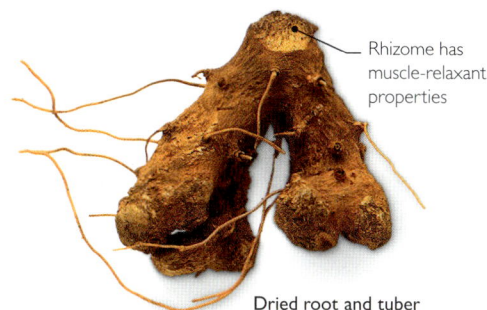

Rhizome has muscle-relaxant properties

Dried root and tuber

Key preparations & their uses

Decoction (to make, p. 301). For irritable bowel syndrome, take ⅓ cup (75 ml) twice a day.

Tincture (to make, p. 302). For arthritis, take ½ tsp with water twice a day.

Caution Do not take during pregnancy.

Muscle spasms & pain Wild yam helps relieve cramps, muscle tension, and colic.

Digestive problems The root can be valuable in digestive problems, including irritable bowel syndrome, and diverticulitis.

Self-help use

Period pain, p. 325.

Echinacea spp. (Asteraceae)

Echinacea, Purple coneflower

A key medicinal herb, echinacea has a tonic action on the body's immune system. Known by 19th-century Americans as Indian Snakeroot (due to its ability to treat snake bites), the herb has a potent ability to counter infection, especially viral and bacterial, and to aid the clearance of toxins from the body. It is commonly taken as a preventative and treatment for upper respiratory infections such as colds, flu, and coughs.

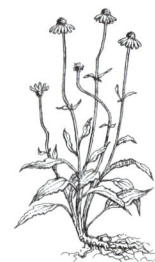

A perennial growing to 4 ft (1.2 m) with upright stems and pink to purple daisylike flowers.

Habitat & cultivation

Native to central parts of the US, three species of echinacea are used medicinally: *E. angustifolia*, *E. purpurea*, and *E. pallida*. All are threatened in the wild and only commercially grown plants should be used. *E. purpurea* is cultivated widely in the US and Europe. Grown from seed in spring or by root division in winter, it thrives in rich, sandy soil. The leaves and flowers are gathered during flowering; the roots of 4-year-old plants are lifted in the fall.

Key constituents

• (*E. purpurea*) • Alkylamides (mostly isobutylamides) • Caffeic acid esters (mainly echinacoside and cynarin) • Polysaccharides

Key actions

• Immune modulator • Antimicrobial
• Anti-inflammatory • Detoxifying
• Heals wounds • Stimulates saliva

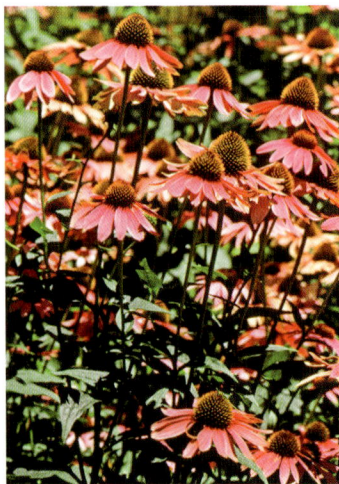

Echinacea is a name derived from the Greek word for hedgehog and was inspired by the appearance of the flower's central cone.

Research

Immune systems Clinical research into echinacea has confirmed that it increases the number of white blood cells and their strength of action, although its precise mode of action on immune function is not well understood. The polysaccharides inhibit the ability of viruses to take over cells, while the alkylamides are antibacterial and antifungal. Research supports the use of echinacea to prevent colds and respiratory infections resulting from air travel. Not all clinical trials have found positive effects, possibly because in some cases too low a dose of echinacea was used.

Traditional & current uses

Indigenous medicine The Comanche people used echinacea as a remedy for toothache and sore throats and the Sioux people took it for rabies, snake bite, and septic conditions.

Western uses Echinacea is a key remedy in Western herbal medicine, and is used to treat many health problems, notably viral and fungal infections, and skin infections such as acne and boils. It makes an excellent gargle for throat infections, and is typically prescribed by herbalists wherever the immune system is underperforming.

Allergies The herb is a helpful remedy for treating allergies such as asthma.

Self-help uses

• Acne & boils, p. 315. • Bites & stings, p. 313. • Chilblains, p. 312. • Cold sores, p. 314. • Coughs & bronchitis, p. 320. • Earache, p. 322. • Flu, sore throats, & tonsillitis, p. 321. • Canker sores, p. 316. • Urinary & fungal infections, p. 324

Parts used

Flower of *E. purpurea* is occasionally used for infections.

Roots of all three species have valuable immune-stimulating properties.

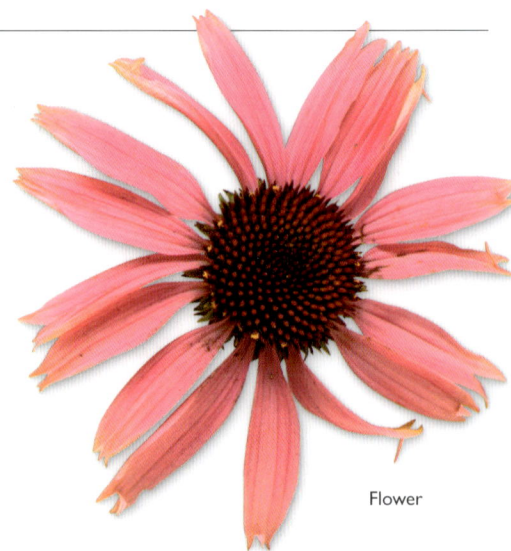

The best-quality root leaves a tingling sensation on the tongue

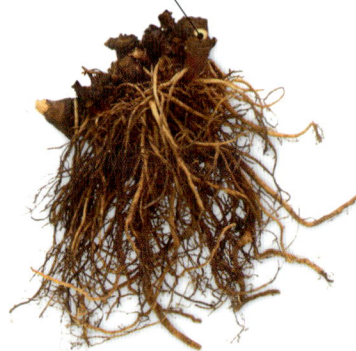

Flower

Fresh *E. purpurea* root

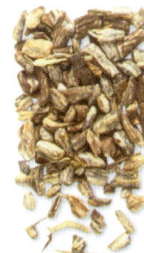

Dried root

Key preparations & their uses

Tincture of root (to make, p. 302). For chronic infections, take ½ tsp in water 3 times a day

Decoction of root (to make, p. 301). To treat throat infections, gargle with 2½ tbsp 3 times a day.

Capsules of powdered root (to make, p. 302). For colds, take a 500 mg capsule 3 times a day.

Tablets Take as an immune-stimulant for infections.

Caution Can cause allergic reactions in rare cases.

Elettaria cardamomum (Zingiberaceae)

Cardamom, *Elaci* (Hindi)

Cardamom is one of the oldest spices in the world and was used extensively in ancient Egypt to make perfumes. Its medicinal uses, however, are less well known. Cardamom has been employed in Ayurvedic medicine for thousands of years, and is an excellent remedy for many digestive problems, helping to soothe indigestion and gas. It has an aromatic and pungent taste and combines well with other herbs.

A perennial growing to 16 ft (5 m), with mauve-marked white flowers and very long, lance-shaped leaves.

Habitat & cultivation

Cardamom is native to southern India and Sri Lanka, where it grows profusely in forests at 2,600–4,900 ft (800–1,500 m) above sea level. It is also widely cultivated in India, southern Asia, Indonesia, and Guatemala. Cardamom is propagated from seed in the fall or by root division in spring and summer, and needs a shady position and rich and moist, but well-drained soil. The seed pods are harvested just before they start to open in dry weather during the fall and are dried whole in the sun.

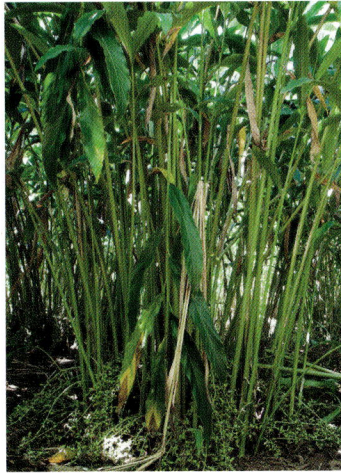

Cardamom seed pods are harvested by hand. Each pod contains up to 20 aromatic, dark red-brown seeds.

Key constituents

• Volatile oil • Alkaloids • Flavonoids
• Saponins • Sterols

Key actions

• Digestive tonic • Protects liver
• Mild stimulant • Antispasmodic

Research

Antispasmodic A 2009 Indian clinical study found that cardamom successfully lowered blood pressure in 20 adults over a 3-month period. Those taking part in the trial had "a feeling of well-being without any side-effects." The herb has a long-established antispasmodic action.

Traditional & current uses

Ancient herb Cardamom has been highly valued both as a spice and a medicine and was known in Greece in the 4th century BCE.

Digestive problems Throughout history, cardamom has been used for the relief of digestive problems, especially indigestion, gas, cramping, and irritable bowel syndrome. The seed's pleasant taste means that cardamom is often added to digestive remedies to improve their flavor.

Current Indian uses Cardamom is used in India for many conditions, including asthma, bronchitis, kidney stones, anorexia, debility, and weakened vata (see p. 41)

Chinese remedy In China, the herb is taken for urinary incontinence and as a tonic.

Bad breath Cardamom is an effective treatment for bad breath, and when taken with garlic helps reduce its smell.

Aphrodisiac The herb contains androgenic compounds and has a long-standing reputation as a tonic and aphrodisiac. A traditional Arabian recipe blends cardamom with coffee..

Self-help use

Wind & bloating, p. 326.

Parts used

Seeds are crushed for use in infusions or have their volatile oil extracted.

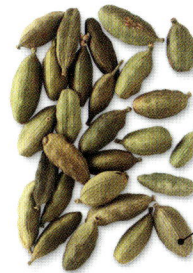

Green seed pods indicate that the seeds are good quality

Seed pods

Opened seed pods

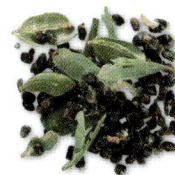

Crushed seeds and seed pods

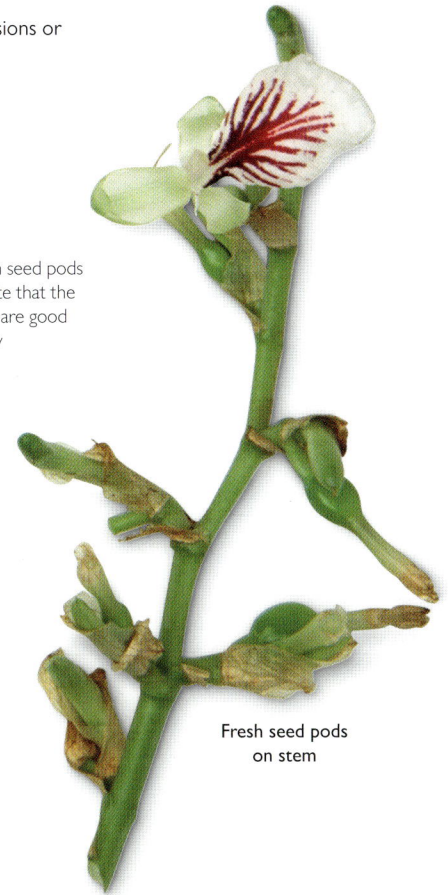

Fresh seed pods on stem

Key preparations & their uses

Essential oil For digestive pain, dilute 10 drops with 4 tsp carrier oil (see p. 307). Gently rub into the abdomen.

Tincture (to make, p. 302) improves the appetite. For poor appetite, combine 5 drops with 15 drops gentian tincture and take 3 times a day.

Infusion (to make, p. 301) is a pleasant drink. For indigestion, drink ¾ cup (150 ml) after meals.

Crush cardamom seeds using a mortar and pestle just before you are about to use them.

Caution Do not take the essential oil internally

Eleutherococcus senticosus (Araliaceae)

Siberian ginseng, Eleuthero

Siberian ginseng is a powerful tonic herb with an impressive range of health benefits. Unlike many plant medicines, Siberian ginseng is generally more useful in maintaining good health than in treating ill health. Research shows that extracts aid the body in coping with both physical and mental stress, including overwork and extreme cold or heat, and the herb is taken to support performance during periods of ongoing pressure or stress.

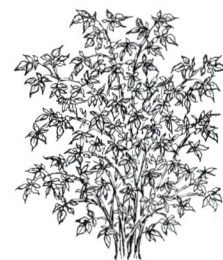

A deciduous, hardy shrub growing to 10 ft (3 m). It has 3–7 toothed leaflets on each stem.

Habitat & cultivation

Siberian ginseng is native to eastern Russia, China, Korea, and Japan. It can be grown from seed, but it is a difficult plant to germinate. The root is lifted in the fall and dried.

Related species

Wu jia pi (*Acanthopanacis gracilistylus*) is a very close relative of Siberian ginseng, used in Chinese herbal medicine to treat "cold, damp" conditions.

Key constituents

• Eleutherosides, 0.6–0.9%
• Polysaccharides • Triterpenoid saponins • Glycans

Key actions

• Adaptogenic • Tonic • Protects the immune system

Research

Russian studies There has been much research into Siberian ginseng in Russia since the 1950s, although the exact method by which it stimulates stamina and resistance to stress is not yet understood.

Tonic herb Siberian ginseng appears to have a general tonic effect on the body, in particular on the adrenal glands, helping the body withstand heat, cold, infection, other physical stresses, and radiation. It has even been given to astronauts to counter the effects of weightlessness.

Stamina Athletes have experienced as much as a 9% improvement in stamina when taking Siberian ginseng.

Traditional & current uses

Enhancing resilience Siberian ginseng is taken to improve mental resilience, such as in preparation for tests, and to reduce the impact of physical training and stress on the body.

Exhaustion Siberian ginseng can be highly beneficial in relieving exhaustion and debilitated states resulting from overwork or long-term stress. It can also prove helpful in treating chronic fatigue, although in some cases it may be overly stimulating.

Cancer treatment A valuable remedy during conventional cancer treatment, Siberian ginseng supports vitality and healthy function when taking chemotherapy, and may reduce side effects. Russian studies suggest that it helps reduce the harmful effects of radiation.

Self-help uses

• Convalescence, p. 329.
• Stress, p. 318.

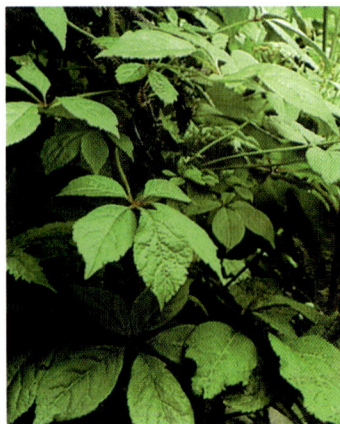

Siberian ginseng can help those exposed to toxic chemicals and radiation and was given to people following the nuclear disaster at Chernobyl in 1986.

Parts used

Root is unearthed in the fall, dried whole, and then chopped up for use in medicinal preparations.

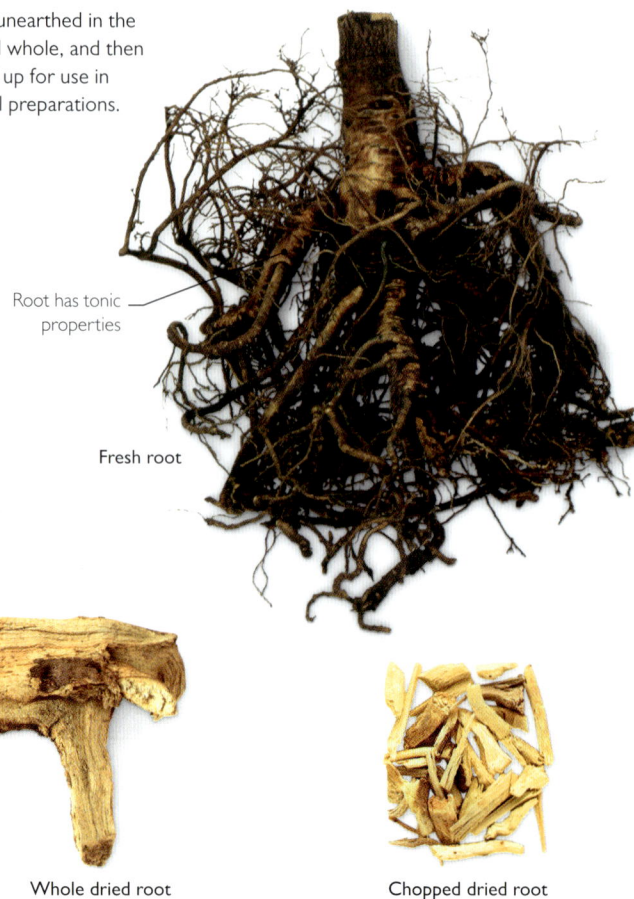

Root has tonic properties

Fresh root

Whole dried root

Chopped dried root

Key preparations & their uses

Decoction (to make, p. 301). Take 2 tbsp twice a day as a general tonic.

Tincture (to make, p. 302). During busy periods, take ½ tsp with water 3 times a day.

Capsules Make with powder (see p. 302) and for long-term stress take 1 g of capsules daily.

Tablets are a convenient way of taking Siberian ginseng. Use before tests or other stressful events.

Cautions Healthy young adults should not take for more than 6 weeks. Can be taken long term with professional advice. Avoid caffeine when taking Siberian ginseng. Side effects are rare, but more likely if the standard dose is exceeded.

Ephedra sinica (Ephedraceae)

Ephedra, *Ma huang* (Chinese)

Ephedra is a strongly stimulant, acrid-tasting herb that has a central place in Chinese and other herbal traditions. According to legend, the bodyguards of Genghis Khan, threatened with beheading if they fell asleep on sentry duty, used to take a tea containing ephedra to stay alert. Today, ephedra is used in the West and in China for problems ranging from chills and fevers to asthma and hay fever.

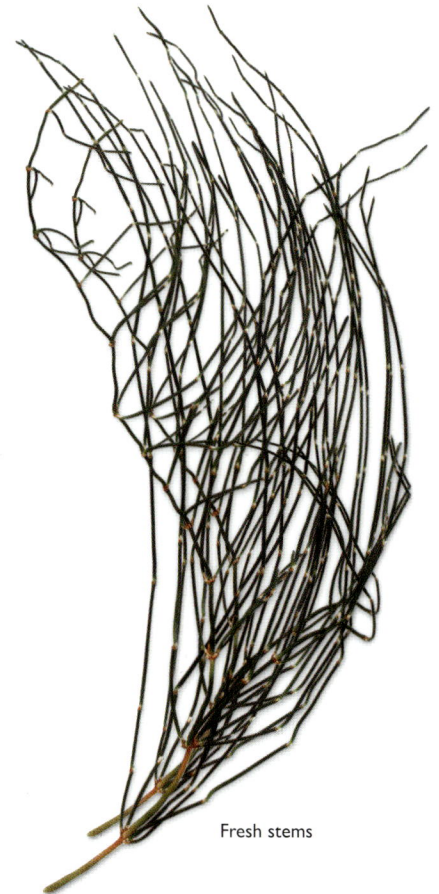

An evergreen shrub growing to 20 in (50 cm), with long, narrow, sprawling stems and tiny leaves.

Habitat & cultivation

Native to northern China and Inner Mongolia, ephedra often grows in desert areas. It is propagated from seed in the fall or by root division in the fall or spring and needs well-drained soil. The stems are gathered throughout the year and dried.

Related species

Other *Ephedra* species with similar medicinal properties to ephedra grow throughout the northern hemisphere. In North America, related species were used to treat fevers and relieve kidney pain, while in India, *Ephedra* species were taken for asthma, hay fever, and rheumatism.

Key constituents

• Protoalkaloids (ephedrine, pseudoephedrine) • Tannins
• Saponin • Flavone • Volatile oil

Key actions

• Increases sweating • Dilates the bronchioles (small airways in the lungs) • Dries mucus membranes
• Diuretic • Stimulant • Raises blood pressure

Research

Active constituents Most of the active constituents mimic the effect of adrenaline within the body, increasing alertness. Ephedrine, extracted originally from ephedra, was first synthesized in 1927 and is used as a decongestant and anti-asthmatic.

Whole herb When used at the correct dosage, the whole herb has significant therapeutic effects—including dilating the bronchial airways—and a very low incidence of side effects.

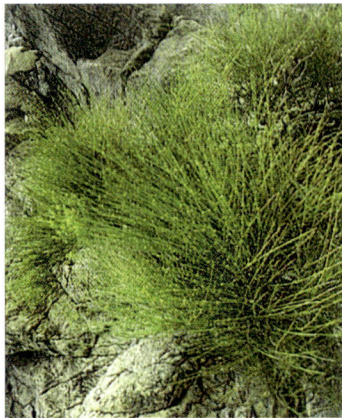

Ma Huang was found in a Middle Eastern neolithic grave, indicating that it may have been used as a medicine 60,000 years ago.

Ephedra abuse Ephedra has been banned in the US due to frequent abuse of the herb, as an amphetamine-type "high" and, at excessive dosage, in weight-loss regimens. At therapeutic dosage, and with professional guidance, ephedra rarely gives rise to side effects.

Traditional & current uses

Historical uses Traditionally, Zen monks used ephedra to promote calm concentration during meditation.

Chinese herb In China, ephedra is popular for chills and fevers, coughs and wheezing, and in combination with rehmannia (*Rehmannia glutinosa*, p. 270) it is given to treat kidney yin deficiency (see pp. 44–45).

Current Western uses Ephedra is used principally in current Western herbal medicine as a treatment for asthma and hay fever, and for the acute onset of colds and flu. It also helps raise blood pressure, cool fevers, and alleviate rheumatism.

Parts used

Stems are collected throughout the year. Ma Huang is best known in medicine for the ephedrine that it contains.

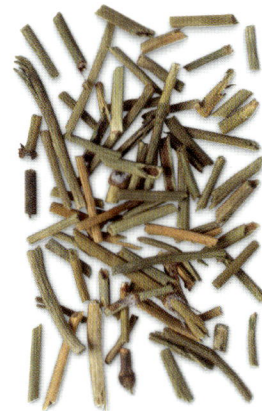

Dried stems

Fresh stems

Key preparations & their uses

Decoction Prescribed by herbalists for asthma.

Powder Used by the Chinese to treat kidney energy deficiency.

Tincture Used in treatments to alleviate the aches and pains of rheumatism.

Cautions Take only under professional supervision. Do not take if suffering from angina, glaucoma, high blood pressure, enlarged prostate gland, or overactive thyroid gland. Ephedra occasionally causes side effects, including headaches, tremors, and insomnia. Restricted herb in some countries.

Eucalyptus globulus (Myrtaceae)

Eucalyptus, Blue gum

Eucalyptus, a traditional Aboriginal remedy, is a powerful antiseptic used all over the world for relieving coughs and colds, sore throats, and other infections. It is warming and stimulating, and for many people its scent conjures up days spent in bed during childhood with eucalyptus and other oils smothered on the chest. Eucalyptus is a common ingredient in many over-the-counter cold remedies.

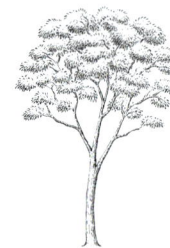

An evergreen tree growing to 195 ft (60 m), with a blue-gray trunk and green leaves.

Habitat & cultivation

Native to Australia, eucalyptus is cultivated on plantations in tropical, subtropical, and temperate areas of the world. Planting can cause ecological problems because the trees absorb huge quantities of water and prevent the growth of native plants. This can be beneficial, however, drying up marshy areas and so reducing the risk of malaria. The leaves are harvested as required and are either dried or distilled for oil.

Related species

Many other *Eucalyptus* species contain valuable essential oils, including *E. smithii* (p. 212).

Key constituents

• Volatile oil (cineole, up to 80%)
• Flavonoids • Tannins • Resin

Key actions

• Antiseptic • Analgesic
• Expectorant • Stimulates local blood flow • Insect repellent

Research

Essential oil Extensive research into eucalyptus essential oil during the last 50 years has shown it to have a marked antiseptic action and the ability to dilate the bronchioles (small airways) of the lungs. The action of the essential oil as a whole is stronger than that of its main constituent, cineole.

Traditional & current uses

Infections Eucalyptus is a traditional Aboriginal remedy for infections and fevers. It is now used throughout the world for these ailments.
Antiseptic The herb is an antiseptic and is very helpful for colds, flu, and sore throats.

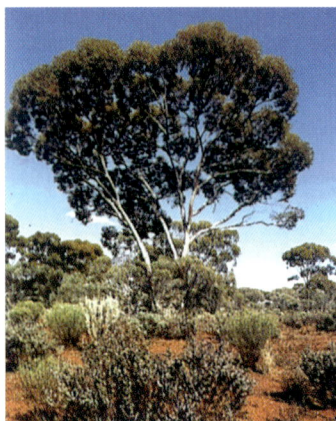

Eucalyptus was first introduced to the West from Australia in the 19th century.

Expectorant Eucalyptus is a strong expectorant, suitable for chest infections, including bronchitis and pneumonia.
Warming The diluted essential oil, applied to the skin as a chest or sinus rub, has a warming and slightly anesthetic effect, helping to relieve respiratory infections. The same effect occurs when the infusion or tincture is used as a gargle.
Pain relief Diluted essential oil applied to the affected area can help relieve rheumatic joints characterized by aching pains and stiffness, as well as neuralgia and some bacterial skin infections.

Self-help uses

• Congestion, sinus problems, & earache, p. 322. • Coughs & bronchitis, p. 320.

Parts used

Leaves, which contain antiseptic chemicals, are either dried or used for essential oil.

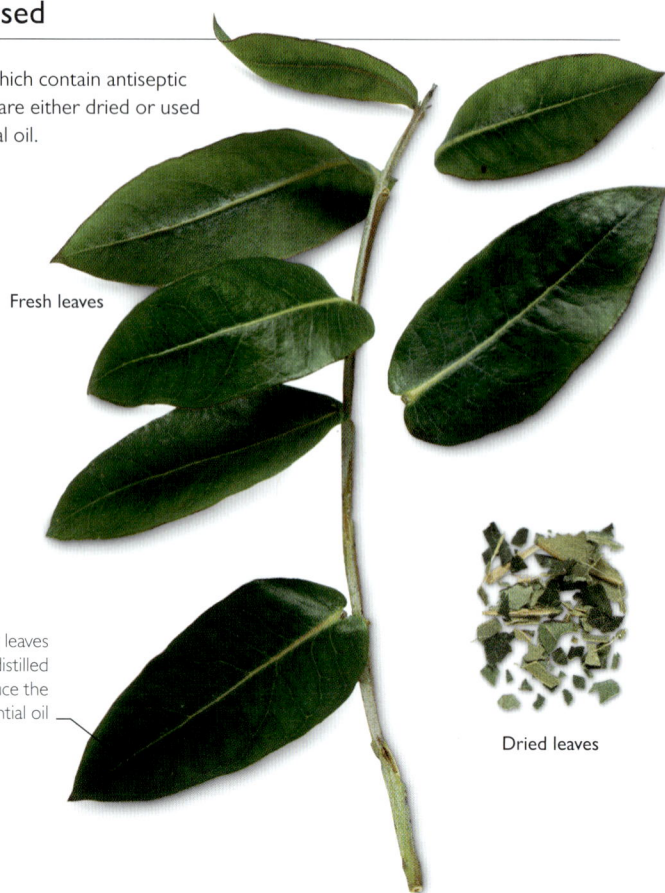

Fresh leaves

Fresh leaves are distilled to produce the essential oil

Dried leaves

Key preparations & their uses

Capsules, (to make, p. 302). For bronchitis, take a 200 mg capsule 3 times a day.

Lozenges, containing eucalyptus. Take for sore throats.

Inhalation For colds, add 10 drops essential oil to boiling water (p. 307).

Essential oil (to use, p. 307). Use 5 drops diluted with 2 tsp carrier oil as a chest or sinus rub.

Tincture (to make, p. 302). For chest coughs, add ½ tsp tincture to ½ cup (100 ml) water and take twice a day.

Caution Do not take essential oil internally except under professional supervision. Do not give to small children or infants.

Eugenia caryophyllata syn. Syzgium aromaticum (Myrtaceae)

Clove

Cloves, the dried flower buds of the clove tree, are best known as a spice, but are also highly valued as an herbal medicine, particularly in India and Southeast Asia. Native to the Molucca Islands, cloves were one of the earliest spices to be traded and were imported into Alexandria in 176 CE. The cloves contain the best essential oil, but the stems and leaves of the tree can also be distilled for their oil.

An evergreen, pyramid-shaped tree growing to 49 ft (15 m). The tree is strongly aromatic.

Habitat & cultivation

Originally from the Molucca Islands (Indonesia) and the southern Philippines, cloves are now grown extensively in Tanzania and Madagascar, and to a lesser extent in the West Indies and Brazil. The tree is grown from seed in spring or from semi-ripe cuttings in summer. Twice a year, the unopened flower buds are picked as they develop, and then sun-dried.

Key constituents

• Volatile oil containing eugenol (up to 85%), acetyleugenol, methyl salicylate, pinene, vanillin • Gum • Tannins

Key actions

• Antiseptic • Carminative
• Stimulant • Analgesic • Prevents vomiting • Antispasmodic
• Eliminates parasites

Research

Volatile oil Argentinian research in 1994 showed clove's volatile oil to be strongly antibacterial. Eugenol (a phenol) is the largest and most important component of the volatile oil. It is strongly anesthetic and antiseptic, and therefore useful in pain relief for toothache, and as an antiseptic for many conditions.
Acetyleugenol Acetyleugenol, another component of the volatile oil, has been shown to be strongly antispasmodic.

Traditional & current uses

Ancient all-purpose remedy Cloves have been used in Southeast Asia for thousands of years and were regarded as a panacea for almost all ills.
Antiseptic The antiseptic property of cloves makes them useful for treating certain viral conditions. In tropical Asia, they have often been given to treat infections such as malaria, cholera, and tuberculosis, and parasites such as scabies.
Antispasmodic Digestive discomfort, such as gas, colic, and abdominal bloating, can be relieved with cloves. Their antispasmodic property also eases coughs and, applied topically, relieves muscle spasms.
Mind & body stimulant Cloves are a stimulant, both to the mind (improving memory) and to the body as a whole, and have been used as an aphrodisiac in India and in the West. The herb has also been used to prepare for childbirth. It helps stimulate and strengthen uterine muscle contractions in labor.
Additional uses Besides all their other uses, cloves can be used to treat acne, skin ulcers, sores, and styes. They also make a potent mosquito and clothes moth repellent. Oranges that had been studded with cloves were used in the Moluccas as insect repellents.

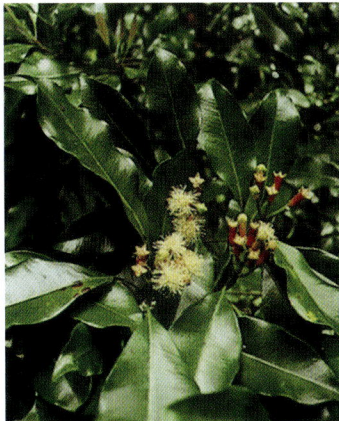

Cloves are pink when unripe, but later turn brown when they are dried outside in the sun.

Parts used

Flower buds are picked unopened and dried for use in infusions or powders and for oil extraction.

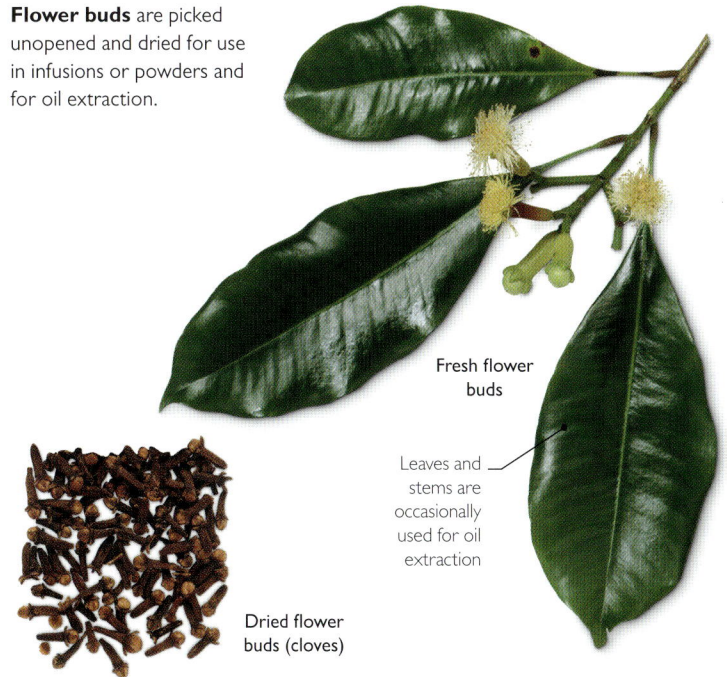

Fresh flower buds

Leaves and stems are occasionally used for oil extraction

Dried flower buds (cloves)

Key preparations & their uses

Infusion For colic, infuse 2 cloves in 1 cup (150 ml) of water (*see* p. 301). Take 3 times daily.

Tincture (to make, p. 302). For flatulence, take 20 drops with water 3 times a day.

Essential oil For toothache, dab 1–2 drops of oil onto a cotton ball and rub over the affected tooth.

Cautions External use can cause dermatitis. Do not take essential oil internally except under professional supervision.

Western herbalism Despite the bewildering variety of their therapeutic uses, cloves are underrated in the West. They are used regularly only in mouthwashes, and for their local anesthetic effect, for example in relieving toothache.

Self-help uses

• Acne & boils, p. 315. • Fever, p. 321.
• Fungal skin infections, p. 314.
• Neuralgia, p. 318. • Toothache, p. 318.

Filipendula ulmaria (Rosaceae)

Meadowsweet, Queen of the meadow

In medieval times, meadowsweet was a favorite strewing herb—Gerard wrote in his *Herball* (1597) that "the smell thereof makes the heart merry and joyful and delighteth the senses." Salicylic acid isolated from the plant was first synthesized in 1860 and later used to develop aspirin. Nowadays, meadowsweet is taken for gastric problems and inflammatory conditions, such as arthritis.

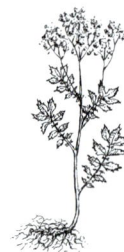

A perennial reaching 5 ft (1.5 m), with toothed leaves and clusters of creamy, scented flowers.

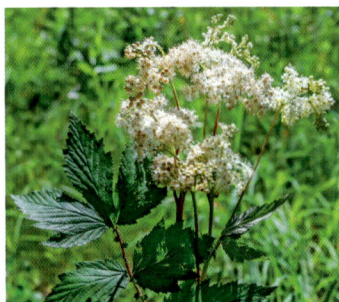

Meadowsweet was called "meadwort" in the Middle Ages, as it was used to flavor mead.

Habitat & cultivation

Native to Europe, meadowsweet grows easily in damp places, preferring ditches and the banks of streams and rivers. It seeds itself freely, but can also be propagated by root division in fall or spring. Leaves and flowering tops are harvested in summer when the flowers open.

Key constituents

- Flavonol glycosides (approximately 1%), mainly glycosides of quercetin
- Phenolic glycosides (salicylates)
- Volatile oil (salicylaldehyde)
- Polyphenols (tannins)

Key actions

- Anti-inflammatory • Antirheumatic
- Astringent • Diuretic
- Stimulates sweating

Research

Salicylates The salicylates are aspirin-type substances that help reduce inflammation and relieve pain, for example in arthritic conditions. However, meadowsweet and its salicylates should not be seen as an equivalent of aspirin. Unlike aspirin, salicylates do not irritate the stomach lining or cause ulceration—key conditions for which meadowsweet is commonly taken—and salicylates do not have blood-thinning properties. **Radiation** A 2015 Russian laboratory study found that meadowsweet significantly protected against radiation-induced cancer.

Traditional & current uses

Acid indigestion The herb is a key remedy for acid indigestion, gastritis, and gastro-oesophogeal reflux and can be taken long term to help relieve these common digestive problems. Its mode of action is not well understood, though its anti-inflammatory action is clearly important.

Urinary remedy It has mild urinary antiseptic activity and has been used to treat cystitis and urethritis.

Arthritis Meadowsweet is commonly taken as a remedy for rheumatic and arthritic problems such as osteoarthritis, gout, lumbago, and sciatica. It is a mild diuretic and is thought to help the kidneys clear acid residues from the body, thereby relieving joint inflammation, which is often associated with acidity.

Digestive remedy Meadowsweet is a safe remedy for diarrhea, even in children, and is used with other herbs for irritable bowel syndrome.

Other uses Meadowsweet has traditionally been taken in much the same way as aspirin—to ease the pain and discomfort of headache, colds and flu, and toothache.

Self-help uses

- Acidity with gastritis, p. 317. • Arthritis associated with acid indigestion or a peptic ulcer, p. 323. • Heartburn, p. 327.

Parts used

Flowering tops and leaves contain salicylates that reduce inflammation. They are harvested in summer.

Fresh flowering tops and leaves

Creamy white flowers smell of almonds

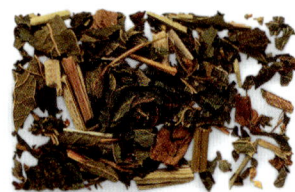

Dried flowering tops and leaves

Key preparations & their uses

Tincture (to make, p. 302). For painful joints, soak a pad in 5 tsp (25 ml) tincture and apply to the area.

Tablets Take for rheumatic aches.

Infusion Add freshly boiled water to the herb (*see* p. 301). For indigestion, take ½ cup (100 ml) every 2 hours.

Decoction (to make, p. 301). For diarrhea, take ¾ cup (150 ml) 2–3 times a day.

Powder For acidity, take ½ tsp mixed with a little water 3 times a day.

Caution Do not take if allergic to aspirin.

Gentiana lutea (Gentianaceae)

Gentian

Gentian is a powerful bitter, and the herb is an essential ingredient of traditional aperitifs and bitters such as Angostura bitters. The customary aperitif about half an hour before a meal is more than a social nicety—the bitter constituents stimulate gastric juices and prime the stomach, enabling it to cope effectively with a heavy meal. Medicinally, gentian strengthens a weak or underactive digestive system.

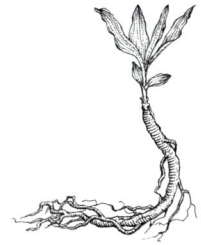

An erect perennial growing to 4 ft (1.2 m), with star-shaped yellow flowers and oval leaves.

Habitat & cultivation

This largest member of the diverse gentian family is native to the Alps and other mountainous regions of central and southern Europe from Spain to the Balkans, flourishing at altitudes of 2,300–7,900 ft (700–2,400 m). The large root crowns can be split or the plant grown from seed. Due to overharvesting from the wild, this is now a threatened species, so buy only cultivated root. It needs a loamy soil and a sheltered site. The root is dug up in early fall and dried.

Related species

Many gentian species are bitter-tasting plants and a number are used in herbal medicine as a result, for example Japanese gentian (*G. scabra*) and the Chinese *qin jiao* (*G. macrophylla*).

Key constituents

• Bitter principles (gentiopicroside, amarogentin) • Gentianose • Inulin
• Phenolic acids

Key actions

• Bitter • Digestive stimulant •
Eases stomach pain

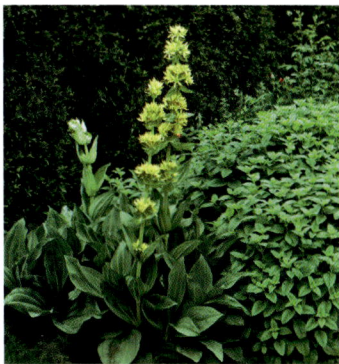

Gentian is a tall, attractive plant and has been cultivated in gardens at least since the time of the 16th-century herbalist Gerard.

Research

• **Amarogentin** Although present in much smaller quantities than gentiopicroside, amarogentin is the constituent largely responsible for the bitterness of gentian. It is 3,000 times more bitter than gentiopicroside, and tasted at dilutions of 1:50,000 it is possibly the most bitter substance on the planet.

Traditional & current uses

• **Origin of the name** Gentius, king of Illyria in the 2nd century BCE, reputedly discovered the virtues of the plant. The name gentian attests to its use in classical times.

• **Action of bitter principles** There are 5 main taste receptors on the tongue—sweet, sour, salt, bitter, and umami. It has been shown that the bitter principles in gentian stimulate the bitter taste receptors on the tongue, causing an increase in the production of saliva and gastric secretions. This in turn stimulates the appetite and improves the action of the digestive system in general.

• **Digestive stimulant** By stimulating the action of the stomach, many symptoms associated with weak digestion, such as gas, indigestion, and poor appetite, are relieved. Stomach and other secretions are improved, which in turn helps increase the absorption of nutrients. The herb also acts as a stimulant on the gallbladder and liver, encouraging them to function more efficiently. Gentian is therefore useful in almost any condition where the digestive system needs to be toned up. It is often taken as a digestive tonic in old age.

• **Nutrient absorption** By improving digestive function, gentian increases the absorption of

Parts used

Root is harvested in the fall for use in remedies to improve digestion.

Root contains
bitter principles

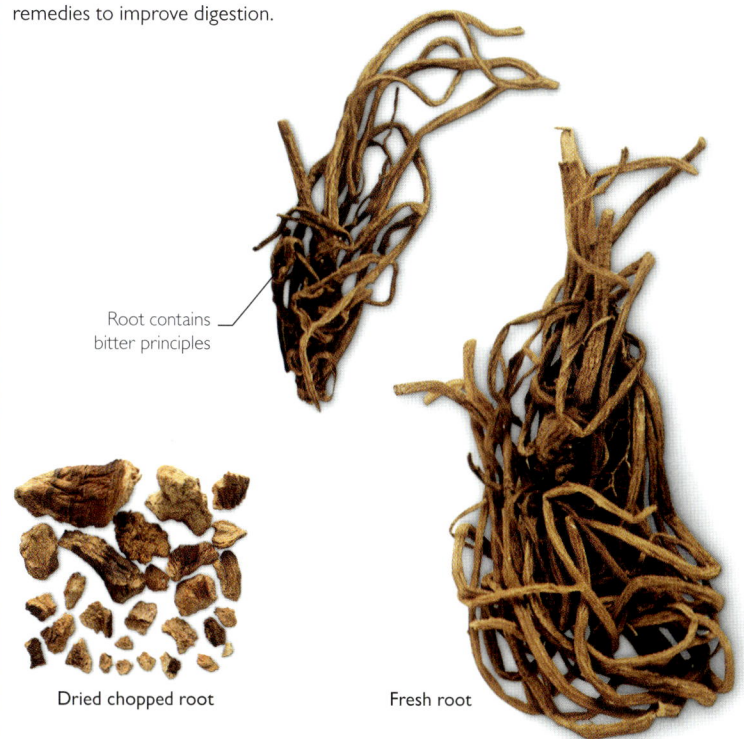

Dried chopped root

Fresh root

Key preparations & their uses

Tincture (to make, p. 302). For poor appetite, take 2–5 drops with water before meals.

Decoction (to make, p. 301). For anemia and weakened digestion,

take 5 tsp 3–5 times a day.

Caution Do not take if suffering from acid indigestion or a peptic ulcer.

nutrients across the gut wall. It aids the absorption of a wide range of nutrients, including iron and vitamin B_{12}, and is therefore useful for iron-deficiency anemia (usually resulting from blood loss). It is often added to prescriptions for women

with heavy menstrual bleeding.

Self-help uses

• Anemia, p. 311. • Fever, p. 321.
• Weakened digestion, p. 329.
• Gas & bloating, p. 316.

Ginkgo biloba (Ginkgoaceae)

Ginkgo, Maidenhair tree, *Bai guo* (Chinese)

Ginkgo is thought to be the oldest tree on the planet, first growing about 190 million years ago. Though long used as a medicine in its native China, its therapeutic properties have only recently been understood. The leaves (and their extract) are used to treat poor circulation and to maintain a plentiful blood flow to the central nervous system. Ginkgo is also valuable for asthma and other allergic problems.

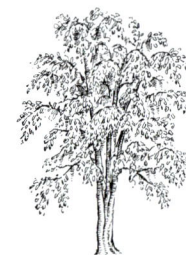

A deciduous tree with one or several main trunks and spreading branches. It grows to 100 ft (30 m).

Habitat & cultivation

Native to China, ginkgo trees are grown on large-scale plantations in China, France, and in South Carolina. They produce green to yellow fan-shaped leaves with radiating veins, and round fruits about 1 in (3 cm) across. Leaves and fruit are harvested in the fall.

Key constituents

• Flavonoids • Ginkgolides
• Bilobalides

Key actions

• Circulatory tonic • Anti-inflammatory • Anti-asthmatic
• Anti-allergenic • Antispasmodic

Research

Clinical trials Extensive research since the 1960s has established the importance of ginkgo in improving poor cerebral circulation and aiding memory and concentration.

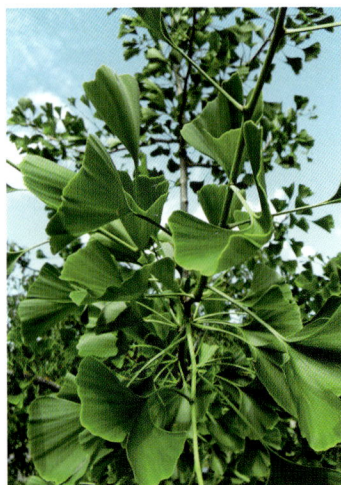

Ginkgo trees are widely cultivated for their leaves, which are an excellent herbal remedy for poor circulation and asthma.

Clinical trials have produced variable results in terms of ginkgo's use as a treatment for dementia, including Alzheimer's disease, though the majority indicate that extracts are valuable in supporting memory and cognition and slowing the impact of mild to moderate dementia. In a 2019 review of clinical trials, ginkgo extract was found "to improve the cognitive function in patients who suffered from mild dementia during long-term administration (more than 24 weeks)." Ginkgo extracts are routinely prescribed for mild to moderate dementia in several countries, including Germany, Switzerland, and China.
Anti-inflammatory action Ginkgo's ability to reduce inflammation makes it valuable in conditions where nerve tissue is damaged by inflammation, for example multiple sclerosis.
Platelet activating factor (PAF) Ginkgo inhibits PAF, a substance released by a range of blood cells that causes the blood to become stickier and more likely to produce clots.

Traditional & current uses

Chinese herbal medicine Ginkgo seeds are used to relieve wheezing and to lessen phlegm. They are also given to treat vaginal discharge, a weak bladder, and incontinence. The leaves are traditionally used for treating asthma.
Western herbal medicine Western interest in ginkgo has concentrated on the remarkable ability of the leaves to improve the circulation, especially poor circulation to the brain, and the herb's anti-allergenic and anti-inflammatory actions, which make it a particularly useful herbal remedy for the treatment of asthma. Ginkgo is a best-selling herbal medicine in France and Germany, where it is taken daily by

millions of people from middle age onward to maintain and improve cerebral circulation and the memory, and to reduce the possibility of a stroke. It is also a valuable medicine to take after a stroke, where it is thought to support nerve tissue and strengthen the circulation.

Parts used

Leaves improve the circulation. They are used to make tinctures, tablets, and fluid extract.

Seeds are prescribed by the Chinese for urinary problems and wheezing.

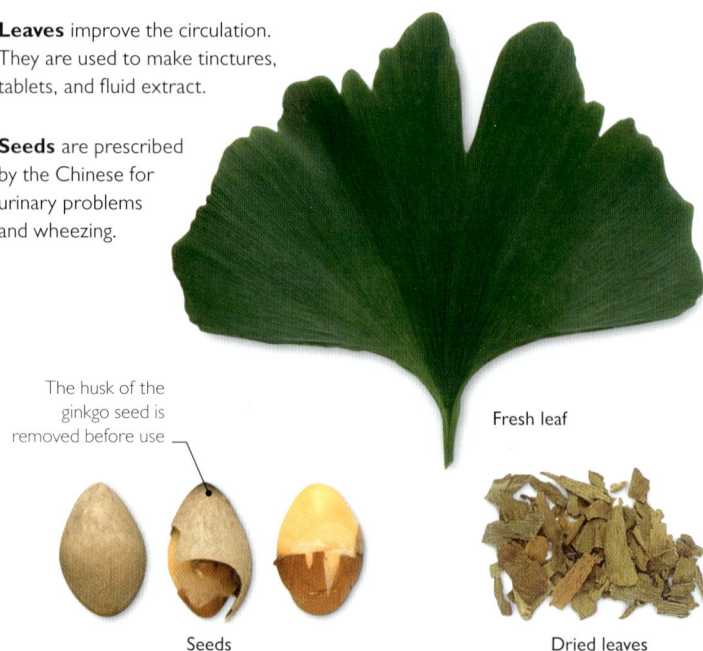

The husk of the ginkgo seed is removed before use

Fresh leaf

Seeds

Dried leaves

Key preparations & their uses

Tincture of leaves (to make, p. 302). For poor circulation, take 1 tsp 2–3 times a day with water.

Tablets Take for poor circulation and memory loss.

Decoction of the seeds is used by herbalists to treat wheezing.

Fluid extract made from the fresh leaves is prescribed by medical herbalists for asthma.

Cautions Do not exceed the dose. May cause toxic reactions if taken to excess. Take only with professional advice if using blood-thinning medication. Restricted herb in some countries.

Self-help uses

• Failing memory, p. 329.
• High blood pressure & arteriosclerosis, p. 311.

Glycyrrhiza glabra (Fabaceae)

Licorice, *Gancau* (Chinese), *Nadyapaan* (Hindi)

With a constituent—glycyrrhizic acid—that is 50 times sweeter than sugar, it is not surprising that licorice is mainly thought of as a candy. Yet it is also one of the most valuable of all herbal medicines, a powerful anti-inflammatory that is effective in conditions as varied as arthritis and canker sores. It is among the most used herbs in European medicine, and has been taken medicinally for several thousand years.

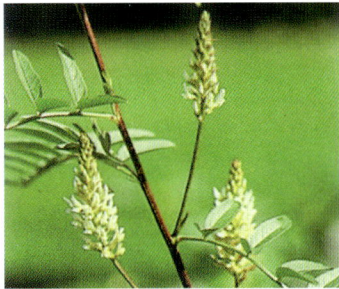

A woody-stemmed perennial growing to 6½ ft (2 m), with dark leaves and cream to mauve flowers.

Licorice has pealike flowers in summer. It is cultivated commercially for its roots.

Habitat & cultivation

Licorice grows wild in southeastern Europe and southwestern Asia, but it is now extensively cultivated. It is propagated by dividing the roots in the fall or spring. The root of 3–4-year-old plants is unearthed in late fall.

Related species

Various *Glycyrrhiza* species are used medicinally in a similar way to licorice, for example the Chinese gan cao (*G. uralensis*).

Key constituents

• Triterpene saponins (glycyrrhizin, up to 6%) • Isoflavones (liquiritin, isoliquiritin, formononetin)
• Polysaccharides • Phytosterols

Key actions

• Anti-inflammatory • Expectorant
• Demulcent • Adrenal agent
• Mild laxative

Research

Adrenal agent Research shows that on being broken down in the gut, glycyrrhizin has an anti-inflammatory and anti-arthritic action similar to hydrocortisone and other corticosteroid hormones. It stimulates production of hormones by the adrenal glands and reduces the breakdown of steroids by the liver and kidneys.
Clinical trials Licorice has a wide range of therapeutic applications, and this is reflected in the varied clinical trials into extracts of the herb. Positive outcomes have been found for: hepatitis B and nonalcoholic fatty liver disease; peptic ulcer and *Helicobacter pylori* infection; dry mouth, mouth ulcers and dental caries; insulin resistance; and skin conditions, including atopic dermatitis and vitiligo. It should be noted though, that at clinical trial dosages, long term licorice extract treatment led to raised blood pressure and reduced potassium levels.

Traditional & current uses

Traditional uses Licorice has long been valued for its medicinal uses. It was taken in ancient Greece for asthma, chest problems, and canker sores.
Soothing herb Inflammatory conditions of the digestive system such as canker sores, gastritis, peptic ulceration, and excessive acid problems benefit from licorice's demulcent and anti-inflammatory properties, as do many chest complaints, arthritis, inflamed joints, and some skin problems. Licorice is also soothing for inflamed eyes.
Adrenal stimulation Licorice stimulates the adrenal glands, helping in Addison's disease, where the adrenal glands cease to function normally.
Constipation Licorice is useful as a gentle laxative.

Self-help uses

• Constipation, p. 317. • Coughs & bronchitis, p. 311. • Loss of appetite & vomiting, p. 316. • Canker sores, p. 316. • Oral thrush, p. 324.

Parts used

Root is harvested in the fall. It has valuable anti-inflammatory properties.

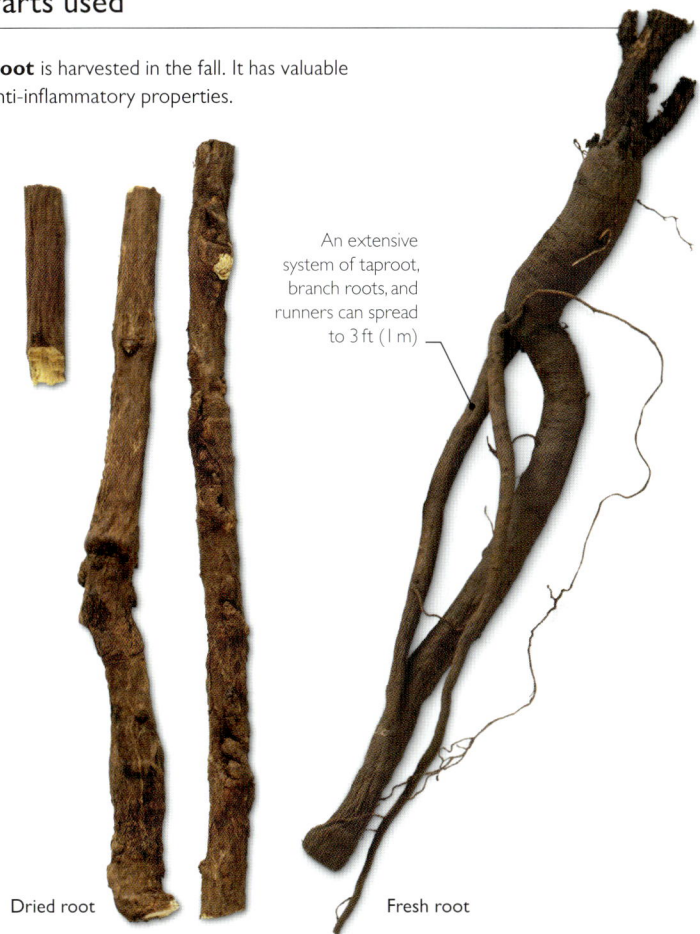

An extensive system of taproot, branch roots, and runners can spread to 3 ft (1 m)

Dried root

Fresh root

Key preparations & their uses

Tincture (to make, p. 302). For gastritis, add ½ tsp to ½ cup (100 ml) water and take twice a day.

Dried juice stick Chew for indigestion.

Powder Gently rub onto canker sores.

Decoction For constipation, make a decoction (see p. 301) with 1 part licorice and 3 parts dandelion root. Drink ¾ cup (150 ml) twice a day.

Fluid extract is prescribed for peptic ulcers.

Cautions Excessive doses can cause serious side effects, including high blood pressure. Do not take large doses with high blood pressure. During pregnancy, or for long-term use, take with professional advice.

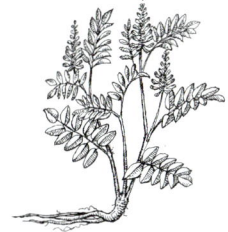

Hamamelis virginiana (Hamamelidaceae)

Witch hazel

Witch hazel was a traditional remedy of many Indigenous peoples of North America. They used poultices soaked in a decoction of bark to treat tumors and inflammations, especially of the eye, and took the herb internally for hemorrhaging and heavy menstrual bleeding. By the mid-18th century, Europeans had begun to value witch hazel for its astringency, and its use spread to Europe and beyond.

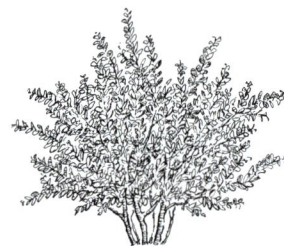

A small, deciduous tree growing to 16 ft (5 m), with coarsely toothed, broadly oval leaves.

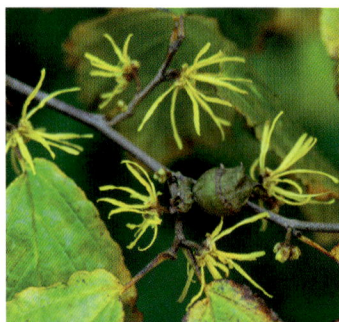

Witch hazel produces distinctive flowers in winter followed by brown fruit capsules that, when ripe, eject 2 seeds up to 13 ft (4 m) away from the tree.

Habitat & cultivation

Witch hazel is a woodland tree, indigenous to Canada and eastern parts of the US. Today it is commonly cultivated in Europe. The trees are grown from hardwood cuttings or from seed, both of which are planted in the fall. The leaves are gathered in summer and dried. The bark is harvested during the fall and dried as quickly as possible in the shade.

Related species

European hazel (*Corylus avellana*) is a similar herb. It is used occasionally in European herbal medicine as an astringent to treat diarrhea. The oil is nutritious and can be used to treat threadworms in children.

Key constituents

• Tannins (8–10%) • Flavonoids
• Bitter principle • Volatile oil (leaves only)

Key actions

• Astringent • Anti-inflammatory
• Stops external and internal bleeding

Traditional & current uses

Established properties Witch hazel contains large quantities of tannins. These have a drying, astringent effect, causing the tightening up of proteins in the skin and across the surface of abrasions. This creates a protective covering that increases resistance to inflammation and promotes healing of broken skin. Witch hazel also appears to help damaged blood vessels beneath the skin. It is thought that this effect may be due to the flavonoids as well as to the tannins. When witch hazel is distilled it retains its astringency, suggesting that astringent agents other than tannins are present.

Skin problems Witch hazel is a very useful herb for inflamed and tender skin conditions, such as eczema. It is mainly used where the skin has not been significantly broken and helps protect the affected area and prevent infection.

Damaged veins Witch hazel is valuable for damaged facial veins, varicose veins, and hemorrhoids, and is an effective remedy for bruises. Due to its astringent properties, it helps tighten distended veins and restore their normal structure.

Other uses A lotion can be applied to the skin for underlying problems such as cysts or tumors. Witch hazel also makes an effective eyewash for inflammation of the eyes. Less commonly, it is taken internally to alleviate diarrhea, helping to tighten up the mucous membranes of the intestines, and for bleeding of any kind.

Self-help uses

• Bruises, p. 314. • Cleansing wounds, p. 314. • Eczema, p. 310.
• Hemorrhoids, p. 312. • Skin rashes, p. 313. • Varicose veins, p. 312.

Parts used

Leaves and young twigs are distilled to make "witch hazel."

Bark is used in tinctures and ointments

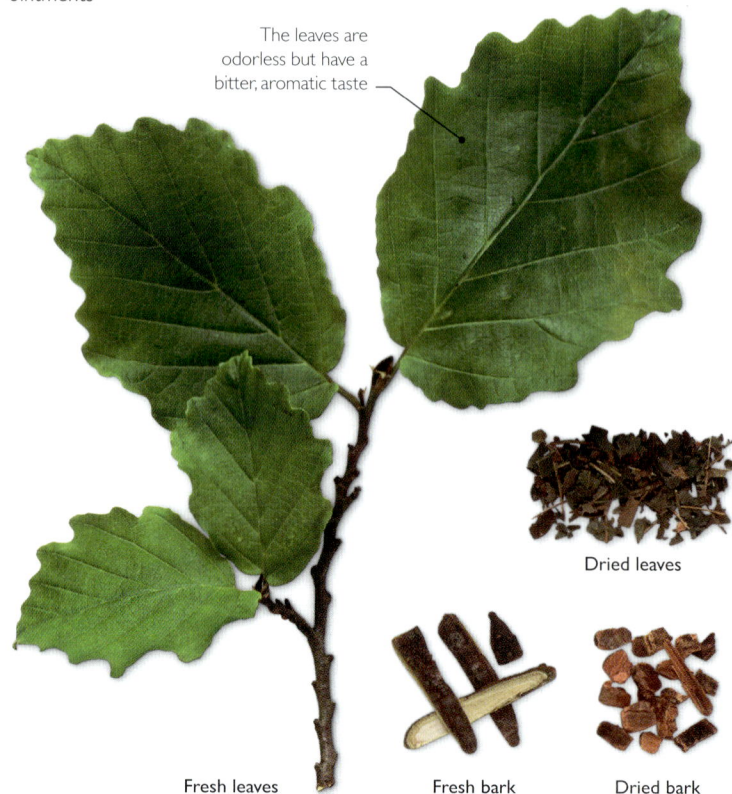

The leaves are odorless but have a bitter, aromatic taste

Dried leaves

Fresh leaves

Fresh bark

Dried bark

Key preparations & their uses

Tincture of bark (to make, p. 302). Dilute 1 tbsp in ½ cup (100 ml) cold water and sponge onto varicose veins.

Distilled witch hazel Dab onto insect stings, sore skin, and broken veins.

Ointment of bark (to make, p. 305). Apply to hemorrhoids twice a day.

Infusion of the leaves (to make, p. 301). Use as a lotion (see p. 306) for broken veins and cysts.

Caution If using internally, take only under professional supervision.

Harpagophytum procumbens (Pedaliaceae)

Devil's claw

The colorful name of this African plant is derived from the appearance of its tough, barbed fruit. The medicinal properties of devil's claw were first discovered by various southern African peoples, who used a decoction of the tuber to treat digestive problems and arthritis. The herb is now widely available in pharmacies and health food stores in the West as a remedy for arthritis and rheumatism.

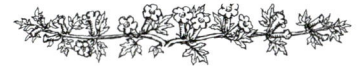

A trailing perennial, reaching 5 ft (1.5 m) in length, with fleshy lobed leaves and barbed, woody fruit.

Habitat & cultivation

Devil's claw is native to Namibia, Botswana, and South Africa, where it is a protected species due to over-harvesting of wild plants. It thrives in clay or sandy soils, preferring roadsides and waste grounds, especially places where natural vegetation has been cleared. Propagated from seed in spring, the young tubers are unearthed in the fall and cut into pieces about ¾ in (2 cm) long. Care is taken not to mix the tubers, which contain the active constituents, with the roots, as this can render the herb ineffective.

Related species

Two related species, both growing in Africa, are used medicinally in a more or less similar way to devil's claw.

Key constituents

- Iridoid glycosides (harpagoside)
- Sugars (stachyose) • Phytosterols
- Flavonoids

Key actions

- Anti-inflammatory • Analgesic
- Digestive stimulant • Anti-arthritic

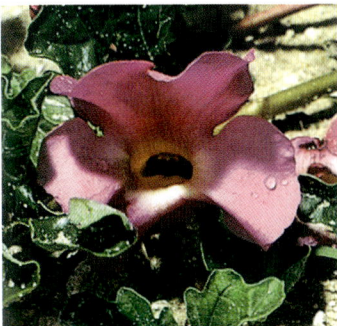

Devil's claw, found growing in the Transvaal, has bright purple flowers in spring.

Research

Anti-inflammatory French research (1992) indicated that devil's claw is anti-inflammatory, but opinion is divided on its effectiveness in practice.

Pain relief There is some evidence to confirm devil's claw's use as an analgesic as it seems to be effective in easing the symptoms of joint pain.

Bitter The strongly bitter action of devil's claw stimulates and tones the digestive system. Many arthritic conditions are associated with poor digestion and absorption of food, and the stimulant effect of this herb on the stomach and gallbladder contributes to its overall therapeutic value as an anti-arthritic remedy.

Traditional & current uses

African traditional remedy Devil's claw is used by various peoples in southern Africa, including the Khoisan and Bantu. Traditionally it has been used as a tonic, especially for digestive problems; for arthritis and rheumatism; to reduce fevers; and as an ointment for sores, ulcers, and boils.

Western uses Current Western use of devil's claw is broadly in line with its traditional application. It is commonly available over the counter in tablet form for arthritic and rheumatic conditions and can bring relief from pain arising from a range of joint and muscular problems, including gout, back pain, fibrositis, and rheumatoid arthritis.

Self-help uses

- Arthritis & inflamed joints, p. 323.
- Back pain due to joint inflammation, p. 323.

Parts used

Tuber is harvested in the fall and used in a variety of anti-arthritic preparations.

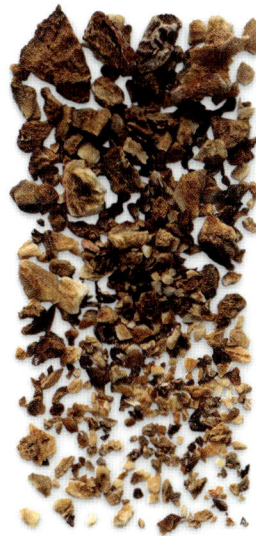

Chopped dried tuber

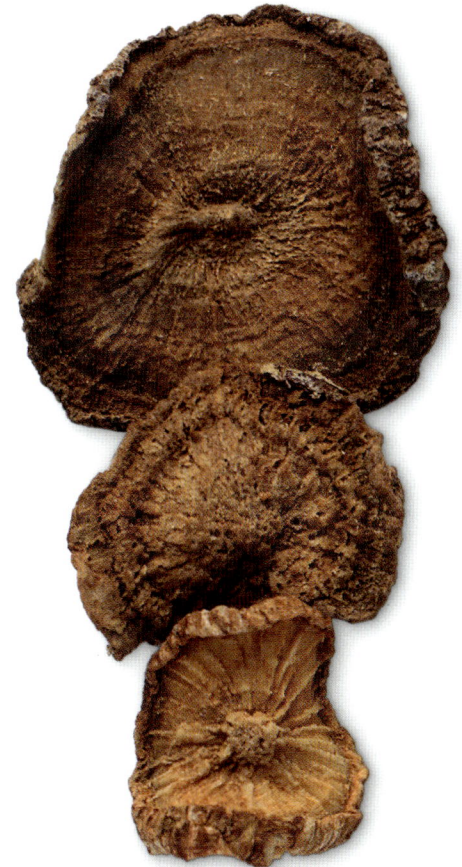

Sliced dried tuber

Key preparations & their uses

Decoction (to make, p. 301). For rheumatism, simmer 1 tsp root in ¾ cup (150 ml) water for 15 minutes. Take in small doses over 1–2 days.

Tincture (to make, p. 302). For arthritis associated with poor digestion, take 30 drops with water twice daily.

Tablets Take for arthritis and rheumatism.

Cautions Do not take if suffering from gallstones or peptic ulcer. Do not take during pregnancy. May interact with anticoagulants.

Humulus lupulus (Cannabaceae)

Hops

The bitter taste of hops, which is well known to beer drinkers, largely accounts for this herb's ability to strengthen and stimulate the digestion. Hops are also sedative and make a valuable remedy for sleeplessness and excitability. When the plant was first used to brew beer in England in the 16th century, it aroused great opposition: a petition to Parliament described it as "a wicked weed" that would "endanger the people."

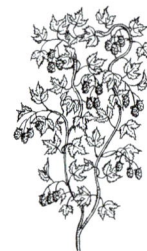

A tall, climbing perennial growing to 23 ft (7 m). Hops plants are either male or female.

Habitat & cultivation
Indigenous to Europe and Asia, hops flourish along roadsides and in open areas. They are grown commercially throughout northern Europe and the northern United States. Flowers of the female plant (strobiles) are picked in early fall and dried at a low temperature.

Related species
Hops are related to marijuana (*Cannabis sativa*, p. 78).

Key constituents
• Bitter principles (lupulin containing humulon, lupulon and valerianic acid)
• Volatile oil (1%), humulene
• Flavonoids • Polyphenolic tannins
• Estrogenic substances

Key actions
• Sedative • Soporific
• Antispasmodic • Aromatic bitter

Research
Hops bitter principles strongly stimulate digestive secretions. They have antimicrobial activity and have potential value in aiding late onset diabetes, metabolic syndrome, and osteoporosis. Numerous laboratory studies indicate that hops have significant anticancer activity. Extracts of the herb also have marked estrogenic activity, and are now marketed for the relief of menopausal symptoms such as hot flashes. Most of these effects will be only marginally present in hoppy beers.

Traditional & current uses
Historical uses Hops feature only occasionally in early herbals, and the health benefits ascribed to them are similar to our understanding today.

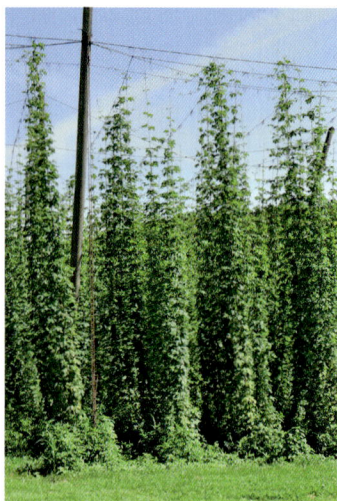

Hops have been cultivated for brewing beer since at least the 11th century. The bines (stems) are trained up raised wire runners.

Sedative The herb is used mostly for its sedative effect. A sachet placed inside a bed pillow releases an aroma that calms the mind. Hops help to reduce irritability and restlessness and promote a sound night's sleep.
Tension Blended with other herbs, hops are good for stress, anxiety, tension, and headaches, though they should not be used if depression is a factor. Their antispasmodic action makes hops useful for certain types of asthma and for period pain.
Aid to digestion Hops are beneficial for the digestion, increasing stomach secretions and relaxing spasms and colic.

Self-help uses
• Insomnia, p. 319.

Parts used

Strobiles (female flowers) are leafy cone-like catkins. Ripe strobiles may be used fresh but are more commonly dried for their sedative and bitter action.

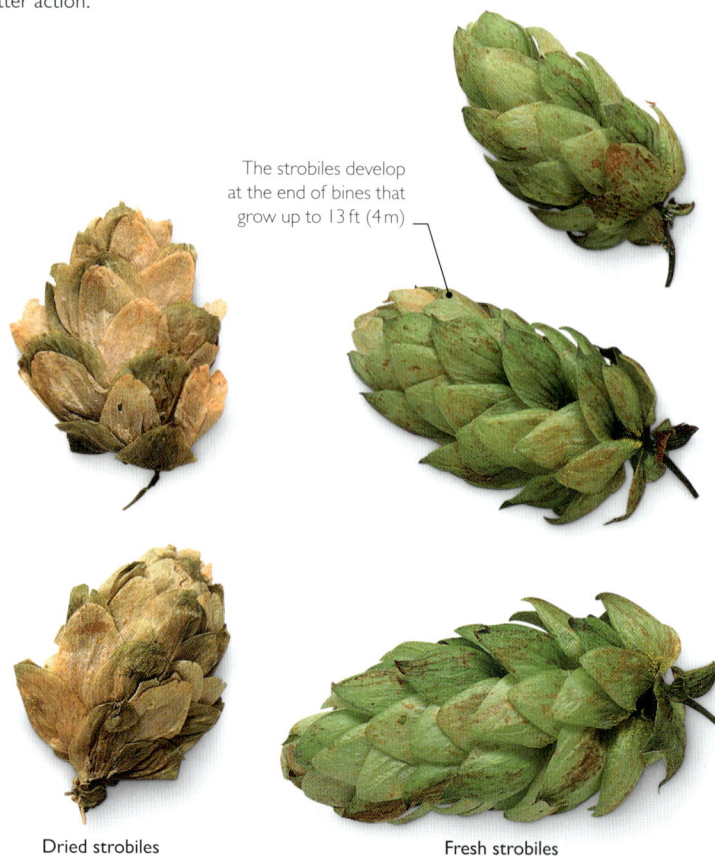

The strobiles develop at the end of bines that grow up to 13 ft (4 m)

Dried strobiles

Fresh strobiles

Key preparations & their uses

Sachet Make a sachet with 100 g dried herb. Put inside a pillow to aid sleep.

Infusion (to make, p. 301). For insomnia, drink ¾ cup (150 ml) at night.

Tablets usually contain other herbs. Take for stress or sleeplessness.

Tincture (to make, p. 302). For excessive anxiety, take 20 drops diluted in a glass of water 3 times a day. For digestive headaches, take 10 drops with water up to 6 times a day.

Capsules (to make, p. 302). To stimulate the appetite, take a 300 mg capsule 2 times a day before meals.

Hydrastis canadensis (Ranunculaceae)

Goldenseal

Goldenseal is a North American remedy, prized during the 19th century as a cure-all. The Cherokee used it—mixed with bear fat—as an insect repellent, and they also made it into a lotion for wounds; ulcers; and sore, inflamed eyes. It was given internally for stomach and liver problems. Today it is chiefly employed as an astringent, antibacterial remedy for infections of mucus membranes within the body.

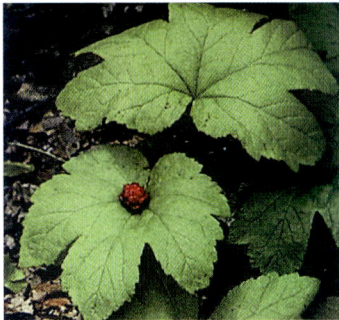

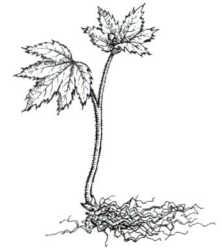

A small, herbaceous perennial, with a thick yellow root and an erect stem growing to 1 ft (30 cm).

Goldenseal is an unusual looking plant with a single, red, inedible fruit.

Habitat & cultivation
Goldenseal grows wild in moist mountainous woodland areas of North America and prefers soil that is well covered with dead leaves. Due to excessive harvesting in the wild, instances of goldenseal in its natural habitat have become very rare. In 1997 it was listed as an endangered species, and so only cultivated produce should be used. Goldenseal is propagated by root division. Rhizomes from 3-year-old plants are dug up in the fall and dried in the open air on cloth.

Key constituents
• Isoquinoline alkaloids (hydrastine, berberine, canadine) • Volatile oil
• Resin

Key actions
• Bitter tonic • Anti-inflammatory
• Antibacterial • Uterine stimulant
• Stops internal bleeding

Research
Alkaloids For an herb with such a high medicinal reputation, there has been very little research into its pharmacology, but it is known that goldenseal's medicinal actions are due largely to the isoquinoline alkaloids.
Hydrastine Research in Canada in the late 1960s showed that hydrastine constricts the blood vessels and stimulates the autonomic nervous system.
Antibacterial Although this herb's mode of action and degree of effectiveness is not fully known, it has been found that the herb's constituents collectively have a stronger antibacterial activity than berberine alone.
Berberine Berberine is bitter, antibacterial, and amebicidal. Recent research has established that it can be used to lower harmful blood-fat levels and stabilize blood glucose levels.
Canadine Research shows that this alkaloid stimulates the muscles of the uterus.

Traditional & current uses
Mucous membranes Most authorities agree that goldenseal is a potent remedy for disorders affecting mucous membranes of the body, notably of the eye, ear, nose, and throat; the stomach and intestines; and the vagina.
Countering infection As a dilute infusion, goldenseal can be used as an eyewash, as a mouthwash for infected gums, and as an extremely effective wash or douche for vaginal yeast and vaginal infections generally. The infusion is also valued as a remedy for psoriasis.
Digestive problems Taken internally, goldenseal increases digestive secretions, astringes the mucous membranes that line the gut, and checks inflammation. It should not be taken for extended periods of time as it reduces the gut's capacity to absorb certain nutrients, notably B vitamins.
• **Gynecological uses** Goldenseal helps reduce heavy menstrual bleeding and is used by herbal practitioners and midwives to help stop bleeding following childbirth (postpartum hemorrhage). Goldenseal stimulates the uterus and should not, therefore, be taken during pregnancy.

Parts used

Rhizome contains alkaloids that help soothe and astringe the mucous membranes.

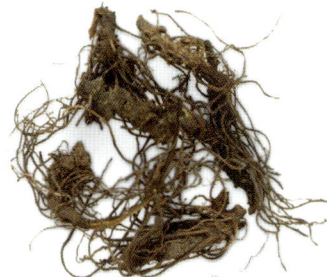

Dried rhizome

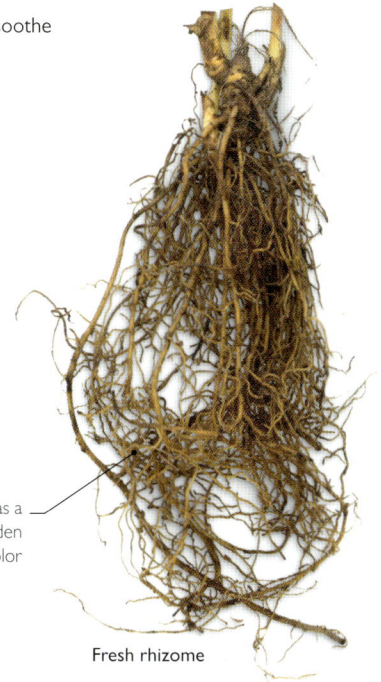

Rhizome has a characteristic golden yellow color

Fresh rhizome

Key preparations & their uses

Capsules For gastritis, take a 300 mg capsule 3 times a day.

Tincture (to make, p. 302). For excess mucus, take 20 drops with water 3 times a day.

Powder is used to make capsules (see p. 302).

Decoction (to make, p. 301). For sore throats, gargle 2½ tbsp 3–4 times a day.

Infusion of powder (to make, p. 301). For yeast infections, apply ¾ cup (150 ml).

Cautions Toxic if taken to excess. Do not take if suffering from high blood pressure. Do not take during pregnancy or while breastfeeding. Not suitable for children.

Hypericum perforatum (Hypericaceae)

St. John's wort

St. John's wort flowers at the summer solstice. In medieval Europe it was considered to have the power to protect against ill health and evil influences. Medicinally it was thought to heal wounds and "all down-heartedness." In the 19th century the herb fell into disuse, but recent research has brought it back into prominence as a key herb for nervous exhaustion and depression. It is now one of the most used herbal medicines in the world.

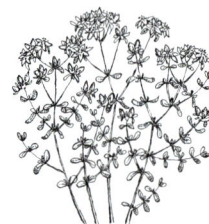

An erect perennial growing to 32 in (80 cm), with bright yellow flowers in a flat-topped cluster.

Habitat & cultivation

St. John's wort thrives in temperate regions worldwide. It prefers a sunny site and well-drained, chalky soil. It can be grown from seed or by root division in the fall. The flowering tops are harvested in summer.

Related species

A number of other *Hypericum* species have a roughly similar medicinal action.

Key constituents

- Phloroglucinols (hyperforin)
- Polycyclic diones (hypericin)
- Flavonoids

Key actions

- Antidepressant • Anxiolytic
- Antiviral • Wound healer
- Anti-inflammatory

Research

Depression Clinical research since the 1970s has established St. John's wort as an effective treatment for mild to moderate depression. A review in 2009 also concluded that the herb was helpful in treating severe depression. Research shows that St. John's wort works on neurotransmitter levels (e.g. serotonin) in several different ways.

Viral infection St. John's wort extracts (particularly hypericin, the red pigment found in the petals and leaves) have strong antiviral activity, notably against influenza, herpes, and hepatitis B and C.

Safety St. John's wort rarely causes side effects itself, but it does interact with certain conventional medicines, mostly increasing the rate at which they are broken down by the liver. This changes the amount of the drug present in the bloodstream, significantly reducing its effectiveness. In rare situations, this can be life threatening.

Traditional & current uses

Nerve tonic The herb acts as a restorative and neuroprotective, helping reverse long-term nervous exhaustion and lowered mood. It can prove useful in seasonal affective disorder and chronic anxiety, and improves sleep quality.

Menopause The herb is considered a specific for the lowered mood that can accompany menopause, often combined with black cohosh (*Cimicifuga racemosa*, p. 61) in such cases.

Tissue healing The red infused oil has potent wound-healing properties and historically has been used to heal knife and stab wounds. Nowadays, St. John's wort oil is more commonly used to promote healing after surgery and minor burns. The oil can be particularly helpful in relieving neuralgia—shingles, sciatica, and toothache being common applications.

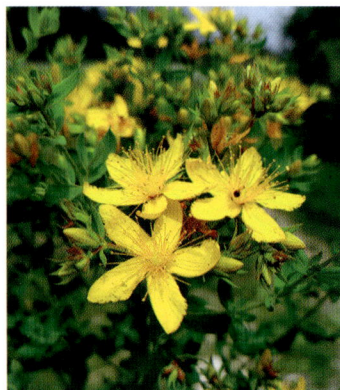

St. John's wort was a folk remedy for mental disorders in the Middle Ages.

Parts used

Flowering tops are picked when the flowers have opened.

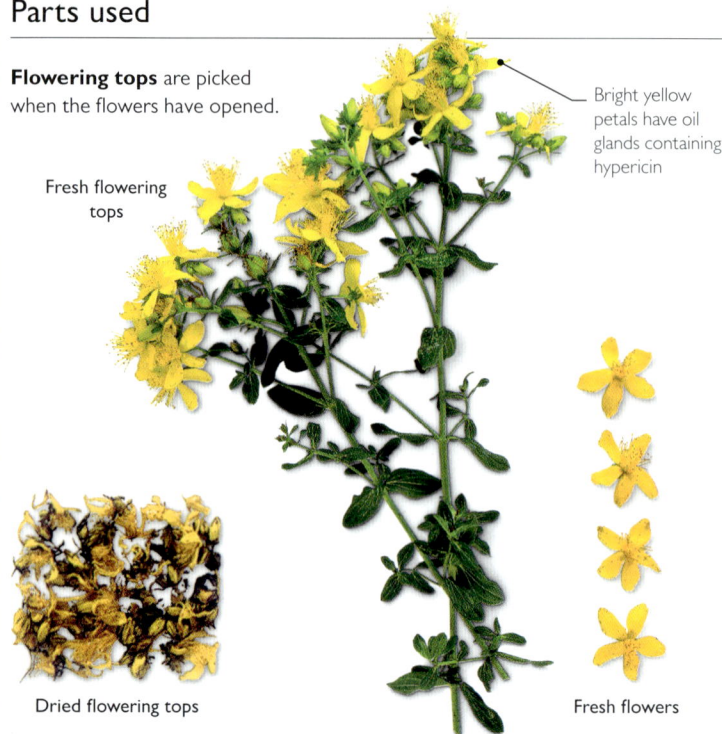

Bright yellow petals have oil glands containing hypericin

Fresh flowering tops

Dried flowering tops

Fresh flowers

Key preparations & their uses

Infused oil Make by steeping the herb in oil for 6 weeks (*see* p. 304). Dab onto minor wounds and burns.

Cream (to make, p. 306). For cramps or neuralgia, rub onto the affected part.

Tincture (to make, p. 302). For depression, take ½ tsp with water 3 times a day.

Infusion (to make, p. 301), Drink ½ cup (100 ml) daily as a digestive tonic.

Cautions Can cause sensitivity to sunlight. Due to possible interactions, seek professional advice if taking a prescribed medicine, including blood thinners. Restricted in some countries. Do not combine with other antidepressants.

Self-help uses

- Anxiety, depression, & tension, p. 318. • Back pain, p. 323. • Bites & stings, p. 313. • Cold sores, chicken pox, & shingles, p. 314. • Depression & decreased vitality due to menopause, p. 326. • Neuralgia, p. 318. • Stiff & aching joints, p. 323. • Tired & aching muscles, p. 322.

Inula helenium (Asteraceae)

Elecampane, *Tumu xiang* (Chinese)

Prized by the Romans as a medicine and as a food, this herb derives its botanical name from Helen of Troy, who, according to legend, was holding elecampane in her hand when she set off with Paris to live with him in Troy. The root of the plant has long been seen as a gently warming and tonic herb, and is particularly useful for chronic bronchitis and other chest problems.

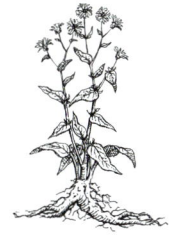

A perennial growing to 10 ft (3 m), with golden yellow, daisylike flowers and large, pointed leaves.

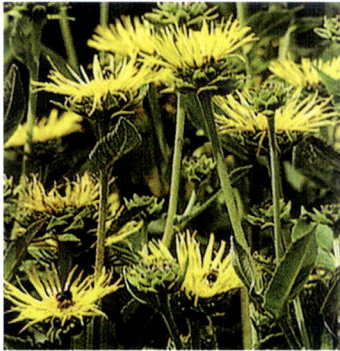

"Elecampane will the spirits sustain," is a medieval saying. It reflects the herb's tonic properties.

Habitat & cultivation

Native to southeastern Europe and western Asia, elecampane now grows in many temperate regions, including parts of the US. It is also cultivated. Propagated from seed in spring or by root division, it prefers moist, well-drained ground. The root is unearthed in the fall, cut up, and then dried at a high temperature.

Related species

Xuan fu hua (*I. japonica*) grows in China and Japan. Other relatives used medicinally include sunflower (*Helianthus annuus*), common fleabane (*Pulicaria dysenterica*), and echinacea (*Echinacea* spp., p. 96).

Key constituents

• Inulin (up to 44%) • Volatile oil (up to 4%), containing alantol and sesquiterpene lactones (including alantolactone)
• Triterpene saponins • Phytosterols

Key actions

• Expectorant • Soothes coughing
• Increases sweating • Mildly bitter
• Eliminates worms • Antibacterial

Research

Inulin Inulin was first isolated from elecampane in 1804 and took its name from the herb. It has mucilaginous qualities that help soothe the bronchial linings.

Antimicrobial Alantolactone has been shown to have significant activity against the tuberculosis mycobacterium. Researchers in Ireland found that the root had potent effect against MRSA, an antibiotic-resistant "superbug."

Whole herb As a whole, the root has a stimulant, expectorant effect, encouraging the coughing up of mucus from the lungs. The volatile oil is known to be partly responsible for this and also for the herb's antiseptic properties.

Traditional & current uses

Chest infections Elecampane has long been valued for its tonic, strengthening effect on the respiratory system and for its ability to resolve chest infections. Its warming effect on the lungs, combined with its ability to gently stimulate the clearing of mucus from the chest, makes it safe for young and old. It can be used in almost all chest conditions, and is very useful when the patient is debilitated.

Chronic chest complaints Elecampane's qualities have led to its specific use for chronic bronchitis and bronchial asthma. It is particularly useful because it both soothes the bronchial tube linings and is an expectorant. In addition, the herb is mildly bitter, helping recovery by improving digestion and the absorption of nutrients.

Digestive problems Elecampane has been taken traditionally as a tonic herb for the digestion. It stimulates the appetite and relieves dyspepsia. It is a useful remedy for the treatment of worms.

Infection In the past, elecampane was used in the treatment of tuberculosis. It works well with other antiseptic herbs and is given for infections such as tonsillitis. Its restorative, tonic action complements its ability to counter infection.

Parts used

Root contains inulin, a mucilaginous (jellylike) substance that soothes and relieves coughing.

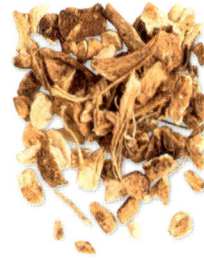

Dried root

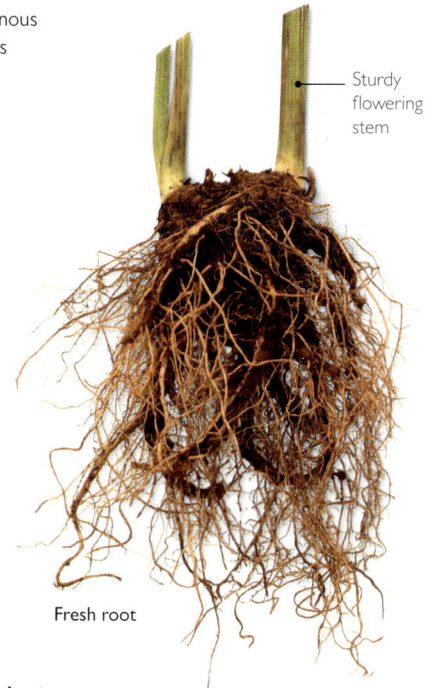

Sturdy flowering stem

Fresh root

Key preparations & their uses

Decoction (to make, p. 301). For irritable coughs, take ⅓ cup (75 ml) 2–3 times a day.

Tincture (to make, p. 302). For bronchitis, mix 2½ tbsp with 2½ tbsp thyme tincture. Take 1 tsp 3 times a day.

Syrup For coughs, make an infusion (*see* p. 301) and simmer until it has reduced to half its volume, before adding the sugar or honey (to make, p. 303). Take 1–2 tsp every 2 hours.

Cautions Can cause skin reactions. Do not take internally during pregnancy or if breastfeeding.

Self-help use

• Coughs & bronchitis, p. 320.

Lavandula angustifolia syn. *L. officinalis* (Lamiaceae)

Lavender

Lavender is an important relaxing herb, but it is better known for its sweet-scented aroma than for its medicinal properties. It became popular as a medicine during the late Middle Ages, and in 1620 it was one of the medicinal herbs taken to North America by the Pilgrims. It was described by the herbalist John Parkinson (1640) as being of "especially good use for all griefes and paines of the head and brain."

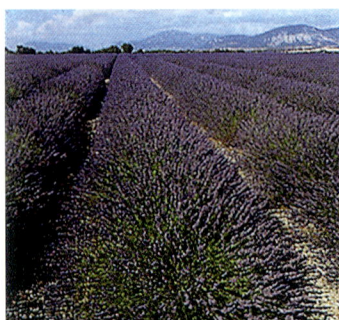

A perennial shrub growing to 3 ft (1 m), with spikes of violet-blue flowers extending above the foliage.

Lavender is widely cultivated for perfume and medicinal use.

Habitat & cultivation

Native to France and the western Mediterranean, lavender is cultivated worldwide for its volatile oil. It is propagated from seed or cuttings and needs a sunny position. The flowers are picked in the morning in high summer and are dried, or distilled to produce essential oil.

Related species

Spike lavender (*L. spica*) yields more oil than *L. officinalis*, but of an inferior quality. *L. stoechas* is used as an antiseptic wash for wounds, ulcers, and sores in Spain and Portugal.

Key constituents

• Volatile oil (up to 3%) containing over 40 constituents, including linalyl acetate (30–60%), cineole (10%), linalool, nerol, borneol • Flavonoids

Key actions

• Antispasmodic • Relieves anxiety
• Antidepressant • Neuroprotective
• Antimicrobial

Research

Lavender oil A 2014 clinical trial found lavender oil taken internally to be more effective than both a placebo and a conventional tranquilizer in relieving generalized anxiety. It also showed antidepressant activity. Other studies have found similar benefits and tended to confirm relaxant, antidepressant, and gently sedative activity. The oil is thought to have low toxicity and significant antibacterial and antifungal activity.

Flowers Lavender flowers and oil have similar properties. Although little research has been conducted, it is likely the flowers have a significantly greater carminative and neuroprotective activity. Applied externally, flower extracts are insecticidal and rubefacient (irritant and stimulating to the local circulation).

Traditional & current uses

Nervous system Lavender is well known for its soothing and calming effect and is combined with other sedative herbs to relieve sleeplessness, irritability, headaches, and migraine. It also helps alleviate depression.

Digestion Like many herbs with a significant volatile oil content, lavender soothes indigestion and colic, and relieves gas and bloating.

Asthma Lavender's relaxing effect makes it helpful for some types of asthma, especially where excessive nervousness is a feature.

Essential oil The oil is an invaluable first aid remedy. It is strongly antiseptic, helping to heal burns, wounds, and sores. Rubbed onto insect stings, it relieves pain and inflammation, and can be used to treat scabies and head lice. Massaging a few drops on the temples eases headaches, and five drops added to a bath at night relieves muscle tension, tones the nervous system, and encourages sleep.

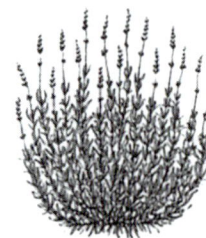

Parts used

Flowers are harvested toward the end of flowering, when the petals have begun to fade.

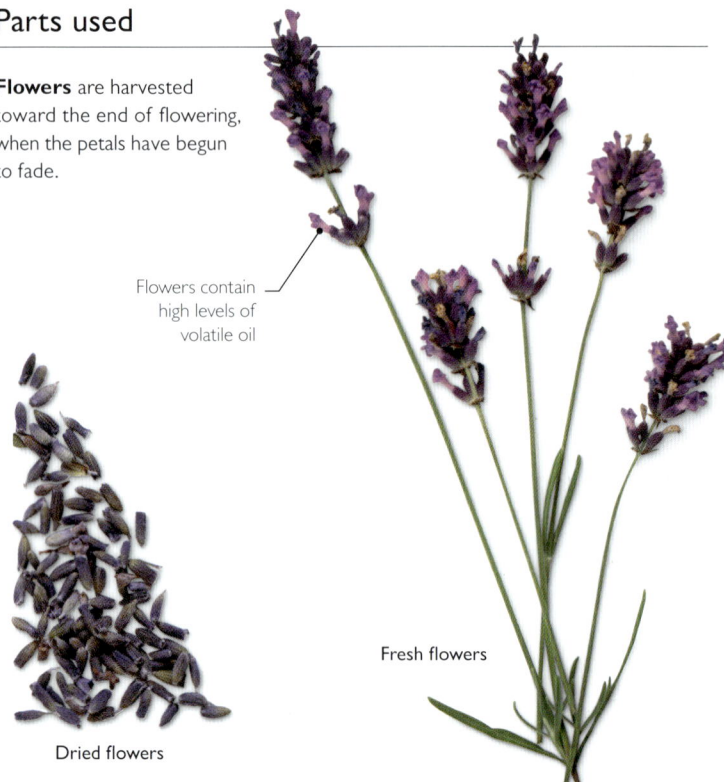

Flowers contain high levels of volatile oil

Fresh flowers

Dried flowers

Key preparations & their uses

Tincture (to make, p. 302). For insomnia, take ½ –1 tsp with water at night.

Massage oil For headaches, combine 20 drops with 1 tbsp carrier oil and apply (see p. 307).

Essential oil Apply undiluted to insect stings.

Infusion (to make, p. 301) is a calming remedy for digestive problems. For indigestion, take ⅓ cup (75 ml) twice a day.

Caution Do not take essential oil internally except under professional supervision.

Self-help uses

• Back pain, p. 323. • Bites & stings, p. 313. • Burns & sunburn, p. 319. • Earache, p. 322. • Headaches & migraine, p. 319. • Insomnia, p. 319. • Neuralgia, p. 318. • Stiff & aching joints, p. 323.

Linum usitatissimum (Linaceae)

Flaxseed, Linseed

Flaxseed or linseed has been cultivated in the Middle East for at least 7,000 years, and its seed and fiber have been put to innumerable uses—both medicinal and industrial—throughout history. Flaxseed has been shown to have very high levels of polyunsaturated essential fatty acids, making it valuable in maintaining a healthy heart and circulation, and in preventing chronic inflammatory diseases.

A slender annual growing to 3 ft (1 m) tall, with narrow leaves, blue flowers, and spherical seed capsules.

Habitat & cultivation

Originally native to temperate zones in Europe and Asia, flaxseed is now widely cultivated in temperate regions, including Canada and the US, Argentina, and northern Europe. It is grown from seed in spring and harvested when the seed is ripe in late summer or early fall.

Related species

Purging flax (*L. catharticum*), native to western Europe, is a purgative, but no longer used.

Key constituents

• Fixed oil (approximately 35%) mostly alpha-linolenic acid (omega-essential fatty acid) • Protein (about 26%) • Fiber (about 14%) • Mucilage (about 12%) • Sterols • Lignans

Key actions

• Demulcent • Emollient • Laxative
• Phytoestrogenic • Anticancer

Research

Omega-3 oils Flaxseed is unusual in that it has very high levels of alpha-linolenic acid, an omega-3 polyunsaturated fatty acid, similar to those most commonly found in fish oils. Research indicates that omega-3 oils have significant anti-inflammatory activity. They also help protect the heart and circulation, and reduce heart irregularities. The seed, rather than the oil, helps to lower cholesterol levels.

Anticancer Ground flaxseed appears to be specifically useful against endometrial, breast, and prostate cancer: it is rich in omega-3 oils, which are deficient in most Western diets; in lignans, which are phytoestrogenic and reduce the impact of estradiol (a potentially harmful type of estrogen); and in mucilage and fiber, which prevent reabsorption of unwanted estrogens from the intestines. Flaxseed added to the diet lowers PSA levels (used to measure prostate cancer risk) and thus is thought to protect against prostate cancer.

Traditional & current uses

Laxative Flaxseed has mostly been used as a bulk laxative, especially valuable in chronic constipation. The seeds soak up fluid in the gut, helping to make the stool softer and encouraging easier bowel movements. They should be taken with about 5 times their volume of water. With their significant mucilage content, the seeds are also soothing and anti-inflammatory, reducing irritation and inflammation in the gut in such conditions as colitis, irritable bowel, and hemorrhoids.

Respiratory & urinary disorders The seeds, which need to be split or ground up before being swallowed, soothe the chest and, to a lesser extent, the urinary tract. They have proved helpful in chronic or paroxysmal coughs, bronchitis, and emphysema, and in urinary troubles such as chronic cystitis.

External uses A poultice of the crushed seeds or of flaxseed flour is applied to painful or tender boils and carbuncles, softening the skin and drawing out the purulent material. A Portuguese recipe recommends combining flaxseed oil with red wine as an effective topical remedy for wounds.

Menopause Adding flaxseed to the diet can support estrogen balance in menopause and reduce associated symptoms. Flax and other seeds can be made into a "menopause cake."

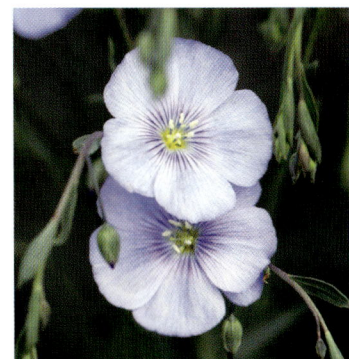

Flaxseed is the best vegetable source of omega-3 essential fatty acids.

Parts used

Whole seeds gently support elimination and cleanse the colon. Cracked or ground seeds need to be used for other medicinal benefits. Golden linseed varieties are usually preferred.

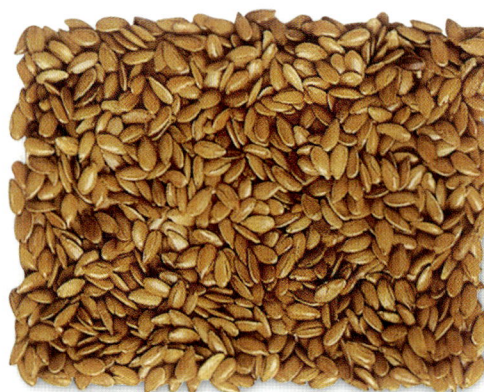

Seeds

Key preparations & their uses

Oil from the seed is convenient to use but goes rancid easily. Take 1–2 tsp daily as a nutritional supplement.

Cracked or ground seed Take 1–2 tbsp daily with water to help relieve menopausal symptoms.

Flour is mixed with water and used as a poultice, and used in baking as a phytoestrogenic food during menopause.

Caution Do not use immature seeds, which may be toxic. Store cracked or ground seed in a closed container and keep in the fridge.

Self-help uses

• Constipation, p. 327.
• Menopause, p. 326.

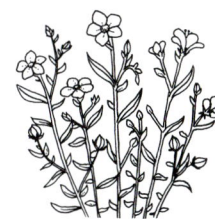

Lobelia inflata (Campanulaceae)

Lobelia, Indian tobacco, *Banbian* (Chinese)

Lobelia is a powerful antispasmodic used for respiratory and muscle disorders and was a traditional remedy used by Indigenous peoples in North America for many conditions. It was used as a "puke weed" to induce vomiting, as a remedy for worms and venereal disease, and as an expectorant. Lobelia was also smoked as a substitute for tobacco, and was reputed to share some of its magical qualities.

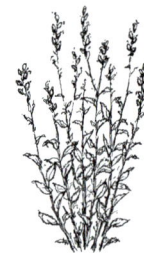

An annual growing to 20 in (50 cm), with lance-shaped leaves and pale blue, pink-tinged flowers.

Habitat & cultivation

An indigenous American plant, lobelia is found in much of North America, especially in eastern parts of the US. It grows by roadsides and in neglected areas, and prefers acid soil. The aerial parts are harvested in early fall, when the seed capsules are most numerous, and are carefully dried.

Related species

At least 4 other *Lobelia* species were traditionally used by Indigenous peoples. One, great lobelia (*L. siphilitica*), as its Latin name suggests, was credited by Indigenous peoples and European colonizers with the power to cure syphilis. Chinese lobelia (*ban bian lian*, *L. chinensis*) is used in Chinese herbal medicine mainly as a diuretic and for snake bite.

Key constituents

- Pyridine alkaloids (6%)—principally lobeline • Flavonoids • Terpenes
- Coumarins

Key actions

- Respiratory stimulant
- Antispasmodic • Expectorant
- Induces vomiting • Increases sweating

Traditional & current uses

Indigenous remedy Lobelia was a traditional Indigenous remedy with a wide range of applications. Its use was later championed by the American herbalist Samuel Thomson (1769–1843), who made the herb the mainstay of his therapeutic system (*see* p. 27). He mainly used it to induce vomiting.

Therapeutic properties The whole herb is strongly antispasmodic. The constituent lobeline stimulates the

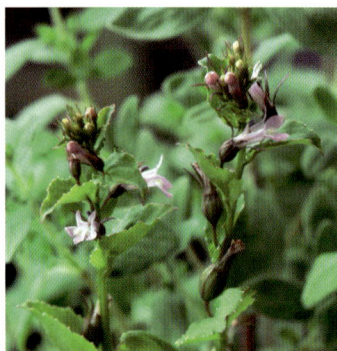

Lobelia's pale blue flowers were believed to have magical properties and were used to ward off ghosts.

respiratory center within the brain stem, producing stronger and deeper breathing. Laboratory investigations during the 1990s suggest that lobeline has antidepressant activity.

Respiratory problems A powerful antispasmodic and respiratory stimulant, lobelia is valuable for asthma, particularly bronchial asthma, and chronic bronchitis. The herb helps to relax the muscles of the smaller bronchial tubes, thereby opening the airways, stimulating breathing, and promoting the coughing up of phlegm. In the Anglo-American herbal tradition, lobelia has always been combined with cayenne (*Capsicum frutescens*, p. 79); the heating, stimulant action helps to push blood into areas that lobelia has relaxed.

External applications Some constituents, especially lobeline, break down rapidly in the body, and lobelia is often most effective applied externally. Its antispasmodic action helps to relax muscles, particularly smooth muscle, making it useful for sprains, and for back problems where muscle tension is a key factor. In combination with

Parts used

Aerial parts have important antispasmodic properties and help relieve respiratory complaints.

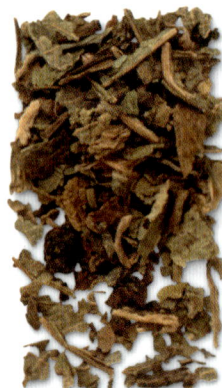

Dried aerial parts

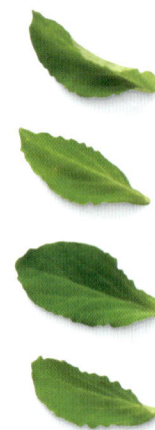

Fresh leaves

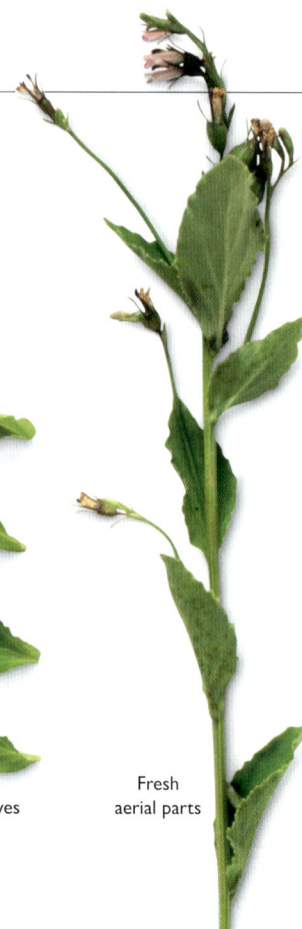

Fresh aerial parts

Key preparations & their uses

Infusion is prescribed for bronchitis.

Tincture is given to relieve asthma.

Tablets containing lobelia in combination with other herbs are used to treat bronchial asthma.

Cautions Take only when prescribed by a medical herbalist or doctor and do not eat the fresh plant. Excessive ingestion is rare (vomiting normally occurs first) but can be fatal. Restricted herb in some countries.

cayenne, lobelia has been used as a chest and sinus rub.

Tobacco addiction The piperidine alkaloids, especially lobeline, have similar chemical effects to nicotine, found in tobacco (*Nicotiana tabacum*, p. 247), and lobelia is employed by herbalists to help patients give up smoking.

Lycium chinense syn. *L. barbarum* (Solanaceae)

Goji berry, Chinese wolfberry

Goji berry is a major Chinese tonic herb, first mentioned in the *Divine Husbandman's Classic (Shen'nong Bencaojing)* written in the 1st century CE. Traditionally it is believed to promote long life—a Chinese herbalist, said to have lived for 252 years, ascribed his longevity to tonic herbs, including goji berry. Today, both the berries and the root have a wide range of medicinal uses.

A deciduous shrub growing to 13 ft (4 m), with bright green leaves and scarlet berries.

Habitat & cultivation

Goji berry grows throughout much of China, and is cultivated extensively across the country's central and northern regions. It is grown from seed in the fall. The root can be unearthed at any time of the year, but is most commonly harvested in spring. The berries are picked in late summer or early fall.

Key constituents

• Beta-sitosterol
Berries only: Polysaccharides
• Flavonoids—principally rutin
• Essential fatty acids • Carotenoids—mostly zeaxanthin • Sterols
• Vitamin C
Root only: Cinnamic acid
• Psyllic acid

Key actions

• Tonic • Protects liver
• Neuroprotective • Lowers blood pressure • Anti-aging

Research

Immune modulation Research that has been carried out over the past 30 years indicates goji berry supports immune function, in part countering the reduction of white blood cell

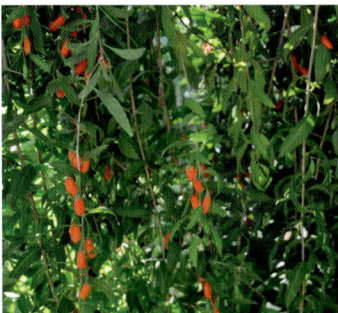

production resulting from aging. It also appears to prevent infection by preventing bacteria and viruses from attaching to cell membranes, particularly in the liver. The polysaccharides have anticancer activity.

Zeaxanthin This compound, occurring in higher concentration in goji berry than any other food, is taken as a supplement to support eyesight and the health of the retina. It is thought to protect against age-related macular degeneration.

Tonic and neuroprotective Several clinical trials in China have found that goji berry juice promotes general well-being, reducing signs of fatigue, weakness, depression, and stress. In early-stage research, goji berry has shown promise as a neuroprotective agent, and seems to act within the brain to prevent some aspects of the degenerative processes associated with Alzheimer's disease.

Traditional & current uses

Circulation In China, goji berry is taken as a blood tonic and to improve the circulation. It is also taken in order to help lower blood pressure and treat a range of symptoms that include dizziness and tinnitus.

Slowing aging The traditional use of goji berry as a tonic of key importance to the elderly is gradually being endorsed by research. Combined effects that protect immune, liver, cardiovascular, and brain function from deterioration suggest that goji berry has a place in the diet of anyone seeking to keep healthy in their later years. A small handful of berries taken on a daily basis (eaten raw or as part of a larger dish) makes a useful contribution to long-term good health.

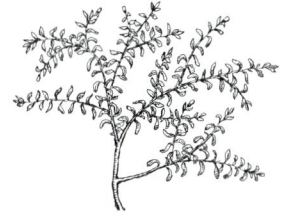

Goji berry produces berries that are a blood tonic.

Parts used

Root is used in preparations to relieve fevers.

Berries can be eaten raw or dried, or used in cooking, e.g. soups.

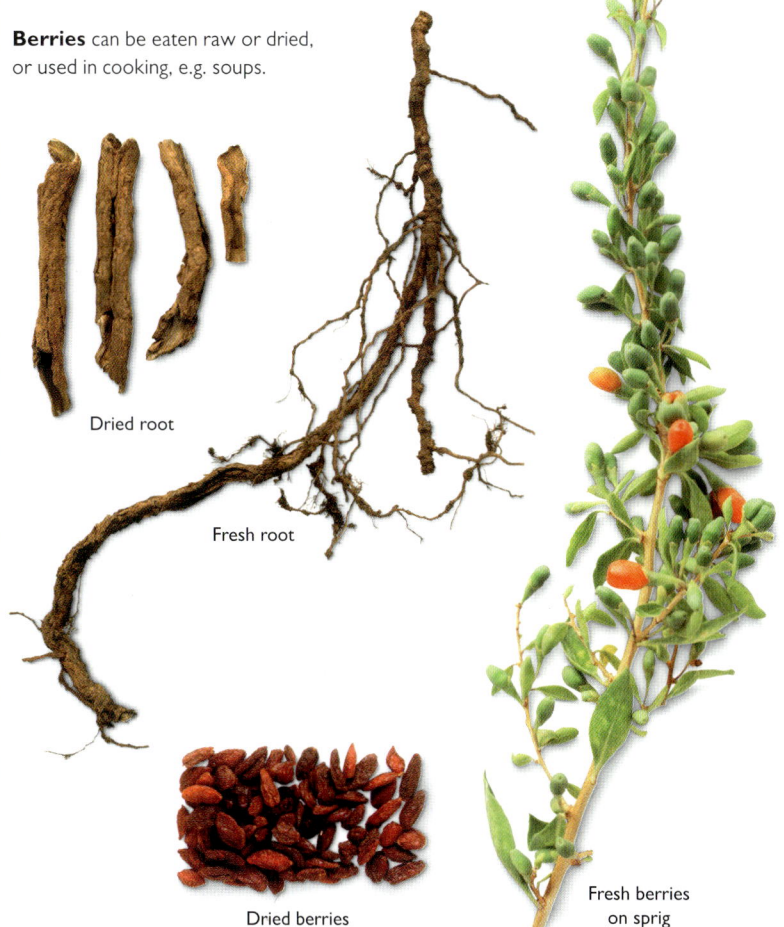

Dried root

Fresh root

Dried berries

Fresh berries on sprig

Key preparations & their uses

Decoction of the root (to make, p. 301). For fevers, take ½ cup (100 ml) daily.

Tincture of the root (to make, p. 302). For coughs and wheezing, take ½ tsp diluted with water 3 times a day.

Making a decoction with berries Chop dried berries and simmer (*see* p. 301). For poor eyesight, take ½ cup (100 ml) daily.

Cautions Avoid during pregnancy. It can interact with some prescribed medicines: do not take with warfarin.

Melaleuca alternifolia (Myrtaceae)

Tea tree

Tea tree, and in particular its essential oil, is one of the most important natural antiseptics. Useful for stings, burns, wounds, and skin infections of all kinds, the herb merits a place in every medicine chest. Tea tree is native to Australia and is a traditional remedy of the Aboriginal People. Western researchers studied its therapeutic properties during the 1920s, and it is now widely used in Europe and the US as well as in Australia.

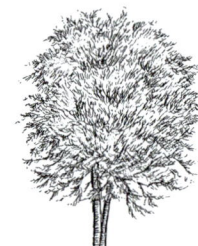

An evergreen reaching 23 ft (7 m), with layers of papery bark, pointed leaves, and white flower spikes.

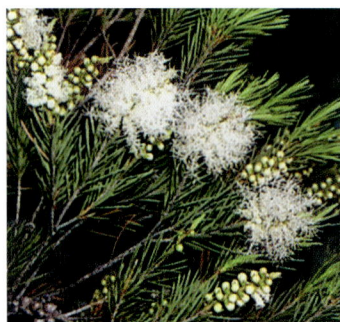

Tea tree provides one of the most effective natural antiseptics.

Habitat & cultivation

Tea tree is native to Australia, flourishing in moist soils in northern New South Wales and Queensland. It is now cultivated extensively, especially in New South Wales. Tea tree is grown from cuttings in summer. The leaves and small branches are picked throughout the year and distilled to produce essential oil.

Related species

Other *Melaleuca* species that provide valuable essential oils include cajuput (*M. leucadendron*, p. 240), broad-leaved paperbark tree (*M. viridiflora*) and *M. linariifolia*, the essential oil of which is very similar to tea tree.

Key constituents

• Volatile oil containing terpinen-4-ol (40%), gamma-terpinene (24%), alpha-terpinene (10%), cineo (5%) (percentages are variable).

Key actions

• Antiseptic • Antibacterial • Antifungal
• Antiviral • Immune stimulant

Research

Antiseptic properties Tea tree essential oil was first researched in 1923 in Australia. Since the 1960s it has been intensively investigated, and its antiseptic properties are well established. Clinical trials, mainly in Australia, have shown that it is effective at treating a broad range of infectious conditions.

Active constituents One of the most important constituents is known to be terpinen-4-ol, which is significantly antiseptic and well tolerated by the skin. The oil also contains cineol, which can irritate the skin. The cineol content varies—poor-quality oil has more than 10%; in some cases up to 65%.

Traditional & current uses

Traditional remedy Tea tree is a traditional Aboriginal remedy. The leaves are crushed and either inhaled or used in infusions for coughs, colds, and skin infections.

Skin problems Tea tree can be applied to skin infections such as athlete's foot and ringworm, as well as to corns, warts, acne, boils, infected burns, wounds, insect bites and stings, and other skin conditions.

Chronic infections Tea tree may be taken internally as a treatment for chronic, and some acute, infections, notably cystitis, glandular fever, and chronic fatigue syndrome.

Oral infections The herb is effective in mouthwashes, countering oral infection and gum disease, and it can also be used as a gargle for sore throats.

Vaginal infections Tea tree is an excellent remedy for vaginal irritation and infection, including thrush. It may be used as a pessary or can be diluted in a carrier cream and then applied.

Self-help uses

• Acne & boils, p. 315. • Athlete's foot, p. 314. • Vaginal yeast infection, p. 324.

Parts used

Leaves have high levels of a strongly antiseptic volatile oil and are used in preparations for skin problems and infections.

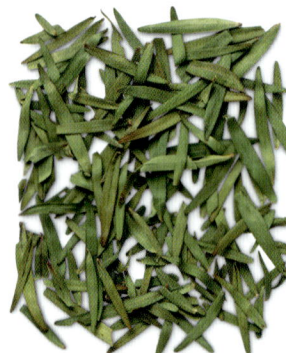

Dried leaves

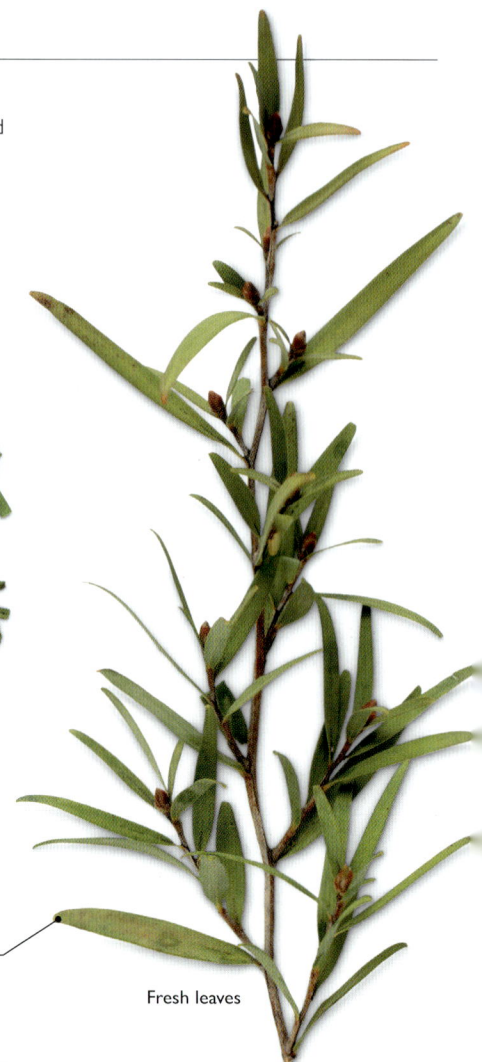

Leaves have a strong aroma when crushed

Fresh leaves

Key preparations & their uses

Cream Add 5 drops essential oil to 1 tsp base cream and apply to pimples 3 times a day.

Infusion (to make, p. 301). For chronic infections, infuse ½ tsp herb in ¾ cup (150 ml) of water. Take twice a day.

Essential oil Add 3 drops to 12 drops carrier oil and dab onto athlete's foot.

Pessaries (to make, p. 307). For vaginal infections, insert one a day.

Caution Do not take the essential oil internally except under professional supervision.

Melissa officinalis (Lamiaceae)

Lemon balm, Melissa

In writing that "Balm is sovereign for the brain, strengthening the memory and powerfully chasing away melancholy," John Evelyn (1620–1706) neatly summarized lemon balm's long tradition as a tonic remedy that raises the spirits and comforts the heart. Today, this sweet-smelling herb is still widely valued for its calming properties, and new research shows that it can help significantly in the treatment of cold sores.

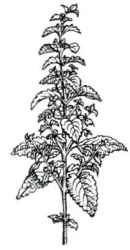

A perennial growing to 5 ft (1.5 m), with tiny white flowers and deeply veined, toothed leaves.

Habitat & cultivation

Native to southern Europe, western Asia, and northern Africa, lemon balm now grows throughout the world. The plant is propagated from seed or cuttings in spring. The aerial parts are picked from early summer onward and are best harvested just before the flowers open, when the concentration of volatile oil is at its highest.

Key constituents

• Flavonoids • Flavones
• Polyphenols, including rosmarinic, caffeic, and chlorogenic acids
• Triterpenes • Essential oil
(up to 0.2%—mainly citral, linalool)

Key actions

• Neuroprotective • Cardiotonic
• Relaxant • Antispasmodic
• Antiviral

Research

Dementia treatment A 4-month-long clinical study in Iran in 2003 concluded that a lemon balm extract is "of value in the management of mild to moderate Alzheimer's disease and has a positive effect on agitation in such patients." The herb has been shown to have anticholinesterase activity, maintaining levels of cholinergic neurons that become depleted in Alzheimer's.

Anxiety and depression A 2021 review of clinical trials into the herb noted that the lemon balm may be effective in improving anxiety and depressive symptoms, particularly in the acute setting.

Polyphenols Polyphenols are antiviral. In particular, they combat the herpes simplex virus, which produces cold sores. In one research study, the average healing time of cold sores was halved to about 5 days and the time between outbreaks doubled.

Traditional & current uses

Traditional uses This herb has always been taken to lift the spirits. Taken regularly, it was believed to encourage longevity. Other traditional uses include healing wounds, relieving palpitations, and treating toothache.

Modern relaxing tonic Lemon balm is a relaxing tonic for anxiety, mild depression, restlessness, and irritability. It reduces feelings of nervousness and panic and will often quiet a racing heart, being a valuable remedy for palpitations of a nervous origin. Lemon balm is also useful when over-anxiety is causing digestive problems such as indigestion, acidity, nausea, bloating, and colicky pains.

Cold sores Lemon balm relieves cold sores and reduces the chances of further outbreaks.

Hormonal herb Following the discovery of its antithyroid effect, the herb is given to people with an overactive thyroid.

Lemon balm's botanical name, Melissa, comes from the Greek for bee and refers to the great attraction the plant holds for bees.

Parts used

Aerial parts are used in a variety of preparations as a calming remedy.

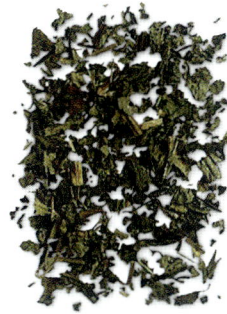

Dried aerial parts

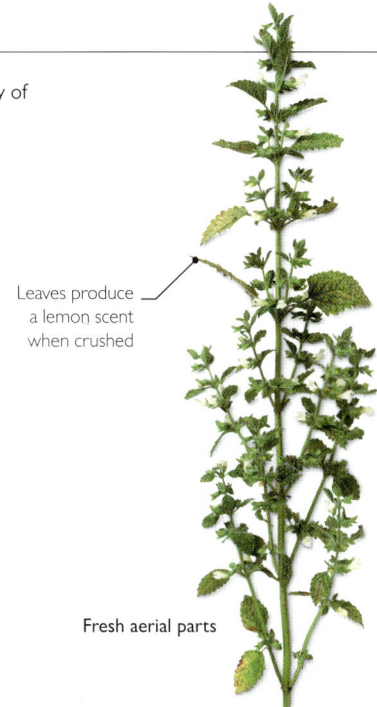

Leaves produce a lemon scent when crushed

Fresh aerial parts

Key preparations & their uses

Essential oil For shingles, add 5 drops to 1 tsp olive oil and massage the painful area gently (see p. 307).

Infusion (to make, p. 301). For nervous headaches, drink ¾ cup (150 ml) 3 times a day.

Tincture (to make, p. 302). For anxiety and mild depression, take ½ tsp with water 3 times a day.

Lotion For cold sores, make an infusion (see p. 301) and apply regularly (see p. 306).

Juice Apply as needed to cuts and scrapes.

Ointment (to make, p. 305). Apply to insect stings.

Caution Do not take the essential oil internally except under professional supervision.

Other uses Lemon balm is a first-aid remedy for cuts and insect stings and is good for fevers.

Self-help uses

• Anxiety, depression, & tension, p. 318. • Cold sores, chicken pox, & shingles, p. 314. • Flu with muscle aches & pains, p. 321. • Nausea due to emotional problems, p. 316. • Stomachache, p. 315.

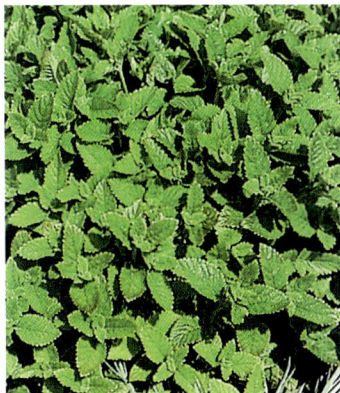

Mentha × piperita (Lamiaceae)

Peppermint

Peppermint's origin is a mystery, but it has been in existence for a long time—dried leaves were found in Egyptian pyramids dating from around 1000 BCE. It was highly valued by the Greeks and Romans, but only became popular in Western Europe in the 18th century. Peppermint's chief therapeutic value lies in its ability to relieve gas, flatulence, bloating, and colic, though it has many other applications.

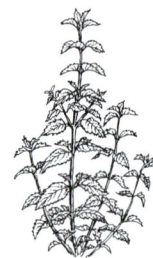

A strongly aromatic, square-stemmed annual, growing to 32 in (80 cm) with serrated leaves.

Habitat & cultivation

Peppermint is grown commercially and in gardens throughout Europe, Asia, and North America. It is propagated from seed in spring and is harvested just before it flowers in summer, in dry sunny weather.

Related species

Peppermint is a hybrid of water mint (*M. aquatica*) and spearmint (*M. spicata*), which have similar, though milder, therapeutic properties.

Key constituents

• Volatile oil (up to 1.5%), including menthol (35–55%), menthone (10–40%) • Flavonoids (luteolin, menthoside) • Phenolic acids
• Triterpenes

Key actions

• Antispasmodic • Stimulates sweating • Antimicrobial
• Analgesic • Carminative

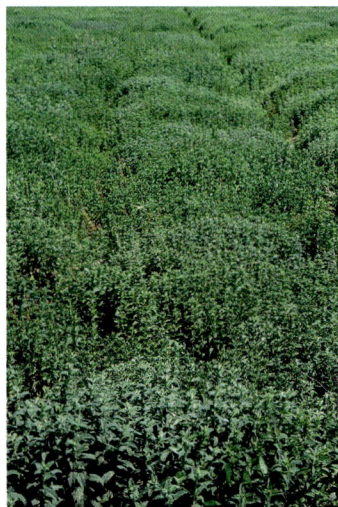

Peppermint is cultivated in many parts of the world for its oil.

Research

Volatile oil Research has shown that the volatile oil is strongly antibacterial. Menthol (a constituent of the oil) is antiseptic, antifungal, cooling, and anesthetic to the skin, although it is also an irritant.

Whole herb The whole plant has an antispasmodic effect on the digestive system. Clinical trials in Denmark and the UK during the 1990s point to the herb's value in the treatment of irritable bowel syndrome.

Traditional & current uses

Digestive problems Peppermint is excellent for the digestive system, increasing the flow of digestive juices and bile and relaxing the gut muscles. It reduces nausea, colic, cramps, and gas, and soothes an irritated bowel. In soothing the lining and muscles of the colon, it helps diarrhea and relieves a spastic colon (often the cause of constipation).

Pain relief Applied to the skin, peppermint relieves pain and reduces sensitivity. It also relieves headaches and migraines linked to digestive weakness.

Infection Diluted oil is used as an inhalant and chest rub for respiratory infections. The whole herb is important for digestive infections.

Self-help uses

• Digestive headaches, p. 319.
• Eczema, p. 310. • Nausea with headache, p. 316. • Neuralgia, p. 318.
• Gas & bloating, p. 316.

Parts used

Aerial parts are distilled for their volatile oil and used in a variety of preparations.

Leaves have high levels of volatile oil, which has important digestive properties

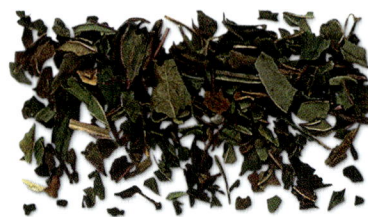

Dried aerial parts

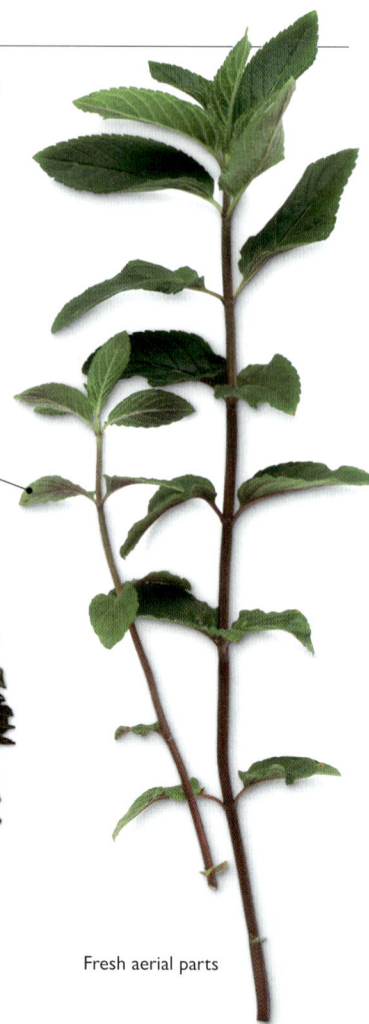

Fresh aerial parts

Key preparations & their uses

Lotion made with infusion (*see* p. 306). Apply to irritated skin.

Essential oil Dilute to 2% (*see* p. 307) and dab onto temples to ease headaches.

Infusion (to make, p. 301). To improve digestion, drink ¾ cup (150 ml) after meals.

Tincture mixed with other herbs, is prescribed mainly for digestive problems.

Capsules are prescribed for irritable bowel syndrome.

Cautions Do not give peppermint to children under 5. The essential oil is best taken internally on the advice of a health care practitioner; it is not suitable for children under 12.

Myristica fragrans (Myristicaceae)

Nutmeg & mace, *Rou dou kou* (Chinese)

Nutmeg and mace both come from the nutmeg tree and have very similar medicinal properties. Because of their toxicity at high dosages, they are infrequently used in the West despite being important medicines, employed principally to stimulate digestion and to treat infections of the digestive tract. Nutmeg also has long been valued as an aphrodisiac and as a remedy for eczema and rheumatism.

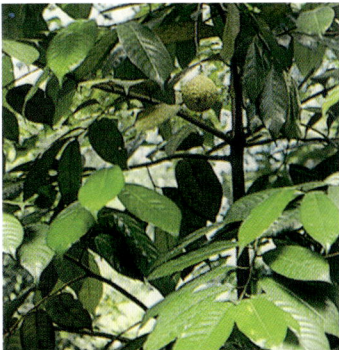

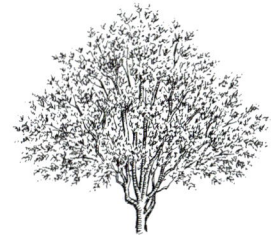

An evergreen tree growing to 39 ft (12 m), with aromatic leaves and clusters of small, yellow flowers.

Nutmeg and mace are cultivated commercially in the tropics.

Habitat & cultivation

Native to the Molucca Islands of Indonesia, nutmeg trees are now widely cultivated. They are propagated from seed, sown when ripe. The tree yields fruit after about 8 years, and can continue to fruit for over 60 years. The fruit is picked when ripe and the nutmeg and mace are separated and dried.

Key constituents

Nutmeg:
• Volatile oil (up to 15%), including alpha-pinene, beta-pinene, alpha-terpinene, beta-terpinene, myristicin, elincin, safrole • Fixed oil ("nutmeg butter"), myristine, butyrin

Mace:
• Volatile oil (similar to nutmeg but with a higher concentration of myristicin)

Key actions

Nutmeg:
• Carminative • Relieves muscle spasms • Prevents vomiting
• Stimulant

Mace:
• Stimulant • Carminative

Traditional & current uses

Digestive problems Nutmeg essential oil has an anesthetic and stimulating effect on the stomach and intestines, increasing appetite and reducing nausea, vomiting, and diarrhea. It is a helpful remedy for many digestive problems, especially gastroenteritis.

Sleep aid Though nutmeg is a stimulant, it has narcotic and anticonvulsant properties and can be successfully used at low dose (a pinch of powder will do) as a sleep aid for short- or long-term sleep problems. Laboratory studies also indicate that nutmeg has antidepressant activity.

Aphrodisiac In India, nutmeg has a long reputation as an aphrodisiac. It is believed to increase sexual stamina.

External uses Ointments based on the fixed oil (nutmeg butter) are used to treat rheumatic conditions. They have a counterirritant effect, stimulating blood flow to the area. In India, nutmeg is ground into a paste and applied directly to areas of eczema and ringworm.

Safety Low medicinal doses and culinary amounts of nutmeg and mace are safe. In excess, however, the herbs are strongly stimulant, hallucinogenic, and toxic. The consumption of just two whole nutmegs has been known to cause death.

Parts used

Aril (mace) surrounds the seed casing. It is used in cooking and as a medicine.

Seed kernel (nutmeg) is a stimulant remedy for intestinal infections and rheumatic conditions. In China, nutmeg is known as *rou dou kou.*

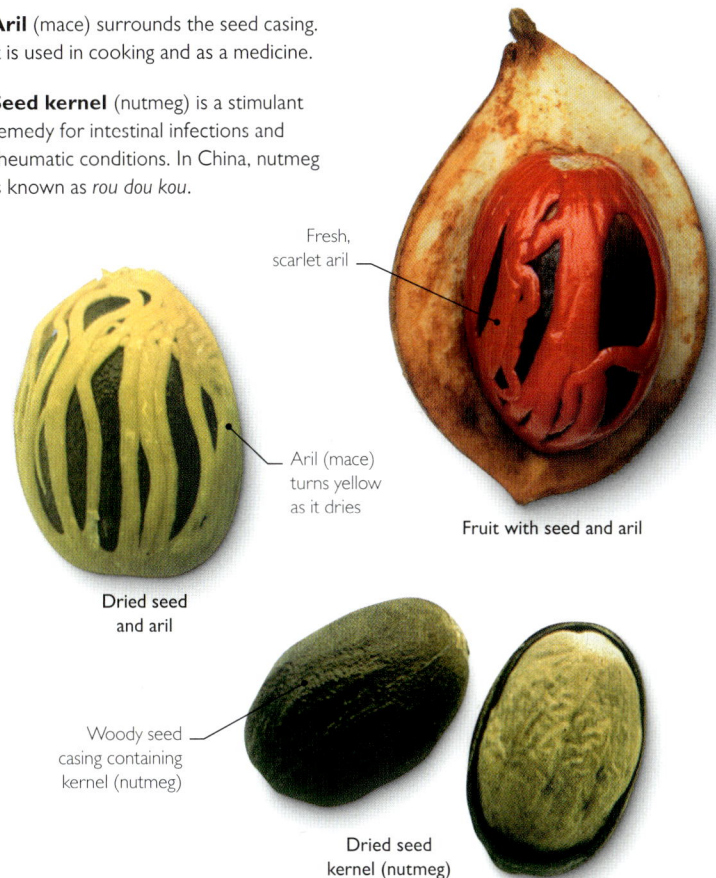

Fresh, scarlet aril

Aril (mace) turns yellow as it dries

Fruit with seed and aril

Dried seed and aril

Woody seed casing containing kernel (nutmeg)

Dried seed kernel (nutmeg)

Key preparations & their uses

Powdered mace is prescribed to treat gas and bloating.

Grated nutmeg For eczema, mix 2 tsp with a little water into a paste and apply.

Essential oil of nutmeg is occasionally used by herbalists to treat vomiting.

Infusion For gastroenteritis, add a pinch of nutmeg to ¾ cup (150 ml) of peppermint infusion (see p. 301). Take 3 times a day.

Ointment made from fixed oil (nutmeg butter). For rheumatic conditions, apply several times a day.

Caution Take the essential oil internally only under professional supervision. Do not take more than 3 g of either herb a day. Do not use during pregnancy.

Ocimum tenuiflorum syn. *O. sanctum* (Lamiaceae)

Holy basil, *Tulsi* (Hindi)

Holy basil, like sweet (culinary) basil, comes from India, where it is revered as the herb sacred to the goddess Lakshmi, wife of Vishnu, the god who preserves life. *Tulsi* means "matchless," and the herb has very important medicinal properties—notably its ability to reduce blood-sugar levels. In Indian herbal medicine, holy basil has a wide range of uses, relieving fevers, bronchitis, asthma, stress, and mouth ulcers.

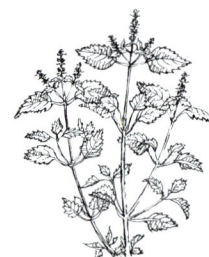

An aromatic annual growing to about 28 in (70 cm), with small, purple-red or white flowers.

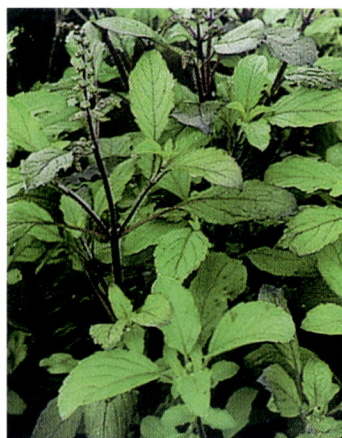

Holy basil is so called because it is often planted around temples and courtyards in India.

Habitat & cultivation

Holy basil is native to India and other tropical regions of Asia. It is also grown extensively in Central and South America, mainly for its medicinal properties. Holy basil can be grown from seed and is often cultivated as a potted plant. The aerial parts are picked before the flowers open, in early summer.

Related species

The familiar culinary species, sweet basil (*O. basilicum*, p. 248), is a close relative.

Key constituents

- Volatile oil (1%) including eugenol (70–80%) • Flavonoids (apigenin, luteolin) • Triterpene (ursolic acid)
- Polyphenols • Saponins

Key actions

- Antispasmodic • Analgesic
- Lowers blood-sugar levels
- Reduces fever • Adaptogenic
- Anti-inflammatory

Research

Diabetes Research into holy basil's ability to reduce blood-sugar levels, and thus help diabetes, has been going on for some decades. It has now been established as a useful medicine for some types of diabetes.

Indian research Research in India has shown that holy basil helps lower blood pressure and has anti-inflammatory, pain-relieving, and fever-reducing properties. Preliminary research also indicates that the herb strengthens immune resistance, protects against radiation, has anticancer properties, and inhibits sperm production.

Traditional & current uses

Traditional use Holy basil has always been considered to be a tonic, invigorating herb, useful for improving vitality.

Ayurvedic remedy In Ayurvedic medicine, holy basil is chiefly employed for fevers. A classical Indian recipe mixes holy basil, black pepper (*Piper nigrum*, p. 258), ginger (*Zingiber officinale*, p. 159), and honey in a remedy that prevents infection and controls high fever.

Heart & stress Holy basil is thought to have an affinity with the heart, protecting it from stress and lowering blood pressure and cholesterol levels. It has a reputation for reducing stress and is regarded as adaptogenic—helping the body adapt to new demands and stresses.

Diabetic remedy The herb's ability to help stabilize blood-sugar levels makes it useful in the treatment of diabetes.

Respiratory problems Holy basil is valuable for respiratory infections, especially colds, coughs, bronchitis, and

Parts used

Aerial parts are tonic and invigorating and have a wide range of other properties.

Leaves are serrated and covered in fine hairs

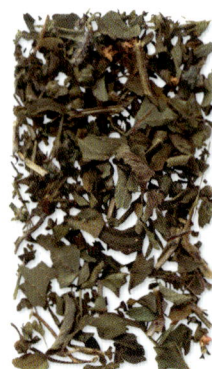

Dried aerial

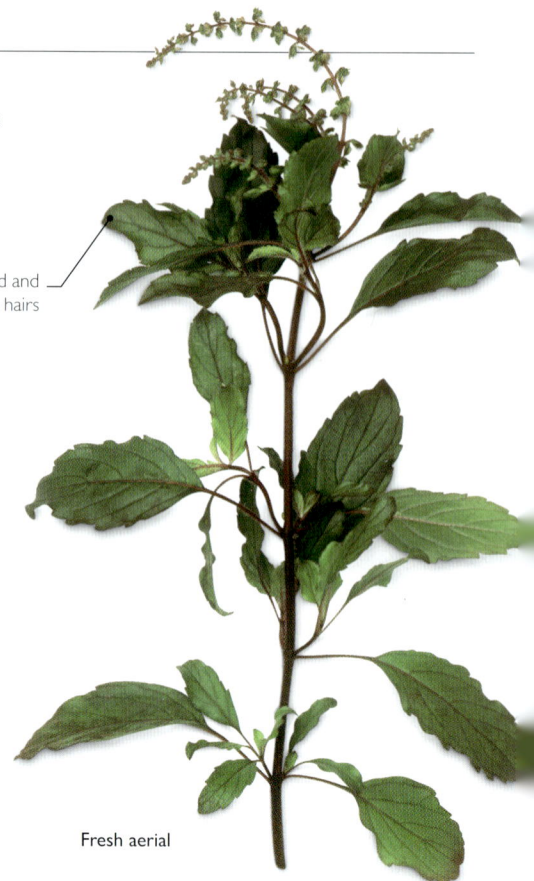

Fresh aerial

Key preparations & their uses

Juice For skin infections, apply ½ tbsp to the affected part twice a day.

Decoction (to make, p. 301) is used for fevers and as a tonic. Take ¾ cup (150 ml) daily as a general tonic.

Powder For mouth ulcers, rub powder gently into sore areas several times a day.

Cautions Do not take during pregnancy. Do not take if trying to conceive.

pleurisy. It also treats asthma.

Other uses Juice is extracted and applied to insect bites, ringworm, and skin diseases. It is also used as ear drops for ear infections. Juice or

powdered herb helps mouth ulcers to heal.

Self-help use

- Bites & stings, p. 313.

Olea europaea (Oleaceae)

Olive

The olive was first cultivated about 6,000–7,000 years ago in the eastern Mediterranean and has been valued as food and medicine ever since. The olive branch is an emblem of peace, and the leaves crowned victors in the ancient Olympic Games. The Bible states that olive "fruit shall be for food, the leaf for medicine," a summary as accurate today as in ancient times. Olive oil and leaf offer multiple health benefits.

Evergreen tree growing to 33 ft (10 m), with leathery leaves and clusters of small greenish-white flowers.

Habitat & cultivation

Olive trees grow wild in the Mediterranean region and are cultivated in Mediterranean countries and in regions with a similar climate in the Americas. The leaves may be gathered throughout the year, the fruit in late summer.

Key constituents

- Secoiridoids—oleuropein
- Flavonoids • Phenolic acids, including caffeic acid • Triterpenes, including oleanolic acid • Oleic acid (fruit)

Key actions

- Anti-inflammatory • Antimicrobial
- Bitter • Cardiovascular tonic
- Lowers raised blood pressure, blood sugar, and blood fat levels

Research

Olive oil Olive oil, rich in monounsaturated fatty acids (oleic acid 75%), is a key element in the traditional Mediterranean diet and is thought to be a major factor in the reduced incidence of cancer found in those eating a Mediterranean diet.
Oleuropein Both olive oil and leaf contain the bitter, oleuropein, thought responsible for many of the olive's medicinal benefits. The dry leaves have far greater medicinal activity as they contain 6–14% oleuropein, roughly 100 times levels found in the oil.
Olive leaf Laboratory studies indicate that olive leaf has wide-ranging health benefits, including anti-inflammatory; antiatherogenic; anticancer; heart-, liver-, and nerve-protective; and antimicrobial activity. Clinical trials support the traditional use of olive leaf as a treatment for high blood pressure.
Cold and flu A small clinical study (2019) in New Zealand tested olive leaf extract in the frequency of colds and flu in high school athletes. No reduction in the incidence of upper respiratory infection was found but in those taking the olive leaf extract there was a 28% reduction in sick day absences.

Traditional & current uses

Traditional use The olive was probably first cultivated in Crete in around 4500 BCE. The leaves have been used since those times to clean wounds.
Heart Olive leaves lower blood pressure and help improve the function of the cardiovascular system.
Diabetic remedy Possessing some ability to lower blood sugar levels, the leaves have been taken for diabetes.
Other uses The oil is nourishing and improves the balance of fats within the blood. It is traditionally taken with lemon juice to treat gallstones. The oil is useful topically for dry skin, cradle cap and dandruff, and excess ear wax.

Self-help uses

Cradle cap, p. 328; • Stretch marks, p. 327.

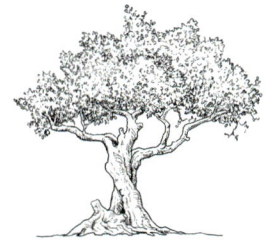

Olive harvesting is carried out in many groves much as it was centuries ago.

Parts used

Fruit (oil) Pressed oil is used in cooking and topically on the skin.

Leaf is a powerful antioxidant that aids the body in controlling inflammation.

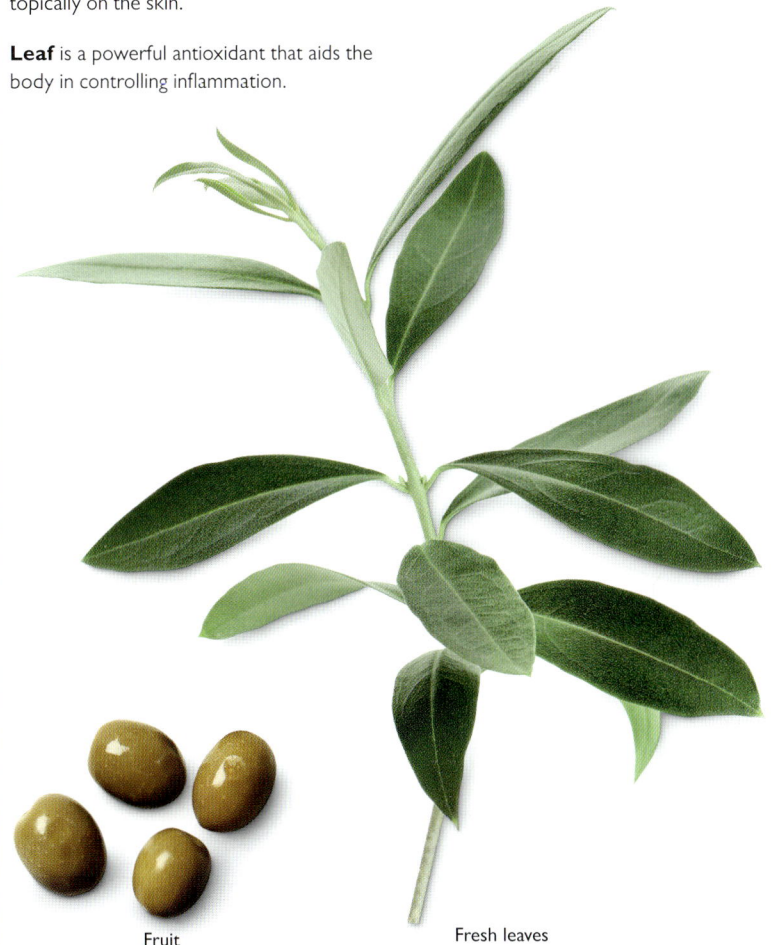

Fruit

Fresh leaves

Key preparations & their uses

Oil Highly nutritious and a mild laxative. Useful topically on dry and irritated skin.

Infusion (to make, p. 301) take 1–3 cups a day for colds and flu.

Tincture (to make, p. 302) take 2.5 ml twice a day for high blood pressure.

Capsule (to make, p. 302) take 1–2 capsules a day to support cardiovascular health.

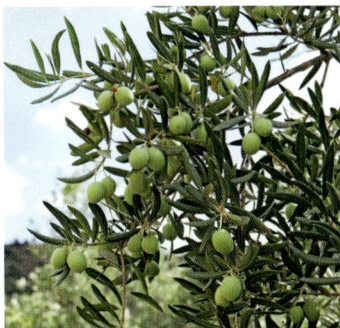

Paeonia lactiflora syn. *P. albiflora* (Paeoniaceae)

White peony, Chinese peony, *Bai shao yao* (Chinese)

White peony's history of medicinal use in China stretches back for at least 1,500 years. It is known most widely as one of the herbs used to make "Four Things Soup," a female tonic, and it is also a remedy for gynecological problems and for cramps, pain, and dizziness. Traditionally, it is considered that women who take the herb on a regular basis become as radiant as the flower itself.

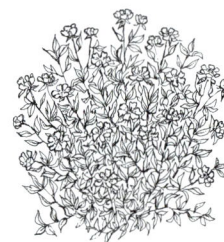

An upright perennial growing to 6½ ft (2 m), with large, white flowers and divided, dark green leaves.

Habitat & cultivation

White peony is cultivated throughout northeastern China and Inner Mongolia. It is propagated from seed in spring, or from root cuttings taken in winter. The root of 4- or 5-year-old plants is harvested in spring or fall.

Related species

P. suffruticosa and peony (*P. officinalis*, p. 250), a European species, have similar properties to white peony.

Key constituents

• Monoterpenoid glycosides (paeoniflorin, albiflorin) • Benzoic acid • Pentagalloyl glucose

Key actions

• Antispasmodic • Anti-inflammatory • Enhances cognition • Lowers blood pressure

Research

Paeoniflorin White peony has anti-inflammatory and antispasmodic properties, and preclinical research indicates that its traditional use for problems such as rheumatoid arthritis is justified. Paeoniflorin, the

constituent most responsible for these effects, is also thought to lower blood pressure and support blood flow to the heart.

Polycystic ovary syndrome (PCOS) White peony has a hormone-balancing activity that helps reverse the symptoms of PCOS, which include irregular menstruation and infertility. In combination with licorice (*Glycyrrhiza glabra*, p. 105) it has been shown to support regular ovulation and lower the raised testosterone levels that typically occur in PCOS.

Supports cognition There is accumulating evidence that white peony supports mental function, including spatial awareness and memory. Although no clinical trials have yet been published, white peony appears to have a strong neuroprotective effect within the brain.

Cold sores Pentagalloyl glucose may have an antiviral action against the cold sore virus, herpes simplex.

Traditional & current uses

Four Things Soup Together with rehmannia (*Rehmannia glutinosa*, p. 270), *chuan xiong* (*Ligusticum wallachii*), and *dong quai* (*Angelica sinensis*, p. 67), white peony is an ingredient in "Four Things Soup," the most widely used women's tonic in China.

Gynecological remedy White peony helps menstrual disorders, including heavy bleeding and bleeding between periods, and is used to treat period pain and cramps. It is a blood and *yin* tonic (see pp. 44–45) and will help "blood deficiency" states, as well as hot flashes and night sweats.

Self-help uses

• Heavy menstrual bleeding, p. 325.
• Hot flashes & night sweats, p. 326.
• Period pain, p. 325.

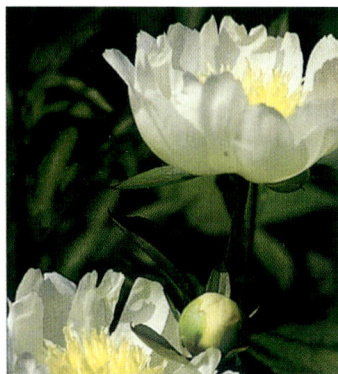

White peony *is cultivated for its root, which is a hormonal tonic, and for its flowers.*

Parts used

Root has important tonic and pain-relieving properties. It is boiled and dried for use in a wide range of preparations.

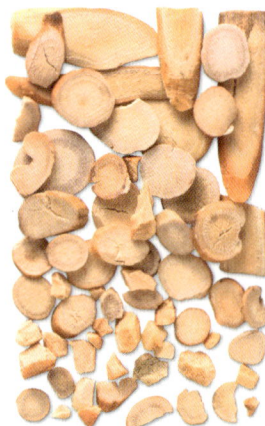

Dried root

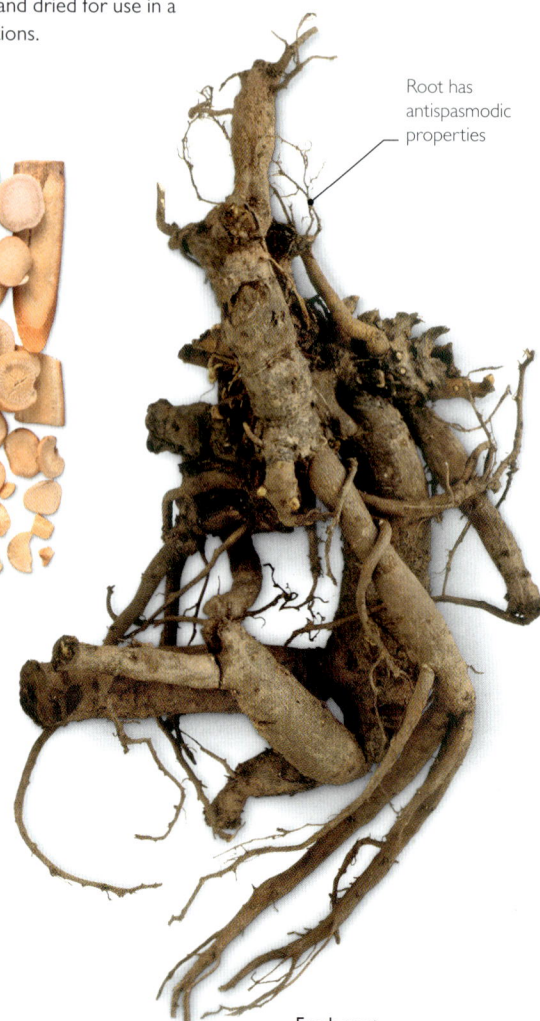

Root has antispasmodic properties

Fresh root

Key preparations & their uses

Decoction (to make, p. 301) helps relieve period pain, heavy bleeding, and other menstrual disorders. To relieve period pain, take ⅓ cup (75 ml) 3 times a day.

Four Things Soup (to make, see p. 325). Drink ¾ cup (150 ml) daily as a general tonic.

Caution Do not take during pregnancy.

Panax ginseng (Araliaceae)

Ginseng, Chinese ginseng, *Ren shen* (Chinese)

Ginseng is the most famous Chinese herb of all. It has been prized for its remarkable therapeutic benefits for about 7,000 years, and was so revered that wars were fought for control of the forests in which it thrived. An Arabian physician brought ginseng back to Europe in the 9th century, yet its ability to improve stamina and resistance to stress became common knowledge in the West only from the 18th century.

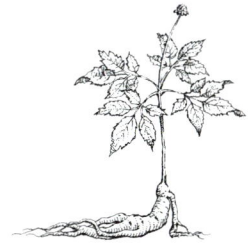

A perennial growing to 3 ft (1 m), with oval, toothed leaves and a cluster of small, green-yellow flowers.

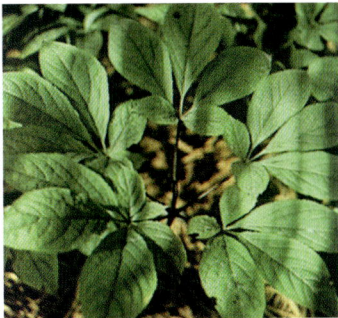

Ginseng has always been valued as a tonic in old age.

Habitat & cultivation

Ginseng is native to northeastern China, eastern Russia, and North Korea, but is now extremely rare in the wild. Ginseng cultivation requires great skill. It is propagated from seed in spring and requires rich, well-drained soil. The plant takes at least 4 years to mature. The root is then normally harvested in the fall and washed and steamed before being dried.

Related species

San qi (*P. notoginseng*, p. 250), *P. pseudoginseng*, and American ginseng (*P. quinquefolium*, p. 250) all have significant benefits.

Key constituents

• Triterpenoid saponins (0.7–3%), ginsenosides—at least 25 have been identified • Acetylenic compounds • Panaxans • Sesquiterpenes

Key actions

• Adaptogen • Tonic

Research

Adaptogen Ginseng has been researched in detail over the last 50 years in China, Japan, Korea, Russia, and many other countries. Its remarkable adaptogenic quality (helping the body adapt to stress, fatigue, and cold) has been confirmed. Trials show that ginseng significantly improves the body's capacity to cope with hunger, extremes of temperature, and mental and emotional stress.

Hormonal support The ginsenosides, which are similar in structure to the body's own hormones, can be adapted within the body to tone up deficient hormonal states. Clinical trials support the root's traditional use by men as they age, to maintain vitality and virility. There is also evidence it helps with both impotence and erectile dysfunction. Research indicates that ginseng is equally valuable for women and is a useful medicine at menopause and beyond, aiding hot flashes and lowered mood, and improving sexual arousal.

Other research Ginseng increases immune function and resistance to infection and improves liver function. Taken long term, it has been shown to improve cognition and enhance visual memory.

Traditional & current uses

Chinese remedy It is a tonic for old age and in China is taken to help endure long, cold winters.

Western tonic In the West, ginseng is seen mainly as a remedy to promote vitality and endurance, helpful in coping with stressful events, such as exams.

Self-help uses

• Impotence & premature ejaculation, p. 326. • Maintaining vitality, p. 329. • Poor sleep & nervous exhaustion, p. 319. • Short-term stress, p. 318.

Parts used

Root is harvested after 4 years, when the active constituents are most concentrated.

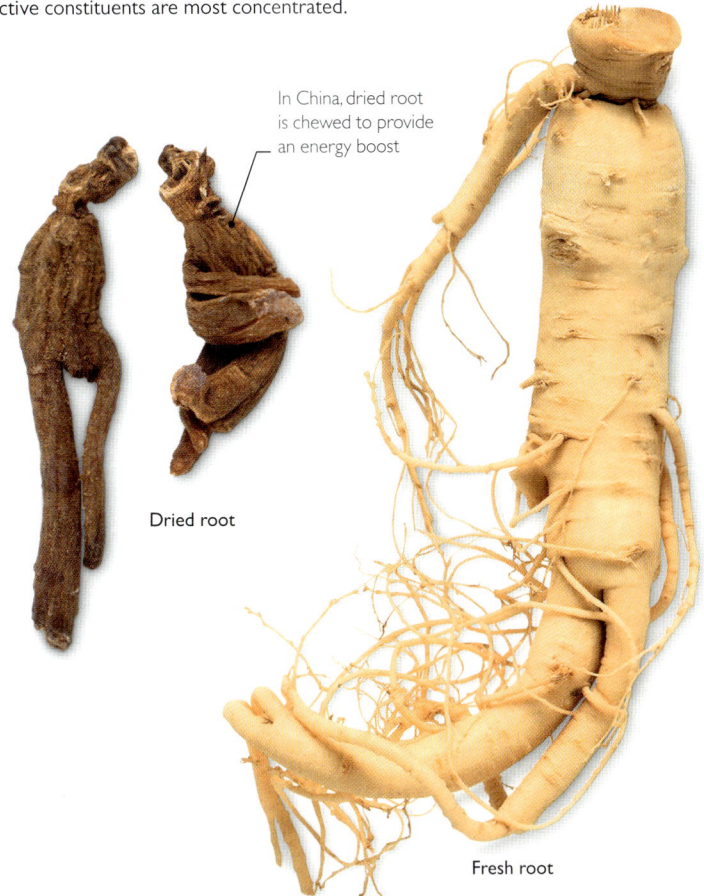

In China, dried root is chewed to provide an energy boost

Dried root

Fresh root

Key preparations & their uses

Capsules For nervous exhaustion, take a 500 mg capsule once a day.

Soup is a common way of taking ginseng in China. Add 1 g dried root per portion of vegetable soup. Take daily.

Tablets are a convenient way of taking ginseng. Take for short-term stressful events, such as moving a household.

Cautions Do not exceed dose (can cause insomnia and high blood pressure). Take with professional advice if using blood-thinning medication. Young healthy adults should not take ginseng more than 6 weeks. Avoid caffeine while taking it. Do not take if pregnant.

Passiflora incarnata (Passifloraceae)

Passion flower, Passiflora, Maypop

Passionflower's name comes from its beautiful flowers, thought to represent Christ's crucifixion—5 stamens for the 5 wounds, 3 styles for the 3 nails, and white and purple-blue colors for purity and heaven. The herb has valuable sedative and tranquilizing properties and has a long use as a medicine in Central and North American herbal traditions. In Mexico, it was taken for insomnia, epilepsy, and hysteria.

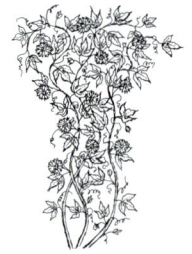

A climbing vine growing to 30 ft (9 m), with 3-lobed leaves, ornate flowers, and egg-shaped fruit.

Habitat & cultivation

Native to the southern US (Virginia, Texas, and Tennessee) and to Central and South America, passion flower is now extensively cultivated in Europe, notably in Italy, as well as in North America. It is propagated from seed in spring and needs plenty of sun. The aerial parts are gathered when the plant is flowering or in fruit.

Related species

There are approximately 400 *Passiflora* species, some of which are popular garden plants. A number have a similar sedative action to passion flower. *P. quadrangularis* has been found to contain serotonin, one of the main chemical messengers within the brain.

Key constituents

- Flavonoids (apigenin) • Amino acids
- Cyanogenic glycosides (gynocardin)
- Indole alkaloids (trace)

Key actions

- Sedative • Antispasmodic
- Tranquilizing

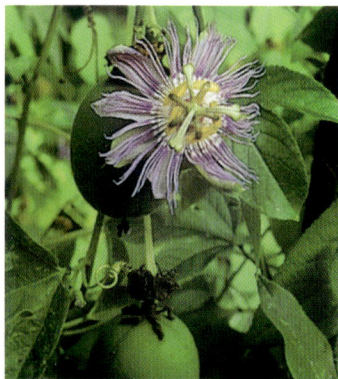

Passion flower was used by the Algonquin people of North America as an herbal tranquilizer.

Research

Tranquilizing properties

Pharmacological research shows the herb to have sedative, tranquillizing, and sleep-inducing properties. A 2001 clinical trial found that passion flower was as effective in relieving anxiety as oxazepam, a conventional tranquillizer, and had fewer reported side-effects. A clinical study in 2011 found improvement in subjective sleep quality in those taking the passion flower. A 2020 clinical trial monitored the sleep patterns of 110 adults with sleep disorder. Those taking a passion flower extract had a significantly increased "total sleep time" compared with those taking a placebo.

Indole alkaloids Research has not yet conclusively established that passionflower contains indole alkaloids.

Traditional & current uses

Insomnia Passion flower is best known as a remedy for insomnia and disturbed sleep patterns, and is useful for short-term bouts of sleeplessness.

Gentle sedative This herb is widely acknowledged to be a good medicine for anxiety, tension, irritability, and insomnia. Its gentle sedative properties produce a soothing and relaxing effect, reducing nervous activity and panic, and making it a mild and nonaddictive herbal tranquilizer, comparable in some ways to valerian (*Valeriana officinalis*, p. 152). Occasionally, it is prescribed for convulsions.

Pain relief Passion flower has valuable painkilling properties and is given for toothache, period pain, and headaches.

Tranquilizing effects Its ability to reduce anxiety makes passion flower valuable for many nervous states, and it is used to treat conditions as diverse as asthma, palpitations, high blood pressure, and muscle cramps. In each case, its antispasmodic and tranquilizing properties are the key to its usefulness, reducing the overactivity responsible for the disorder.

Parts used

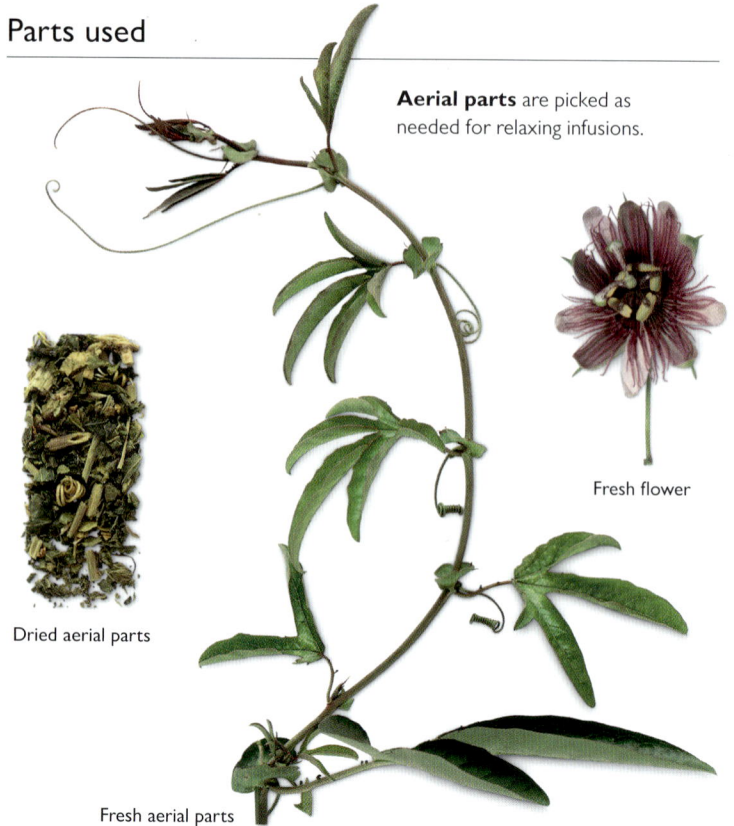

Aerial parts are picked as needed for relaxing infusions.

Fresh flower

Dried aerial parts

Fresh aerial parts

Key preparations & their uses

Tincture (to make, p. 302) is a useful sedative for an overactive mind. Take 1 tsp with water daily.

Infusion (to make, p. 301). For occasional sleeplessness, drink up to 1½ cups (300 ml) during the evening.

Tablets are a common over-the-counter remedy for insomnia and stress.

Cautions Passion flower can cause drowsiness. Do not take high doses in pregnancy.

Self-help uses

- Insomnia, p. 319.
- Sleeplessness due to backache, p. 323.

Pelargonium sidoides (Geraniaceae)

Pelargonium, Umckaloabo

Known as umckaloabo (thought to mean "heavy cough" in Zulu), pelargonium has been used for centuries by traditional South African healers as a key remedy for coughs and respiratory infections and for gastrointestinal disorders. The herb came to the attention of Europeans in the early 1900s after an Englishman named Charles Stevens was cured of his tuberculosis by a Basuto traditional healer who had given him large doses of pelargonium root.

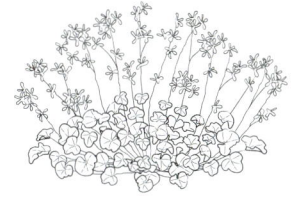

An evergreen herb growing to 10 in (25 cm), pelargonium forms a rosette of long-stalked, heart-shaped leaves with striking purple-black flowers.

Habitat and Cultivation
Pelargonium is still collected from the wild in the eastern parts of South Africa where it is native, though demand for the root has led to increased commercial cultivation. The root is harvested at the end of the growing season, sliced, and then kiln dried. The plant is mostly propagated from seed.

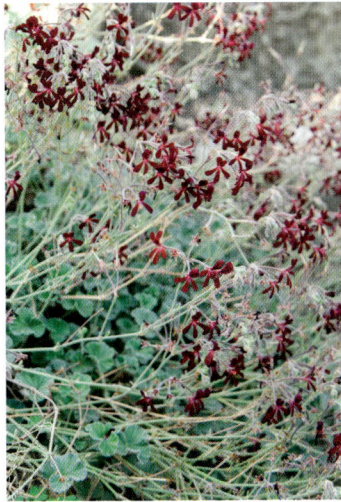

Related species
Many other geranium species have medicinal activity, including another South African species, *P. reniforme*, which is often used for the same indications. The closely related American cranesbill and herb robert (*Geranium maculatum* and *Geranium robertianum*, both p. 221) are strongly astringent in action.

Key constituents
• Polyphenols (including high levels of proanthocyanidins) • Coumarins

Key actions
• Antibacterial • Antiviral • Immune enhancing • Expectorant

Research
Antimicrobial Pelargonium extracts have been shown to have strong activity against a wide range of bacteria, notably those commonly responsible for ear, nose, throat, and chest infections. Extracts have also been shown to act against herpes viruses. The root exerts a tonic effect on the immune system.

Upper respiratory tract problems German research over the last 20–25 years has established conclusively that pelargonium is a safe and effective treatment for problems affecting the upper respiratory tract and chest. Clinical trials have shown

Pelargonium is a potent medicine for coughs, colds, and sore throats.

that it is an effective treatment for acute and chronic bronchitis, tonsillitis, sinusitis, and the common cold, reducing the intensity of symptoms and speeding recovery.

Children's remedy Unusually, several clinical trials have focused on treating respiratory infections in children, and the results of these indicate that pelargonium is a very safe and well-tolerated medicine for children (from 1 year old) with coughs, colds, sore throats, and sinus problems.

Traditional & current uses
Respiratory infections Now commonly available in health stores and pharmacies, pelargonium can be considered a front-line home treatment for upper respiratory problems and chest infections. It combines well with elderberry extract, also easily found and very safe for children.

Parts used

Root is used for its strong antimicrobial activity.

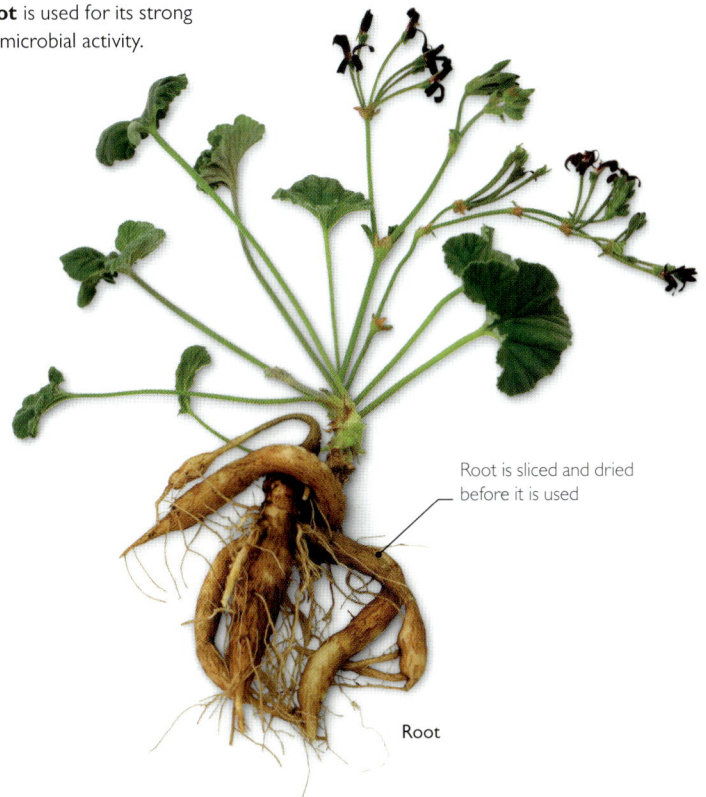

Root is sliced and dried before it is used

Root

Key preparations & their uses

Tincture (to make, p. 302) is a valuable remedy for acute and chronic bronchitis.

Tablets can be taken to support and strengthen immune function.

Fluid extract is best for children with upper respiratory tract infections.

Cautions Give to children under 1 year of age only on professional advice.

Traditional African remedy
Pelargonium has a much wider range of uses in South Africa, where the root has been used to treat not only respiratory infections, including tuberculosis, but conditions as diverse

as painful periods, liver disease, and gastroenteritis.

Self-help uses
• Colds & congestion in children, p. 328.

Persea americana (Lauraceae)

Avocado

Many parts of the avocado tree have a use in herbal medicine. The leaves and bark are effective remedies for digestive problems and coughs. As well as being extremely nutritious, the fruit has a wide range of medicinal uses. Indigenous peoples of Guatemala, for example, use the pulp to stimulate hair growth, the rind to expel worms, and the seeds to treat diarrhea. The fruit pulp is used as a baby food in West Africa.

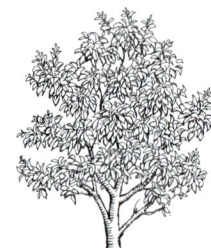

An evergreen tree growing to 65 ft (20 m), with dark green, leathery leaves and white flowers.

Habitat & cultivation
Indigenous to Central America, avocado is widely cultivated for its fruit in tropical and subtropical areas, including Israel, Spain, and South Africa. It is propagated from seed. The leaves are harvested as needed; the unripe fruit is picked when fully grown.

Related species
Other *Persea* species have similar fruits to avocado and are used in a similar way.

Key constituents
Leaves & bark:
• Volatile oil (methyl chavicol, alpha-pinene) • Flavonoids • Tannins
Fruit pulp:
• Unsaturated fats • Protein (about 25%) • Sesquiterpenes • Vitamins A, B_1, and B_2

Key actions
Leaves & bark:
• Astringent • Carminative • Relieve coughs • Promote menstrual flow
Fruit pulp:
• Emollient • Carminative
Rind:
• Eliminates worms

Research
Avocado has long been recognized as a healthy and health-giving food. A 2021 research review of the fruit that included 19 clinical trials has taken this understanding a major step further. The review concluded that avocado protected the heart and circulation in overweight and obese individuals with disordered blood fats/raised cholesterol levels, supported weight loss in the overweight and obese, lowered the risk of becoming overweight, and improved cognitive

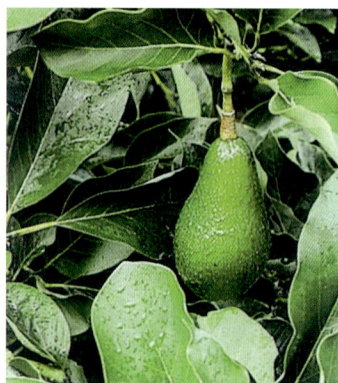

Avocado *is very nutritious and makes an excellent baby food.*

function in older adults. The fruit is also associated with a reduced risk of developing metabolic syndrome.
Poisons Livestock that have grazed on avocado leaves, fruit, or bark have been observed to suffer less toxic effects from snake bite and other poisons.

Traditional & current uses
Leaves & bark Avocado leaves and young bark stimulate menstruation and can induce abortion. The leaves are taken for diarrhea, bloating, and gas and are valuable for relieving coughs, for liver obstructions, and for clearing high uric acid levels.
Fruit The rind is used to expel worms. The fruit pulp is considered to have aphrodisiac properties. Used externally, it soothes the skin. It is applied to suppurating wounds and to the scalp to stimulate hair growth.
Oil The expressed oil of the avocado seed nourishes the skin. It softens rough, dry, or flaking skin and, massaged into the scalp, it improves hair growth.

Parts used

Leaves are an astringent remedy for diarrhea.

Bark is stripped from the tree for use in treating diarrhea and dysentery.

Seed contains good-quality oil.

Fruit is nutritious and is used to "draw" wounds.

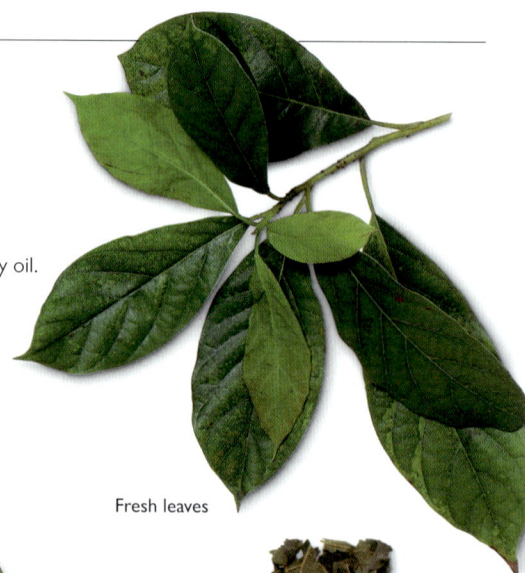

Fresh leaves

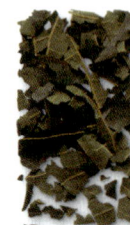

Dried leaves

Rind has the ability to expel worms

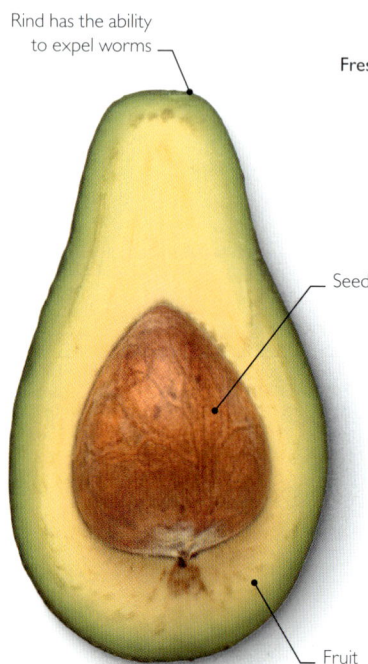

Seed

Fruit

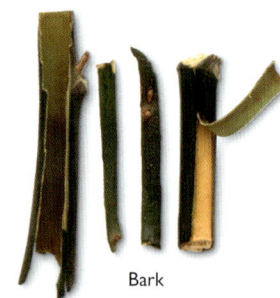

Bark

Key preparations & their uses

Decoction of leaves or bark (to make, p. 301). For diarrhea, take ⅓ cup (75 ml) 3 times daily.

Mashed pulp To help wounds heal, apply a little mashed pulp 3 times a day.

Oil from the seed. For skin blemishes, rub a little oil on the area daily 3 times a day.

Caution The leaves and bark should not be used during pregnancy.

Piper methysticum (Piperaceae)

Kava, Kava kava

Kava has major ritual and cultural significance among the peoples of the Pacific Islands, where it is as much a part of daily social life as coffee is in the West. In modest doses, kava is calming and tranquilizing. In large doses, it leads to intoxication and euphoria, though without a hangover the next day. It has a hot, slightly aromatic and bitter taste and leaves the mouth feeling slightly numb.

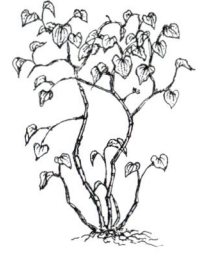

An evergreen shrub climbing to 10 ft (3 m), with fleshy stems and heart-shaped leaves.

Habitat & cultivation

Kava is an indigenous Polynesian vine and grows throughout the Pacific Islands as far east as Hawai'i. It is cultivated commercially in parts of the US and in Australia. Kava is propagated from runners in late winter or early spring and is usually grown on frames. It needs well-drained, stony soil and a shady position. The root is harvested at any time of year.

Related species

The closely related *P. sanctum* is native to Mexico. It is similar to kava in many ways; for example, it also contains kava lactones and is traditionally taken as a stimulant. Other related species include matico, betel, cubeb, and pepper (*P. angustifolia, P. betle, P. cubeba,* and *P. nigrum,* pp. 257–258).

Key constituents

• Resin containing kava lactones, including kawain • Piperidine alkaloid (pipermethysticine)

Key actions

• Tonic • Reduces anxiety • Urinary antiseptic • Analgesic • Induces sleep

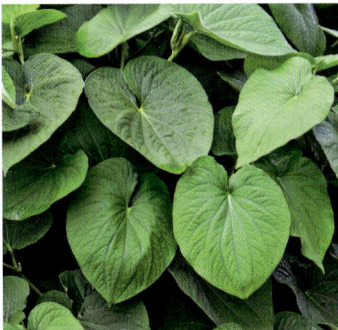

Kava has huge, tapering leaves, growing to 10 in (25 cm) across. Its root is used medicinally to relieve pain.

Research

German ban In 2002, German regulators banned kava products due to concerns that extracts were toxic to the liver and had led to 20 deaths. Many other countries followed Germany's example. The ban was repealed by the German authorities in 2015. Those campaigning against it had long maintained that the traditional use of kava, especially water-based extracts of kava, were inherently safe. Australian regulators had adopted this approach in 2003 by allowing the sale of water-based extracts of kava. A rigorous reexamination of the 20 fatal cases found that only two cases could in any way be attributed to the use of kava.

Anxiety A 2003 review of kava found that "compared with placebo, kava extract is an effective symptomatic treatment for anxiety." The authors commented that "few adverse events were reported in the reviewed trials." Kava is nonaddictive, and clinical evidence suggests it is also a safe and effective treatment for anxiety linked with depression, for insomnia, and for pain relief.

Traditional & current uses

Traditional aphrodisiac Kava is valued in the South Sea Islands as a calming and stimulating intoxicant. It produces a euphoric state when taken in large quantities.

Relaxing remedy Kava is a safe and proven remedy for anxiety that does not cause drowsiness or affect the ability to operate machinery. It is valuable for treating muscle tension as well as emotional stress.

Pain relief With its tonic, strengthening, and mildly analgesic properties, kava is a good remedy for chronic pain, helping reduce

Parts used

Root relieves pain and counters urinary infections.

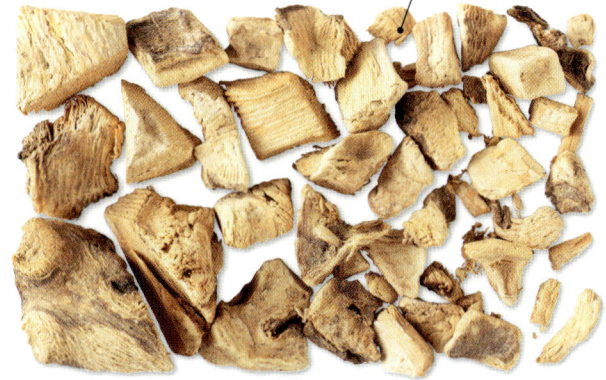

Traditionally the root is chewed and fermented with saliva

Dried root

Key preparations & their uses

Infusion (to make, p. 301). To relieve anxiety and muscle tension, drink ⅓ cup (75 ml) a day.

Tablets containing a water-based extract can be taken for anxiety.

Cautions Do not exceed recommended dosage or take for more than 2 months at a time. Use water-based extracts. Do not take during pregnancy. If there is a history of liver disease, take only with professional advice. Subject to legal restrictions in many countries.

sensitivity and relax muscles that are tensed in response to pain.

Arthritic conditions The analgesic and cleansing diuretic effect of Kava often makes it a beneficial herb for treating rheumatic and arthritic problems such as gout. It helps bring relief from pain and remove waste products from the affected joint.

Antiseptic Kava is routinely used by peoples of the South Pacific to treat infection, especially where pain is a key symptom. In New Guinea, it is taken to soothe and treat sore throats and to relieve toothache. It makes a valuable urinary antiseptic and will help in treating cystitis, urethritis, urinary frequency, and bladder irritability.

External uses The herb makes a useful analgesic mouthwash for treating toothache and mouth ulcers.

Plantago spp. (Plantaginaceae)

Psyllium, *Ispaghula* (Hindi), Flea seed

Produced by several *Plantago* species—*P. ovata*, *P. psyllium,* and *P. indica*—psyllium has been used as a safe and effective laxative for thousands of years in Europe, North Africa, and Asia. Given their small size and brown color, psyllium husks and seeds have been mistaken for fleas, hence their folk name flea seed. Bland-tasting, they swell when moistened, and have a jellylike consistency in the mouth.

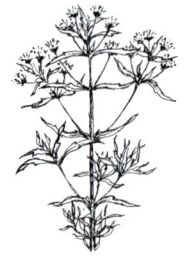

An annual growing to 16 in (40 cm) high, with narrow leaves and clusters of minute white-brown flowers.

Habitat & cultivation

The three species that produce psyllium grow throughout southern Europe, North Africa, and Asia, especially in India, and are extensively cultivated. They are propagated from seed in spring and require plenty of sun. The seeds are harvested when ripe in late summer and early fall.

Related species

Common plantain (*P. major*, p. 251) is prescribed for diarrhea and irritable bowel syndrome. *Che qian zi* (*P. asiatica*) is used in China as a diuretic, for diarrhea, and for bronchial congestion. The powdered husk is given late in pregnancy to aid normal presentation of the fetus (head-down position in the uterus).

Key constituents

• Mucilage (arabinoxylan) • Fixed oil (2.5%)—mainly linoleic, oleic, and palmitic fatty acids • Starch

Key actions

• Demulcent • Bulk laxative
• Antidiarrheal

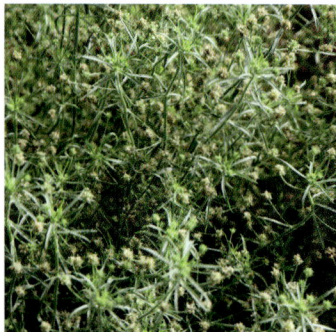

Psyllium is widely cultivated for its husks and seeds, which are used as a remedy for bowel problems.

Research

Regulating bowel function

Clinical trials in the US, Germany, and Scandinavia during the 1980s have shown that psyllium has both a laxative and an antidiarrheal action.

Effect on the microbiome Part of psyllium's effects are due to the positive influence it exerts on the microbiome (gut bacteria). A recent study found that in constipated patients, psyllium increased levels of specific gut bacteria, which in turn led to increased fluid levels within the colon.

Diabetes A 1998 clinical trial with 125 patients concluded that 5 g of psyllium taken 3 times a day helped lower blood-fat and -glucose levels in people with type 2 diabetes.

Traditional & current uses

Laxative Psyllium is prescribed in conventional as well as herbal medicine for constipation, especially when the condition results from an over-tensed or over-relaxed bowel. Both husks and seeds contain high levels of fiber (the mucilage) and expand, becoming highly gelatinous when soaked in water. By maintaining a high water content within the large intestine, they increase the bulk of the stool, easing its passage.

Other bowel problems Contrary to expectation, psyllium is a useful remedy for diarrhea. It is also an effective treatment for many other bowel problems, including ulcerative colitis, irritable bowel syndrome, and Crohn's disease. In India, psyllium is commonly used to treat dysentery.

Hemorrhoid relief Psyllium is valuable for hemorrhoids, helping to soften the stool and reduce irritation of the veins.

Parts used

Seeds should be soaked in water before they are used.

Seeds

Husks are generally powdered for use in a variety of preparations.

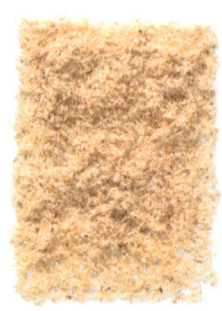

Powdered husk

Key preparations & their uses

Cold maceration For constipation, soak 20 g of seeds in ¾ cup (200 ml) water for 10 hours. Take the whole dose at night.

Capsules of powdered husk (p. 302). For hemorrhoids, take a 200 mg capsule 3 times a day.

Poultice For boils, mix 5 g of powdered husks with sufficient infusion of calendula to make a thick paste. Apply (*see* p. 305) 3 times a day.

Cautions Do not exceed the stated dose. Always take with plenty of water.

Detoxifying herb The jellylike mucilage produced when psyllium is soaked in water has the ability to absorb toxins within the large intestine. Psyllium is commonly taken to reduce autotoxicity (the toxins are expelled from the body with the husks and seeds in the feces).

Digestive ailments The soothing, protective effect imparted by the mucilage-rich husks and seeds benefits the whole gastrointestinal tract. Psyllium is taken for stomach and duodenal ulcers, and for acid indigestion.

Urinary infections The demulcent action of psyllium extends to the urinary tract. In India, an infusion of the seeds (the only time this preparation is used) is given for urethritis.

External uses When psyllium husks are soaked in an infusion of calendula (*Calendula officinalis*, p. 77), they make an effective poultice for external use, drawing out infection from boils, abscesses, and whitlows (pus-filled swellings on the fingertips).

Self-help uses

• Chronic diarrhea & irritable bowel syndrome, p. 317. • Constipation, p. 327. • Difficult passage of the stool & hemorrhoids, p. 312.

Polygonum multiflorum (Polygonaceae)

Fo Ti, *He shou wu* (Chinese)

A Chinese tonic herb with a bittersweet taste, *fo ti* is thought to concentrate *qi* (vital energy) in its root, so that taking this herb gives vitality to the body. It has always been considered a rejuvenating herb, helping prevent aging and encouraging longevity. Traditionally, much folklore is attached to this herb, and large, old roots are thought to have remarkable powers.

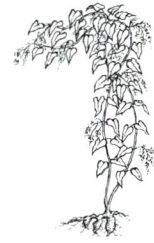

A perennial climber growing to 33 ft (10 m), with red stems, light-green leaves, and white or pink flowers.

Habitat & cultivation

Fo ti is native to central and southern China, and is cultivated throughout that region. It is propagated from seed or by root division in spring, or from cuttings in summer. The plant requires well-fertilized soil and plenty of protection from winter weather. The roots of 3- to 4-year-old *fo ti* plants are unearthed and dried during the fall. Older, larger roots are prized for their therapeutic properties, but are generally not available to obtain commercially.

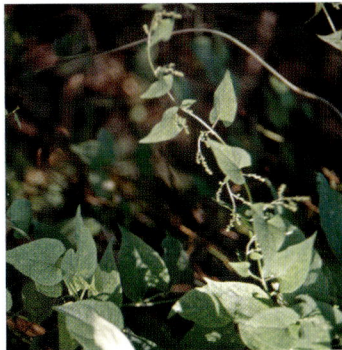

Fo ti is one of the oldest Chinese tonic herbs. It is used to help lower blood cholesterol levels.

Related species

Bistort (*P. bistorta*, p. 261), one of the most strongly astringent of all herbs, and knotgrass (*P. aviculare*, p. 260) are used in European herbal medicine. They do not have the same tonic therapeutic properties as *P. multiflorum*. In Chinese herbal medicine, *P. cuspidatum* is used to treat amenorrhea (absence of periods).

Key constituents

- Anthraquinone glycosides
- Stilbene glycoside • Polyphenols
- Phospholipids, including lecithin

Key actions

- Tonic • Antioxidant • Mild sedative
- Lowers cholesterol levels
- Neuroprotective

Research

Cholesterol levels In animal experiments in China, *fo ti* was shown to significantly reduce raised blood cholesterol levels. Also, in a clinical trial, over 80% of patients with high blood cholesterol who had been taking decoctions of the root showed an improvement.

Blood-sugar levels Chinese research has revealed that *fo ti* helps increase the levels of sugar in the blood.

Neuroprotective Preclinical research points to *fo ti* having a stabilizing effect on brain function, and that it might—as traditional use would suggest—prove valuable in slowing aging processes within the central nervous system.

Traditional & current uses

Popular tonic Although *fo ti* is not the earliest tonic herb listed in Chinese herbal medicine (it is first mentioned in 713 CE), it has become one of the most widely used. It is taken regularly by millions of people in the East for its rejuvenating and toning properties, and to increase fertility in both men and women.

Liver & kidney remedy In Chinese herbal medicine, *fo ti*'s most important use is as a tonic for the liver and kidneys. By strengthening liver and kidney function, it helps cleanse the blood, enabling the *qi* to circulate freely around the whole body.

Nerve & blood tonic *Fo ti* is given in Chinese herbal medicine to people with symptoms, such as dizziness,

Parts used

Root is highly valued in Chinese medicine for its tonic properties. It is unearthed in the fall.

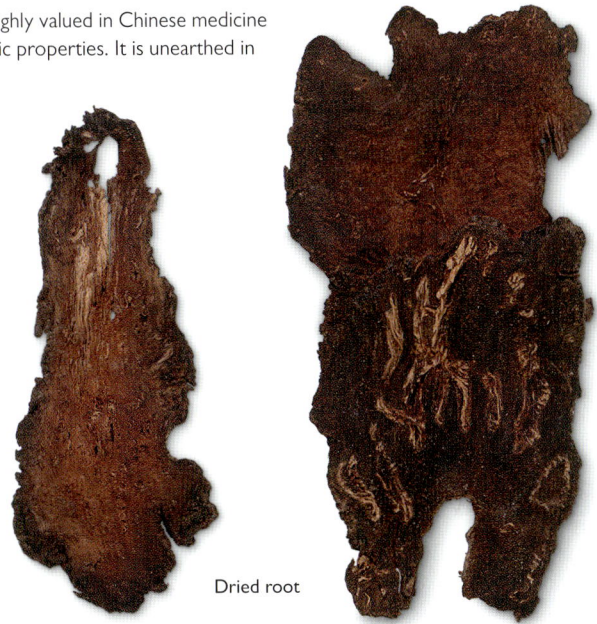

Dried root

Key preparations & their uses

Decoction (to make, p. 301). As a general tonic, take the decoction over 2 days.

Tablets, known as *shou wu pian*, are taken in China for their rejuvenating properties.

Tincture (to make, p. 302). To reduce

blood cholesterol levels, take 1 tsp twice a day with water.

Powder may be added to food for its tonic effect. Take 5 g a day.

Caution Only the prepared root from Chinese herbal shops should be used.

weakness, numbness, and blurred vision, that indicate inefficient nerves and "blood deficiency."

Premature aging *Fo ti* is prescribed in China for people showing signs of premature aging. This suggests it helps the body function in a balanced, healthy way. In particular, there is a lot of evidence to support the root's use

to aid reversing hair loss and graying of the hair.

Malaria The herb is prescribed in the treatment of chronic malaria, when it is often combined with ginseng (*Panax ginseng*, p. 123), dong quai (*Angelica sinensis*, p. 67), as well as green tangerine peel (*Citrus reticulata*).

Rheum palmatum (Polygonaceae)

Chinese rhubarb, *Da huang* (Chinese)

Chinese rhubarb has long been prized as the most useful purge in herbal medicine, safe even for young children due to its gentle action. It has been used in China for over 2,000 years and is an extremely effective treatment for many digestive problems. Paradoxically, it is a laxative when taken in large doses but has a constipating effect in small measures. The rhizome has an astringent, unpleasant taste.

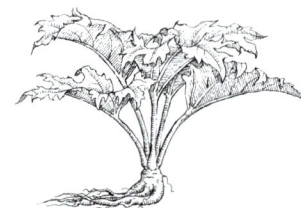

A thick-rhizomed perennial growing to 10 ft (3 m), with large palm-shaped leaves and small flowers.

Habitat & cultivation

Native to China, where the best-quality herb is still found, Chinese rhubarb now also grows in the West. It is found in the wild and is widely cultivated. It is grown from seed in spring or by root division in spring or fall and requires a sunny position and well-drained soil. The rhizomes of 6–10-year-old plants are dug up in the fall after the stem and leaves have turned yellow.

Related species

R. tanguticum and *R. officinale* have similar uses to *R. palmatum*. These 3 species are considered to be superior in action to other rhubarbs. The familiar, edible rhubarb is *R. rhaponticum*.

Key constituents

• Anthraquinones (3–5%), rhein, aloe-emodin, emodin • Flavonoids (catechin) • Phenolic acids • Tannins (5–10%) • Calcium oxalate

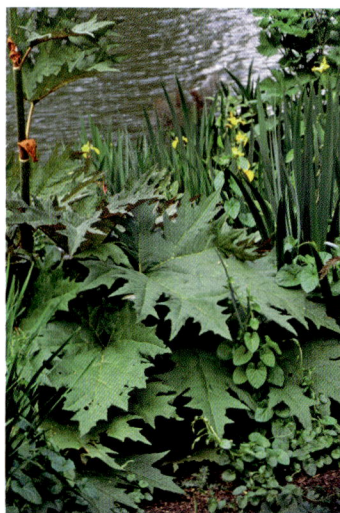

Chinese rhubarb grows best close to water. In summer it produces clusters of red flowers.

Key actions

• Laxative • Anti-inflammatory
• Astringent • Stops bleeding
• Antibacterial

Research

Anthraquinones & tannins

Chinese rhubarb's medicinal value is largely due to the irritant, laxative, and purgative properties of the anthraquinones, and in large doses the rhizome is strongly laxative. A 2007 Chinese study concluded that the anthraquinones in rhubarb "possess promising anticancer properties and could have a broad therapeutic potential."

Antibacterial properties

Decoctions of the root have been shown to be effective against *Staphylococcus aureus*, an infectious bacterium that causes mouth ulcers and folliculitis (an acne-type infection of the beard area). In laboratory studies, rhubarb has been found to have notable activity against *Helicobacter pylori*, a bacterium that causes stomach ulcers.

Traditional & current uses

History Chinese rhubarb was first mentioned in the 1st century CE Chinese text *The Divine Husbandman's Classic*, and has been grown in the West since 1732. It is one of the few herbs still used today in conventional as well as herbal medicine, and is listed in the *British Pharmacopoeia* of 1988.

Constipation Large doses of Chinese rhubarb are combined with carminative herbs and taken as a laxative, helping to clear the colon without causing excessive cramping. This is useful for treating constipation where the muscles of the large intestine are weak.

Parts used

Rhizome contains anthraquinones, which are laxative, and tannins, which are astringent.

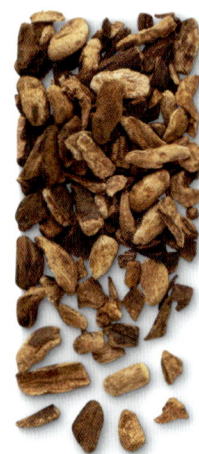

Rhizome is a mild appetite stimulant and helps improve digestion

Dried rhizome

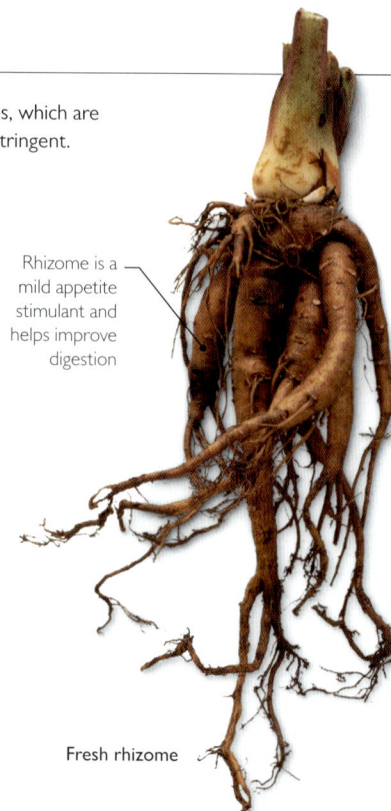

Fresh rhizome

Key preparations & their uses

Decoction (to make, p. 301). For an occasional bout of constipation, take ½ cup (100 ml) each evening.

Tincture (to make, p. 302). To stimulate the appetite, take 20 drops with water twice a day.

Tablets are one of the most convenient ways of taking the herb. Take for occasional bouts of constipation.

Cautions Do not take during pregnancy or while breastfeeding. Do not take during menstruation or if prone to gout or kidney stones. Not suitable for children.

Diarrhea Small doses of the root are astringent, relieving irritation of the inner lining of the gut, thus reducing diarrhea.

Other uses Chinese rhubarb can be applied to burns, boils, and carbuncles. The herb acts as a tonic and mild appetite stimulant and serves as a useful mouthwash for mouth ulcers.

Self-help use
• Constipation, p. 317.

Rhodiola rosea (Crassulaceae)

Rhodiola, Golden root

An Arctic plant that thrives in extreme environments, rhodiola's rose-colored roots have pronounced medicinal activity, enhancing the ability of the body to deal with stresses of all kinds. An adaptogen, similar to ginseng (*Panax ginseng*, p. 123), rhodiola also acts on the central nervous system, supporting memory and concentration under conditions of stress, and helping to relieve nervous exhaustion and mild to moderate depression.

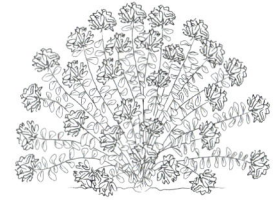

A fleshy perennial growing to 16 in (40 cm) in height with thick oblong leaves and clusters of yellow flowers.

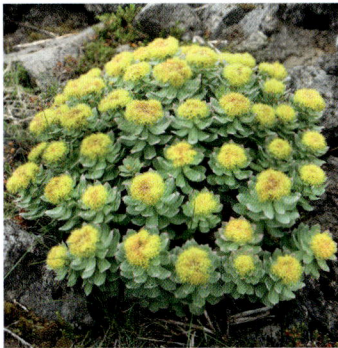

Rhodiola root is most commonly taken to improve mental and physical performance.

Habitat and Cultivation

Rhodiola is indigenous to mountainous and Arctic regions of the northern hemisphere, including Canada, Scotland, Scandinavia, Russia, and Alaska. Rhodiola is still mostly collected from the wild, threatening its long-term survival in some regions, though it is now cultivated in Canada, Norway, and Finland.

Related species

The central Asian *R. quadrifida* is used in Mongolia to enhance strength and vigor. *R. crenulata* and *R. rosea* are used in Chinese medicine, though across China many different species of *Rhodiola* are used to alleviate fatigue and protect against the cold. Chinese research into *R. crenulata* indicates that this species aids endurance and has a protective activity against radiation.

Key constituents

- Phenylpropanoids (rosavins—occurring only in *Rhodiola rosea*)
- Salidroside • Flavonoids
- Monoterpenes (including rosiridin)
- Triterpenes

Key actions

- Adaptogen • Antidepressant
- Aids mental performance
- Anti-inflammatory

Research

Adaptogen Rhodiola is an unusual medicine—an adaptogen that combines the ability to promote physical and mental endurance with antidepressant and anti-inflammatory activity. Though large-scale clinical trials are lacking, research shows that rhodiola root increases the capacity to resist physical and mental fatigue.

Clinical trials In a 2000 Armenian clinical trial, young, healthy doctors working night shifts in hospitals were given a rhodiola extract. After 2 weeks, those taking the extract showed significantly fewer signs of mental fatigue, including better levels of concentration and short-term memory, than those taking a placebo. In a 2015 US clinical trial, 57 adults with moderate depression were given rhodiola or sertraline, a conventional antidepressant. Both medicines proved effective, but those taking rhodiola reported fewer side effects.

Traditional & current uses

Key traditional uses In Europe and Asia, the central core of rhodiola's use in traditional medicine has always been its power to increase endurance and work rate, and the capacity to cope with high altitude and winter cold. The roots have also been taken to promote longevity, ease depression, and treat infection. Rhodiola is now most commonly taken to improve mental and physical performance and protect against the harmful effects of ongoing stress.

Russian medicine Rhodiola became an official medicine in Russia in 1969,

Parts used

Root helps support physical and mental endurance and counter the effects of stress.

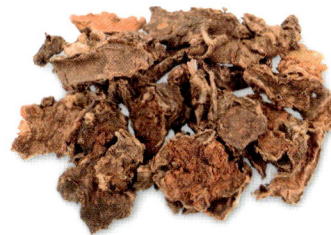

Dried rhizome

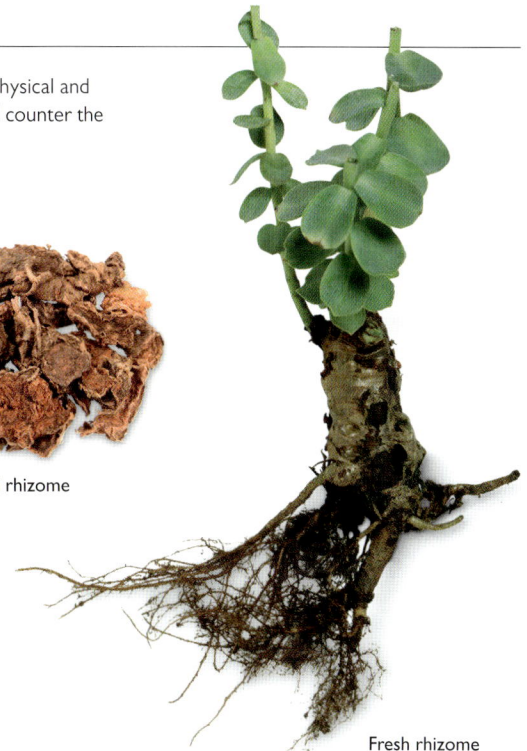

Fresh rhizome

Key preparations & their uses

Decoction Take 2½ tsp twice a day to promote physical endurance.

Tablets take as recommended by supplier for lowered mood and vitality.

Tincture (to make, p. 302). To

support memory and concentration, take ½ tsp 2–3 times a day.

Cautions Can cause irritability and sleep disturbance. Not advisable with manic and bipolar disorders.

being recommended for a wide range of health problems, not only as an adaptogen (*see Research*), but for psychiatric and neurological problems, such as depression and schizophrenia.

Other uses Rhodiola is traditionally considered to help improve fertility in both men and women. In Siberia, rhodiola roots are given to marrying

couples to promote fertility and the health of their future children. In Mongolia, alongside its use as a tonic, rhodiola is given for infections such as bronchitis and pneumonia, and is also used as a mouthwash for bad breath.

Self-help use

- Maintaining vitality, p. 329.

Rosmarinus officinalis (Lamiaceae)

Rosemary

Rosemary is a well-known and greatly valued herb that is native to southern Europe. It has been used since antiquity to improve and strengthen the memory. To this day it is burned in the homes of students in Greece who are about to take exams. Rosemary has a longstanding reputation as a tonic, invigorating herb, imparting a zest for life that is to some degree reflected in its distinctive aromatic taste.

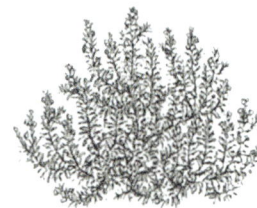

A strongly aromatic evergreen shrub growing to 6½ ft (2 m), with narrow, dark green, pine-like leaves.

Habitat & cultivation

Native to the Mediterranean, rosemary grows freely in much of southern Europe and is cultivated throughout the world. It is propagated from seed or cuttings in spring and prefers a warm, moderately dry climate and a sheltered site. The branches are gathered during the summer after flowering and dried in the shade.

Key constituents

- Volatile oil (1–2%) containing borneol, camphene, camphor, cineole
- Flavonoids (apigenin, diosmin)
- Tannins • Rosmarinic acid
- Diterpenes (including carnosic acid and carnosol)

Key actions

- Antiaging • Antidepressant
- Anti-inflammatory •
Neuroprotective • Bitter tonic
- Circulatory stimulant

Research

Neuroprotection and cognitive enhancement Several of rosemary's active constituents, notably rosmarinic acid and carnosol, are known to have beneficial effects on the brain.

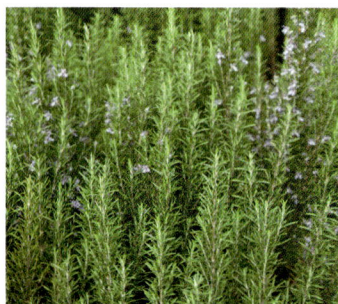

Rosemary was a symbol of fidelity between lovers, on account of its ability to improve the memory.

Rosemary is now thought to have neuroprotective activity and, in line with traditional usage, to enhance memory and cognition—in young and old alike. A double-blind clinical trial (2017) investigated the effects of rosemary on cognition and sleep in university students. Rosemary leaves, the study concluded, can be used to boost memory, reduce anxiety and depression, and improve sleep quality. A small 2012 study tested the immediate impact of rosemary leaf powder on mental performance in 28 adults with an average age of 75. Their cognitive performance improved, and the lowest dose of leaf (750 mg) proved to be the most effective. Small amounts of rosemary leaf, taken regularly, are thought to be the most effective way to use the herb.

Low blood pressure A small 2006 clinical trial in Germany concluded (in line with traditional usage) that rosemary raised blood pressure in people suffering from low blood pressure. All those taking rosemary also reported feeling better at the end of the trial.

Other actions Japanese laboratory research in 2003 found that diterpenes within rosemary (carnosic acid and carnosol) strongly stimulated nerve growth factor, suggesting that rosemary may stimulate nerve repair. A 2015 review in *Cancer Letters* stated that these constituents also had "promising results of anticancer activity."

Traditional & current uses

Circulatory stimulant Rosemary has a central place in European herbal medicine as a warming, tonic remedy that stimulates blood flow throughout the body, especially low blood pressure. It is thought to promote blood to the head, improving memory. It may be taken to relieve migraine and headaches and encourages hair growth and health.

Poor circulation Thought to raise low blood pressure, the herb is valuable for fainting and weakness associated with deficient circulation.

Restorative Rosemary aids recovery from long-term stress and chronic illness. It is thought to stimulate the adrenal glands and is used specifically for debility, especially when accompanied by poor circulation and digestion.

Uplifting herb Valued as an herb that raises the spirits, rosemary is useful for mild to moderate depression.

Other uses Applied as a lotion or diluted essential oil, rosemary eases aching, rheumatic muscles. Add the infusion, or essential oil, to bathwater for a reviving soak.

Self-help uses

- Migraine, p. 319. • Premenstrual syndrome, p. 325. • Sore throats, p. 321. • Tired & aching muscles, p. 322.

Parts used

Leaves are gathered in summer and used in preparations or distilled for their oil.

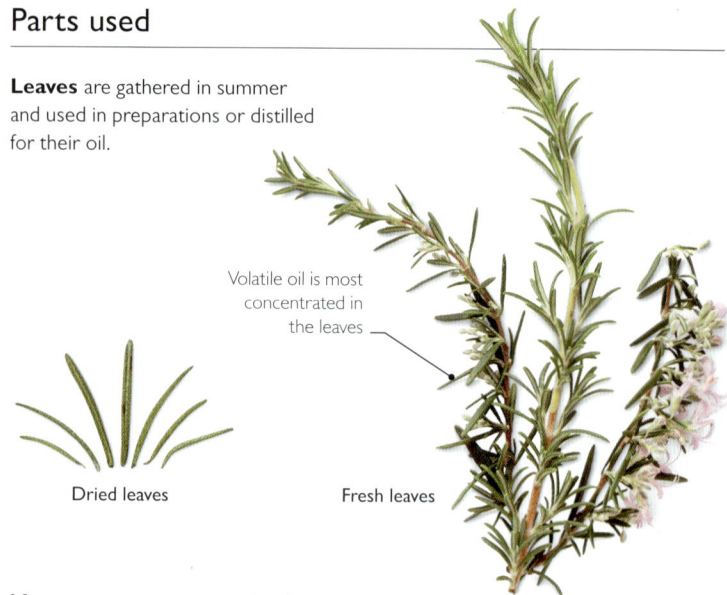

Volatile oil is most concentrated in the leaves

Dried leaves

Fresh leaves

Key preparations & their uses

Tincture (to make, p. 302) is an excellent tonic. For stress, take 40 drops twice daily with water.

Essential oil To improve concentration, burn several drops in an oil burner (to use, p. 307).

Infusion (to make, p. 301). To relieve headaches, take 2½ tsp every 3 hours. The infusion, rubbed into the scalp, improves hair growth.

Caution Do not take the essential oil internally except under a professional practitioner's supervision.

Salix alba (Salicaceae)

White willow

Justly famous as the original source of salicylic acid (the forerunner of aspirin), white willow and closely related species have been used for thousands of years in Europe, Africa, Asia, and North America to relieve joint pain and manage fevers. Dioscorides, a Greek physician in the 1st century CE, suggested taking "willow leaves, mashed with a little pepper and drunk with wine" to relieve lower back pain.

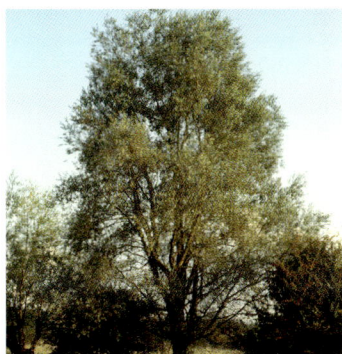

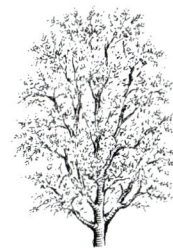

A deciduous tree growing to 80 ft (25 m), with green tapering leaves, and catkins in spring.

White willow is used in Britain to make cricket bats. The bark has anti-inflammatory properties.

Habitat & cultivation

Native to much of Europe, white willow is also found in northern Africa and Asia, thriving in damp areas, such as on riverbanks. It is propagated from semi-ripe cuttings in summer or from hardwood cuttings in winter. The trees are frequently pollarded and bark is stripped from branches of 2- to 5-year-old trees in spring.

Related species

Many *Salix* species, for example crack willow (*S. fragilis*), are used interchangeably with white willow. *S. acmophylla* is used on the Indian subcontinent as a remedy for fevers. In North American herbal medicine, black willow (*S. nigra*) is given as an anaphrodisiac (sexual depressant).

Key constituents

• Phenolic glycosides (up to 11%)
• Salicin • Flavonoids • Polyphenols

Key actions

• Anti-inflammatory • Analgesic
• Reduces fever • Antirheumatic
• Astringent

Research

Salicylic acid & aspirin Salicylic acid, a strongly anti-inflammatory and analgesic compound, was first isolated from salicin in willow bark in 1838. It was the forerunner of aspirin, a chemical drug developed in Germany during 1899. Salicylic acid (and salicin) has many of the properties of aspirin but causes notably fewer side effects. As such, it is now being widely researched as an alternative to aspirin-based anti-inflammatory medicines such as ibuprofen. Unlike aspirin, salicylic acid does not thin the blood, and any problems it might cause within the digestive tract are likely to be minor.

Clinical trials Over the last 15 years, clinical trials have shown that high-strength willow bark extract offers an effective alternative to mainstream anti-inflammatory medicines, particularly in treating conditions such as osteoarthritis and lower back pain. In a 2008 clinical trial published in *Phytomedicine*, among people with arthritis of the hip or knee, aged between 50 and 75, those taking willow bark extract, after 6 weeks, were rated by doctors as doing significantly better than those taking standard aspirin-based medication. Those taking willow bark reported far fewer side effects.

Traditional & current uses

Joint remedy White willow is an excellent remedy for arthritic and rheumatic pain affecting the back and joints such as the knees and hips, though large doses may be required, such as a standardized tablet. In combination with other herbs and dietary changes, it relieves inflammation and swelling, and improves mobility in painful or creaky joints.

Fevers & pain White willow is taken to manage high fevers. It may also be used to ease headaches and head pain.

Menopause A cooling herb that reduces sweating, willow bark can be helpful in controlling symptoms such as hot flashes and night sweats.

Parts used

Bark is stripped from young branches and used fresh or dried.

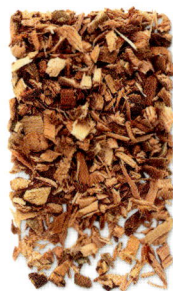

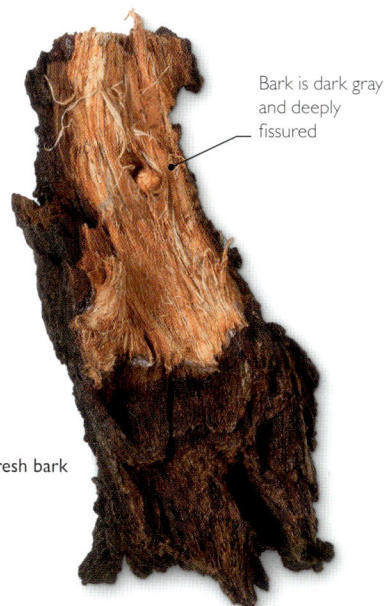

Bark is dark gray and deeply fissured

Dried bark

Fresh bark

Key preparations & their uses

Tincture (to make, p. 302). For rheumatism, take ½ tsp with water 3 times a day.

Remedy Make a decoction (*see* p. 301) with 10 g each of white willow, St. John's wort, and cramp bark. For aching muscles, drink ¾ cup (150 ml) twice a day.

Tablets often also contain other herbs. Take for arthritis.

Decoction (to make, p. 301). For painful joints and aching rheumatic muscles, take ⅓ cup (75 ml) 3 times a day.

Caution Avoid if allergic to aspirin. Do not take during pregnancy or if breastfeeding. Not suitable for young children. Rarely, may cause gastrointestinal upset.

Self-help uses

• Arthritis & inflamed joints, p. 323.
• Back pain due to joint inflammation, p. 323. • Hot flashes & night sweats, p. 326.

Salvia miltiorrhiza (Lamiaceae)

Dan shen, Chinese sage

Recent scientific research supports *dan shen's* traditional usage as a remedy for heart and circulatory problems such as angina and palpitations. *The Divine Husbandman's Classic* (*Shen'nong Bencaojing*), the earliest of all Chinese herbal texts, listed *dan shen* as an herb that "invigorates the blood," and it is still used as a circulatory remedy. In particular, it is taken for period pain and other conditions resulting from circulatory congestion.

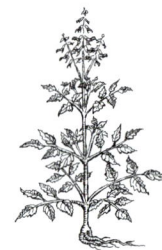

A hardy perennial growing to 32 in (80 cm), with toothed oval leaves and clusters of purple flowers.

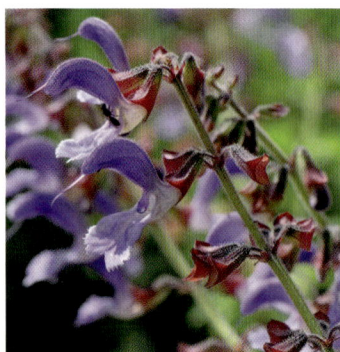

Dan shen is an important circulatory stimulant. It is sold in herbal markets across China for use in medicinal formulas.

Habitat & cultivation

Native to China, *dan shen* is now cultivated in northeastern China and Inner Mongolia. It requires moist, sandy soil and is propagated by root division in spring. The root is harvested from late fall through early spring.

Related species

Sage (*S. officinalis*, p. 135) is closely related, but is used for an entirely different range of medical problems. In Mexico, the related species *S. divinorum* is used as a hallucinogen.

Key constituents

• Diterpenes (tanshinones)
• Phenolic compounds • Volatile oil
• Vitamin E

Key actions

• Tonic to heart and circulation
• Anticoagulant • Dilates the blood vessels • Sedative • Antibacterial

Research

Tanshinones There has been extensive research into *dan shen* in China, and the tanshinones have been shown to have a profound effect on coronary circulation, reducing the symptoms of angina and improving heart function.

Heart attack The whole herb (rather than isolated constituents) has been used in China to assist patients who are recovering from a heart attack and it appears to support heart function at this critical time. Clinical trials in China, however, have shown that *dan shen* is most effective when taken as a preventative, rather than as a remedy after the heart attack has taken place.

Other research Many recent clinical trials involving *dan shen* have used Chinese herbal combinations, rather than *dan shen* alone, so it is hard to draw conclusions. However, they do provide further evidence of *dan shen's* usefulness in cardiovascular problems such as high blood pressure, angina, and heart disease. Unusually, two clinical trials in China (2012) found that injected extracts of *dan shen* were helpful in preeclampsia, a serious condition during pregnancy which involves fluid retention and high blood pressure.

Traditional & current uses

Circulatory stimulant *Dan shen* has been esteemed by the Chinese for thousands of years as a circulatory stimulant. Like hawthorn (*Crataegus oxyacantha*, p. 91), it is a safe, effective remedy for many circulatory problems. It particularly benefits coronary circulation, opening up the arteries and improving blood flow to the heart, and is therefore helpful in treating coronary heart disease. Though it does not lower blood pressure, *dan shen* relaxes the blood vessels and improves circulation throughout the body.

Circulatory congestion *Dan shen* is used traditionally to treat conditions caused by blood stagnation, primarily those affecting the lower abdomen, such as absent or painful periods and fibroids.

Sedative The sedative action of *dan shen* helps calm the nerves, and it is therefore helpful in treating angina, a condition made worse by anxiety and worry. Palpitations, insomnia, and irritability also benefit from *dan shen's* sedative properties.

Parts used

Root is an ancient Chinese remedy for circulatory disorders.

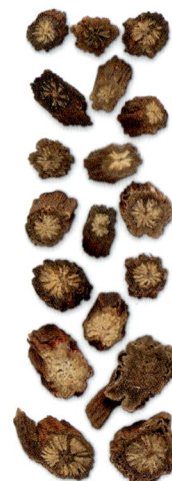

Dried chopped root

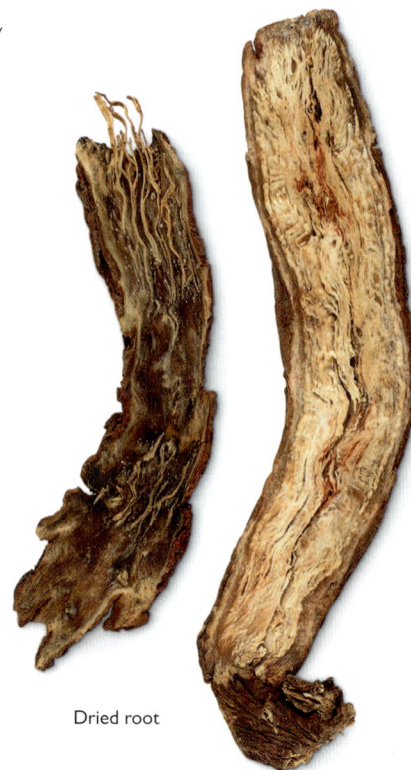

Dried root

Key preparations & their uses

Tincture is used by herbalists to treat angina and other circulatory problems.

Decoction (to make, p. 301). For painful periods, take 1/3 cup (75 ml) up to 3 times a day.

Self-help Use

• Migraine, p. 319. • Premenstrual tension, p. 325. • Sore throats, p. 321.
• Tired & aching muscles, p. 322.

Salvia officinalis (Lamiaceae)

Sage

Sage's botanical name is a clue to its medicinal importance: *Salvia* comes from *salvare*, meaning "to cure" in Latin. A medieval saying echoes this: "Why should a man die while sage grows in his garden?" Today, sage is an excellent remedy for sore throats, poor digestion, and irregular periods, and it is also taken as a gently stimulating tonic. It has a slightly warm, noticeably bitter, and astringent taste.

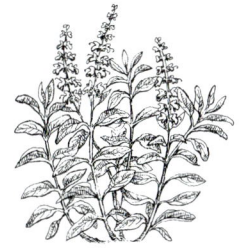

An evergreen growing to 32 in (80 cm), with square stems and hairy gray-green or purple leaves.

Habitat & cultivation

Native to the Mediterranean, sage is cultivated all around the world, thriving in sunny conditions. It is grown from seed in spring and the plants are replaced after 3 to 4 years. The leaves are picked in summer.

Related species

In all, there are about 500 species of *Salvia*. Spanish sage (*S. lavandulifolia*) is the most familiar culinary variety and does not contain thujone. Two close relatives of *S. officinalis* are *dan shen* (*S. miltiorrhiza*, p. 134) and clary sage (*S. sclarea*, p. 274).

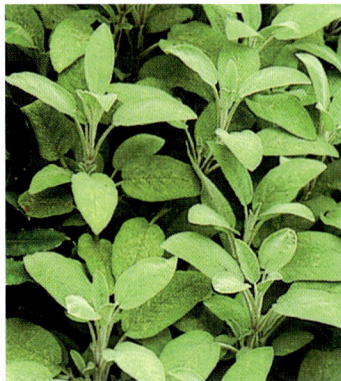

Key constituents

• Essential oil (1–2%) • Diterpenes
• Triterpenes • Phenolic compounds including rosmarinic acid • Tannins

Key actions

• Antiseptic • Astringent • Clears mucus • Nerve tonic • Estrogenic

Research

Nerve tonic Ongoing research taking place in the UK provides strong support for the traditional use of sage to enhance memory. In the most recent study (2008), healthy volunteers averaging 73 years of age showed a significant improvement in memory processing and accuracy of attention after taking a single dose of sage extract. Interestingly, a moderate dose, equivalent to 2.5 g of sage, proved most effective, more so than higher doses.
Sore throat In a randomized trial published during 2006, a sage throat spray was found to relieve throat pain in people who had acute throat infection.
Hormonal activity The herb's

Sage is known most commonly as a culinary herb, but it is also of great medicinal importance.

longstanding use during menopause has also been researched. In the most recent study, undertaken in Switzerland (2011), women with at least 12 months of hot flashes reported an average 64% decrease in symptoms after 8 weeks of taking sage.
Lowering blood fat levels A clinical trial published in 2011 in *Phytotherapy Research* concluded that "sage may be effective and safe in the treatment of hyperlipidemia." All blood fat markers showed improvement in those taking sage.

Traditional & current uses

Sore throat Sage's combination of antiseptic and astringent action makes it ideal as a gargle for sore throats and throat infections. It can equally be used for mouth ulcers and sore gums.
Hormonal remedy A valuable remedy for irregular and scanty periods, sage encourages better blood flow at menstruation. The herb is thought to reduce or prevent

Parts used

Leaves have valuable antiseptic and astringent properties.

Purple sage, *S. officinalis purpurascens*, is the preferred medicinal variety

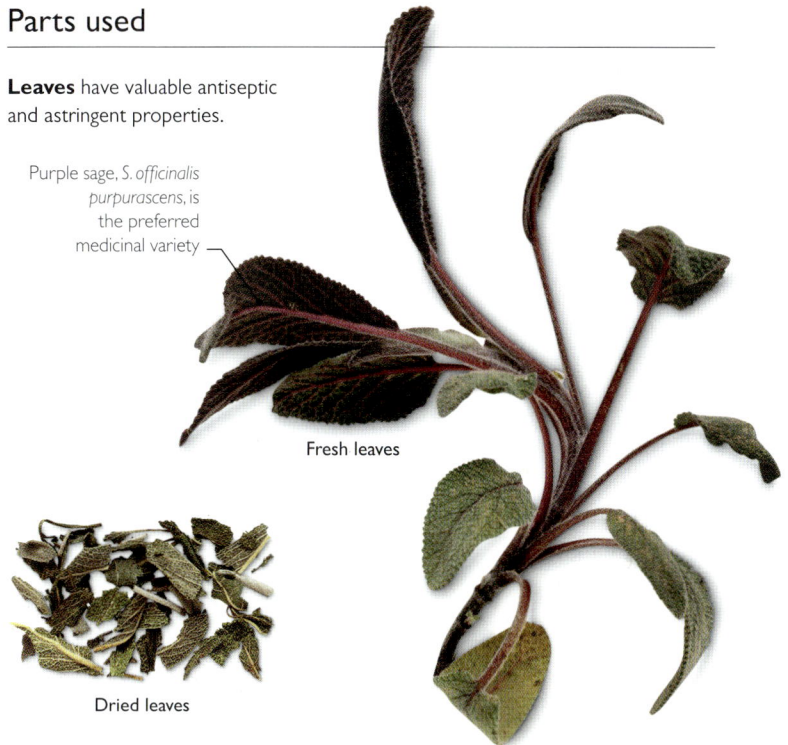

Fresh leaves

Dried leaves

Key preparations & their uses

Infusion (to make, p. 301). Use as a gargle for sore throats up to 3 times a day.

Tincture (to make, p. 302) is a digestive tonic. Take 40 drops with water twice a day.

Fresh sage leaves are a useful first aid remedy. Rub on stings and bites.

Cautions Do not take medicinal doses during pregnancy or while breastfeeding, or if epileptic.

sweating and can prove particularly effective during menopause. It also helps reduce hot flashes and night sweats and it has a calming, relaxant aspect. Sage will decrease breast milk production, and is traditionally taken by a mother while weaning.
Digestive tonic Sage has a long traditional use as a digestive aid,

supporting stomach health and promoting better digestion and absorption.

Self-help uses

• Bites & stings, p. 313. • Diarrhea, p. 317. • Hot flashes & night sweats, p. 326. • Mouth ulcers, p. 316. • Sore throats, p. 321.

Sambucus nigra (Caprifoliaceae)

Elder, European elder

Elder has more folklore attached to it than almost any other European plant, except perhaps mandrake (*Mandragora officinarum*, p. 238). Chopping elder branches was considered dangerous in rural England as it was believed that the tree was inhabited by the Elder Mother, and to avoid her wrath, woodcutters would recite a placatory rhyme. Elder is a valuable remedy for flu, colds, and chest conditions.

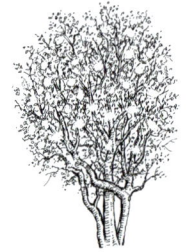

A deciduous tree growing to 33 ft (10 m), with oval leaves, cream flowers, and blue-black berries.

Habitat & cultivation

Native to Europe, elder thrives in woods, hedges, and in waste ground. It is now found in most temperate regions, and is often cultivated. Elder is propagated from cuttings in spring. The flowering tops are harvested in late spring and the berries are picked in early fall.

Key constituents

Berries:
- Flavonoids • Anthocyanins
- Lectins • Vitamins A and C

Flowers:
- Flavonoids • Anthocyanins
- Lectins • Vitamins A and C
- Triterpenes • Volatile oil (0.7%)
- Mucilage • Tannins

Key actions

- Antiviral • Clears mucus
- Anti-inflammatory • Diuretic
- Increases sweating

Research

Elder berries Israeli influenza research from 1995 found 90% of people that were given elderberry extract recovered in 2–3 days, while 90% of those taking the placebo took up to 6 days. Further clinical trials have supported these findings—a 2014 review concluded there was "good scientific evidence" that elderberry extract was an effective treatment for influenza. Although the safety profile of elderberry has not been established, evidence indicates it is a safe influenza remedy for adults and children.

Traditional & current uses

Coughs & colds The berries have an established antiviral activity, helping prevent and speed recovery from upper respiratory infections, such as colds and flu. Following traditional usage, the flowers are taken to stimulate sweating and relieve fever by cooling the body. An elderflower infusion makes a soothing remedy when suffering from cold and flu.

Congestion & allergies The flowering tops tone the mucous linings of the nose and throat (increasing their resistance to infection) and are prescribed for chronic congestion, ear infections, and allergies. Infusions with other herbs can reduce severity of hay fever attacks if taken some months before the season.

Arthritis By encouraging sweating and urine production, elder flowering tops aid removal of waste products and are of value in arthritic conditions.

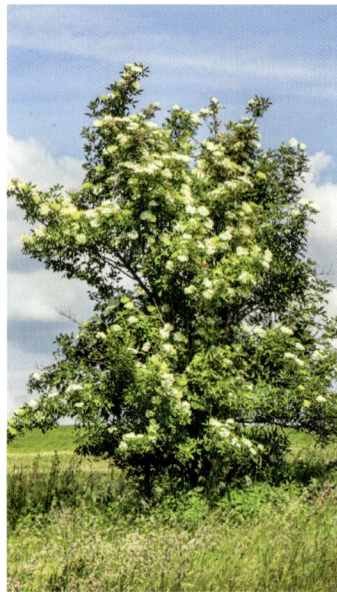

Elder was traditionally known as "Nature's medicine chest."

Parts used

Flowering tops reduce fevers and help coughs, colds, and flu.

Berries are nutritious and may be used as a mild laxative.

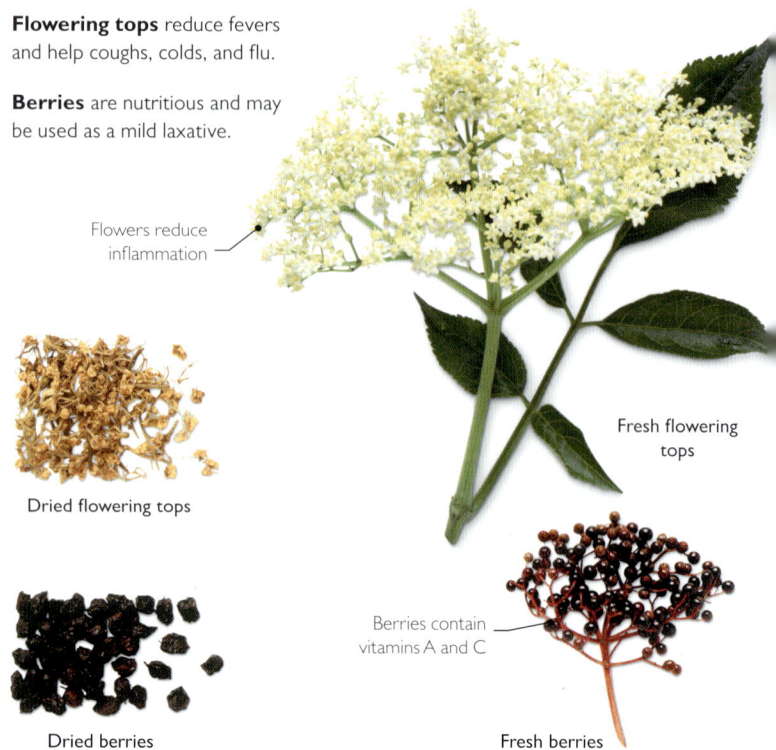

Flowers reduce inflammation

Dried flowering tops

Fresh flowering tops

Berries contain vitamins A and C

Dried berries

Fresh berries

Key preparations & their uses

Infusion of flowering tops (to make, p. 301). For colds, drink ¾ cup (150 ml) 3 times a day.

Cream made with flowering tops (see p. 306). Apply freely to chapped skin.

Tincture of flowering tops (to make, p. 302). For hay fever, take 1 tsp with water 3–4 times a day.

Decoction of berries (to make, p. 301). For rheumatic aches, take ½ cup (100 ml) 3 times a day.

Other uses Flowers and berries are mildly laxative and appear to help lower blood pressure. The flowers are thought to help control diabetes. The berries appear to enhance immune function.

Self-help uses

- Allergic rhinitis, including hay fever, p. 310. • Colds, flu, & fevers, p. 321.
- Colds & congestion in children, p. 328. • Earache due to chronic congestion, p. 322.

Schisandra chinensis (Schisandraceae)

Schisandra, *Wu wei zi* (Chinese)

Schisandra ranks along with other Chinese tonic herbs as an excellent tonic and restorative. It helps in stressful times and increases zest for life. The berries tone the kidneys and sexual organs, protect the liver, strengthen nervous function, and cleanse the blood. The name *wu wei zi* means "5-flavored herb," since this herb reputedly tastes of the 5 main elemental energies (see p. 44). It has a sour, salty, and slightly warm taste.

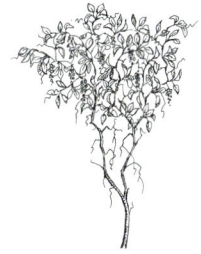

An aromatic, woody vine reaching up to 26 ft (8 m), with pink flowers and spikes of red berries.

Habitat & cultivation

Schisandra is cultivated in northeastern China, especially in the provinces of Jilin, Liaoning, Heilongjiang and Hebei. It is propagated from seed in spring. The fruit is harvested in the fall when it is fully ripe.

Related species

Though less therapeutically active than schisandra, the berries of the related *nan wu wei zi* (*S. sphenanthera*) are commonly used in Chinese medicine for the treatment of acute coughs.

Key constituents

- Lignans (schizandrin, deoxyschizandrin, gomisin)
- Triterpenes • Volatile oil
- Vitamins C and E

Key actions

- Nerve tonic • Adaptogenic
- Protects liver

Research

Aiding performance Healthy adults given schisandra extract showed a marked improvement in both physical and mental stamina. Russian sailors given schisandra had an increased capacity to maintain and endure normal working regimens, and Russian factory workers were reported to have decreased sickness levels.

Protecting the liver The lignans have been shown to have pronounced antihepatoxic (liver-protective) action. Up to 30 different lignans have been identified in schisandra, which all contribute to this effect. One clinical trial reported a 76% success rate in treating patients with hepatitis, with no side effects being noted.

Nervous system Schisandra is known to stimulate the nervous system, increasing the speed of reflex nervous responses and improving mental clarity. The berries have a mild antidepressant activity and are thought to improve nervous irritability and forgetfulness. In Russia, schisandra has been used to treat people with severe mental health disorders including schizophrenia and chronic alcoholism. Clinical studies in 1967 found that those taking a schisandra tincture became more sociable and less emotionally tense.

Traditional & current uses

Tonic Schisandra is a major tonic herb and acts throughout the body, strengthening and toning many different organs.

Sexual stimulant Probably best known as a sexual tonic for both men and women, schisandra reputedly increases the secretion of sexual fluids and, in men, it also improves sexual stamina.

Liver treatment herb Schisandra has proven benefits for the liver and is used in the treatment of hepatitis and poor liver function.

Sedative Although a stimulant, schisandra is used in Chinese medicine to "quiet the spirit and calm the heart." It is given for insomnia and dream-disturbed sleep and is a fine example of how adaptogenic herbs often work in apparently contradictory ways to restore normal body function.

Mental & emotional disorders In Russia and China, schisandra berries have traditionally been prescribed to treat mental illnesses such as neuroses. They are also given to improve concentration and coordination and are a traditional remedy for forgetfulness and irritability.

Respiratory infections The herb is used in the treatment of respiratory infections such as chronic coughs, shortness of breath, and wheezing.

Parts used

Fruit helps the body cope with stress.

Berries are chewed every day for 100 days as a tonic in China

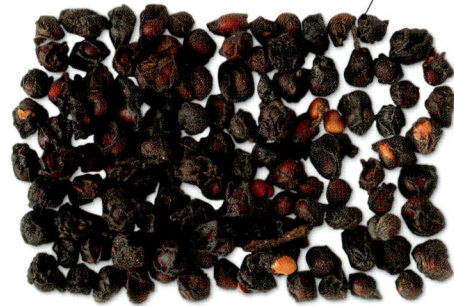

Dried fruit

Key preparations & their uses

Decoction (to make, p. 301). For coughs and shortness of breath, decoct 5 g crushed berries with ½ cup (100 ml) of water. Divide into 3 doses and drink during a 24-hour period.

Balancing fluid levels Schisandra is used to tone and strengthen kidney function and to help the body balance levels of fluid, making it helpful for treating night sweats, thirst, and urinary frequency.

Skin rashes Recently, Chinese herbalists have started to use schisandra to treat urticaria (hives) and other skin problems, including eczema. It is usually given for these conditions in the form of a medicinal wine.

Additional uses Schisandra is used for a wide variety of other physical disorders, including diarrhea and dysentery, as well as to help improve failing sight and hearing.

Self-help use

- Low sex drive, p. 326.

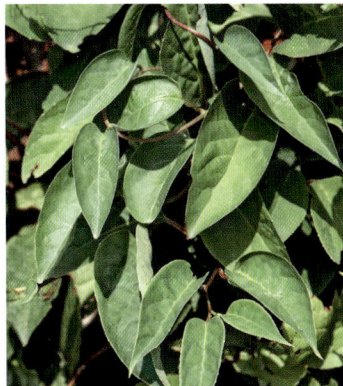

Schisandra is one of China's most important tonic herbs, widely taken as a sexual tonic.

Scutellaria baicalensis syn. *S. macrantha* (Lamiaceae)

Baikal skullcap, *Huang quin*

In 1973, 92 wooden tablets were discovered in a 2nd-century CE tomb in northwestern China. Among other herbs listed in prescriptions for decoctions, tinctures, pills, and ointments was Baikal skullcap. The herb has had an established role in Chinese herbal medicine at least from that time, and is one of the main remedies for "hot and damp" conditions, such as dysentery and diarrhea.

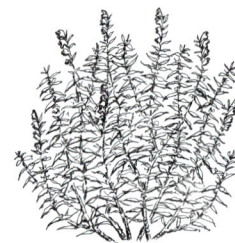

A perennial growing to 1–4 ft (30–120 cm) high, with lance-shaped leaves and purplish-blue flowers.

Habitat & cultivation

Baikal skullcap is found in China, Japan, Korea, Mongolia, and Russia. It thrives on sunny, grassy slopes and waste ground between 330 ft (100 m) and 5,900 ft (1,800 m) above sea level. Baikal skullcap is propagated from seed sown in the fall or spring. The roots of 3- to 4-year-old plants are harvested in the fall or spring.

Related species

Skullcap (*S. lateriflora*, p. 139) is a close relation, used by Indigenous North American peoples for anxiety and stress.

Key constituents

• Flavonoids (about 12%)—baicalin, wogoniside • Sterols • Benzoic acid

Key actions

• Sedative • Anti-allergenic
• Antibacterial • Anti-inflammatory

Research

Flavonoids Baikal skullcap has been quite widely researched in China, and it is clear that it has marked anti-inflammatory, anti-allergy, and antioxidant effects, all 3 actions mostly being due to the flavonoids.
Clinical evidence Clinical studies investigating different applications of Baikal skullcap show the herb has promise in the treatment of infections, including bronchitis, and dysentery, high blood pressure, chronic hepatitis, and allergic rhinitis (hay fever). The root has anticancer activity, with studies showing small-scale positive results in patients with lung and prostate cancer.
Diabetes The herb may be useful for problems arising from diabetes, including cataracts.
Weight-loss aid A South Korean

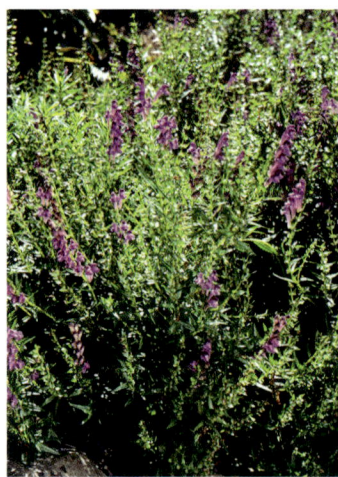

Baikal skullcap is an important medicinal plant in China and is also cultivated as an ornamental.

clinical trial in 2011 looked at the effectiveness of a Baikal skullcap and platycodon (Platycodon grandiflorum) combination in treating obesity. After 2 months, the group taking the herbs had lost significantly more weight than the placebo group.

Traditional & current uses

Cold & bitter herb In traditional Chinese medicine, Baikal skullcap is "cold" and "bitter" (see p. 42). It is prescribed in China for hot and thirsty conditions such as high fevers; coughs with thick, yellow phlegm; and gastrointestinal infections that cause diarrhea, such as dysentery. It is also given to people suffering from painful urinary conditions.
Circulatory remedy Baikal skullcap is a valuable remedy for circulation. In combination with other herbs, it is used to treat high blood pressure, arteriosclerosis, varicose veins, and easy bruising.

Parts used

Root is harvested when the plant is 3–4 years old in the fall or spring.

Root has anti-inflammatory properties

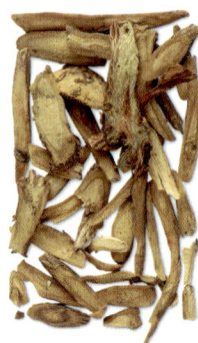

Dried root

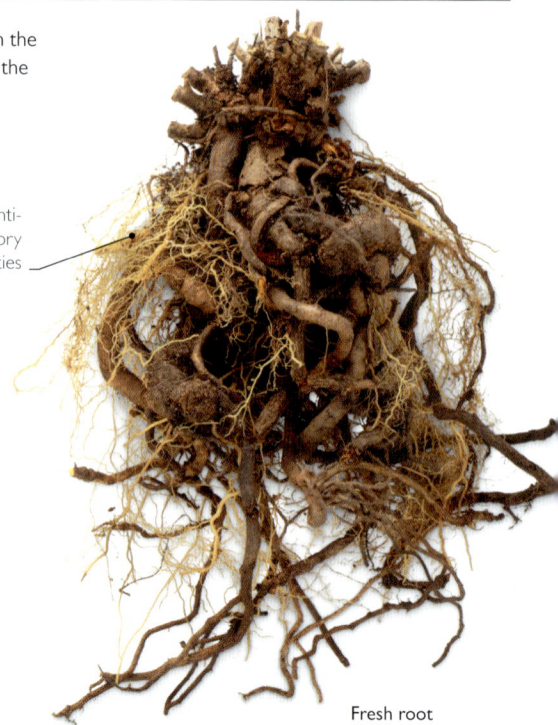

Fresh root

Key preparations & their uses

Decoction (to make, p. 301). For feverish chest colds, drink ⅓ cup (75 ml) 3 times a day.

Remedy For headaches, decoct 15 g root with 10 g self-heal (see p. 301). Drink ⅓ cup (75 ml) 3 times a day.

Tincture (to make, p. 302). For hay fever, take 40 drops with water 3 times a day.

Other uses Applied to the skin, Baikal skullcap treats sores, swelling, and boils. It is also given for circulatory problems that arise from diabetes.
Allergic conditions The herb is useful for treating allergic conditions such as asthma, hay fever, eczema, and

hives. The flavonoids in particular inhibit the inflammatory processes in the body that lead to allergic reactions.

Self-help uses

• Allergic rhinitis including hay fever, p. 310. • Wheezing, p. 311.

Scutellaria lateriflora (Lamiaceae)

Skullcap, Virginian skullcap, Mad dog

A key North American medicinal plant, skullcap has longstanding use as a remedy for menstrual problems. It was also used in purification ceremonies when menstrual taboos had been broken. Skullcap became well-known in 19th-century America as a treatment for rabies, hence its folk name "mad dog." Today, it is mainly used as a tonic and sedative for the nerves in times of stress. It has a bitter, slightly astringent taste.

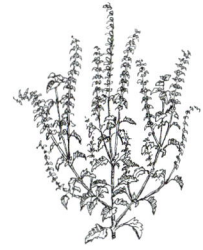

A perennial growing to 2 ft (60 cm), with an erect, many-branched stem and pink to blue flowers.

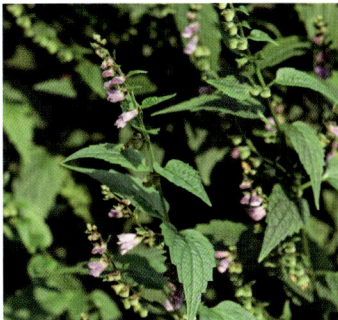

Skullcap is easy to recognize. It has pairs of pink to blue flowers and distinctive seed capsules.

Habitat & cultivation

A native of North America, skullcap still grows wild in much of the US and Canada. It thrives in damp conditions, for example on riverbanks, and needs plenty of sun. Skullcap can be propagated from seed or by root division in spring. The aerial parts of 3- to 4-year-old plants are harvested in summer, when in flower.

Related species

There are around 100 species of Scutellaria. In the past, European skullcap (*S. galericulata*) and lesser skullcap (*S. minor*) have been used in a similar way to S. lateriflora, but today they are considered to have a less important therapeutic action. Baikal skullcap (*S. baicalensis*, p. 138) is also closely related.

Key constituents

• Flavonoids (scutellarin) • Bitter iridoids (catalpol) • Volatile oil
• Tannins

Key actions

• Sedative • Nervine tonic
• Antispasmodic • Mild bitter

Research

Anxiety remedy Little research has been carried out on this species of *Scutellaria* despite its long use in North American and British herbal medicine to ease anxiety and stress. A small English study published in 2011 tested skullcap against placebo in reducing anxiety in 43 "non-anxious" people. Those taking skullcap showed significantly better overall mood levels at the end of the 2 weeks of the study.

Traditional & current uses

Indigenous cure The Cherokee peoples used skullcap to stimulate menstruation, relieve breast pain, and encourage expulsion of the placenta.

19th-century remedy The Physiomedicalists (followers of a 19th-century Anglo-American school of herbal medicine) first discovered skullcap's use as a nervine. They recognized that it has a "deeper" action on the nervous system than many other herbs and used it for hysteria, epilepsy, convulsions, and rabies, as well as for serious mental illnesses such as schizophrenia.

Current uses Today, skullcap is taken mainly as a nerve tonic and for its restorative properties. It helps support and nourish the nervous system, and calms and relieves stress and anxiety. Its antispasmodic action makes it useful for conditions where stress and worry cause muscular tension. Skullcap is often prescribed on its own, or with other sedative herbs, to treat insomnia, and it is also given for period pain.

Self-help uses

• Anxiety, depression, & tension, p. 318. • Migraine, p. 319. • Panic attacks & headaches, p. 318.

Parts used

Aerial parts are harvested in summer for use in a number of calming preparations.

Seed capsules, when dry, look like skullcaps

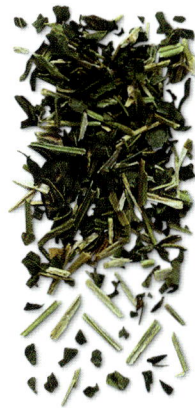

Dried aerial parts

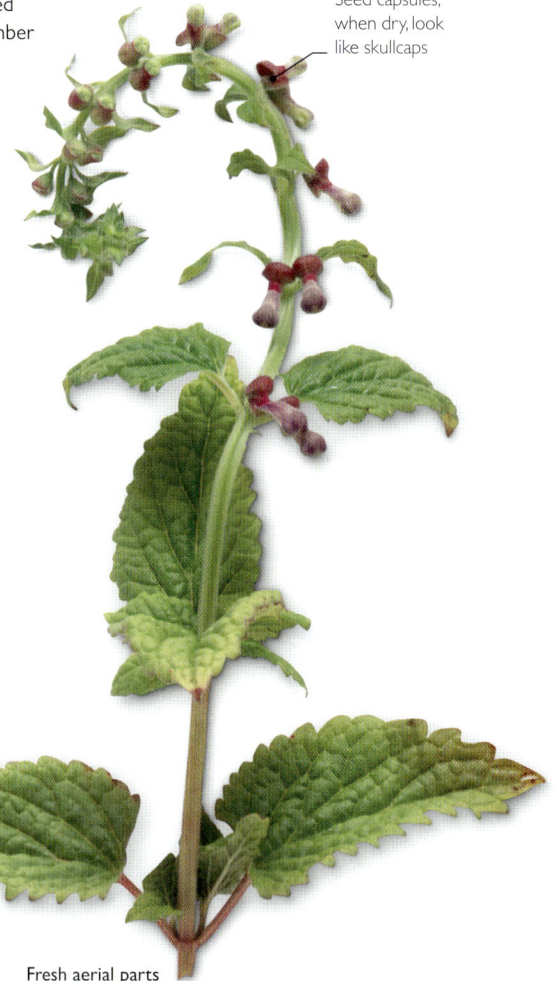

Fresh aerial parts

Key preparations & their uses

Infusion (to make, p. 301). For short-term relief of stress and anxiety, take 2½ tbsp 3 times a day.

Tincture (to make, p. 302). For nervous tension and headaches, take ½ tsp with water twice a day.

Capsules (to make, p. 302). For nervous exhaustion, take a 200 mg capsule twice daily.

Tablets, often containing other sedative herbs, are taken for insomnia.

Serenoa repens syn. *Sabal serrulata* (Palmaceae)

Saw palmetto

Saw palmetto berries were widely eaten as food by indigenous peoples in Florida. European colonizers reported seeing animals consuming the berries grow "sleek and fat", ate the berries and attributed medicinal properties to them. The fruit pulp was used as a tonic from the 19th century onward, and today it is used to help in debility, for urinary tract problems, and for reducing an enlarged prostate gland.

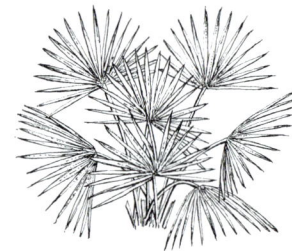

A small palm growing to 20 ft (6 m), with fans of yellow-green leaves and ivory flowers.

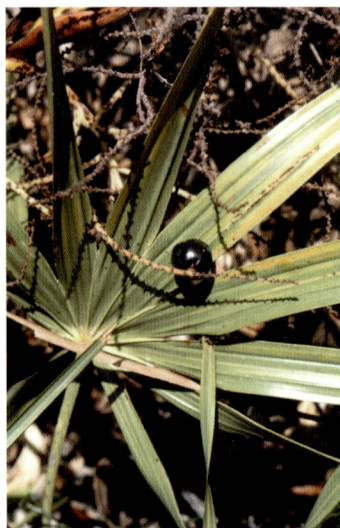

Saw palmetto has dark purple to black berries, growing in the center of the leaf fans.

Habitat & cultivation

Saw palmetto is indigenous to North America and can be found growing in sand dunes along the Atlantic and Caribbean coasts from South Carolina to Texas. It is propagated from seed in spring and needs well-drained soil and plenty of sun. The berries are harvested when ripe in the fall, then dried, often with the seeds removed.

Related species

The Maya of Central America used the roots or leaves of *S. japa,* another small palm, as a remedy for dysentery and abdominal pain. The crushed roots of *S. adamsonii* were used by the Houma, who also lived in Central America, as an eye lotion.

Key constituents

• Lipid (fat) content includes phytosterols • Flavonoids
• Polysaccharides

Key actions

• Anti-inflammatory • Antispasmodic
• Diuretic • Male tonic

Research

Benign prostatic hypertrophy (BPH) Extensive clinical research, mostly in Europe, has shown that a lipid or fat extract of saw palmetto is effective in reversing enlargement of the prostate gland. In the process, the extract reduces urinary retention and eases urine flow. In many European countries saw palmetto extract is a standard treatment for enlarged prostate. It is not clear how extracts of the herb work.

Combination with nettle root In the late 1990s two clinical trials gave men with early stage BPH a combination of saw palmetto and nettle root. One trial compared the herbs with placebo, the other with finasteride, a standard conventional treatment for BPH. Results for the herb combination in both trials were very good, with a clear improvement in symptoms in respect to placebo, and similar outcomes for those taking the herbs or finasteride, but those taking the herbs experienced fewer side effects.

Traditional & current uses

Urinary remedy Saw palmetto has been nicknamed the "plant catheter." This is because it has the ability to strengthen the neck of the bladder, and to reduce an enlarged prostate gland. It can be equally useful in treating lower urinary tract symptoms, such as pain, frequency, and urgency in urination. It is a useful remedy in cystitis and prostatitis (inflammation of the prostate gland).

Anabolic action Saw palmetto is a tonic and is one of the few Western remedies that is considered to be anabolic—it strengthens and builds body tissues and encourages weight gain. Fruit pulp or tincture is given to those suffering from wasting illnesses and for general debility and failure to thrive.

Parts used

Berries have powerful diuretic and tonic properties. They are a traditional North American remedy for a wide range of problems.

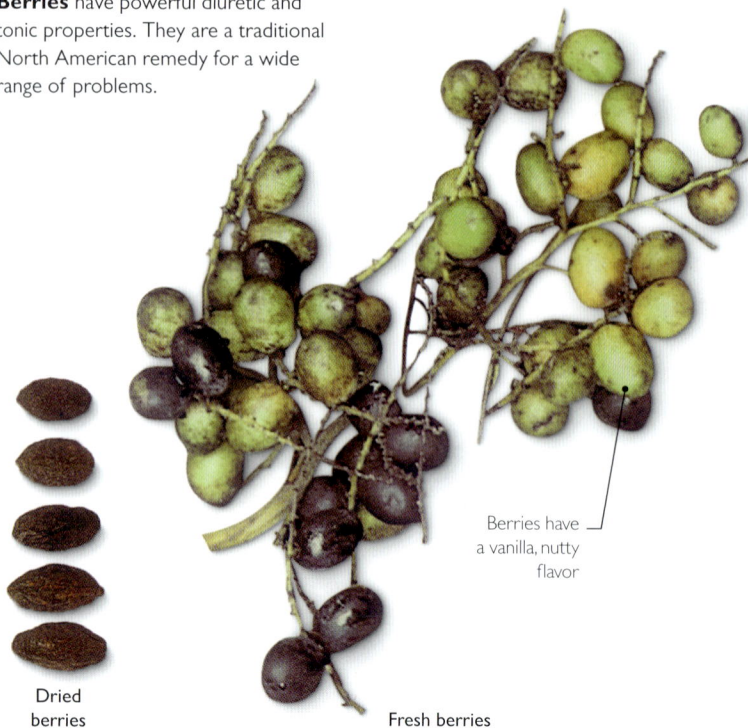

Berries have a vanilla, nutty flavor

Dried berries

Fresh berries

Key preparations & their uses

Infusion (to make, p. 301) is a diuretic. For enlarged prostate, take ¾ cup (150 ml) daily.

Tincture (to make, p. 302) can be taken as a long-term tonic for debility. Take 1 tsp with water daily.

Remedy Make an infusion (see p. 301) with 2 tsp saw palmetto, 2 tsp horsetail, 1 tsp licorice, and ¾ cup (200 ml) water. Take ½ cup (100 ml) as a tonic twice a day.

Self-help use

• Impotence & premature ejaculation, p. 326.

Silybum marianum syn. *Carduus marianus* (Asteraceae)

Milk thistle, Mary thistle

Milk thistle has been used in Europe as a remedy for depression and liver problems for hundreds, if not thousands, of years. Recent research has confirmed traditional herbal knowledge, proving that the herb has a remarkable ability to protect the liver from damage resulting from alcoholic and other types of poisoning. Today, milk thistle is widely used in the West for the treatment of a range of liver conditions.

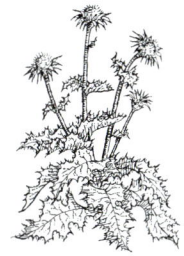

A spiny biennial, growing to 5 ft (1.5 m), with white-veined leaves and purple flower heads.

Habitat & cultivation

Native to the Mediterranean, milk thistle grows throughout Europe but is rare in Britain. It grows wild, thriving on waste ground, and is also cultivated as an ornamental plant. Milk thistle prefers a sunny position and self-seeds readily. The flower heads are picked in full bloom in early summer and the seeds are collected in late summer.

Related species

Other closely related herbs, including holy thistle (*Cnicus benedictus*, p. 195) and globe artichoke (*Cynara scolymus*, p. 203), protect the liver from toxicity and exert a positive restorative action on liver function.

Key constituents

• Flavonlignans (1–4%) (known collectively as "silymarin")
• Bitter principles • Polyacetylenes

Key actions

• Liver protective
• Chemoprotective
• Anticancer • Anti-allergenic
• Increases breast milk production

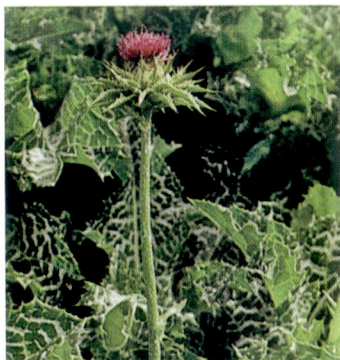

Milk thistle has distinctive white markings on its leaves caused, according to tradition, by the Virgin Mary's milk.

Research

Silymarin German research from the 1970s onward has focused on silymarin, a substance contained in the seeds. This exerts a highly protective effect on the liver, maintaining its function and preventing damage from compounds that are normally highly toxic. It has been shown that severe liver breakdown, resulting from ingesting carbon tetrachloride or death cap mushrooms, can be prevented if silymarin is taken immediately before, or within 48 hours. In Germany, silymarin has been used successfully to treat hepatitis and liver cirrhosis.

Other research In several clinical trials, silymarin extracts protected liver function in people taking chemotherapy for cancer, including, in one trial, children suffering from leukemia. Research so far suggests that silymarin extracts support healthy liver function during chemotherapy and do not reduce the effectiveness of chemotherapy drugs. Laboratory research indicates that silymarin, particularly silybin, has significant anticancer properties. In a 2011 clinical trial in Iran, patients with allergic rhinitis experienced significantly fewer symptoms when taking a silymarin extract.

Traditional & current uses

Traditional uses Milk thistle flower heads, boiled and eaten like artichokes, were useful as a spring tonic after the winter months when people had been deprived of fresh vegetables. They were also taken to increase breast milk production, and were considered excellent for *melancholia* (depression), which was traditionally associated with the liver.

Parts used

Flower heads are eaten as a tonic food and can be used in remedies.

Seeds contain silymarin, which protects the liver. They are the main part used in remedies.

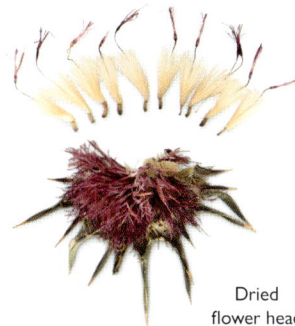

Dried flower head

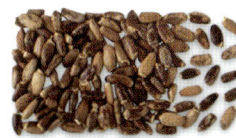

Seeds

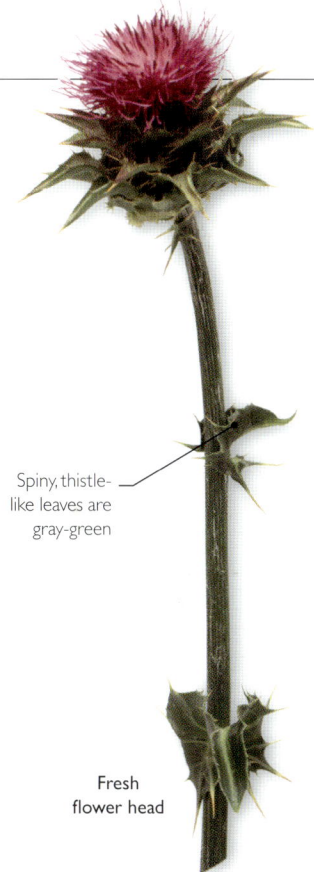

Spiny, thistle-like leaves are gray-green

Fresh flower head

Key preparations & their uses

Decoction of seeds (to make, p. 301). For liver infections, take ⅓ cup (75 ml) a day.

Tincture of seeds may be taken to help hay fever.

Capsules of seeds (to make, p. 302). For a hangover, take a 500 mg capsule.

Tablets are prescribed for long-term treatment of liver disorders.

Gerard states in his *Herball* of 1597, "My opinion is that this [milk thistle] is the best remedy that grows against all melancholy diseases."

Liver disorders Today, milk thistle is the main remedy used in Western herbal medicine to protect the liver and its many metabolic activities, and help renew its cells. The herb is used in the treatment of hepatitis and jaundice, as well as in conditions where the liver is under stress—whether from infection or excess alcohol, or from chemotherapy.

Symphytum officinale (Boraginaceae)

Comfrey, Knitbone

Comfrey's names testify to its traditional use in mending broken bones. "Comfrey" is a corruption of con firma, meaning the bone is "made firm," *Symphytum* is derived from the Greek for "to unite," and knitbone speaks for itself. Comfrey is also a wound herb. K'Eogh in his Irish *Herbal* (1735) wrote that it "heals all inward wounds and ruptures." Today, it is still highly regarded for its healing properties.

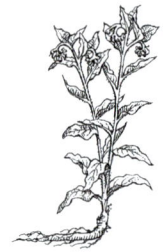

A perennial growing to 3 ft (1 m), with thick leaves and bell-like white to pink or mauve flowers.

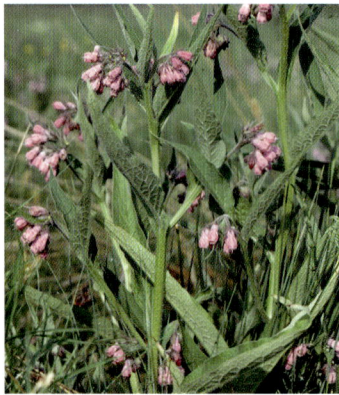

Comfrey was known to the 1st century CE Greek physician Dioscorides, who wrote about it in his Materia Medica.

Habitat & cultivation

A plant native to Europe, comfrey grows in all temperate regions of the world, including western Asia, North America, and Australia. It thrives in moist, marshy places. It can be grown from seed in spring or by root division in the fall, and the leaves and flowering tops are harvested in summer. The root is unearthed in the fall.

Key constituents

• Allantoin (up to 4.7%) • Mucilage (about 29%) • Triterpenoids
• Phenolic acids (rosmarinic acid)
• Asparagine • Pyrrolizidine alkaloids (0.02–0.07%) • Tannins

Key actions

• Demulcent • Astringent
• Anti-inflammatory • Heals wounds and bones

Research

Active constituents Allantoin is a cell-proliferant that stimulates the repair of damaged tissue. The herb's anti-inflammatory activity is partly due to the presence of rosmarinic acid and phenolic acids.

Pyrrolizidine alkaloids Research shows that, as isolated substances, certain pyrrolizidine alkaloids can be highly toxic to the liver. It is still unclear whether they are toxic in the context of the whole plant, as they are only present in minute amounts, often being completely absent from samples of dried aerial parts. The highest concentration is in the root, which should not be used internally. Skin applications, as well as the aerial parts of the plant, are considered safe.

Clinical research In Germany and elsewhere in Europe, comfrey is widely used for sprains, bruises, and sports injuries. Research, mostly in Germany, endorses the traditional knowledge of comfrey's wound-healing ability. In a 2007 study, physicians rated the efficacy of a comfrey leaf cream in healing abrasions. The doctors rated its effectiveness as good or very good in 93% of cases, and complete healing took 4 days with comfrey and 7 days with placebo. Other studies indicate comfrey's value in promoting tissue repair and as an anti-inflammatory in conditions such as sprained ankle, osteoarthritis, and lower back pain.

Traditional & current uses

Injuries Comfrey's ability to promote the healing of bruises, sprains, fractures, and broken bones has been known for thousands of years. It encourages ligaments and bones to knit together firmly. A comfrey compress applied immediately to a sprained ankle can significantly reduce the severity of the injury. The combination of tannins and mucilage helps soothe bruises and grazes.

Other uses Comfrey preparations have many other uses and can be applied to heal problems such as insect bites, scars, skin inflammation, acne, and mastitis.

Parts used

Root is harvested in the fall when the allantoin levels are highest.

Aerial parts are rich in anti-inflammatory and astringent substances.

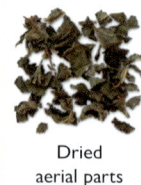

Dried aerial parts

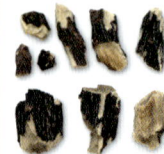

Dried root

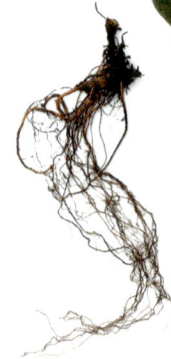

Fresh root

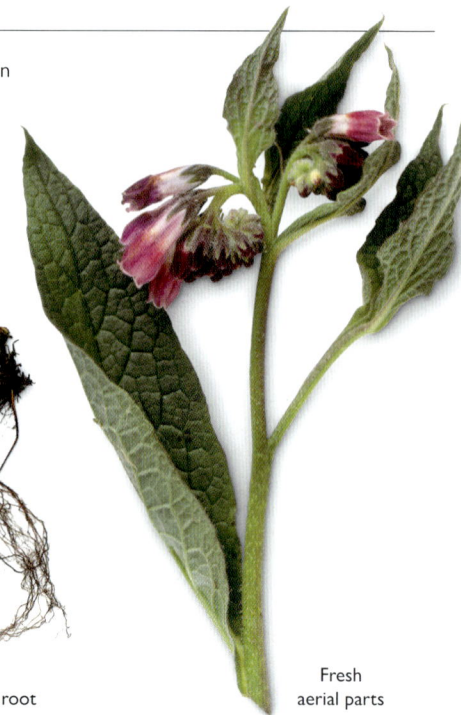

Fresh aerial parts

Key preparations & their uses

Infused oil of leaves (to make, p. 304). Apply to sprains.

Chopping leaves Apply as a poultice (see p. 305) to boils.

Ointment of leaves (to make, p. 305). Apply to bruises.

Tincture of root (to make, p. 302). Apply undiluted to acne.

Cautions Do not use on dirty wounds as rapid healing can trap dirt or pus. Not for internal use. Restricted in some countries. Do not use during pregnancy or while breastfeeding.

Self-help uses

• Acne & boils, p. 315. • Fractures, p. 322. • Fungal skin infections, p. 314. • Healing wounds, p. 314. • Inflamed skin rashes, p. 313. • Stiff & aching joints, p. 323.

Tabebuia spp. (Bignoniaceae)

Pau d'arco (Portuguese), *Lapacho* (Spanish)

Bark from the pau d'arco tree has been valued for centuries in traditional South American herbal medicine for its remarkable health benefits. Today, it is given as a remedy for inflammatory and infectious problems, including conditions such as chronic fatigue and candidiasis. It is also used for other conditions and has a mixed reputation as a treatment for cancer, including leukemia.

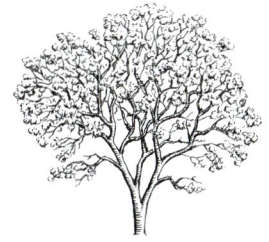

An evergreen tree (deciduous in cold climates) reaching 100 ft (30 m), with pink flowers.

Habitat & cultivation

A tree native to South America, pau d'arco grows well in mountainous terrains. In Peru and Argentina it is found growing high up in the Andes. *Pau d'arco* is also found in low-lying areas (in Paraguay and Brazil), where it is thought to have originated. Many *Tabebuia* species are used in herbal medicine, so quality control of dried bark can be difficult. *T. avellanedae* is considered to be the most therapeutically effective species, while *T. impetignosa* is the species that is most commonly available. *Pau d'arco* is not normally cultivated—the prized inner bark is collected from trees growing in the wild, throughout the year.

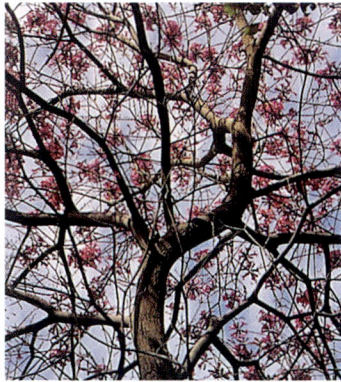

Key constituents

- Napthaquinones (lapachol)
- Anthraquinones • Coumarins
- Flavonoids • Iridoids • Carnosol

Key actions

- Antibacterial • Antifungal
- Antiparasitic • Immunostimulant
- Anti-inflammatory • Tonic
- Antitumor

Research

Antibacterial and antifungal activity A Colombian review (2013) of research data on *Tabebuia* species, much of which was undertaken in South America, highlighted pau d'arco's strong, direct activity against several key bacteria, notably *Staphylococcus aureus* and *Helicobacter pylori*, the latter being the principal cause of stomach ulcers. It also has broad-ranging activity against many fungal agents, including *Candida albicans*.

Antitumor properties *Pau d'arco*'s anticancer action has been established in laboratory experiments, with many of its constituents suppressing the growth of cancer cells. Research in Brazil in the 1960s raised great hopes that pau d'arco might prove to be a major cancer treatment, but clinical research has failed to produce positive results.

Traditional & current uses

Early cure-all The Incas, the Callawaya in Brazil, and other Indigenous South American peoples all prized *pau d'arco* as a cure-all. They used it to treat a variety of conditions, including wounds, fever, dysentery, and intestinal inflammation, as well as certain types of cancer and snake bite.

Infections Given the large number of active constituents in *pau d'arco* it is not surprising that this beneficial herb is used in South America and by herbal practitioners throughout the world. It is an important, natural antibiotic for bacterial and viral infections, especially of the nose, mouth, and throat, and is considered helpful for chronic conditions such as CFS (chronic fatigue syndrome). *Pau d'arco* is also used for fungal conditions, including ringworm and thrush, and is considered especially useful for treating chronic candidiasis.

Anti-inflammatory action *Pau d'arco* reduces and relieves inflammatory problems, especially in the stomach and intestines. It is used to treat a wide range of other inflammatory conditions, including cystitis, inflammation of the cervix, and prostatitis.

Cancer remedy Clinical experience in Brazil, combined with its worldwide use by herbalists as a cancer remedy, suggests that *pau d'arco* may be beneficial in the treatment of cancer, including leukemia. However, more intensive research is needed into its therapeutic value.

Pau d'arco *is valued for its durable wood and for its bark that has important therapeutic properties.*

Parts used

Inner bark is prized for its immunostimulant properties. It is used to treat many inflammatory conditions.

Bark has important antibiotic properties

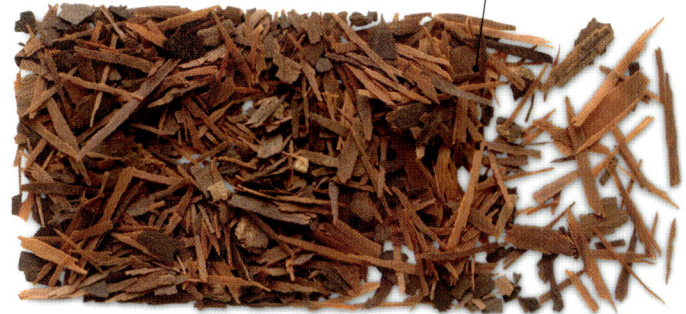

Dried inner bark

Key preparations & their uses

Decoction (to make, p. 301) is a traditional preparation in South America. For candidiasis, drink ¾ cup (150 ml) 3 times a day.

Ointment (to make, p. 305). For wounds, apply freely.

Tincture (to make, p. 302) is suitable for long-term use. For CFS, take 40 drops with water 3 times a day.

Cautions If taking anticoagulant medication, take *pau d'arco* only with professional advice. Do not take during pregnancy. Avoid if trying to conceive.

Tanacetum parthenium (Asteraceae)

Feverfew

Feverfew's main traditional use was as a woman's herb. Nicholas Culpeper in *The English Physitian* (1652) sings its praises as "a general strengthener of [the] womb ... it cleanseth the womb, expelleth the after-birth, and doth the woman all the good she can desire of an herb." Feverfew is now used principally as a treatment for migraine, but has also long been thought of as an herb for arthritis and rheumatism.

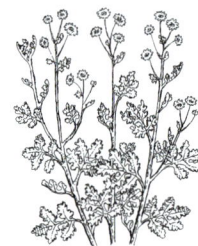

An herbaceous perennial growing to 2 ft (60 cm), with numerous daisylike flower heads.

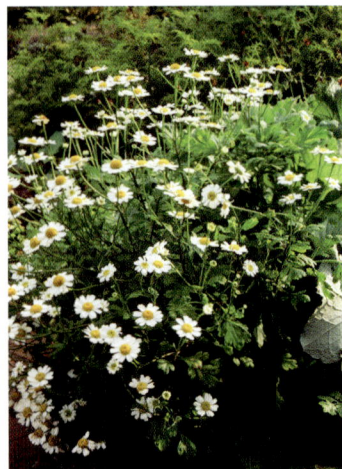

Feverfew has daisylike flowers that bloom all summer.

Habitat & cultivation

Originally from southeastern Europe, feverfew is now common throughout Europe, Australia, and North America. It can be propagated from seed or cuttings, and prefers well-drained soil and sun. The leaves are picked as required and the aerial parts as a whole are harvested in summer when the plant is in flower.

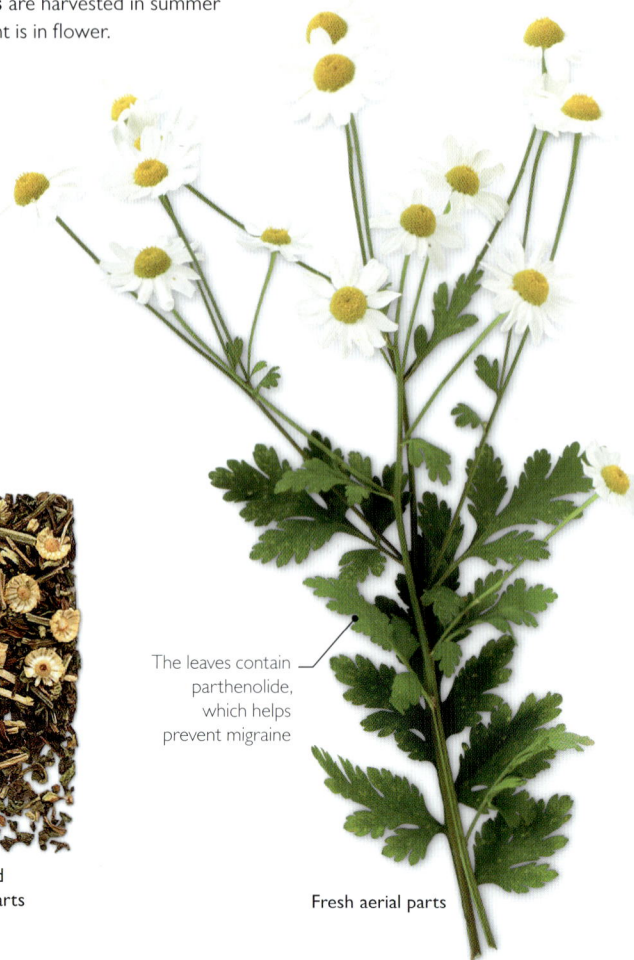

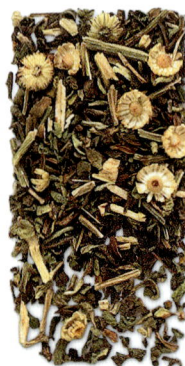

Related species

Feverfew is related to tansy (*Tanacetum vulgare*, p. 284), and chamomile and chrysanthemum.

Key constituents

- Volatile oil (alpha-pinene)
- Sesquiterpene lactones (parthenolide) • Sesquiterpenes (camphor)

Key actions

- Anti-inflammatory • Analgesic
- Reduces fever • Antirheumatic
- Promotes menstrual flow

Research

Migraine When, in 1973, the wife of a Welsh doctor ended her 50-year history of migraine with a course of feverfew, a detailed scientific investigation got underway. In clinical trials in Britain during the 1980s the herb was shown to be an effective remedy for migraine. Further clinical trials across Europe, including one in 2006 that combined feverfew and willow bark (*Salix alba*, p. 133), attest to feverfew's ability to treat migraine. The trials indicate feverfew may need to be taken long term (for 6 months or more) for full effect.

Rheumatoid arthritis Feverfew's effectiveness in the treatment of rheumatoid arthritis is being investigated.

Traditional & current uses

Fevers As its name implies, feverfew may be used to lower temperature and cool the body.

Gynecological uses The herb has been used since Roman times to induce menstruation. It is also given in childbirth to aid expulsion of the placenta.

Migraine & headaches In small quantities, feverfew is now used as a preventative for migraine. It has to be taken regularly, and at the first signs of an attack. It is useful for migraine associated with menstruation, and for headaches.

Arthritis remedy The herb can help arthritic and rheumatic pain, especially with other herbs.

Self-help use

- Migraine prevention, p. 319.

Parts used

Aerial parts are harvested in summer when the plant is in flower.

The leaves contain parthenolide, which helps prevent migraine

Dried aerial parts

Fresh aerial parts

Key preparations & their uses

Fresh leaves To prevent migraine, eat 2–3 leaves daily on a piece of bread.

Tincture (to make, p. 302). For long-term prevention of migraine, take 10 drops a day.

Capsules (to make, p. 302). For symptomatic relief of headaches take a 100 mg capsule daily.

Tablets often contain other herbs. Take for headaches.

Cautions Eating fresh leaves may cause mouth ulcers. Do not take feverfew if taking warfarin or other blood-thinning drugs. Do not take during pregnancy. Can cause allergic reactions in rare cases.

Taraxacum officinale (Asteraceae)

Dandelion

Known principally as a weed, dandelion has an astonishing range of health benefits. In Western folk medicine, the leaves, which can be eaten in salads, have long been used as a diuretic. They were recommended in the works of Arab physicians in the 11th century, and in an herbal written by the physicians of Myddfai in Wales in the 13th century. The root, which has a shorter history of medicinal use, is good for the liver.

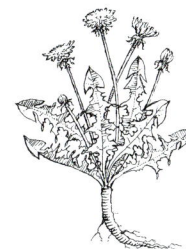

A perennial growing to 20 in (50 cm), with ragged basal leaves, hollow stalks, and golden flowers.

Habitat & cultivation

Dandelion grows wild in most parts of the world and is cultivated in Germany and France. It is propagated from seed in spring. The young leaves are picked in spring for tonic salads, and later as a medicine. The root of 2-year-old plants is unearthed in the fall.

Related species

Pu gong ying (*T. mongolicum*) is used in Chinese herbal medicine to "clear heat" and relieve toxicity, especially of the liver.

Key constituents

• Sesquiterpene lactones
• Triterpenes • Polysaccharides
Leaf only:
• Coumarins • Carotenoids
• Minerals (especially potassium)
Root only:
• Taraxacoside • Phenolic acids
• Minerals (potassium, calcium)

Key actions

• Bitter • Liver protective • Diuretic
• Antiviral • Antibacterial

Research

Leaves Research published in the journal *Planta Medica*, in 1974, confirmed that dandelion leaves are a powerful diuretic, though their exact mode of action is not understood. Many other small-scale studies have confirmed this diuretic, or more accurately, aquaretic effect of dandelion leaf. Aquaretic refers to the fact that many herbal diuretics stimulate just the elimination of water and potassium. As dandelion leaf has very high levels of potassium, it is thought that no net loss of this mineral occurs on taking the leaf.

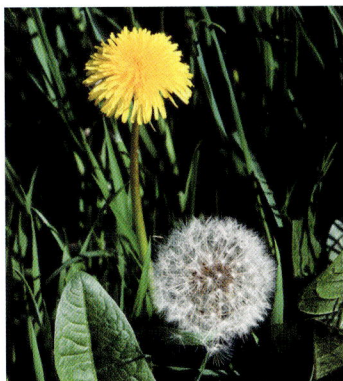

Dandelion's name, which is a corruption of the Latin dens leonis, *meaning "lion's teeth," derives from the appearance of its flowers.*

Root Ongoing research suggests that dandelion root has significant anticancer activity. In laboratory studies extracts increase tumor necrosis factor and stimulate apoptosis (programmed cell death).

Traditional & current uses

Diuretic Dandelion leaf is used as a diuretic and treats high blood pressure by reducing the volume of fluid in the body.

Detoxifying remedy Dandelion root is a key detoxifying herb that stimulates the liver and gallbladder's capacity to clear waste products from the body. This action makes it valuable in the many health conditions that involve chronic toxicity, whether this toxicity is linked to inflammation, infection or dietary or environmental factors. The root is typically taken to treat constipation, skin problems, such as eczema, and arthritic conditions, where improved clearance of waste products can reduce local inflammation.

Other uses Dandelion root is a good prebiotic, supporting the health of the

Parts used

Leaves are juiced, eaten raw in salads, or dried for use in herbal preparations.

Root is harvested after 2 years and is dried or roasted.

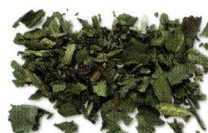

Dried leaves

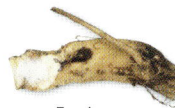

Fresh root

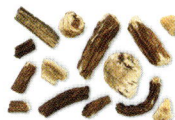

Dried root

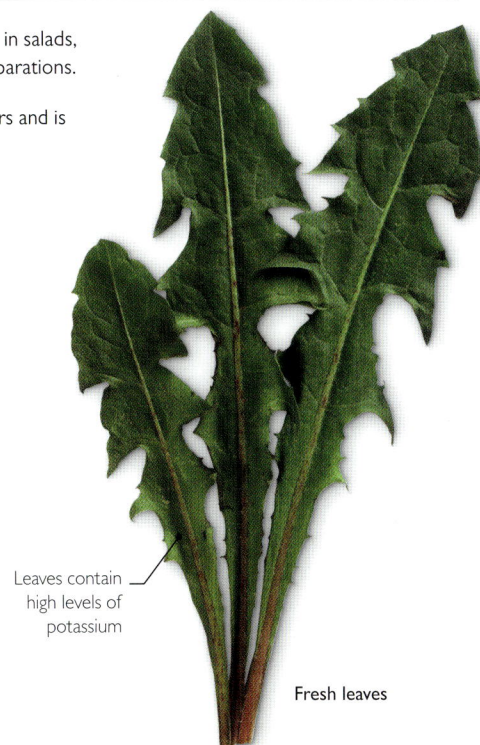

Leaves contain high levels of potassium

Fresh leaves

Key preparations & their uses

Tablets have a diuretic effect. Take for fluid retention.

Tonic salad made with dandelion leaves. Eat regularly for its cleansing benefits.

Tincture of root (to make, p. 302). For eczema, take ½ tsp diluted with ½ cup (100 ml) water 3 times a day.

Decoction of root (p. 301). For acne, take ⅓ cup (75 ml) 3 times a day.

Infusion of leaves (p. 301). For swollen ankles, take 2 cups (500 ml) daily.

Juice made from leaves. For fluid retention, take 1 tbsp 3 times a day.

gut flora. It has traditionally been used in the early stages of type 2 diabetes, stimulating insulin release from the pancreas and supporting stable blood-sugar levels.

Self-help uses

• Acne & boils, p. 315. • Constipation, p. 317. • Detoxification for hangover, p. 319. • Fluid retention, p. 325. • Hives, p. 313.

Terminalia arjuna (Combretaceae)

Arjun

The bark of the arjun tree has been used in Indian herbal medicine for at least 3,000 years, and has always been valued as a remedy for the heart. The first person credited with prescribing arjun for heart disease was Vagbhata, an Indian physician of the 7th century CE. Arjun is an example of an herb for which the traditional use has been confirmed by modern pharmacological research.

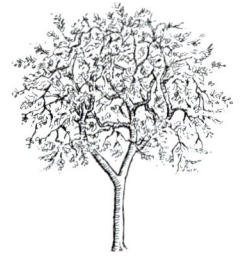

An evergreen tree reaching 100 ft (30 m), with pale yellow flowers and cone-shaped leaves.

Habitat & cultivation

Arjun is found throughout most of the Indian subcontinent, from Sri Lanka to the foothills of the Himalayas. It thrives in wet, marshy areas and on riverbanks. The tree is grown from seed and the bark is cut in late winter.

Related species

A number of other *Terminalia* species are also used medicinally, notably beleric myrobalan and chebulic myrobalan (*T. bellerica* and *T. chebula*, p. 285). Both are close relatives of arjun and are among the most used herbal medicines in India.

Key constituents

• Tannins • Triterpenoid saponins
• Flavonoids • Phytosterols

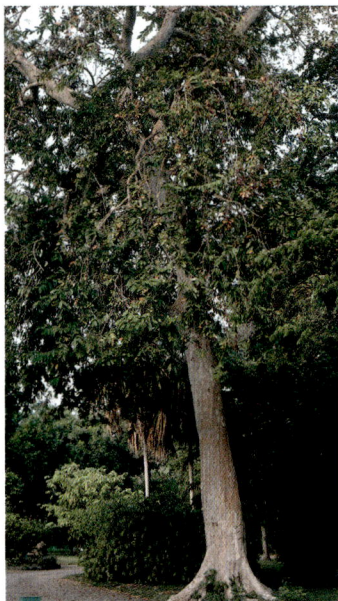

Arjun is a handsome evergreen tree. Its bark is prescribed to help heart and circulation problems.

Key actions

• Cardiac tonic • Lowers blood pressure • Reduces cholesterol levels

Research

Cardiac tonic Research into arjun has been going on in India since the 1930s. The results have been highly conflicting, with some studies indicating that it increases heart rate and blood pressure, and others suggesting the reverse. It seems that the herb is best used to treat conditions where the blood supply to the heart is poor, for example in ischemic heart disease and angina. In a 2002 clinical trial in India, 58 men with angina were given arjun. Results were very positive, with those taking arjun experiencing a marked reduction in angina symptoms and an increased capacity to exercise.

Cholesterol Indian research has demonstrated that arjun reduces blood cholesterol levels.

Traditional & current uses

Traditional heart remedy
In Indian herbal medicine, arjun has always been taken as a heart tonic. It has a long history of treating heart failure and edema (a condition in which fluid accumulates in the ankles and legs because the heart is not pumping adequately).

Ayurvedic medicine Ayurvedic physicians use arjun to restore balance when any of the 3 humors, *kapha*, *pitta*, or *vata* (see p. 41), is present in excess. As a decoction, the bark is given to treat diarrhea and dysentery. Powdered bark is part of a traditional Ayurvedic treatment for asthma. Arjun is also given in Ayurveda for bile duct problems, as well as for poisoning and scorpion stings.

Parts used

Bark has constituents that lower blood pressure and reduce cholesterol levels.

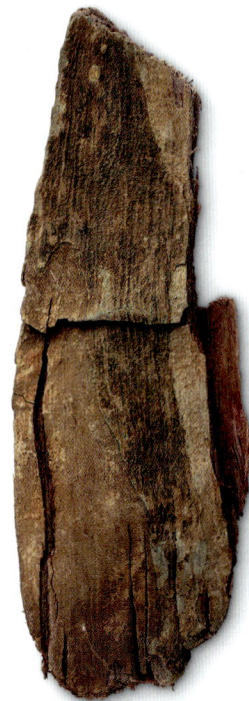

Dried bark

Bark is used to treat heart disease in India

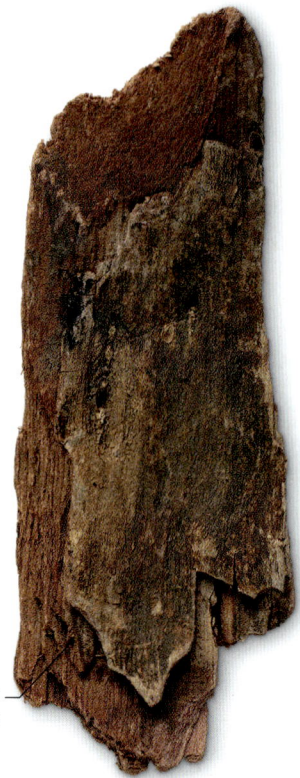

Key preparations & their uses

Decoction is used by herbalists to treat poor circulation to the heart.

Tincture is a valuable cardiac tonic. Herbalists prescribe it to treat angina.

Powder is a traditional Ayurvedic remedy, prescribed for asthma.

Caution Take only under professional supervision.

Modern heart remedy Arjun is beneficial for angina and poor coronary circulation. It is also of benefit if the heart's rate and rhythm are abnormal. By lowering blood cholesterol levels, reducing blood pressure, and supporting normal heart function, arjun improves the health of the circulation and reduces the risk of developing a serious heart problem.

Thymus vulgaris (Lamiaceae)

Thyme, Garden thyme

Thyme was praised by the herbalist Nicholas Culpeper (1616–1654) as "a notable strengthener of the lungs, as notable a one as grows; neither is there a better remedy growing for that disease in children which they commonly call chin-cough [whooping cough]." Thyme is an excellent antiseptic and tonic, and today it is still used as a respiratory remedy, as well as being important for a variety of other ailments.

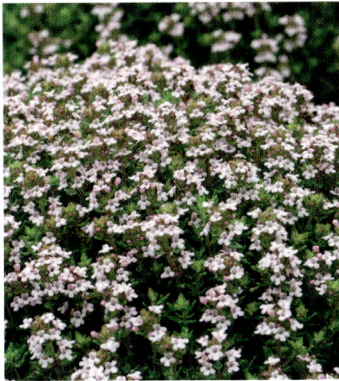

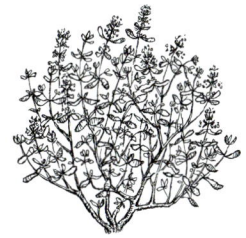

An aromatic shrub growing to 16 in (40 cm), with woody stems, small leaves, and pink flowers.

Thyme's pink flowers attract bees in profusion and give a distinctive flavor to the honey.

Habitat & cultivation

Thyme is a cultivated variety of the wild thyme (*T. serpyllum*, p. 286) of southern Europe and is now grown worldwide. It is raised from seed or by root division in spring and prefers light, chalky soils. The aerial parts are harvested in summer.

Related species

There are many *Thymus* species, each with a different volatile oil content. Wild thyme (*T. serpyllum*, p. 286) is often used in the same way as thyme.

Key constituents

• Volatile oil (mostly thymol and carvacrol) • Flavonoids
• Phenolic acids

Key actions

• Antiseptic • Tonic • Relieves muscle spasms • Expectorant • Expels worms • Antioxidant

Research

Volatile oil Thyme's volatile oil is strongly antiseptic—the constituent thymol, in particular, is a most effective antifungal. The oil is also expectorant and it expels worms.

Antiaging Research in the 1990s in Scotland suggests that thyme and its volatile oil have a markedly tonic effect, supporting the body's normal function and countering the effects of aging. More recent research indicates that thyme is strongly antioxidant and may help maintain higher levels of essential fatty acids within the brain.

Stomach ulcers Extracts of the herb have shown strong antibacterial activity against *H. pylori*, a bacterium often associated with stomach ulcers.

Menstrual pain Many compounds within thyme relieve muscle cramps. A 2014 Iranian clinical trial compared the ability of thyme and ibuprofen to relieve period pains. The findings showed both treatments to be effective.

Traditional & current uses

Infections The antiseptic and tonic properties of thyme make it a useful tonic for the immune system in chronic, especially fungal, infections, as well as an effective remedy for throat and chest infections.

Asthma & hay fever Thyme is prescribed with other herbs for asthma, especially in children. Its invigorating qualities balance the sedative effect of many herbs used for asthma. Thyme is also helpful in hay fever.

Worms Thyme is often used to treat worms in children.

External uses Applied to the skin, thyme relieves bites and stings, and is used for sciatica and rheumatic pains. It helps ringworm, athlete's foot, thrush, and other fungal infections, as well as scabies and lice. Thyme infusion and diluted oil are also massaged into the scalp to encourage hair growth and reverse hair loss.

Self-help uses

• Allergic rhinitis, p. 310. • Back pain, p. 323. • Bites & stings, p. 313. • Colds & flu, p. 321. • Coughs & bronchitis, p. 320. • Earache, p. 322. • Fungal infections, pp. 314 & 324.
• Maintaining vitality, p. 329. • Mild asthma, p. 311. • Tired & aching muscles, p. 322.

Parts used

Aerial parts, harvested in summer, contain antiseptic volatile oil.

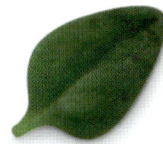

Leaves have an aromatic, bitter taste

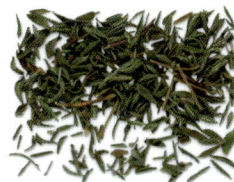

Fresh leaves

Dried aerial parts

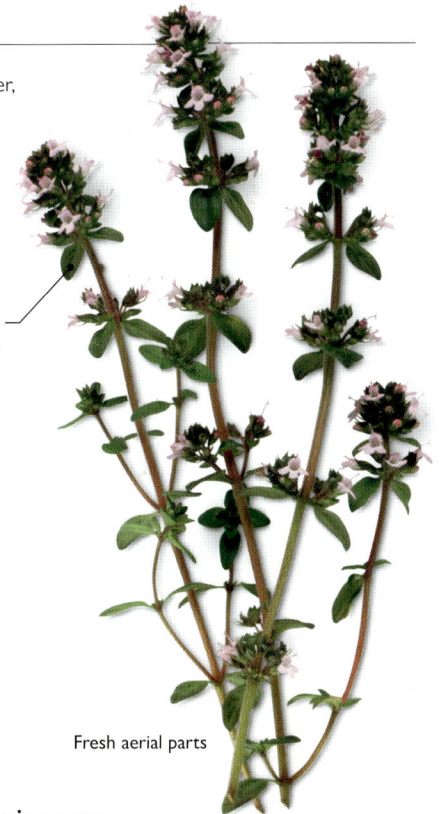

Fresh aerial parts

Key preparations & their uses

Infusion (to make, p. 301). For colds, take ½ cup (100 ml) 3 times daily.

Essential oil for acne, dilute to 5% and dab onto inflamed spots.

Syrup (to make, p. 303) is a traditional cough remedy. Take 1 tbsp 3 times a day.

Tincture (to make, p. 302). For thrush, apply 40 drops, 2–3 times daily.

Cautions Do not take the essential oil internally. Do not use the essential oil externally during pregnancy.

Turnera diffusa syn. *T. diffusa* var. *aphrodisiaca* (Passifloraceae)

Damiana

Damiana is a traditional aphrodisiac of the Maya people in Central America. It continues to be considered valuable as an aphrodisiac and general tonic, and its stimulant, tonic action also makes it a valuable remedy for those suffering from mild depression. Damiana has a strongly aromatic, slightly bitter taste. The leaves are used to flavor liqueurs and are taken in Mexico as a substitute for tea.

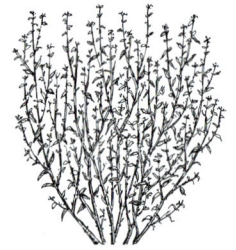

An aromatic shrub growing to 6½ ft (2 m), with smooth, pale green leaves and small, single yellow flowers.

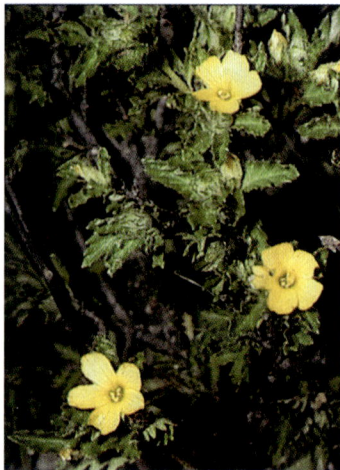

Damiana is an excellent tonic herb for physical weakness and nervous exhaustion.

Habitat & cultivation

Damiana is native to the Gulf of Mexico, southern California, the northern Caribbean Islands, and Namibia. It is also cultivated in these areas. Damiana is grown from seed in spring and prefers a hot, humid climate. The leaves are harvested when the herb is in flower in summer.

Related species

T. opifera and *T. ulmifolia* are used as tonics in Brazil and Central America, respectively.

Key constituents

• Volatile oil (about 0.5–1%), including caryophyllene, thymol, and cadinene
• Flavonoids • Hydroquinones (arbutin) • Tannins

Key actions

• Tonic • Nerve tonic • Aphrodisiac
• Mild stimulant • Mild antidepressant • Mild laxative
• Urinary antiseptic

Research

Initial research The first study into the aphrodisiac activity of damiana (published in 1999) found that male rats with low sexual activity became more sexually active when given damiana extract. One cannot generalize from animals to humans, but this does correspond with traditional views of the herb. Other recent research suggests that damiana helps prevent raised blood-sugar levels in diabetics.

Traditional & current uses

Tonic Damiana is a tonic and restorative for the nervous system, and has always been considered an aphrodisiac. Its tonic action is partly due to the constituent thymol, which is antiseptic and tonic.

Antidepressant Technically, damiana is a thymoleptic (having a stimulating action on the body and mind). It is given to people suffering from mild to moderate depression or nervous exhaustion. Its stimulating and restorative properties make it valuable when anxiety and depression happen together.

Sexual restorative Due to its reputed testosterogenic activity, damiana has always been seen as an herb for men, helpful in treating premature ejaculation and impotence. It is, however, beneficial for both men and women, being considered restorative to the reproductive organs of both sexes.

Gynecological problems Damiana is often given for painful and delayed periods, and is used specifically for headaches connected to menstruation.

Urinary antiseptic Being a diuretic and urinary antiseptic, damiana is

Parts used

Leaves are harvested in summer. They make a pleasant-tasting tea and are used for a wide range of medicinal preparations.

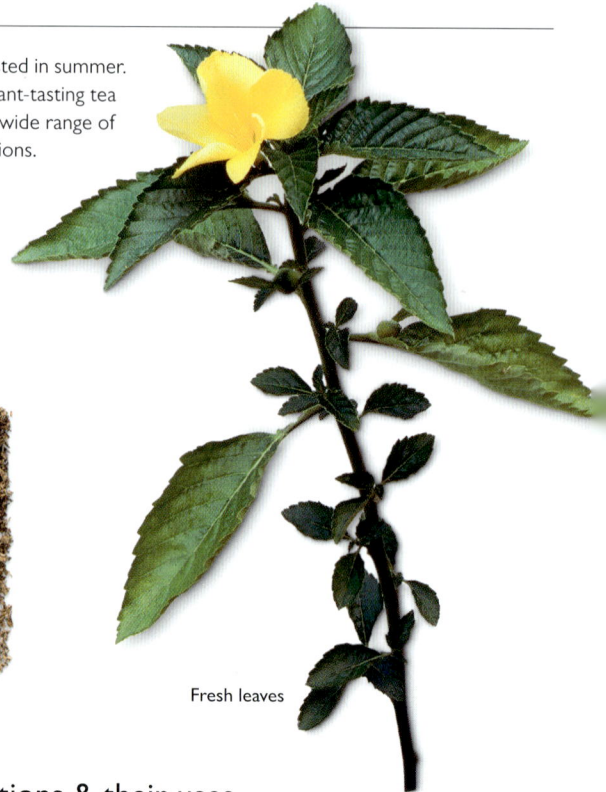

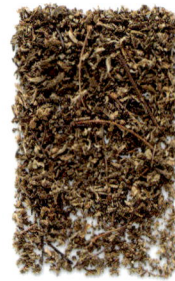

Dried leaves

Fresh leaves

Key preparations & their uses

Tablets usually also contain other herbs. Take as a relaxing tonic.

Tincture (to make, p. 302) is a nerve tonic and antidepressant. For mild depression, take 30 drops with water 4 times a day.

Infusion (to make, p. 301) is a tonic and is useful for urinary infections. Drink ¾ cup (150 ml) daily as a general tonic.

useful in the treatment of urinary infections such as cystitis and urethritis. This action is partly due to the constituent arbutin, which is converted into hydroquinone, a strong urinary antiseptic, in the urinary tubules. This constituent is also found in a number of other

plants, notably uva-ursi (*Arctostaphylos uva-ursi*, p. 174).

Laxative Damiana is a mild laxative, useful in the treatment of constipation due to poor bowel muscle tone.

Self-help use

Anxiety, depression, & tension, p. 318.

Ulmus rubra (Ulmaceae)

Slippery Elm

This marvelous herb is a gentle and effective remedy for irritated states of the mucous membranes of the chest, urinary tubules, stomach, and intestines. It was used in many different ways by the Indigenous peoples in North America—as a poultice for wounds, boils, ulcers, and inflamed eyes, and internally for fevers, colds, and bowel complaints. Slippery elm has a strongly mucilaginous "slippery" taste and texture.

A large tree growing to 59 ft (18 m) with a brown trunk and rough gray-white bark on the branches.

Habitat & cultivation

Slippery elm is native to the US and Canada, and is most commonly found growing in the Appalachian Mountains. The tree thrives on high ground and dry soil. The inner bark of the trunk and branches is collected in spring.

Related species

White elm (*U. americana*) is used in a similar way to slippery elm, and was taken for coughs by the Mohicans. In Europe, the dried bark of elm (*Ulmus* spp.) was used as a demulcent, and was first mentioned by Dioscorides in the 1st century CE.

Key constituents

• Mucilage • Starch • Tannins

Key actions

• Demulcent • Emollient • Nutritive
• Laxative

Research

Mucilage There is limited research into slippery elm, but its action as an herb with large quantities of mucilage is well understood. When the herb comes into direct contact with inflamed surfaces such as the skin or the intestinal membranes, it soothes and coats the irritated tissue, protects it from injury, and draws out toxins or irritants.

Reflex action When slippery elm is taken internally, it is thought likely that it causes a reflex stimulation of nerve endings in the stomach and intestines that leads to secretion of mucus by the membranes of the urinary tract.

Traditional & current uses

Nourishing Taken regularly, slippery elm is a nutritious and soothing food that acts as a prebiotic, supporting beneficial bacterial growth within the gut. It is excellent as a baby food and during convalescence.

Digestive disorders Slippery elm is a particularly soothing herb and can bring instant relief to acidity, diarrhea, and gastroenteritis. It will also help alleviate conditions such as colic, inflammation of the gut, constipation, hemorrhoids, diverticulitis, and irritable bowel syndrome.

Urinary problems This herb is a useful remedy for urinary problems such as chronic cystitis.

Respiratory conditions Slippery elm has been used to treat all manner of chest conditions and has a soothing effect on everything from coughs and bronchitis to pleurisy and tuberculosis.

External uses Applied externally, the herb softens and protects the skin. It also works very well as a "drawing" poultice for boils and splinters.

Self-help uses

• Acidity & indigestion, p. 317. • Acne & boils, p. 315. • Constipation in children, p. 328. • Hemorrhoids, p. 312.

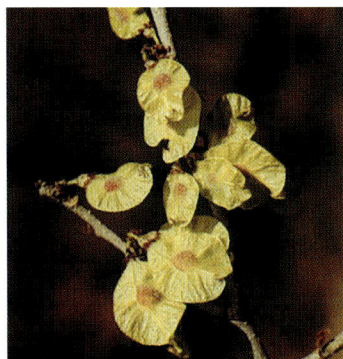

Slippery elm produces red-brown fruit, each consisting of a single seed, in summer.

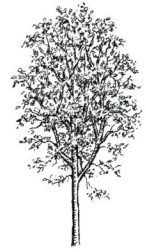

Parts used

Inner bark of 10-year-old slippery elm trees is collected in spring and powdered.

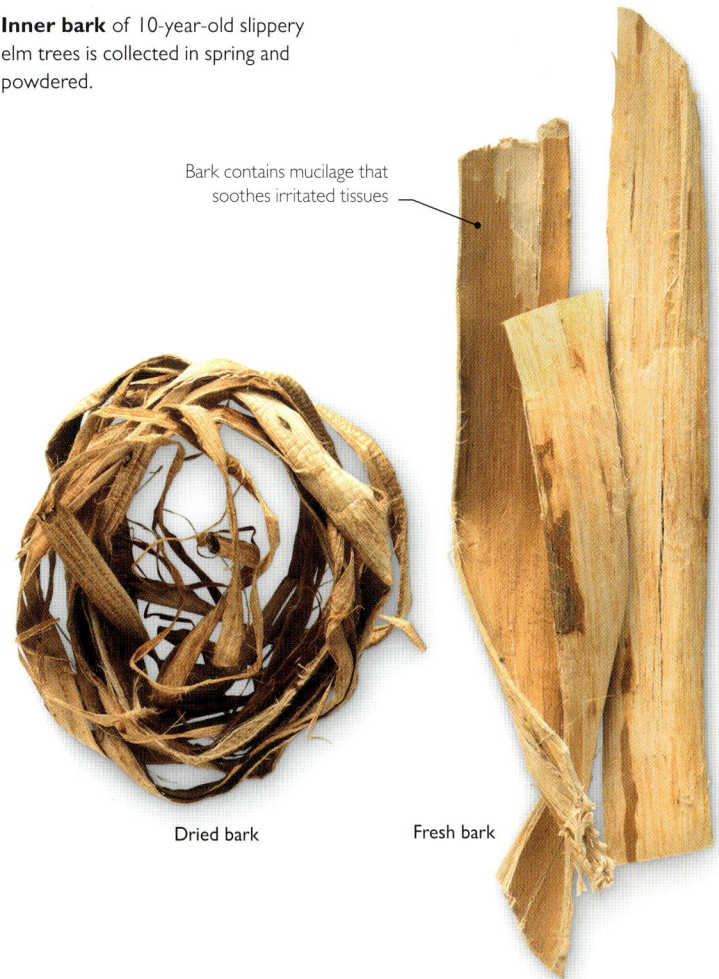

Bark contains mucilage that soothes irritated tissues

Dried bark

Fresh bark

Key preparations & their uses

Infusion Mix 1 heaped tsp with 3 cups (750 ml) of warm water. Infuse for 5 minutes. For diarrhea, drink a whole dose 1–2 times a day.

Poultice For wounds, add several drops of calendula tincture to 1 tsp of powder. Mix into a paste and apply (*see* p. 305).

Capsules (to make, p. 302) For bronchitis, take a 200 mg capsule 2–3 times a day.

Powder For acid indigestion, take 1 tsp with water 2–3 times daily.

Tablets Take for diarrhea.

Urtica dioica (Urticaceae)

Nettle, Stinging nettle

Known for its sting, nettle has long been appreciated for its medicinal uses. In the 1st century CE, the Greek physician Dioscorides listed a range of uses—the fresh chopped leaves as a bandage for septic wounds, the juice for nosebleeds, and the cooked leaves mixed with myrrh to stimulate menstruation. Today, nettle is used for hay fever, arthritis, anemia, and, surprisingly, even for some skin conditions.

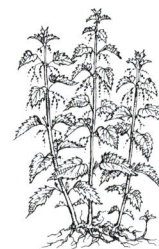

A perennial growing to 5 ft (1.5 m), with lance-shaped leaves and green flowers with yellow stamens.

Habitat & cultivation

Nettle grows in temperate regions worldwide. The shoots are picked in spring for use as a tonic and a vegetable. Aerial parts are picked in summer when the plant is in flower. The root is harvested in the fall.

Related species

The annual nettle (*U. urens*) is used in similar ways to *U. dioica*. Roman nettle (*U. pilulifera*) was the species most used by the Romans for "urtication" (beating with nettles to encourage blood to the surface), which they did to keep themselves warm.

Key constituents

Aerial parts:
• Flavonoids (quercitin) • Amines (histamine, choline, acetylcholine, serotonin) • Glucoquinone
• Minerals (calcium, potassium, silicic acid, iron)

Root:
• Plant sterols (stigmast-4-en-3-one and stigmasterol) • Phenols

Key actions

• Diuretic • Tonic • Astringent
• Prevents hemorrhaging
• Anti-allergenic • Reduces prostate enlargement (root)
• Anti-inflammatory

Research

Root Clinical trials over the past 20 years have supported the root's use in treating an enlarged prostate and easing lower urinary tract symptoms, though several tested it in combination with saw palmetto (*Serenoa repens*, p. 140) rather than on its own.
Anti-arthritic Studies into nettle's benefit in osteoarthritis have had mixed results, though a 2009 French

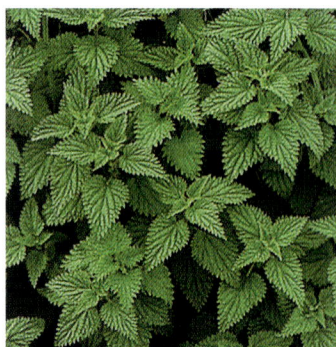

Nettle can be cooked as a vegetable and tastes like spinach.

trial found it reduced patients' required daily intake of anti-inflammatories when combined with Vitamin E, zinc, and fish oil.
Seeds Results of a 2009 Iranian laboratory study suggested that the seeds are antioxidant and protect liver function.

Traditional & current uses

Cleansing Nettle's key traditional use is as a cleansing, detoxifying herb. It has a diuretic action, possibly due to its flavonoids and high potassium content, and increases urine production and the elimination of waste products. It helps many skin conditions and arthritic problems.
Astringent Nettle slows or stops bleeding from wounds and nosebleeds, and is good for heavy menstrual bleeding.
Allergies Nettle is anti-allergenic. It treats hay fever, asthma, itchy skin conditions, and insect bites. The juice can be used as a treatment for nettle stings.
Enlarged prostate Following research, nettle root has now become a common treatment

Parts used

Aerial parts are eaten as a tonic vegetable and used to make medicinal preparations.

Root has important diuretic properties that make it useful for prostate problems.

Seeds are thought to act to protect the liver.

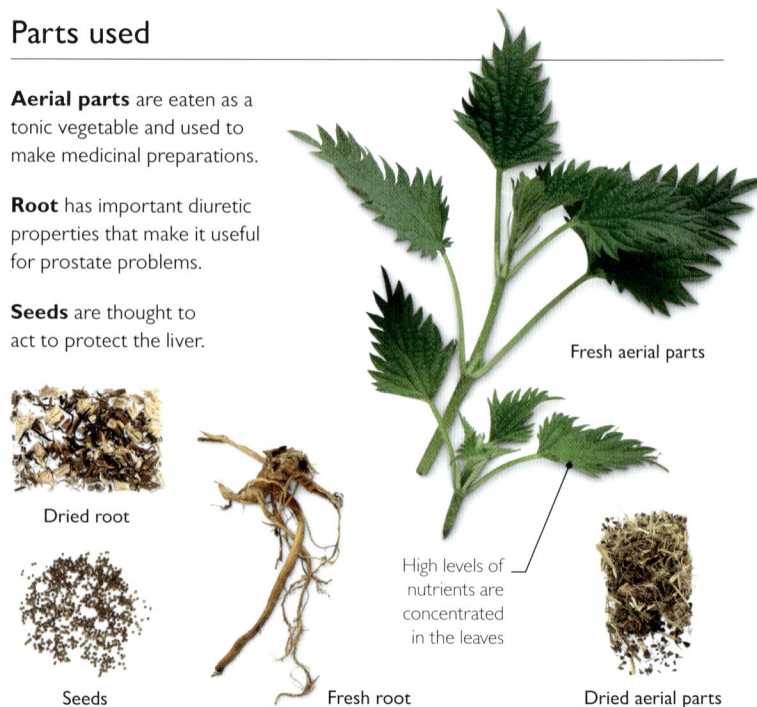

Fresh aerial parts

Dried root

High levels of nutrients are concentrated in the leaves

Seeds

Fresh root

Dried aerial parts

Key preparations & their uses

Decoction of root (see p. 301). For enlarged prostate, drink ¾ cup (150 ml) daily.

Ointment of leaves (to make, p. 305). For eczema, rub liberally.

Soup with nettle leaves, carrots, and onions is rich in iron. Drink regularly.

Capsules of leaf, (to make, p. 302). For enlarged prostate take a 300 mg

capsule 2–4 times a day. For heavy periods, take a 100 mg capsule 3 times a day.

Infusion of leaves (to make, p. 301). Drink ¾ cup (200 ml) daily as a tonic.

Tincture of root (to make, p. 302) helps allergies and skin conditions. For hay fever, take 1 tsp diluted with ½ cup (100 ml) water twice a day.

for symptoms linked to having an enlarged prostate.

Self-help uses

• Allergic rhinitis including hay fever, p. 310. • Anemia due to heavy

menstrual bleeding, p. 311. • Bites & stings, p. 313. • Mild asthma, p. 311.
• Diaper rash, p. 328. • Hives, p. 313.
• Nosebleeds, p. 320.

Vaccinium myrtillus (Ericaceae)

Bilberry, Blueberry

Bilberry fruit first came to attention in World War II (1939–1945) when pilots found that their night vision improved on eating bilberry jam. Since then research has shown that bilberries help the eyes adjust to the dark, and stimulate the part of the retina most involved in seeing clearly, especially in dim or dark conditions. There is also the suggestion that bilberry fruit helps correct nearsightedness.

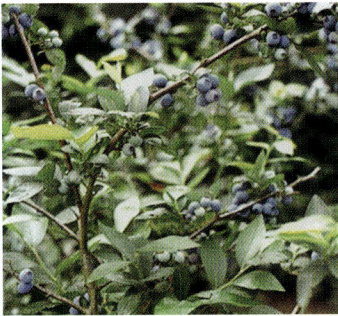

A deciduous shrub growing to 16 in (40 cm) tall, with white or pink flowers and purple-black berries.

Bilberry fruit can be used as a natural antioxidant supplement.

Habitat & cultivation

Bilberry thrives in moist undergrowth on moors, hillsides, and heathland, throughout temperate regions of the northern hemisphere—Asia, Europe, and North America. Widely cultivated around the world, bilberry is propagated from seed in the fall, or from cuttings. The leaves are collected in summer, the fruit when ripe in late summer or early fall.

Related species

Other members of the Ericaceae, such as bearberry (*Arctostaphyllos uva-ursi*, p. 174), lingonberry (*V. vitis-idaea*), and cranberry (*V. macrocarpon*, p. 290) are used principally as urinary antiseptics.

Key constituents

- Tannins (approximately 7%)
- Proanthocyanins • Flavonoids
- Fruit acids • Phenolic acids • Pectin
- Vitamin B_2, C, and carotene

Key actions

- Circulatory tonic • Antioxidant
- Anti-inflammatory • Astringent
- Urinary antiseptic

Research

Circulation Clinical trials from 1964 onward have shown that bilberry fruits protect peripheral circulation and capillaries. Symptoms that have been shown to improve with bilberry extracts include fluid retention, pain, pins and needles (paresthesia), and cramps—all resulting from impaired peripheral blood flow.

Eyesight Different trials have also shown improvement to eyesight in the nearsighted, in those with retinal damage due to diabetes, and to high blood pressure in patients taking bilberry extracts, beta-carotene, and retinol. Other conditions such as period pain and recovery from hemorrhoid operations may improve with bilberry.

Traditional & current uses

Digestive problems Bilberry fruit has long been used as a mild laxative (because of its sugars), and to relieve diarrhea (due to the tannins). It is also moderately antibacterial and, since it tastes pleasant, is useful for treating diarrhea and indigestion in children.

Circulatory disorders Many circulatory disorders will benefit from the fruit's ability to improve capillary function and heal inflammation. These include intermittent claudication; Raynaud's disease; varicose veins; hemorrhoids; easy bruising; and all conditions impairing blood flow to the eyes, particularly diabetes and high blood pressure.

Antioxidant The fruit is used to protect against tissue damage (it may prevent cataract formation) and to promote tissue healing, for example in the gastrointestinal tract or in rheumatoid or osteoarthritis.

Parts used

Leaves make a useful urinary antiseptic and astringent for urinary tract problems such as cystitis and irritable bladder.

Berries have a strong healing effect on capillaries, especially on the microcirculation within the eye.

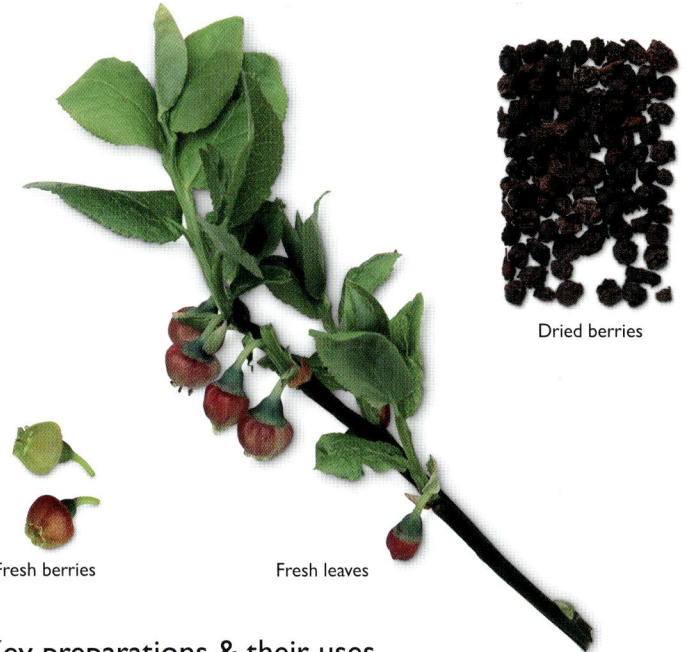

Dried berries

Fresh berries

Fresh leaves

Key preparations & their uses

Capsules Take up to 4 x 500 mg capsules a day to improve circulation within the eye.

Tincture (to make, p. 302). Take ½ tsp a day for poor circulation.

Decoction (to make, p. 301) is pleasant-tasting and useful for short-term treatment of diarrhea in children.

Tablets, like capsules, are convenient for long-term use.

Caution If taking anticoagulants or diagnosed with a bleeding disorder, take medicinal doses with professional advice only.

Antiseptic The leaves have a marked antiseptic effect within the bladder and urinary tubules, and can be used to treat urinary infections such as cystitis.

Antidiabetic The leaves and fruit have antidiabetic activity, helping especially in prediabetic states. There is growing evidence that the fruit can help promote weight loss.

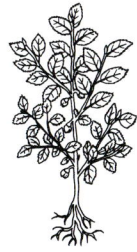

Valeriana officinalis (Valerianaceae)

Valerian

Valerian has been used as a sedative and relaxant at least since Roman times. It was known to Dioscorides in the 1st century CE, who named it *phu*, the sound of the word reflecting its unpleasant smell. Valerian helps relieve stress and has become an increasingly popular remedy in recent decades. It is a safe, nonaddictive relaxant that reduces nervous tension and anxiety and promotes restful sleep.

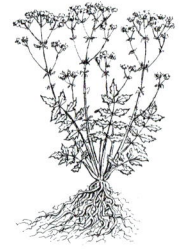

Erect perennial growing to 4 ft (1.2 m), with pinnate divided leaves and pink flowers.

Habitat & cultivation
Native to Europe and northern Asia, valerian grows wild in damp conditions. It is cultivated in central and eastern Europe. The plant is grown from seed in spring, and the root and rhizome of 2-year-old plants are unearthed in the fall.

Related species
V. capensis is given in South Africa for hysteria and epilepsy; *V. hardwickii*, found in China and Indonesia, is taken as an antispasmodic; *V. uliginosa* was used for cramps and menopausal symptoms by the Menominee people in North America; and *V. wallichii* is used in the Himalayas in almost exactly the same way as valerian.

Key constituents
• Volatile oil (up to 1.4%), including bornyl acetate, beta-caryophyllene
• Iridoids (valepotriates)—valtrate, isovaltrate • Alkaloids

Key actions
• Sedative • Relaxant • Relieves muscle spasms • Relieves anxiety
• Lowers blood pressure

Research
Therapeutic properties Extensive research in Germany and Switzerland has endorsed the use of valerian to aid sleep, improve sleep quality, and lower blood pressure. A German trial carried out in 2002 that tested valerian and oxazepam (a conventional sleep treatment) found both to be effective—83% of those taking valerian rated the treatment as very good compared to 73% of those taking oxazepam. A 2020 Japanese systematic review examined 60 studies investigating valerian and

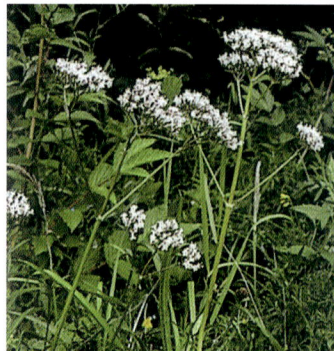

Valerian helps reduce stress. Its name is thought to be derived from the Latin valere, *"to be well."*

found it to be a safe and effective herb to promote sleep and reduce anxiety.

Traditional & current uses
Historical uses Known as "all-heal" in the Middle Ages, valerian was credited with many virtues, in particular with healing epilepsy. In 1592, Fabius Calumna published a detailed work on herbal medicine in which he claimed to have cured his epilepsy with the herb.
Stress-related disorders Valerian reduces mental over-activity and nervous excitability, helping people who find it hard to "switch off." It is beneficial for almost any stress-related condition, and, in general, has a calming, rather than directly sedative, effect on the mind.
Anxiety & insomnia Many symptoms of anxiety, including tremors, panic, palpitations, and sweating, can be relieved with valerian. It is a useful remedy for insomnia, whether caused by anxiety or overexcitement.
Effective relaxant Valerian relaxes

Parts used

Root and rhizome are harvested in the fall when they contain the highest level of active ingredients.

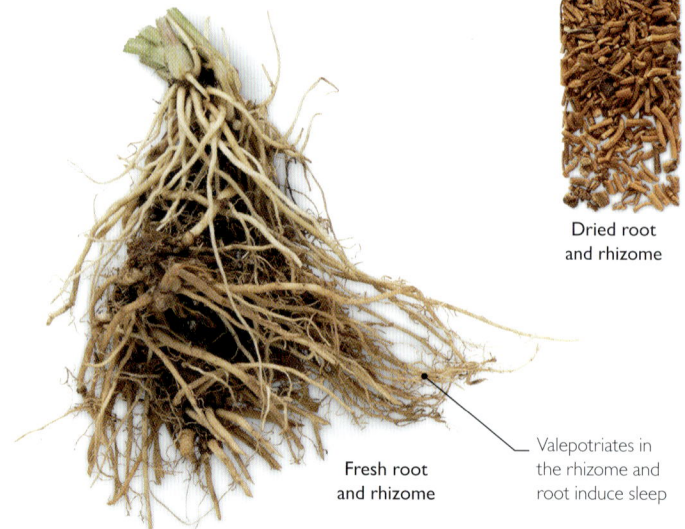

Dried root and rhizome

Fresh root and rhizome

Valepotriates in the rhizome and root induce sleep

Key preparations & their uses

Tablets often also contain other herbs. Take for stress or anxiety.

Powder can be taken as capsules (to make, p. 302). For insomnia, take 1–2 doses of 500 mg at night.

Tincture (to make, p. 302). For anxiety, take 20 drops in hot water up to 5 times a day.

Decoction (to make, p. 301). Take 1–5 tbsp as a sedative at night.

Cautions Can cause drowsiness. Do not take valerian if already taking sleep-inducing drugs.

over-contracted muscles, and is helpful for shoulder and neck tension, asthma, colic, irritable bowel syndrome, period pain, and muscle spasms.
High blood pressure Valerian is used with other herbs in remedies for high blood pressure caused by stress and anxiety.

Self-help uses
• Chronic anxiety, p. 318. • Insomnia, p. 319. • Nervous exhaustion, p. 319. • Premenstrual syndrome, p. 325. • Sleeplessness due to backache, p. 323.

Verbena officinalis (Verbenaceae)

Vervain, *Ma bian cao* (Chinese)

Vervain has long been credited with magical properties and was used in ceremonies by the Druids of ancient Britain and Gaul. It is a traditional herbal medicine in both China and Europe. Dioscorides in the 1st century CE called vervain the "sacred herb," and for many centuries it was taken as a cure-all. It has tonic, restorative properties, and is used to relieve stress and anxiety and to improve digestive function.

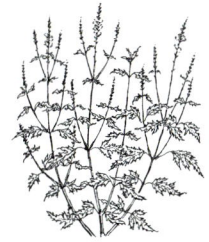

A slender perennial growing to 3 ft (1 m), with stiff, thin stems and spikes of small lilac flowers.

Habitat & cultivation

Vervain grows wild throughout much of Europe and North Africa as well as in China and Japan. It is propagated from seed in spring or fall and thrives in well-drained soil in a sunny position. The aerial parts are harvested in summer when the plant is in flower.

Related species

Blue vervain (*V. hastata*), which is native to North America, is used medicinally in the same way as vervain.

Key constituents

• Bitter iridoids (verbenin, verbenalin)
• Volatile oil • Alkaloids • Triterpenes (beta-sitosterol) • Flavonoids

Key actions

• Nervine • Tonic • Mild bitter
• Mild antidepressant

Research

Hormonal effects Early indications from research into vervain are that it has both estrogenic and progestogenic activity. It also stimulates the muscles of the womb, and production of breast milk.

Lack of research For an herb with such long traditional use, surprisingly little research into vervain has occurred to date. Laboratory studies indicate that vervain has significant anti-inflammatory activity. In Pakistani research published in 2016, the herb was found to have anticonvulsant, anxiolytic, and sedative activities. Vervain also appears to have antimicrobial, antiviral, and liver protective properties.

Traditional & current uses

Digestive tonic Vervain improves the function of the digestive system and absorption of food.

Nervous system Vervain is prized as a restorative for the nervous system and is especially helpful for nervous tension. It is thought to have a mild antidepressant action, and is used specifically to treat anxiety and the nervous exhaustion that follows long-term stress.

Convalescence By aiding digestion and restoring the nervous system, vervain is an ideal tonic for people recovering from chronic illness.

Headaches & migraines Vervain alleviates headaches, and in Chinese herbal medicine it is used for migraines connected with the menstrual cycle.

Other uses Among its other medicinal uses, vervain is given for jaundice, gallstones, asthma, insomnia, premenstrual syndrome, flu, and fevers.

Self-help uses

• Nervous exhaustion, p. 319.
• Premenstrual syndrome, p. 325.

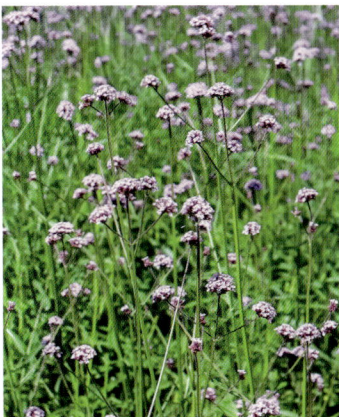

Vervain was carried in the Middle Ages to bring good luck.

Parts used

Aerial parts have a tonic effect on the nervous system and digestion, and have been used medicinally for thousands of years in Europe and China.

Vervain has slender, almost "wand-like," flowering stems

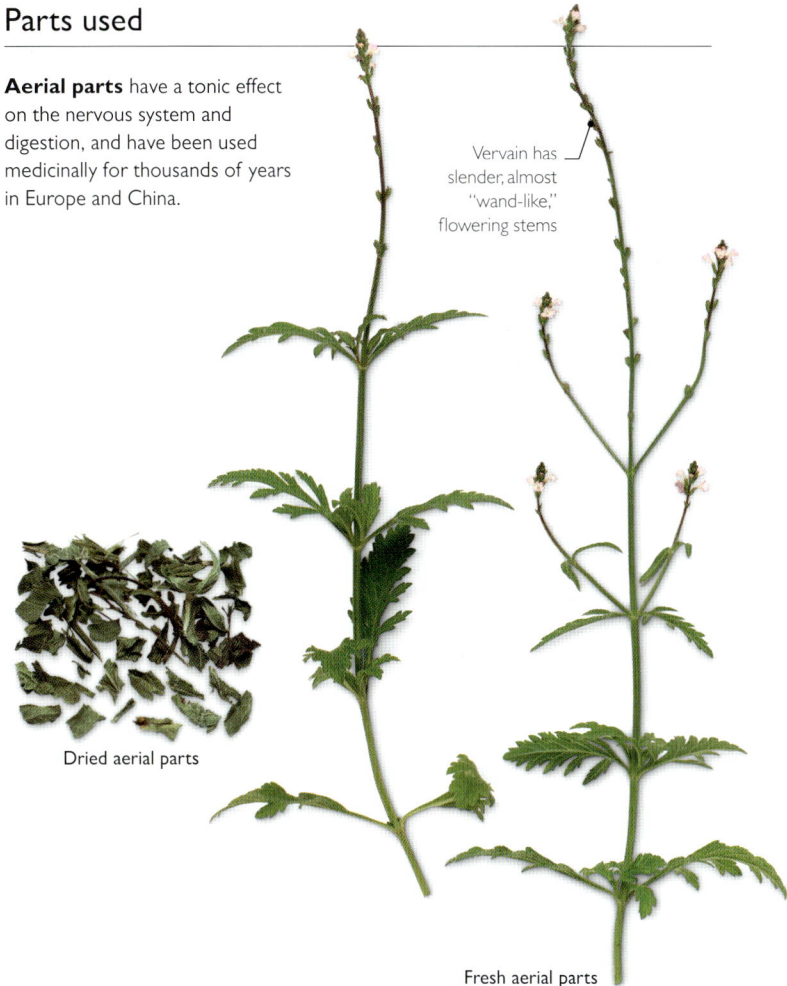

Dried aerial parts

Fresh aerial parts

Key preparations & their uses

Tincture (to make, p. 302) is a relaxing, calming tonic. For stress and anxiety, take ½ tsp diluted in a glass of water 3 times a day.

Infusion (to make, p. 301) helps stimulate digestion and improves effective absorption of food. Drink ¾ cup (150 ml) regularly, particularly after heavy meals.

Powder can be used as a toothpaste. Rub on the teeth regularly to clean and protect them.

Cautions Do not exceed the stated dose. Vervain can cause vomiting if taken in excess. Do not take during pregnancy.

Viburnum opulus (Caprifoliaceae)

Cramp bark, Guelder rose

Native to both North America and Europe, cramp bark was recognized as recently as 1960 in the *US National Formulary* as a sedative remedy for nervous conditions and as an antispasmodic in the treatment of asthma. As its name implies, the herb's primary medicinal use is to relieve cramps and other conditions, such as colic or painful menstruation, caused by over-contraction of muscles.

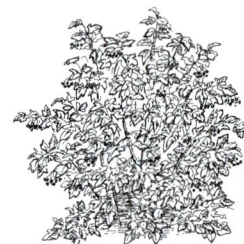

A deciduous shrub or tree growing to 13 ft (4 m), with lobed leaves, white flowers, and red oval fruit.

Habitat & cultivation
Cramp bark grows in woodlands, hedges, and thickets in Europe and eastern North America. It is propagated from seed sown in the fall. Bark from the branches is collected in spring and summer, when the plant is in flower.

Related species
Black haw (*V. prunifolium*, p. 291) is often used interchangeably with cramp bark, but it is thought to have a more specific action on the uterus.

Key constituents
- Hydroquinones (arbutin)
- Coumarins (scopoletin)
- Tannins (3%) • Proanthocyanidins
- Polysaccharides

Key actions
- Antispasmodic • Sedative
- Astringent • Relaxant

Research
Antispasmodic activity in kidney stones A Turkish hospital urology department tested the ability of

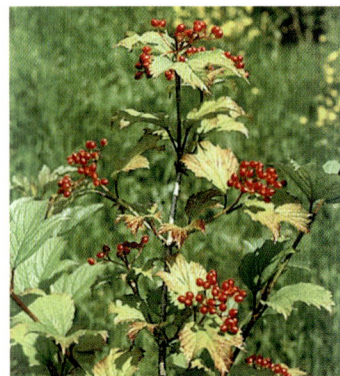

Cramp bark has distinctive bright red berries in the fall.

cramp bark to ease the passage of kidney stones up to ⅓ in (1 cm) in diameter—an extremely painful condition. 103 patients were given diclofenac (an analgesic) alone or with cramp bark. The rate of stone expulsion and time taken was significantly shorter in the cramp bark group, who also required less analgesic and less additional treatment. The 2019 study noted that cramp bark facilitated the passage of ureteral stones—evidence indeed of the herb's antispasmodic activity. A further 2022 study produced similar results.

Traditional & current uses
Indigenous remedy Cramp bark has a history of use in Indigenous herbalism. The Meskwaki people took cramp bark for cramps and pains throughout the body, while the Penobscot used it to treat swollen glands and mumps.

Muscle relaxant Cramp bark is effective at relieving any tense muscle, whether smooth muscle in the intestines, airways, or uterus, or striated muscle (attached to the skeleton) in the limbs or back. It may be taken internally, or applied topically to relieve muscle tension. The herb also treats symptoms arising from excess muscle tension, including breathing difficulties in asthma, and menstrual pain caused by excessive contraction of the uterus. For night cramps and back pain, lobelia (*Lobelia inflata*, p. 114) is often mixed with cramp bark. The herb also relieves constipation, colic, and irritable bowel syndrome, as well as the physical symptoms of nervous tension.

Arthritis In some cases of arthritis, where joint weakness and pain have

Parts used

Bark is peeled off the tree in strips during spring and summer. Care must be taken to leave enough bark for the tree to stay alive.

Berries are astringent, bitter, and rich in vitamin C.

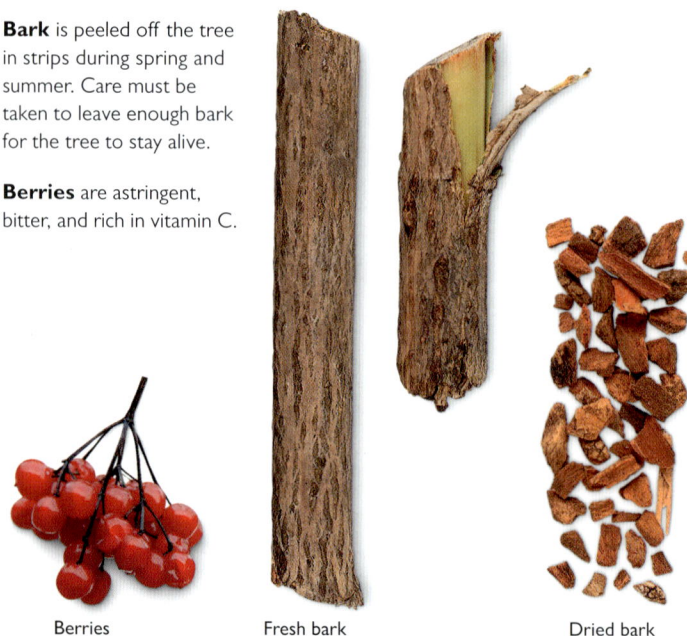

Berries   Fresh bark   Dried bark

Key preparations & their uses

Decoction (to make, p. 301). For period pain, take ⅓ cup (75 ml) every 3 hours.

Tincture (to make, p. 302) is used for long-term treatment of muscular tension. For irritable bowel syndrome,

take ½ tsp diluted with hot water twice a day.

Lotion (to make, p. 306) relieves aching muscles. Rub into tense neck and shoulders.

caused muscles to contract until they are almost rigid, cramp bark can bring remarkable relief. As the muscles relax, blood flow to the area improves, waste products such as lactic acid are removed, and normal function can return.

Berries The berries and juice have been used to treat a wide range of illnesses, including heart disease, high

blood pressure, coughs and colds, neurosis, and diabetes.

Self-help uses
- Back pain, p. 323. • Breathing difficulties, p. 311. • Cramps & muscle spasms, p. 322. • Period pain, p. 325.
- Poor circulation to the hands & feet, p. 312. • Spastic constipation, p. 317.
- Stomach spasm, p. 315.

Vitex agnus-castus (Verbenaceae)

Chaste tree, Agnus castus, Vitex, Chasteberry

Chaste tree was well known in ancient times and featured in Homer's 6th-century BCE epic, the *Iliad*, as a symbol of chastity capable of warding off evil. As the name "chaste tree" implies, it was thought to reduce sexual desire, and traditionally it was chewed by monks to reduce unwanted libido. Research has confirmed that chaste tree has a hormonal action, and today it is used for menstrual problems and infertility.

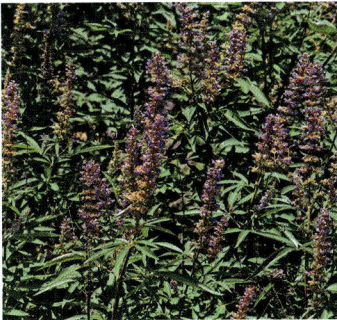

A deciduous aromatic tree growing to 23 ft (7 m), with palm-shaped leaves and small, lilac flowers.

Chaste tree has small, fragrant, lilac flowers in summer that grow in whorls on long spikes.

Habitat & cultivation

Chaste tree is native to the Mediterranean region and western Asia. It is cultivated in subtropical areas around the world, and has become naturalized in many regions. It is grown from seed in spring or fall. The ripe berries are collected in the fall.

Related species

As a member of the Verbenaceae genus, chaste tree is a distant relative of vervain (*Verbena officinalis*, p. 153) and lemon verbena (*Lippia citriodora*, p. 168).

Key constituents

• Volatile oil (cineol) • Flavonoids (casticin) • Iridoids (aucubin, agnoside, eurostoside) • Diterpenes

Key actions

• Regulates hormones
• Progestogenic • Increases breast-milk production • Aids sleep

Research

Hormonal properties The berries are thought to induce subtle hormonal effects within the brain, leading to increased levels of the neurotransmitters dopamine and melatonin. These changes are thought to promote better hormonal regulation of the menstrual cycle, notably through raised progesterone levels. In some people, the raised melatonin levels may aid sleep quality. The diterpenes are thought to be chiefly responsible for these effects.

Gynecological problems Clinical research by and large supports the use of chaste tree in many female hormonal problems, including premenstrual syndrome (PMS), irregular menstruation, breast tenderness, and infertility. A 2001 clinical trial tested chaste berry against placebo in 178 women with PMS. After 3 months, those taking chaste tree had a 50% reduction in symptoms compared to placebo.

Sleep aid Since researchers found that chasteberry increases melatonin levels, chasteberry has been thought of as a possible sleep aid. Some small studies indicate that chasteberry might help people with insomnia due to unhealthy melatonin levels, such as shift workers or those who are jet lagged.

Traditional & current uses

Menstrual problems Chaste tree is probably the most used herb in Western herbal medicine for regulating the menstrual cycle. With its progestogenic action, chaste tree is often helpful in relieving premenstrual symptoms, including irritability and lowered mood, headache, acne, and breast tenderness. Chaste tree also promotes greater menstrual regularity, and this use extends to more significant hormonal problems

Parts used

Berries, harvested in the fall, are used to treat female fertility problems.

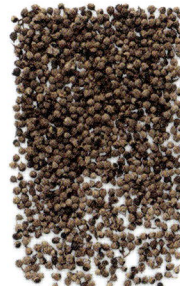

Tiny yellow-red berries contain hormonal substances

Dried berries

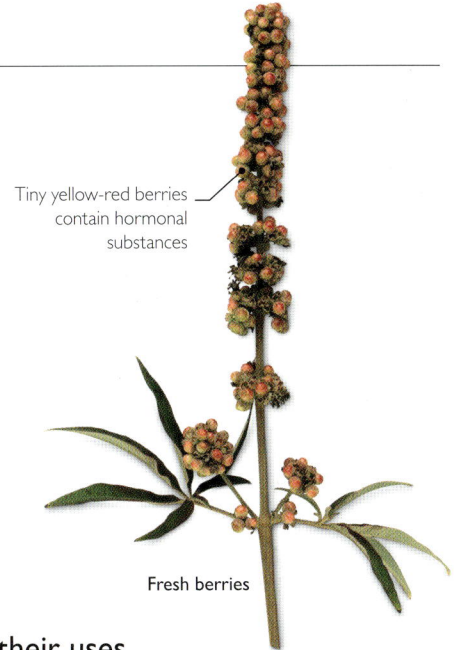

Fresh berries

Key preparations & their uses

Tablets Take for premenstrual syndrome.

Tincture (to make, p. 302). For an irregular cycle, take 40 drops with water daily for 3 months.

Caution Excess can cause formication (a sensation of ants crawling on the skin). Concurrent use with the contraceptive pill or fertility treatment is not advisable. Avoid in pregnancy. In rare cases may cause gastrointestinal upset, headache, or dizziness.

including polycystic ovary syndrome, fibroids, and endometriosis.

Irregular periods The herb helps regulate irregular periods, tending to shorten a long cycle and lengthen a short one.

Infertility Chaste tree can be of help to some women trying to conceive if infertility is due to low progesterone levels.

Difficulty in breastfeeding The berries are taken to increase breast milk production.

Acne Though rarely used on its own, chaste tree can be extremely helpful in treating acne in both men and women. Used in combination with herbs such as echinacea (*Echinacea* spp., p. 96), it will often reduce the frequency and intensity of acne blemishes where hormonal imbalance is a major factor.

Self-help uses

• Aiding conception, p. 326.
• Decreased estrogen & progesterone levels, p. 326.
• Irregular cycle, p. 325.

155

Withania somnifera (Solanaceae)

Ashwagandha

Ashwagandha has been called "Indian ginseng" because it is used in Ayurveda in much the same way that ginseng is used in Chinese medicine: to improve vitality and to aid recovery after chronic illness. Today, ashwagandha seems to be an herb designed to deal with the busy nature of modern life. It invigorates when fatigued, eases the impact of stress and anxiety, and aids sleep—all traditional uses largely supported by clinical research.

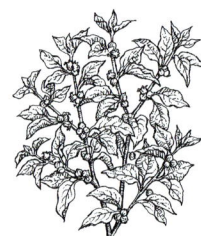

A stout shrub growing to 5 ft (1.5 m), with oval leaves and greenish or yellow flowers.

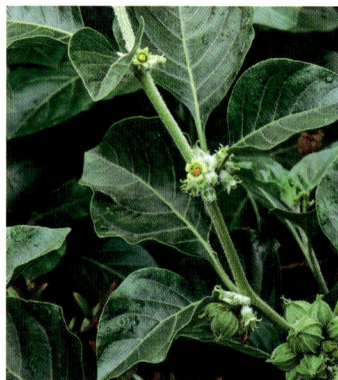

Ashwagandha has powerful medicinal properties proven by research.

Habitat & cultivation

Ashwagandha is found in India, the Mediterranean, and the Middle East. It is propagated from seed or cuttings in spring. The leaves are harvested in spring, and the fruit and root in the fall.

Key constituents

• Alkaloids • Steroidal lactones (withanolides) • Iron

Key actions

• Adaptogenic • Tonic • Mild sedative

Research

Chronic stress Clinical research has been wide-ranging and examined many aspects of ashwagandha's potential medicinal uses, many linked to the withanolides, compounds similar to the body's own steroid hormones. A 2012 Indian clinical trial noted that those taking withania had lower stress levels and an increased sense of well-being, as well as lower cortisol and blood pressure levels.

Anxiety and tension Ashwagandha has been proven to reduce anxiety

and tension in at least 6 clinical trials. In a 2009 Canadian trial, ashwagandha, paired with dietary advice and a multivitamin supplement, was found more effective in decreasing anxiety than psychotherapy and a placebo. Those taking ashwagandha also reported improved concentration and less fatigue.

Sleep aid Ashwagandha root's ability to promote restorative sleep has consistently been endorsed in clinical trials. A 2020 Indian study, where 150 healthy adults took a root extract to aid sleep for 6 weeks, found that ashwagandha improved sleep quality and promoted restorative sleep.

Male fertility Two clinical trials testing ashwagandha's role as a male sexual tonic indicate that the herb markedly improves semen quality. Another clinical trial failed to find any benefit in aiding erectile dysfunction.

Other actions Ashwagandha has also been researched for its use as a tonic suitable for children, to improve muscle strength and mental function in the elderly, for arthritis, and to enhance immune function. Ashwagandha is thought to have anticancer activity.

Traditional & current uses

Ayurvedic tonic Ashwagandha has always been valued in Ayurveda for its tonic, strengthening, and relaxing properties. Robert Svoboda in *Ayurveda: Life, Health, and Longevity* states that it "clarifies the mind, calms and strengthens the nerves, and promotes sound restful sleep."

Restorative Today, the herb is still prized as a tonic, but valued also for its unusual combination of actions. As a tonic, it strengthens and supports physical and mental performance, yet

Parts used

Leaves contain the most withanolides, constituents that inhibit cancer cell growth.

Root is powdered or made into decoctions and taken as a strengthening and calming tonic.

Berries are chewed in India to help in convalescence.

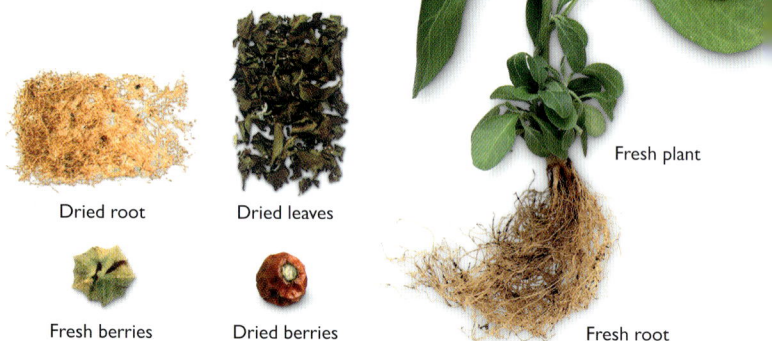

Dried root

Dried leaves

Fresh berries

Dried berries

Fresh plant

Fresh root

Key preparations & their uses

Decoction of the root (to make, p. 301). For stress, decoct 5 g with ⅓ cup (75 ml) water and take over 2 days.

Powder made from the leaves. For anemia, take ½ tsp in a little water once a day.

Capsules of powdered root (to make, p. 302). For nervous exhaustion, take 1–2 g a day with water.

at the same time it relieves anxiety and, as its botanical name suggests, encourages better sleep quality. It is an excellent herb for convalescence.

Inflammatory conditions Ashwagandha can be a useful addition to treatment for chronic inflammatory diseases such as rheumatoid arthritis and psoriasis.

Long-term stress By reducing

overactivity and encouraging rest and relaxation, ashwagandha is useful in countering the debility that accompanies long-term stress.

Anemia Ashwagandha's high iron content makes it useful in anemia.

Self-help uses

• Long-term stress & convalescence, pp. 318 & 329. • Male fertility, p. 326.

Zanthoxylum americanum (Rutaceae)

Prickly ash, Toothache tree

Indigenous to North America, prickly ash is a warming, stimulating herb for circulation. It was held in high regard by Indigenous peoples in North America for its medicinal properties, and both the bark and berries were chewed to alleviate rheumatism and toothache. Today, prickly ash is mainly given for arthritic and rheumatic conditions, but it is also helpful for certain digestive problems and for leg ulcers.

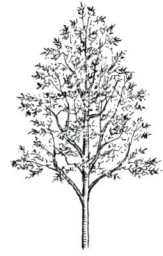

A deciduous shrub growing to 10 ft (3 m), with thorny, gray branches and compound leaves.

Habitat & cultivation

Prickly ash is native to southern Canada and northern, central, and western parts of the US, preferring moist, shady sites such as woodlands. It is propagated from seed in the fall. The bark is harvested in spring and the berries are collected in summer.

Related species

Southern prickly ash (*Z. clava-herculis*) grows in the central and southern US, where it is used interchangeably with prickly ash. *Chuan jiao* (*Z. bungeanum*) is given in Chinese herbal medicine for "cold" patterns of illness causing abdominal pain. *Z. capense* is taken for colic in South Africa. *Z. zanthoxyloides* is a traditional West African herb for rheumatic conditions.

Key constituents

• Isoquinoline alkaloids
• Furanocoumarins • Lignans
• Volatile oil • Tannins

Key actions

• Circulatory stimulant • Increases sweating • Antirheumatic • Antifungal

Research

Antifungal Research into prickly ash is limited, though a 2005 study found extracts from prickly ash fruit and leaf demonstrated antifungal activity.

Traditional & current uses

North American herb Northern prickly ash has longstanding traditional use in North America as a remedy for toothache and rheumatism. It was used in the US during the 19th century as a circulatory stimulant and to treat arthritis.

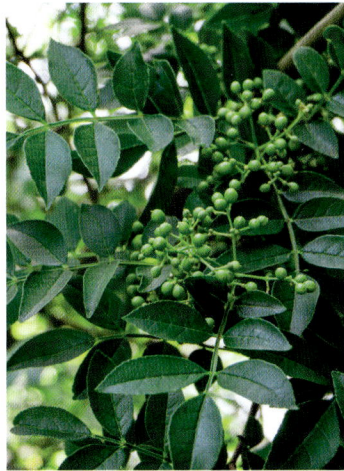

Prickly ash is antirheumatic and improves circulation.

Arthritic conditions Western herbalists regard northern prickly ash as a prime remedy for rheumatic and arthritic problems. It stimulates blood flow to painful and stiff joints, promoting the supply of oxygen and nutrients to the area and removing waste products.

Circulation The herb improves circulation in intermittent claudication and Raynaud's disease, conditions where the arteries of the limbs have narrowed, preventing sufficient blood reaching the hand or leg muscles.

Other uses Prickly ash relieves gas and diarrhea and tones the digestive tract. It is applied topically to treat leg ulcers and chronic pelvic inflammatory disease.

Self-help uses

• Back pain, p. 323. • Poor circulation, p. 312

Parts used

Bark is considered to have a stronger effect than the berries. It is used in preparations to stimulate blood flow.

Berries are made into remedies for poor circulation.

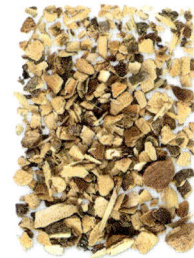

Dried chopped bark

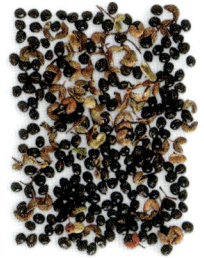

Dried berries

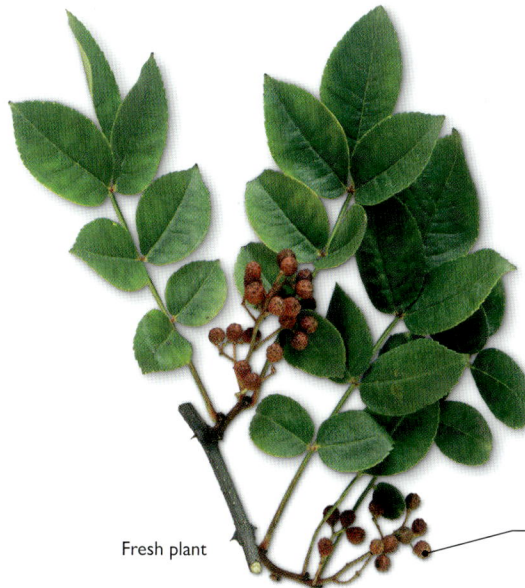

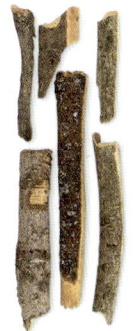

Fresh bark

Fresh plant

Berries and bark were chewed for toothache

Key preparations & their uses

Tincture of bark (to make, p. 302). For arthritis, take 20 drops with water 3 times a day.

Decoction For poor circulation, decoct 3 tsp ginger and 3 tsp prickly ash berries with 3 cups (750 ml) water (*see* p. 301). Take ¾ cup (150 ml) twice a day.

Tablets Take tablets, which often contain other herbs, for arthritis and rheumatism.

Lotion For poor circulation in the legs, make a decoction of bark (p. 301) and apply.

Cautions Avoid in pregnancy and while breastfeeding.

Zea mays (Poaceae)

Corn, Maize, corn silk, *Yu mi shu* (Chinese)

The staple food of Central and South America for at least 4,000 years, corn is also used medicinally in countless different ways. The Aztecs gave a corn meal decoction for dysentery and "heat in the heart," and to increase breast milk production. Corn silk (the silky fronds wrapped around the cob) has always been the part most used medicinally, and it is of particular value in treating urinary conditions.

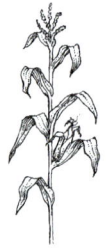

An annual grass reaching 10 ft (3 m), with plumelike male flowers. Female flowers produce cobs.

Habitat & cultivation

Cultivated almost universally as a food crop, corn is native to the Andes and Central America, possibly originating in Peru. It is propagated from seed in spring. The corn silk is harvested with the ripe cob in summer, then separated and dried.

Related species

Corn smut (*Ustilago zeae*), a fungus that grows on corn, is used by the Zuni of New Mexico to speed childbirth and stop uterine hemorrhage.

Key constituents

• Flavonoids • Carotenoids

Cob:

• Anthocyanins (purple corn)

Corn silk:

• Carotenoids • Volatile oil

• Sterols

Key actions

• Urinary demulcent • Diuretic

• Mildly stimulates bile secretion

• Gently lowers blood pressure

Research

Purple corn Purple corn contains unusually high levels of anthocyanins, dark red or blue plant pigments that have strong antioxidant and protective effects within the body. A 2007 paper reported that, weight for weight, purple corn contained nearly four times more anthocyanins than blueberries, suggesting that purple corn could be a key dietary source of anthocyanins.

Carotenoids Corncob and corn silk contain high levels of carotenoids (including lutein and zeaxanthin), compounds that are thought to protect the eye from oxidative damage. Zeaxanthin in particular is

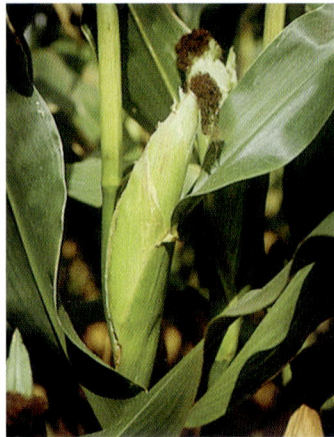

Corn's Latin name reflects its value— zea *means "cause of life" and* mays *means "our mother."*

thought to protect against age-related macular degeneration.

Traditional & current uses

Traditional herb Corn meal is both food and medicine for indigenous peoples in the Americas. In Mayan, Incan, and American traditional medicine, it has been used as a poultice to treat bruises, swellings, sores, boils, and similar conditions. Virgil J. Vogel writes that "the Chickasaw [people] treated itching skin, followed by sores when scratched, by burning old corncobs and holding the affected part over the smoke."

Urinary remedy Corn silk is a gentle-acting diuretic with mild antibiotic activity. It can help in acute and chronic cases of cystitis and is commonly used in prostate disorders. It may also prove useful in frequent urination and bladder irritability.

Kidney stones Corn silk is thought to have a beneficial effect on the kidneys, reducing kidney stone

Parts used

Corn silk (stamens) can be used fresh or dried as a remedy for urinary disorders.

Meal is used externally to treat bruises and other skin problems.

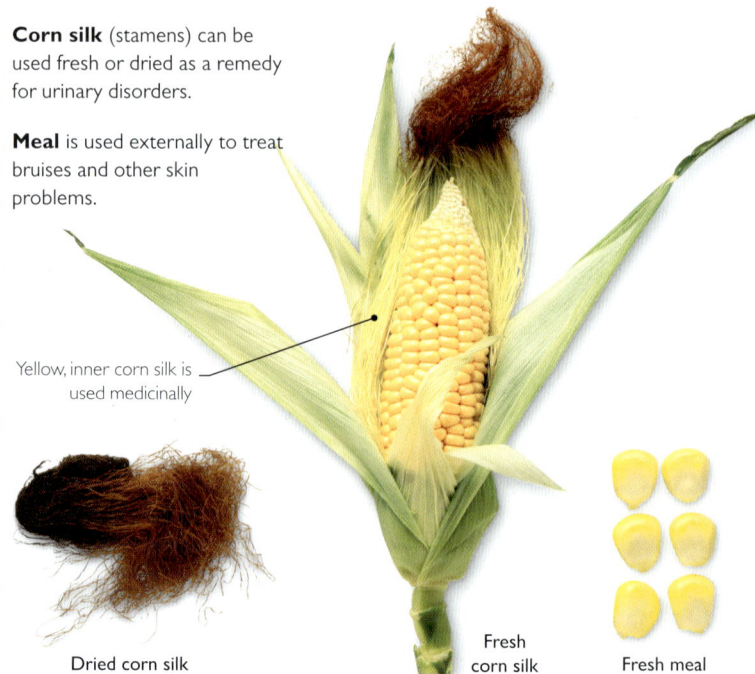

Yellow, inner corn silk is used medicinally

Dried corn silk

Fresh corn silk

Fresh meal

Key preparations & their uses

Infusion of corn silk (to make, p. 301) is soothing. For cystitis, drink 2 cups (500 ml) daily.

Decoction of meal (to make, p. 301). Apply as a poultice (*see* p. 305) to sores and boils.

The outer leaves of corn are stripped to reveal the corn silk and meal.

Capsules of corn silk (to make, p. 302). For edema, take 2 g daily.

Tincture of corn silk (to make, p. 302). For cystitis, combine ⅓ cup (80 ml) with 1 tbsp of buchu tincture and take 1 tsp with water 3 times a day.

formation and relieving some of the symptoms of existing stones.

Chinese remedy In China, corn silk is used to treat fluid retention and to support the liver in jaundice.

Self-help uses

• Fluid retention in pregnancy, p. 327.

• Urinary infections, p. 324.

Zingiber officinale (Zingiberaceae)

Ginger, *Sheng jian* (Chinese), *Singabera* (Sanskrit)

Familiar as a spice and flavoring, ginger is also one of the world's best medicines. It has been revered in Asia since the earliest times, and in medieval Europe it was thought to have derived from the Garden of Eden. Ginger's warming and anti-inflammatory properties can bring relief to problems as varied as headache and migraine, joint pain, indigestion, motion sickness, and morning sickness. Fresh ginger has a pungent, slightly lemony taste.

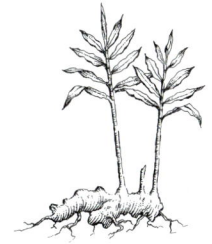

A perennial growing to 2 ft (60 cm), with lance-shaped leaves and spikes of white or yellow flowers.

Habitat & cultivation

Native to Asia, ginger is grown throughout the tropics. It is propagated by dividing the rootstock. Ginger flourishes in fertile soil and needs plenty of rain. The rhizome is unearthed when the plant is 10 months old. It is washed, soaked, and sometimes boiled and peeled.

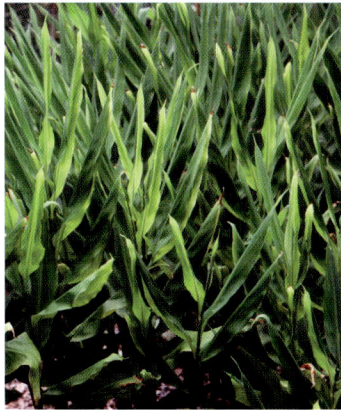

Related species

Various *Zingiber* species are used medicinally, but no other has benefits equal to ginger. Turmeric (*Curcuma longa*, p. 94) is a close relative.

Key constituents

• Volatile oil (1–3%)—zingiberene (20–30%) • Oleoresin (4–7.5%)—gingerol, shogaols

Key actions

• Anti-inflammatory • Circulatory stimulant • Antiemetic • Antiviral • Digestive stimulant

Research

Digestive health Ginger speeds up the rate of gastric emptying and aids the absorption of nutrients from the digestive tract. By improving iron absorption, it helps to treat anemia. Clinical trials indicate that it can relieve nausea and vomiting.

Morning sickness A 2013 Australian review of clinical trials using ginger to relieve morning sickness concluded that "the best available evidence suggests that ginger is a safe and effective treatment for PNV."

Pain relief Several small-scale research studies have found that ginger reduces muscle pain, for example, after exercise. This is because of a potent anti-inflammatory action. One study found that after 2 months

Ginger, widely used as a spice, is also an important digestive remedy.

of treatment, ginger was as effective in relieving menstrual cramps as mefenamic acid (an aspirin-type painkiller). A 2014 Iranian clinical trial compared the effects of ginger and sumatriptan (a painkiller) in relieving migraine, and reported that the two treatments were similarly effective.

Traditional & current uses

Digestive problems Ginger is thought to be helpful for almost all digestive complaints. It is an excellent remedy for symptoms such as indigestion, nausea, gas, bloating, and cramps—whether taken as an infusion, juice, tincture, or powder, or with food. Its antiseptic activity makes it valuable in all gastrointestinal infections, including food poisoning.

Circulatory stimulant Ginger stimulates the circulation, and helps blood to flow to the surface, making it an important remedy for chilblains and poor circulation to the hands and feet. Juice squeezed from fresh ginger root can be applied to chilblains (and cold sores), bringing quick relief.

Parts used

Rhizome contains high levels of a volatile oil that is warming and stimulating.

Yellowish fresh rhizome is strongly aromatic

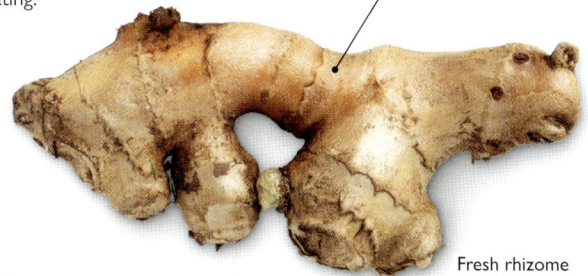

Fresh rhizome

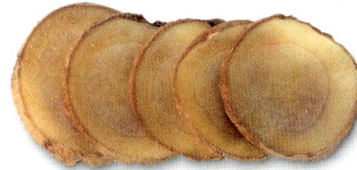

Sliced dried rhizome

Key preparations & their uses

Infusion (to make, p. 301). For nausea, drink ¾ cup (150 ml) 3 times a day.

Essential oil For arthritic aches and pains, dilute 5 drops in 20 drops carrier oil and apply (*see* p. 307).

Capsules (to make, p. 302). For morning sickness, take a 75 mg capsule every hour.

Tincture (to make, p. 302). To improve digestion, take 30 drops with water twice a day.

Cautions Do not take ginger in medicinal doses if suffering from peptic ulcers. Do not take the essential oil internally except under professional supervision. Maximum recommended dose in pregnancy and if taking anticoagulants is 2 g dried (4 g fresh) root a day.

Respiratory conditions Ginger has antiviral activity and is a first-rate remedy for coughs, colds, flu, and other respiratory problems. Despite its warming properties, ginger stimulates sweating and helps cool and control fevers.

Self-help uses

• Chilblains, p. 301. • Colds, flu, & fevers, p. 321. • Cold sores, p. 314. • Constipation, p. 317. • Digestive upsets, gas, & colic, p. 328. • High blood pressure & arteriosclerosis, p. 311. • Morning sickness, p. 327. • Nausea & motion sickness, p. 316.

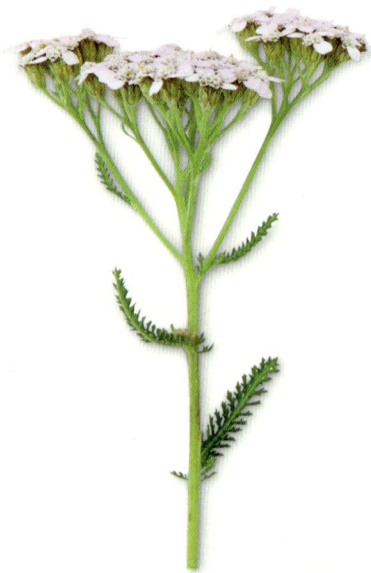

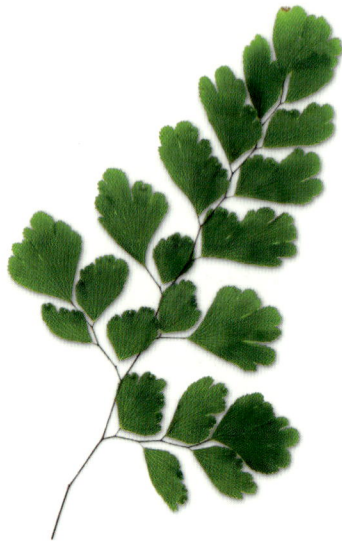

Other medicinal plants

This index of medicinal plants features in Latin name order more than 450 plants that have played a significant role in herbal medicine worldwide. They include familiar plants such as oats (*Avena sativa*, p.179) and exotic herbs like *ylang-ylang* (*Cananga odorata*, p. 185). Some are well researched, while others are known only within their native region. A number of medicinal plants included have fallen out of favor but remain historically significant. In addition, this index features plants such as eucommia bark (*Eucommia ulmoides*, p. 212) that research shows have the potential for a more prominent medicinal role in the future.

Abies balsamea (Pinaceae)

Balsam Fir

Description Conical evergreen tree growing to 90 ft (27 m). Has aromatic needlelike leaves and purple fir cones.

Habitat & cultivation Native to North America, balsam fir is commercially grown for its timber. The resin is tapped from 60- to 80-year-old trees in spring.

Parts used Oleoresin, leaves.

Constituents Balsam fir leaves contain a liquid oleoresin.

History & folklore Balsam fir resin, often known as Canada balsam, was used for many illnesses by both Indigenous peoples and colonizers. The Penobscot smeared the resin on burns, cuts, and sores, while others applied it to the chest and back for colds and chest problems. The Pillagers used the aromatic needles in their sweat lodges, inhaling smoke from the burning leaves. Dr. Wooster Beech (1794–1868), founder of the Eclectic healing movement, regarded balsam fir as stimulating and laxative when taken internally, and emollient and cooling when used externally. Balsam fir leaves, cones, and resin are commonly added to potpourri.

Medicinal actions & uses Balsam fir is antiseptic and stimulant, and has been used in North America and Europe for congestion, chest infections such as bronchitis, and urinary tract conditions such as cystitis and frequent urination. Externally, balsam fir was rubbed on the chest or applied as a plaster for respiratory infections. It is not used much in herbal medicine today.

Abrus precatorius (Fabaceae)

Jequirity

Description Deciduous climber growing to 12 ft (4 m). Has compound leaves, clusters of pink flowers, and seed pods containing scarlet or (rarely) white seeds.

Habitat & cultivation Jequirity is native to India, and now grows in hedges and among bushes in all tropical regions.

Parts used Root, leaves, seeds.

Constituents Jequirity seeds contain abrin, indole alkaloids, triterpenoid saponins, and anthocyanins. The root and leaves contain glycyrrhizin and traces of abrin. Abrin is extremely toxic.

History & folklore Jequirity seeds have been used since ancient times in India to help weigh precious materials, including the famous Koh-i-noor diamond. The seeds are notorious as a poison.

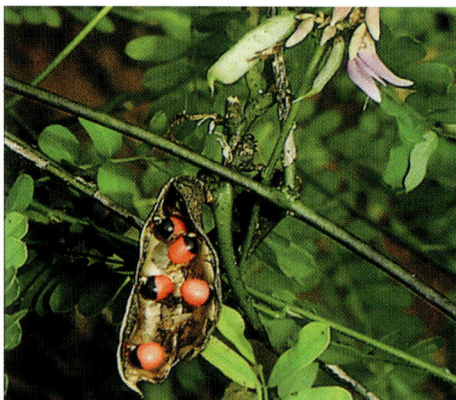

Jequirity seeds were used medicinally in former times, but are also extremely poisonous.

Medicinal actions & uses Jequirity seeds have been used medicinally in the past as a contraceptive, abortifacient (to induce a miscarriage), and as a treatment for chronic conjunctivitis. However, they are so poisonous that even external application can be fatal. In laboratory experiments, extracts of the seeds had a strong antifertility effect on sperm production and fertility. The ground root is traditionally taken to treat worm infestation.

Cautions Never use the seeds. Use the leaves and roots only under professional supervision. Jequirity is subject to legal restrictions in some countries.

Abutilon indicum (Malvaceae)

Kanghi, Indian mallow

Description Upright, woody shrub growing to 5 ft (1.5 m). Has a downy, slightly oily surface, single yellow flowers, and kidney-shaped seeds.

Habitat & cultivation Kanghi grows throughout much of India in addition to Southeast Asia.

Parts used Root, bark, leaves, seeds.

Constituents Kanghi contains mucilage, tannins, and asparagine. Asparagine is diuretic.

Medicinal actions & uses Also known as Indian mallow, kanghi is used in much the same way as marshmallow (*Althaea officinalis*, p. 169), one of the main European demulcent herbs. The root, leaves, and bark of kanghi are mucilaginous and are used to soothe and protect the mucous membranes of the respiratory and urinary systems. A decoction of the root is given for chest conditions such as bronchitis. The mucilaginous effect benefits the skin; an infusion, poultice, or paste made from the powdered root or bark is applied to wounds and used for conditions such as boils and ulcers. A decoction of the root can also be used to good effect as a mouthwash for toothache and sore and infected gums. The seeds are laxative and "useful in killing threadworms, if the rectum of the affected child be exposed to the smoke of the powdered seeds" (*Herbs that Heal*, H. K. Bakhru, 1992). The plant has an antiseptic effect within the urinary tract.

Related species *A. trisulcatum*, native to Central America, is used to treat asthma in children, and is applied as a poultice for treating cancerous sores and ulcers, especially of the mouth and cervix.

Acanthus mollis (Acanthaceae)

Acanthus, Bear's Breeches

Description Perennial growing to 3 ft (1 m). Has a black, branched taproot; white, purple, or blue flowers; and dark green basal leaves up to 3 ft (1 m) in length.

Habitat & cultivation Native to Europe, acanthus is most commonly found as a garden plant. It prefers damp sites and low-lying ground. The leaves are gathered in early summer and the roots in the fall.

Parts used Leaves, roots.

Constituents Acanthus contains large quantities of mucilage and tannin.

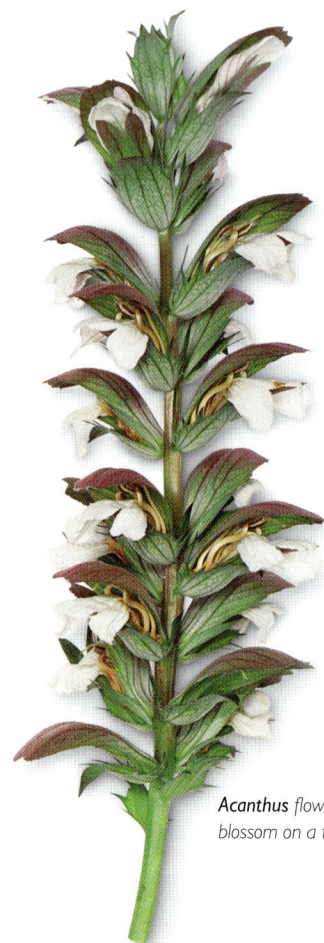

Acanthus flowers blossom on a tall spike.

History & folklore Acanthus was well known in the ancient world. Callimachus, a Greek architect of the 5th century BCE, reputedly created the decorative pattern of foliage at the top of Corinthian columns after being inspired by the perfect symmetry of acanthus leaves. The description of acanthus in *Materia Medica*, written in the 1st century CE by the Greek physician Dioscorides, is one of the most accurate botanical descriptions to survive from the ancient world. Dioscorides recommended the roots in the form of a plaster to treat burns and to wrap around dislocated joints. As an infusion, acanthus was thought to be diuretic. It was also used to relieve gas and spasms and to soothe damaged nerves.

Medicinal actions & uses The herb's appreciable quantities of mucilage and tannin substantiate its traditional use as a treatment for dislocated joints and burns. Its emollient properties make it useful in the treatment of irritated mucous membranes in the digestive and urinary tracts. Acanthus is similar to marshmallow (*Althaea officinalis*, p. 169) in that it can be used externally to ease irritation, and internally to heal and protect.

Achyranthes bidentata (Amaranthaceae)

Chaff flower, Huai niu xi (Chinese)

Description Erect perennial herb growing to 3 ft (1 m). Has slender, rambling branches, elliptical leaves, and greenish-white flowers on terminal spikes.

Habitat & cultivation Chaff flower is found in China at the edge of forests, along streams, and amid bushes. Grown commercially in the eastern provinces, the root is unearthed in winter once the foliage has died back.

Part Used Root.

Constituents *Achyranthes* species contain triterpenoid saponins and sterones.

History & folklore Chaff flower's potent ability to bring on menstruation led the 13th-century Chinese gynecologist Chen Ziming to prohibit its use during pregnancy to avoid causing miscarriage.

Medicinal actions & uses In traditional Chinese medicine, chaff flower is believed to invigorate blood flow. It is used to stimulate menstruation when a period is delayed or scanty. The herb is also prescribed to ease period pain. Chaff flower is used to relieve pain in the lower back, especially where the discomfort is attributable to kidney stones. The herb is also taken as a treatment for canker sores, toothache, bleeding gums, and nosebleeds.

Research Research suggests that chaff flower may lower blood pressure by reducing heart rate and dilating the peripheral arteries. Its constituents are being researched as potential anticancer drugs.

Related species *A. aspera*, found in tropical areas worldwide, is used in Ayurvedic medicine to treat chest conditions and a range of digestive problems.

Caution Do not take chaff flower during pregnancy.

Aconitum napellus (Ranunculaceae)

Aconite, Monkshood

Description Perennial herb growing to 4 ft (1 m). Has dark green lobed leaves with violet or blue delphinium-like flowers on long spikes.

Habitat & cultivation Aconite grows mainly in southern and central Europe. It prefers damp and shady sites, and is cultivated as a garden plant. The root is unearthed in the fall.

Part used Root.

Constituents Aconite contains 0.3–2% terpenoid alkaloids, principally aconitine.

History & folklore *Aconitum* species have traditionally been used as arrow poisons.

Medicinal actions & uses Aconite is poisonous in all but the smallest doses, and is rarely prescribed for internal use. More commonly, it is applied to unbroken skin to relieve pain from bruises or neurological conditions. In Ayurvedic medicine, aconite is used to treat neuralgia, asthma, and heart weakness. Aconite is also used extensively in homeopathy as an analgesic and sedative.

Related species Chinese aconite (*A. carmichaelii*) is used in China for shock and to support the circulatory system in emergencies. Trials in China indicate that it is helpful in congestive heart failure.

Cautions Aconite is highly toxic and is subject to legal restriction in some countries. Use only under professional supervision.

Acorus calamus (Araceae)

Sweet flag, Sweet sedge, calamus, bacc (Hindi)

Description Sweet flag has a long-standing reputation as a tonic and stimulant. An important herb in Ayurvedic medicine, it is also widely used in Europe and the US. The rhizome is a valuable remedy for digestion, and is a tonic for the nervous system. It stimulates the appetite and soothes digestion, relieving gas and calming indigestion and colic. Sweet flag has a strongly aromatic, bitter taste.

Habitat & cultivation Sweet flag, believed to originate from India, now grows in many parts of the world. It prefers wet soil and is found in ditches, beside lakes and rivers, and in marshy places. Propagation is carried out in the fall or early spring by dividing the clumps of rhizomes and replanting them in shallow water. The rhizomes are harvested as needed.

Part used Rhizomes.

Constituents Volatile oil—sesquiterpenes (*A. calamus* var. *americanus* only); asarone (except *A. calamus* var. *americanus*), Saponins, Bitter principle (acorin), Mucilage

History & folklore Sweet flag has been regarded as an aphrodisiac in India and Egypt for at least 2,500 years. In Europe, it was valued as a stimulant, bitter herb for the appetite (if not for the appetites) and as an aid to digestion. In North America, the decoction was used for fevers, stomach cramps, and colic; the rhizome was chewed for toothache, and powdered rhizome was inhaled for congestion. Sweet flag is an important herb in Ayurvedic medicine, and is valued as a "rejuvenator" for the brain and nervous system, and as a remedy for digestive disorders. In Western herbal medicine, the herb is chiefly used for digestive problems such as bloating, gas, colic, and poor digestive function. Sweet flag, particularly *A. calamus* var. *americanus*, which is the most effective antispasmodic, relieves spasm of the intestines. It helps uncomfortable and distended stomachs, and headaches associated with weak digestion. Small amounts are thought to reduce stomach acidity, while larger doses increase deficient acid production—a good example of how different doses of the same herb can produce different results.

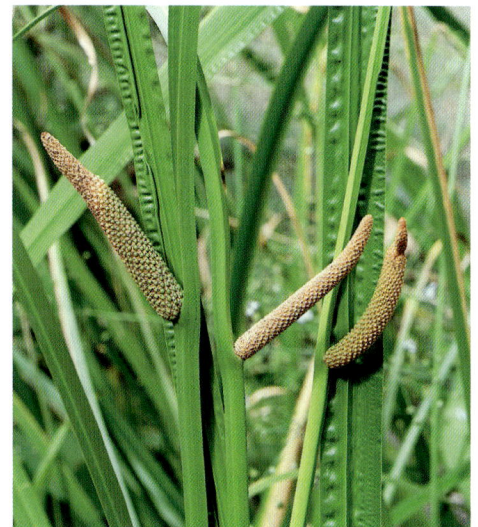

Acorus calamus has been regarded as an aphrodisiac in India and Egypt for at least 2,500 years.

Research Research attention has focused on the constituent beta-asarone in the volatile oil, which has a carcinogenic action when isolated. The American variety of sweet flag (*A. calamus* var. *americanus*), commonly available in Europe, does not contain beta-asarone, and only preparations made from this should be used. In India, sweet flag powder has been taken for thousands of years with no reports of cancer arising from its use. This suggests that use of the whole herb may be safe, but more research is needed.

Related species *A. gramineus* (*shi chang pu*) is a Chinese herb and a close relative that is used medicinally for much the same range of conditions as *A. calamus*.

Adhatoda vasica syn. *Justicia adhatoda* (Acanthaceae)

Malabar nut, Vasaka

Description Evergreen shrub growing to 10 ft (3 m), with lance-shaped leaves, white or purple flowers, and 4-seeded fruit.

Habitat & cultivation Native to tropical India, malabar nut grows in low-lying regions up to the Himalayan foothills.

Parts used Leaves, root, flowers, fruit (nut).

Constituents Malabar nut contains pyrroloquinoline alkaloids and an unidentified volatile oil.

History & folklore The highly bitter-tasting malabar nut is a traditional Ayurvedic remedy for chest problems.

Medicinal actions & uses Due to its expectorant qualities, malabar nut is useful for bronchitis and other chest conditions. An Ayurvedic preparation that includes malabar flowers is used to treat tuberculosis. All parts of the plant are used to expel worms. A poultice of the fresh leaves is applied to wounds and to inflamed joints.

Caution Do not take during pregnancy.

Adiantum capillus-veneris (Polypodiaceae)

Maidenhair fern

Description Fern with delicate fronds growing to 1 ft (30 cm) long.

Habitat & cultivation Native to Europe, Asia, most of the Americas, and Australasia.

Parts used Aerial parts.

Constituents Maidenhair fern contains flavonoids (including rutin and isoquercitin), terpenoids (including adiantone), tannin, proanthocyanidins, and mucilage.

History & folklore Maidenhair fern has been used since ancient times. Pliny the Elder (23–79 CE) states that the herb "is of singular efficacy in expelling and breaking calculi of the bladder."

Medicinal actions & uses Commonly used in Latin America and occasionally in Europe, a decoction or tincture of maidenhair fern is used as an expectorant to treat coughs, bronchitis, sore throat, and chronic nasal congestion. The plant has a longstanding reputation as a remedy for conditions affecting the hair and scalp.

Related species *A. caudatum* has been shown to act as an antispasmodic and could be useful in the treatment of asthma.

Research An Iranian research article (2018) found that maidenhair fern has wide-ranging therapeutic activity, including antidiabetic, anticonvulsant, anti-asthmatic and pain relieving properties.

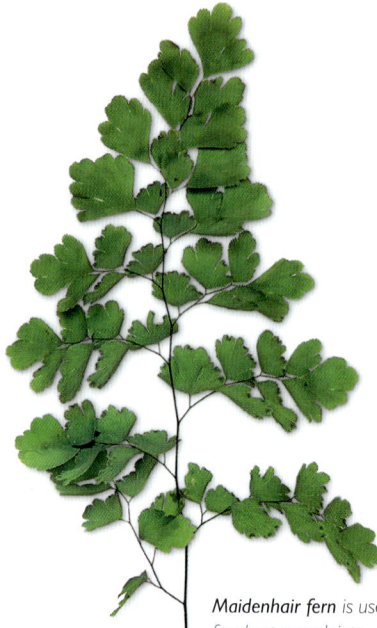

Maidenhair fern is used for chest complaints.

Adonis vernalis (Ranunculaceae)

False hellebore, Yellow pheasant's eye

Description Perennial herb growing to 8 in (20 cm). Has a scaly stem and feathery compound leaves. Stem bears large, bright yellow flowers up to 3 in (8 cm) across.

Habitat & cultivation Originating from the steppes of Russia and from the Black Sea region, this herb is native to much of Europe but not to Britain. It grows in mountain pasture undergrowth. It is rare

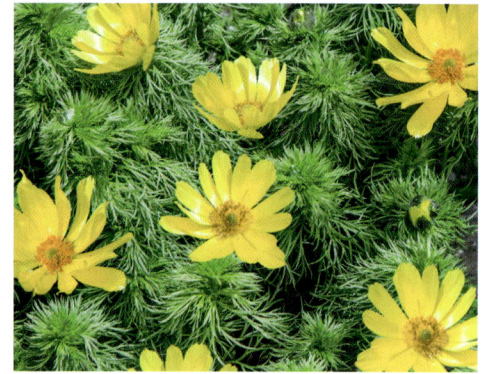

False hellebore's cardiac glycosides help to slow down heart rate.

and legally protected in Western Europe.

Parts used Aerial parts.

Constituents False hellebore contains cardiac glycosides, including adonitoxin.

History & folklore False hellebore's botanical name refers to Adonis, a figure in Greek mythology associated with the seasonal renewal of plant life.

Medicinal actions & uses False hellebore contains cardiac glycosides similar to those found in foxglove (*Digitalis purpurea*, p. 207). These substances improve the heart's efficiency, increasing its output while at the same time slowing its rate. Unlike foxglove, however, false hellebore's effect on the heart is slightly sedative, and it is generally prescribed for patients with hearts that are beating too fast or irregularly. False hellebore is also recommended as a treatment for certain cases of low blood pressure. In common with other plants containing cardiac glycosides, false hellebore is strongly diuretic and can be used to counter water retention, particularly in cases of poor circulatory function. False hellebore is used in homeopathic medicine as a treatment for angina.

Cautions Take only under professional supervision. Gathering wild plants and their medicinal use are subject to legal restrictions in some countries.

Aegle marmelos (Rutaceae)

Bael, Bengal quince

Description Thorny deciduous tree growing to 26 ft (8 m). Has aromatic oval- to lance-shaped leaves, greenish-white flowers, and yellow plum-shaped fruit.

Habitat & cultivation Native to India, bael grows throughout much of Southeast Asia in dry forests. It is also cultivated throughout the region.

Parts used Fruit, leaves, root, twigs.

Constituents Bael contains coumarins, flavonoids, alkaloids, tannins, carotenoids, and volatile oil.

History & folklore The bael tree is sacred to the Hindu deities Lakshmi (the goddess of wealth and good fortune) and Shiva (the god of health), and it is commonly planted near temples. Its medicinal virtues are described in the *Charaka Samhita*, an herbal text written c.400 BCE.

Medicinal actions & uses The astringent half-ripe bael fruit reduces irritation in the digestive tract and is excellent for diarrhea and dysentery. The ripe fruit is demulcent and laxative, with a significant vitamin C content. It eases stomach pain and supports the healthy function of this organ. Bael's astringent leaves are taken to treat peptic ulcers. The tree's most unusual application is for earache. A piece of dried root is dipped in the oil of the neem tree (*Azadirachta indica*, p. 74) and set alight. Oil from the burning end is dripped into the ear. (This is not a recommended practice.)

Self-help use Diarrhea, p. 317.

Agastache rugosa (Lamiaceae)

Korean mint, *Huo xiang* (Chinese)

Description Aromatic perennial or biennial herb growing to 4 ft (1.2 m). Has a square stem, triangular leaves, and purple flowers growing in dense spikes.

Habitat & cultivation Native to China and also found in Japan, Korea, Laos, and Russia, Korean mint grows wild on slopes and roadsides. It is cultivated throughout China and gathered in summer.

Parts used Aerial parts.

Constituents Korean mint contains a volatile oil, including methylchavicol, anethole, anisaldehyde, and limonene.

History & folklore Korean mint was first mentioned in a Chinese medicinal text—Tao Hongjing's revision of the *Divine Husbandman's Classic (Shen'nong Bencaojing)*, which he wrote in about 500 CE.

Medicinal actions & uses The acrid Korean mint is considered a warming herb in Eastern herbal medicine (see pp. 44–47) and is used to treat "dampness" within the digestive system. In Korea, as its name suggests, the leaves are eaten as a condiment to aid digestion. The herb stimulates and warms the digestive tract, relieving symptoms such as abdominal bloating, indigestion, nausea, and vomiting. It is commonly used to relieve vomiting and morning sickness. Korean mint is used to treat the early stages of viral infections that feature symptoms such as stomachache and nausea. A lotion containing

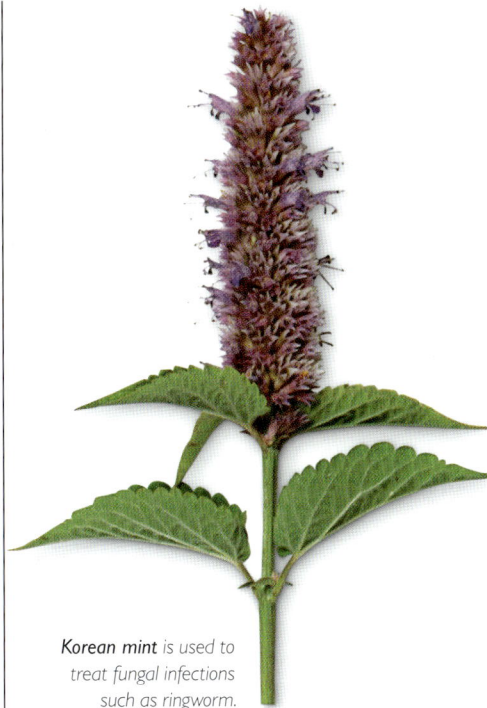

Korean mint is used to treat fungal infections such as ringworm.

Korean mint may be applied to fungal conditions such as ringworm.

Research Laboratory experiments indicate that Korean mint has marked activity against fungal infections.

Related species In southern China, *Pogostemon cablin* is used interchangeably with Korean mint. *P. cablin* is a close relative of the Indian plant *P. patchouli*, from which patchouli oil is produced.

Agave americana (Agavaceae)

Agave, Century plant

Description Succulent perennial with large rosette of 30–60 fleshy, sharply toothed leaves that reach a height of 6½ ft (2 m). After 10 years or more, clusters of yellow flowers, growing to 2¾ in (7 cm) across, bloom on a pole-like stem 26–30 ft (8–9 m) tall.

Habitat & cultivation Agave is native to deserts of Central America. It is now grown as an ornamental plant in tropical and subtropical areas around the world.

Part used Sap.

Constituents Agave sap contains estrogen-like isoflavonoids, alkaloids, coumarins, and vitamins pro-A, B₁, B₂, C, D, and K.

History & folklore Unlike Europeans at the time of the Spanish conquest of the Americas, the Aztec and Maya people were skilled in wound healing. They

used agave sap (often with egg white) to bind powders and gums in pastes or poultices to be applied to wounds. The *Badianus Manuscript* (1552 CE), which was the first herbal text to list the plants of the Americas, describes an Aztec treatment for diarrhea and dysentery, in which agave juice, combined with freshly ground maize (*Zea mays*, p. 158) and extract of bladderwort (*Utricularia* species), is given as an enema, using a syringe made from the bladder of a small animal and a hollow bone or reed. Both tequila and mescal, popular Mexican alcoholic drinks, are distilled from the fermented sap or juice of agaves.

Medicinal actions & uses Demulcent, laxative, and antiseptic, agave sap is a soothing and restorative remedy for many digestive ailments. It is used to treat ulcers and inflammatory conditions affecting the stomach and intestines, protecting these parts from infection and irritation and encouraging healing. Agave has also been employed to treat many other conditions, including constipation, jaundice, liver disease, and tuberculosis.

Related species Agave is a fairly close relative of aloe (*Aloe vera*, p. 64). The two plants have similar medicinal uses. The sisal agave (*A. sisalana*) is cultivated in the subtropical Americas and in Kenya as a source of hecogenin, the substance that is the starting point in the production of corticosteroids (steroid hormones).

Cautions Do not use during pregnancy. Do not exceed the dose as this may cause digestive irritation and eventual liver damage. External use may cause skin irritation.

Agrimonia eupatoria (Rosaceae)

Agrimony

Description Erect, downy, and slightly aromatic perennial growing to 3 ft (1 m). Has paired leaves, green above and silvery-green beneath, and small 5-petaled yellow flowers growing on terminal spikes.

Habitat & cultivation Agrimony is a native European herb commonly found in marshes, wet meadows, and on waste ground. It is harvested when in flower in summer.

Parts used Aerial parts.

Constituents Agrimony contains tannins, coumarins, flavonoids (including luteolin, a volatile oil), and polysaccharides.

History & folklore The species name *Eupatoria* has regal associations. Mithridates Eupator (d.63 BCE), King of Pontus in northern Turkey (Türkiye), was said to have had a profound knowledge of plant lore and antidotes to poisons.

Medicinal actions & uses Agrimony has long been used by herbalists to heal wounds because it staunches bleeding and encourages clot formation. An astringent and mild bitter, it is also a helpful remedy for diarrhea and a gentle tonic for digestion as a whole. Combined with other herbs such as corn silk (*Zea mays*, p. 158), it is a valuable remedy for cystitis and urinary incontinence, and has also been used for kidney stones, sore throats, hoarseness, rheumatism, and osteoarthritis.

Research Ongoing research supports many of the traditional uses of agrimony. The herb has established wound healing, anti-inflammatory and antioxidant activity, as well as indications that it supports healthy liver function and relieves superficial pain.

Related species *Xian he cao* (*A. pilosa*) is used in China for comparable conditions.

Self-help uses Diarrhea, p. 317; Diarrhea in children, p. 328.

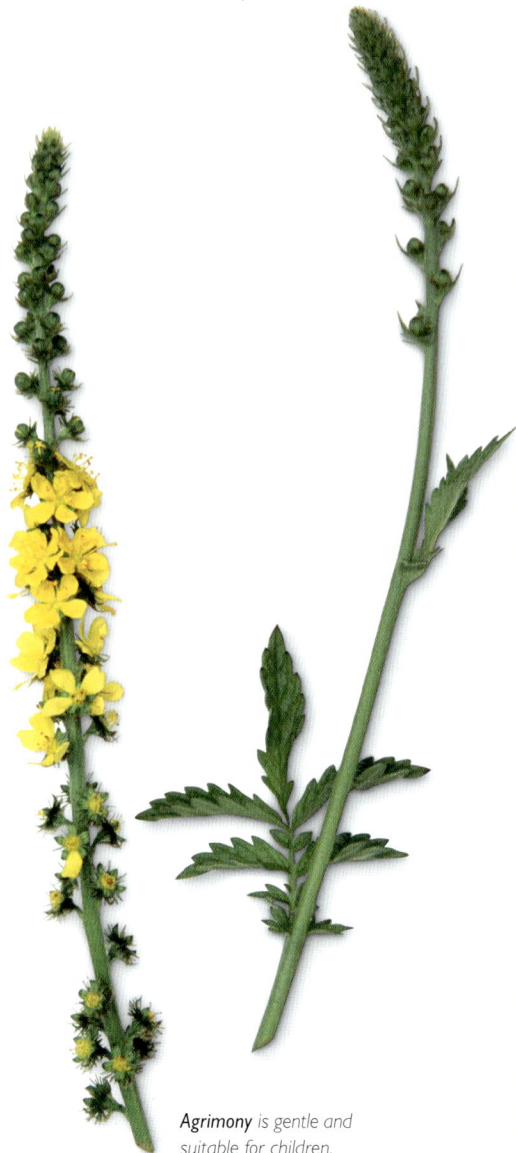

Agrimony is gentle and suitable for children.

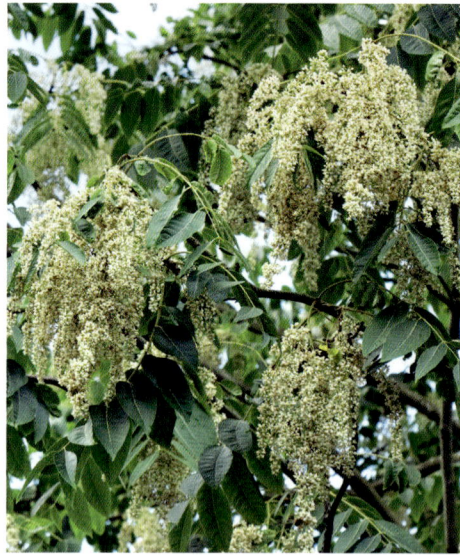

Tree of heaven has an unpleasant, bitter taste.

Ailanthus altissima syn. *A. glandulosa* (Simaroubaceae)

Tree of heaven, *Chun pi*

Description Deciduous tree growing to 65 ft (20 m). Has large leaves with up to 12 lance-shaped leaflets, and small greenish-yellow flowers. It has an unpleasant odor.

Habitat & cultivation Native to China and India, tree of heaven is now naturalized in some parts of Europe, Australia, and North America. It is cultivated as a garden tree. The bark and root bark are harvested in spring.

Parts used Bark, root bark.

Constituents The bark contains quassinoids (such as ailanthone and quassin), alkaloids, flavonols, and tannins. Quassinoids are intensely bitter, antimalarial, and act against cancerous cells.

Medicinal actions & uses In Chinese herbal medicine, tree of heaven is used to treat diarrhea and dysentery, especially if there is blood in the stool. The bark of the tree has been used in Asian and Australian medicine to counter worms, excessive vaginal discharge, gonorrhea, and malaria, and it has also been given for asthma. Tree of heaven has marked antispasmodic properties and acts on the body as a cardiac depressant.

Research Chinese researchers gave tree of heaven to 82 patients with acute dysentery, and cured 81. Abdominal pain generally eased within 2 days. The anticancer properties of quassinoids are being extensively investigated. Laboratory research indicates that the whole plant has a marked antimalarial activity.

Related species *A. malabrica* is used in herbal medicine in Southeast Asia for its tonic properties and to reduce fever.

Caution Use tree of heaven only under professional supervision.

Ajuga reptans (Lamiaceae)

Bugle

Description Low-growing, creeping perennial up to 1 ft (30 cm) in height. Has rooting runners, erect hairy stems, oblong to oval leaves, and purplish-blue flowers.

Habitat & cultivation Native to Europe, North Africa, and parts of Asia, bugle has become naturalized in North America. It prefers damp woods and grassy and mountainous areas, and is usually gathered when in flower in early summer.

Parts used Aerial parts.

Constituents Bugle contains iridoid glycosides, diterpene bitters, phytoecdysone, and caffeic acids.

History & folklore In the European tradition, bugle has long been valued as a wound-healing herb. Nicholas Culpeper praised it in 1652: "The decoction of the leaves and flowers made in wine and taken, dissolveth the congealed blood in those

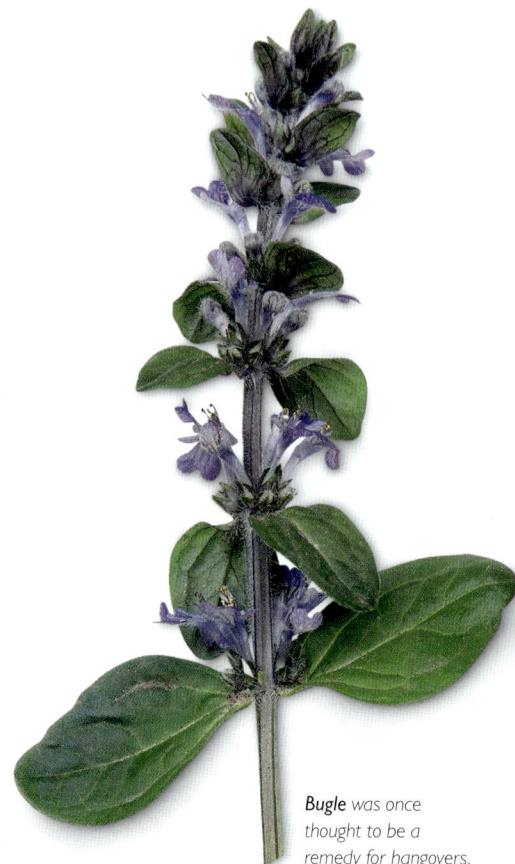

Bugle was once thought to be a remedy for hangovers.

that are bruised inwardly by a fall or otherwise, and is very effectual for any inward wounds, thrusts or stabs into the body or bowels." The herbalist Mrs. Grieve, writing in 1931, reported that it lowers the pulse rate and "equalizes the circulation."

Medicinal actions & uses Bugle is bitter, astringent, and aromatic, but opinion varies as to its value as a medicine. It has mild analgesic properties, and it is still used occasionally as a wound healer. It is also mildly laxative and traditionally has been thought to help cleanse the liver.

Related species Ground pine (*A. chamaepitys*) is used to treat gout and rheumatism. It is believed to have diuretic, menstruation-inducing, and stimulant properties. *A. decumbens* is used in Chinese medicine as an analgesic.

Research A 2019 Romanian laboratory study found that Bugle had potent anti-inflammatory activity, comparable in action to diclofenac, a commonly prescribed anti-inflammatory.

Albizia lebbeck (Fabaceae)

Albizia,
Siris Tree, Pit Shirish

Description Deciduous tree growing to 65 ft (20 m). Has compound leaves, white fragrant flowers, and long, shiny, pale yellow seed pods.

Habitat & cultivation Native to the Indian subcontinent, albizia grows in moist teak-bearing forests. It is also cultivated.

Parts used Stem bark; also flowers and seeds.

Constituents Albizia contains saponins, cardiac glycosides, tannins, and flavonoids.

History & folklore Albizia has been used for several thousand years within Ayurvedic medicine to treat allergies, skin eruptions, glandular disorders, and poisoning.

Medicinal actions & uses Albizia bark has anti-allergenic properties and is used orally (and topically) to relieve problems such as eczema, hives, hay fever, and asthma. The herb helps lower cholesterol and may be useful as part of a broad approach to treating abnormal fat levels in the blood. It is usually taken as a decoction or tincture. In Ayurveda, the bark is given for *pitta* (fire) and *kapha* (water) conditions such as asthma; the flowers for coughs and bronchitis; and the seeds for skin diseases.

Research Laboratory research has shown that the plant helps reduce allergic sensitivity, and one clinical study has indicated potential value in the treatment of asthma. In another clinical study, weeping eczema

improved significantly with a topical application of albizia. Extracts of the plant also have antifungal and antibacterial activity. Saponins from the seed pods have spermicidal and antiprotozoal activity.

Alchemilla mollis, syn. *Alchemilla vulgaris*

Lady's mantle

Description Herbaceous perennial growing to 1 ft (30 cm). Has a basal rosette of lobed leaves and insignificant green flowers ⅛–¼ in (3–5 mm) across in loose clusters.

Habitat & cultivation Lady's mantle is native to Britain and continental Europe. It is gathered in summer.

Parts used Aerial parts, root.

Constituents Lady's mantle contains notable levels of phenolic compounds, such as catechin, quercetin and caffeic acid.

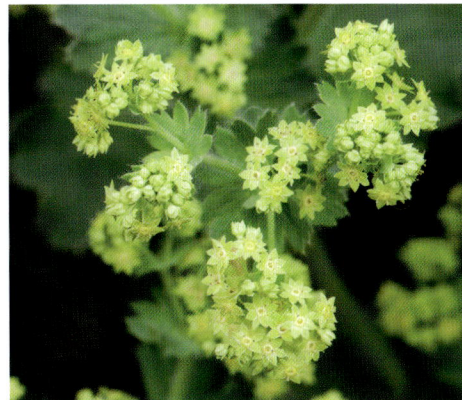

Lady's mantle is chiefly used to reduce heavy menstrual bleeding.

History & folklore Andres de Laguna's translation (1570) of Dioscorides' *Materia Medica* recommends two preparations of lady's mantle—the root, powdered and mixed with red wine, for internal and external wounds, and an infusion of the aerial parts, for "greenstick" fractures and broken bones in babies and young children. When taken regularly for 15 days, lady's mantle was said to reverse sterility due to "slipperiness" of the womb. The plant's astringent effect is sufficiently marked that the infusion was used to contract the female genitalia, and it was "a thousand times sold" to those wishing to appear to be virgins.

Medicinal actions & uses Lady's mantle has always been prized as a wound healer. Its astringency ensures that blood flow is staunched and the first stage of healing soon gets under way. As the name

implies, it is a valuable herb for women's complaints and is thought to have a progesterogenic action. It is commonly taken to reduce heavy menstrual bleeding, to relieve menstrual cramps, and to aid menstrual regularity. Lady's mantle is also prescribed for fibroids and endometriosis. It has been used to facilitate childbirth, and is thought to act as a liver decongestant. Its astringent properties make it a useful herb for the treatment of diarrhea and gastroenteritis.

Research Recent research papers have noted the potent antioxidant and anti-inflammatory activity of lady's mantle. In laboratory studies, extracts have been shown to inhibit cholinesterase, giving the herb "a potential use in prevention of neurodegenerative illnesses".

Caution Do not use lady's mantle when pregnant.

Aletris farinosa (Liliaceae)

Star grass,
True unicorn root, Colic root

Description Perennial growing to 3 ft (1 m). Has a flowering stem; smooth, lance-shaped leaves; and white, bell-shaped flowers that appear to be covered with frost.

Habitat & cultivation Native to eastern North America, star grass grows in swamps and wet sandy woodland, especially near the seashore. It is harvested commercially in Virginia, Tennessee, and North Carolina, but is threatened and should not otherwise be picked.

Parts used Rhizome, leaves.

Constituents Star grass contains steroidal saponins based on diosgenin, as well as a bitter principle, volatile oil, and a resin.

History & folklore The Catawba peoples used a cold-water infusion of star grass leaves for stomachache. Star grass was also advocated for snake bite.

Medicinal actions & uses It is difficult to gain a clear picture of star grass's medicinal value. Due to its estrogenic action, it is employed chiefly for gynecological problems, particularly at menopause. It is also given for period pain and irregular periods. Some authorities hold that it prevents threatened miscarriage. Star grass is also a good digestive herb, proving beneficial in treating loss of appetite, indigestion, flatulence, and bloating.

Cautions Use only under professional supervision. The dried, and especially the fresh, rhizome can be toxic when taken in overdose, causing colic, diarrhea, and vomiting.

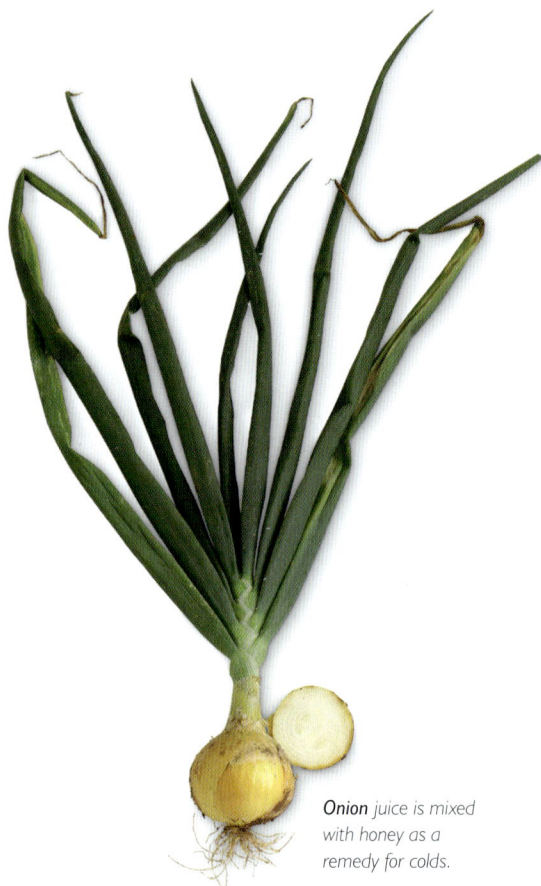

Onion juice is mixed with honey as a remedy for colds.

Allium cepa (Liliaceae)

Onion

Description Bulbous perennial growing to 3 ft (1 m). Has hollow stems and leaves, and white or purple flowers.

Habitat & cultivation Native to the northern hemisphere, onion has been cultivated in the Middle East for millennia. It is now grown worldwide as a vegetable.

Part Used Bulb.

Constituents Onion contains a volatile oil with sulfur-containing compounds such as allicin (an antibiotic) and alliin, flavonoids, phenolic acids, and sterols.

History & folklore Authorities throughout the ancient world recommended onion for a variety of health problems. Bunches were hung on doors to ward off the plague in medieval Europe. Wild onion (*A. sibiricum*) was also used extensively by Indigenous North Americans to treat stings and help relieve colds.

Medicinal actions & uses Onion boasts a long list of medicinal actions—diuretic, antibiotic, anti-inflammatory, analgesic, expectorant, and antirheumatic. It is also beneficial to the circulation. Onions are taken the world over for colds, flu, and coughs, much like garlic (*A. sativum*, p. 63). Onion offsets tendencies to angina, arteriosclerosis, and heart attack. It is also useful in preventing oral infection and tooth decay. The warmed juice can be dropped into the ear for earache, and baked onion is used as a poultice to drain pus from sores. Onion has a longstanding reputation as an aphrodisiac, and it is also used cosmetically to stimulate hair growth.

Related species In Chinese herbal medicine, the scallion (*A. fistulosum*) is given to encourage sweating, to unblock the nose, and to relieve bloating. It is also used to help drain boils and abscesses.

Self-help use Mild fever, p. 321.

Allium ursinum (Liliaceae)

Ramsons

Description Bulbous perennial smelling strongly of garlic, growing to 11 in (28 cm). Has a triangular stem and broad elliptical leaves. Clusters of white, starlike flowers grow from a common stem.

Habitat & cultivation Wild garlic is native to Europe and Asia. It carpets shady sites in damp woods and by streams. The plants are gathered in early summer.

Parts used Bulb, aerial parts.

Constituents Wild garlic contains steroidal glucosides, lecitins, fatty acids, amino acids and an essential oil.

History & folklore Wild garlic (and many other onion-like plants) have been highly regarded as preventative medicines, as an old English rhyme attests: "Eat leeks in Lide and ramsons in May/And all the year after physicians may play!" More prosaically, Gerard (1597) wrote that the leaves "maye very well be eaten in April and Maie with butter [by those of] a strong constitution."

Medicinal actions & uses Used mainly as a folk remedy and as a food, wild garlic is similar to garlic (*A. sativum*, p. 63) but weaker in action. It lowers high blood pressure and helps to prevent arteriosclerosis. As wild garlic eases stomach pain and is tonic to the digestion, it has been used for diarrhea, colic, gas, indigestion, and loss of appetite. The whole herb is used in an infusion against threadworms, either ingested or given as an enema. Wild garlic is also thought to be beneficial for asthma, bronchitis, and emphysema. The juice is used as an aid to weight loss.

Alnus glutinosa syn. *A. rotundifolia* (Betulaceae)

Alder

Description Small tree with fissured bark, growing to 65 ft (20 m). Has notched oval leaves and male and female catkins.

Habitat & cultivation Alder is native to Europe, Asia, and North Africa. It thrives in damp places and along riverbanks. The bark and leaves are gathered in spring.

Parts used Bark, leaves.

Constituents Alder contains diarylheptanoids, polyphenols, flavonoids, terpenoids, and steroidal compounds. It is also reported to contain shikimic acid, a potent antiviral.

History & folklore Water-resistant, alder was used in the construction of Venice. Wooster Beech (1794–1868), founder of the Eclectic healing movement, used a decoction of the bark to "purify the blood."

Medicinal actions & uses Alder is most often used as a mouthwash and gargle for tooth, gum, and throat problems. The drying action of a decoction of the bark helps to contract the mucous membranes and reduce inflammation. A decoction may also be used to staunch internal or external bleeding, and to heal wounds. It is also used as a wash for scabies. In Spain, alder leaves are smoothed and placed on the soles of the feet to relieve aching. Leaves are used to help reduce breast engorgement in nursing mothers.

Aloysia citriodora syn. *Lippia citriodora*

Lemon verbena

Description Deciduous shrub growing to 6½ ft (2 m). Has strongly scented lance-shaped leaves and clusters of tubular, pale green to mauve flowers.

Habitat & cultivation Lemon verbena is native to South America. It is cultivated in temperate climates as an aromatic, ornamental plant and for its leaves, which are used to make herbal tea. The leaves are gathered in late summer.

Parts used Leaves.

Constituents Lemon verbena contains a volatile oil (mainly consisting of citral, cineole, limonene, and geraniol), mucilage, tannins, and flavonoids.

History & folklore Lemon verbena was introduced to Europe in 1784. In Spain, France, and elsewhere in Europe, the infusion is a popular drink.

Medicinal actions & uses An undervalued medicinal herb, lemon verbena shares qualities with lemon balm (*Melissa officinalis*, p. 117). Both herbs contain a strong lemon-scented volatile oil that has calming and digestive properties. Lemon verbena has a gentle sedative action and a reputation for soothing abdominal discomfort. Its tonic effect on the nervous system is less pronounced than that of lemon balm, but it nonetheless helps lift the spirits and counter depression.

Research A 2018 placebo-controlled clinical trial found that a lemon verbena extract improved the rate of recovery after intensive exercise. The researchers noted that those in "the lemon verbena group benefited from less muscle damage as well as faster and full recovery. Lemon verbena extract receiving participants had significantly less exercise-related loss of muscle strength."

Related species Yerba dulce (*L. dulcis*), native to Mexico, is used therapeutically as a demulcent and expectorant remedy. In Mexico, many other *Lippia* species are used for their antispasmodic, period-inducing, and stomach-soothing properties. *L. adoensis* is drunk as a tea in West Africa. See also lippia (*Lippia alba, preceding entry*).

Self-help use Gas & bloating, p. 316.

Alpinia officinarum (Zingiberaceae)

Galangal (Hindi), Gao liang jiang (Chinese)

Description Like other members of the ginger family, galangal is warming and comforting to the digestion. It has a pleasantly aromatic and mildly spicy taste, and is suitable for all conditions where the central areas of the body need greater warmth. It was introduced into Europe in about the 9th century. The German mystic Hildegard of Bingen regarded it literally as the "spice of life," given by God to ward off ill-health.

Habitat & cultivation Native to grassland areas of southern China, and Southeast Asia in general, *galangal* is now cultivated as a spice and as a medicine throughout much of tropical Asia. It is propagated by dividing and replanting the rhizomes in spring, and it requires well-drained soil and a shady position. The rhizomes are harvested from 4- to 6-year-old plants at the end of the growing season and may be used fresh or dried.

Part used Rhizomes.

Constituents Volatile oil (about 1%) containing alpha-pinene, cineole, linalool, Sesquiterpene lactones (galangol, galangin), diterpenes, flavonoids.

History & folklore In traditional Chinese herbal medicine, *galangal* is a warming herb used for abdominal pain, vomiting, and hiccups, as well as for diarrhea due to internal cold. When used for hiccups, it is combined with codonopsis (*Codonopsis pilosula*, p.

83) and *fu ling* (*Poria cocos*). In India and southwestern Asia, *galangal* is considered stomachic, anti-inflammatory, expectorant, and a nervine tonic. It is used in the treatment of hiccups, dyspepsia, stomach pain, rheumatoid arthritis, and intermittent fever. *Galangal* was introduced into Europe by Arabian physicians over 1,000 years ago. It is mainly used in the West for wind, indigestion, vomiting, and stomach pain. An infusion can be used to alleviate mouth ulcers and sore gums. *Galangal* has long been recommended as a treatment for seasickness, which is not surprising given the well-established ability of its relative, ginger (*Zingiber officinale*, p. 155) to relieve motion sickness. It can be used with other antifungal herbs as part of a regime to treat intestinal candidiasis. At a moderate dosage, *galangal* is a warming and gently stimulating herb for a weakened digestive system, but at a higher dosage it can be an irritant.

Research Research indicates that *galangal* has antibacterial activity, notably against *Staphylococcus aureus*, responsible for many ear, nose, and throat infections. *Galangal* has shown pronounced activity against fungi in laboratory research, especially against *Candida albicans*. A 2001 clinical trial found that a concentrated extract of ginger (*Zingiber officinalis*, p. 155) and *galangal* was effective in relieving osteoarthritis symptoms in the knee.

Self-help use Nausea & motion sickness, p. 306.

Alstonia spp. (Apocynaceae)

Fever bark

Description Evergreen trees growing to 49 ft (15 m). Have glossy oblong leaves and creamy-white, star-shaped flowers.

Habitat & cultivation *A. constricta* is native to Australia, and *A. scholaris* to Australia and Southeast Asia. Both are now found in tropical regions around the world.

Parts used Stem bark, root bark.

Constituents The bark of both species contains indole alkaloids. *A. constricta* contains reserpine, a powerful hypotensive.

Medicinal actions & uses Fever bark has been taken to treat malarial fever (and has been called Australian quinine), but its efficacy against malaria remains unclear. The bark is antispasmodic and lowers blood pressure, and is now used mainly to reduce high blood pressure. Strongly bitter, the bark is also used to treat gastrointestinal disorders, jaundice, and diarrhea.

Cautions Take only under professional supervision. Fever bark is toxic in large doses. The herb is subject to legal restrictions in some countries.

Althaea officinalis (Malvaceae)

Marshmallow

Description Downy perennial growing to 7 ft (2.2 m). Has thick white roots, heart-shaped leaves, and pink flowers.

Habitat & cultivation Native to Europe, marshmallow is naturalized in the Americas. It prefers marshy fields and tidal zones and is cultivated for medicinal use. The aerial parts are gathered in summer as the plant begins to flower and the root is unearthed in the fall.

Parts used Root, leaves, flowers.

Constituents Marshmallow root contains about 37% starch, 11% mucilage, 11% pectin, flavonoids, phenolic acids, sucrose, and asparagine.

History & folklore The philosopher Theophrastus (c. 372–286 BCE) reported that marshmallow root was taken in sweet wine for coughs. Marshmallow was once a key ingredient in the confections of the same name.

Medicinal actions & uses Useful whenever a soothing effect is needed, marshmallow protects and soothes the mucous membranes. The root counters excess stomach acid, peptic ulceration, and gastritis. Marshmallow is also mildly laxative and beneficial for

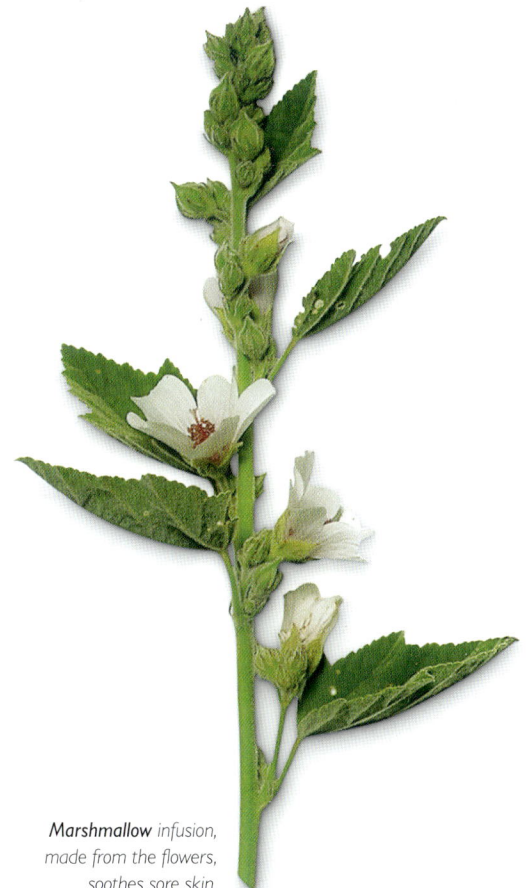

Marshmallow infusion, made from the flowers, soothes sore skin.

many intestinal problems, including regional ileitis, colitis, diverticulitis, and irritable bowel syndrome. The leaves treat cystitis and frequent urination. Marshmallow's demulcent qualities bring relief to dry coughs, bronchial asthma, chronic bronchitis, and pleurisy. The flowers are applied to help soothe inflamed skin. The root is used in an ointment for boils and abscesses, and in a mouthwash for inflammation. The peeled root may be given as a teether to teething babies.

Other Species Hollyhock (*A. rosea*) and common mallow (*Malva sylvestris*, p. 238) are used in a similar fashion.

Self-help uses Allergic rhinitis with mucus, p. 310; Earache due to chronic mucus, p. 322; Urinary infections, p. 324.

Amaranthus hypochondriacus
(Amaranthaceae)

Amaranth

Description Sturdy, upright annual growing to about 3 ft (1 m). Has deeply veined, lance-shaped, purple-green leaves that grow to 6 in (15 cm) and tufts of small, deep crimson flowers on long spikes.
Habitat & cultivation Native to India, amaranth grows wild in many countries, including the US. A common garden plant, it is harvested when in flower in late summer and early fall.

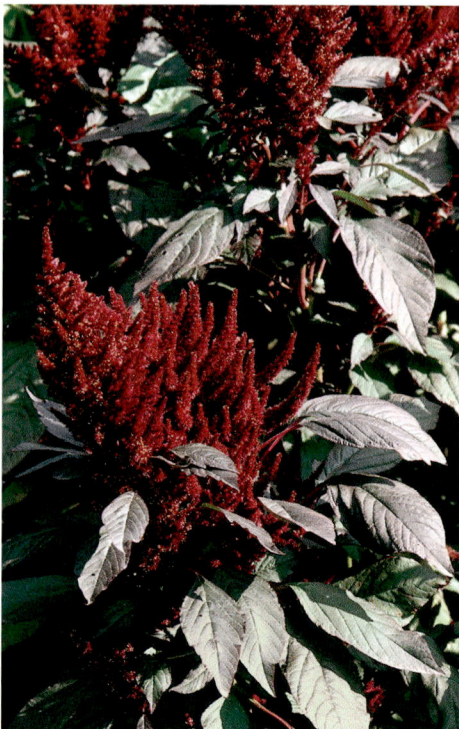

Amaranth's long-lasting flowers gave rise to its name, meaning "unwithering" in Greek.

Parts used Aerial parts.
Constituents Amaranth contains abundant protein, carbohydrates, and dietary fiber, as well as minerals such as magnesium and calcium. It also contains polyphenols, flavonoids including anthocyanins, and carotenoids.
History & folklore Amaranth comes from the Greek word meaning "unwithering." The amaranth was sacred to the goddess Artemis, worshipped at Ephesus, and was thought to have special healing powers. As a symbol of immortality, it was used to decorate tombs and images of the gods.
Medicinal actions & uses Amaranth is an astringent herb that is used primarily to reduce blood loss and to treat diarrhea. A decoction of amaranth is taken as a remedy in cases of heavy menstrual bleeding, excessive vaginal discharge, diarrhea, and dysentery. It is also used as a gargle to soothe inflammation of the pharynx and to hasten the healing of canker sores.
Related species Quinoa (*Chenopodium quinoa*) see p. 192, is another nutritious seed food and a close relative of Amaranth. The seeds of *A. grandiflorus* are used as a foodstuff by Australian Aboriginal people.

Ammi majus (Apiaceae)

Bishop's weed

Description Erect annual herb growing to 32 in (80 cm), with tangled leaflets and umbels of small white flowers.
Habitat & cultivation Bishop's weed is native to the Mediterranean region and as far east as Iran. It is cultivated for its seeds, which are harvested in late summer.
Parts used Seeds.
Constituents The seeds contain furanocoumarins (including bergapten), flavonoids, and tannins.
History & folklore Bishop's weed has been grown as a medicinal plant since the Middle Ages, but has been less often used than visnaga (*A. visnaga*, p. 65).
Medicinal actions & uses Bishop's weed produces strongly aromatic seeds. In an infusion or as a tincture, they calm the digestive system. They are also diuretic, and, like visnaga, have been used to treat asthma and angina. Bishop's weed reputedly helps treat patchy skin pigmentation in vitiligo. It has also been used for psoriasis.
Cautions Bishop's weed increases sensitivity to sunlight and can provoke sunburn and sunlight-related allergic reactions. Side effects can include nausea, vomiting, and headaches. It is subject to legal restrictions in some countries.

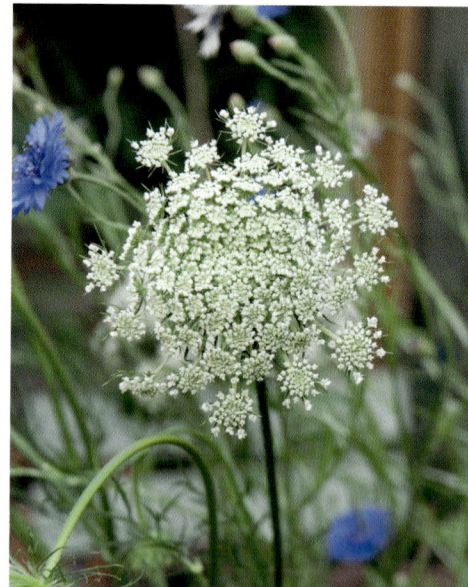

Bishop's weed, like most members of the carrot family, has highly aromatic seeds.

Anacardium occidentale (Anacardiaceae)

Cashew

Description Evergreen tree growing to a height of 49 ft (15 m). Has large oval leaves and pink-streaked yellow flowers on long spikes. Its greenish-gray "fruit" or "apple" is in fact a thickened stem. The true fruit hangs just below this stem and contains the nut, which is encased in red or yellow flesh.
Habitat & cultivation This tree is native to tropical American forests and grasslands. It is now cultivated for its highly prized nuts throughout the tropics, especially in India and eastern Africa.
Parts used Nuts, leaves, bark, root, gum.
Constituents The gum contains anacardic acid, which is bactericidal and fungicidal, and kills worms and protozoa.
History & folklore The "apple" is made into jams, and, in Brazil, into a liquor called *cajuado*. The gum exuded by the stem wards off ants and other insects.
Medicinal actions & uses Though many parts of the plant are used medicinally, cashew nut is chiefly a food—after removal of its toxic lining. The nut is highly nutritious, containing 45% fat and 20% protein. The leaves are used in Indian and African herbal medicine for toothache and gum problems, and in West Africa for malaria. The bark is used in Ayurvedic medicine to detoxify snake bite, while in Brazil it is used to treat rheumatic disease, hemorrhoids and diarrhea. The roots are purgative. The gum is applied externally for skin conditions such as corns and fungal infection. The oil between

the outer and inner shells of the nut is caustic and causes an inflammatory reaction even in small doses. In folk medicine in the tropics, the oil is used very sparingly to eliminate warts, corns, ringworm, and ulcers.

Research Research at the University of Berkeley (California) has shown anacardic acids to have significant antibacterial activity against *Helicobacter pylori*, the bacterium thought to be the main cause of stomach ulcers.

Caution The shell oil and its vapor are highly irritant—do not use in any form.

Anacyclus pyrethrum (Asteraceae)

Pellitory

Description Perennial herb growing to 1 ft (30 cm). Has smooth alternate leaves and large white flowers with yellow centers.

Habitat & cultivation Pellitory is native to the Mediterranean region as far east as the Middle East. It is cultivated in Algeria, and the root is unearthed in the fall.

Parts used Root, essential oil.

Constituents Pellitory contains anacycline, inulin, and volatile oil.

History & folklore The herbalist Nicholas Culpeper wrote in 1652 that pellitory "purgeth the brain of phlegmatic humours … easing pains in the head and teeth." It has been listed in the *British Pharmacopoeia* and was used in the form of lozenges to relieve dryness of the mouth. It was also taken to help ease neuralgia and paralysis of the tongue or lips.

Medicinal Actions & Uses Pellitory root is taken as a decoction or chewed to relieve toothache and increase saliva production. The decoction may also be used as a gargle to soothe sore throats. In Ayurvedic medicine, pellitory root is considered tonic and is used to treat paralysis and epilepsy. Diluted pellitory essential oil is used in mouthwashes and to treat toothache.

Caution Do not take the oil internally except under professional supervision.

Anagallis arvensis (Primulaceae)

Scarlet pimpernel

Description Creeping annual growing to 2 in (5 cm) with oval- to lance-shaped leaves and salmon-red flowers on long stems.

Habitat & cultivation Scarlet pimpernel is found in Europe and in temperate regions generally. It prefers open areas and untended sandy

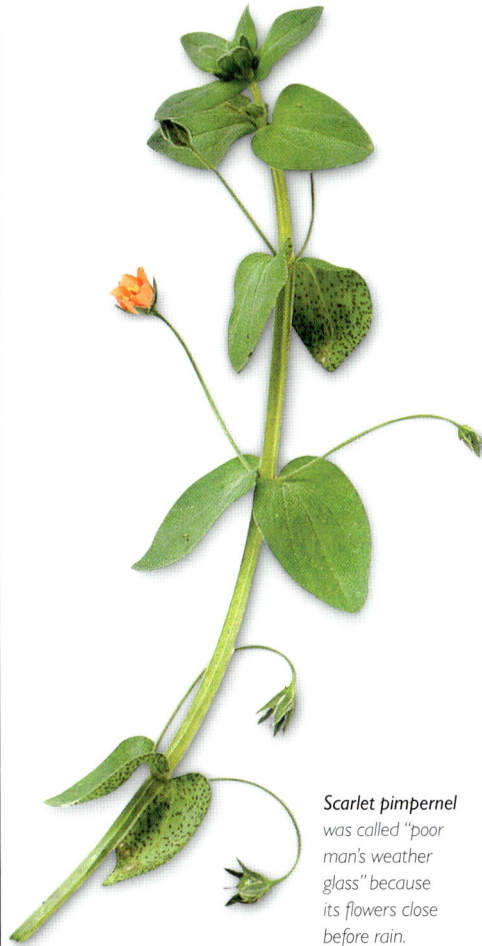

Scarlet pimpernel was called "poor man's weather glass" because its flowers close before rain.

ground, and is gathered in summer toward the end of its flowering period.

Parts used Aerial parts.

Constituents The herb contains saponins (including anagalline), tannins, and cucurbitacins. The latter are cytotoxic (damaging to cells).

History & folklore Classical Greek writers believed scarlet pimpernel helped melancholy. In her *Modern Herbal* (1931), Mrs. Grieve quotes an old saying: "No heart can think, no tongue can tell/The virtues of the pimpernel." It has been employed in European folk medicine as a treatment for gallstones, liver cirrhosis, lung problems, kidney stones, urinary infections, gout, and rheumatism. This pattern of use suggests a detoxifying action for the plant.

Medicinal actions & uses Little used by medical herbalists today, scarlet pimpernel has diuretic, sweat-inducing, and expectorant properties. As an expectorant, it was used to stimulate the coughing up of mucus and help recovery from colds and flu. It has been used to treat epilepsy and mental problems for 2,000 years, but there is little evidence to support its efficacy.

Caution Scarlet pimpernel is not recommended for medicinal use for more than 2–3 weeks.

Ananas comosus (Bromeliaceae)

Pineapple

Description Herbaceous perennial growing to 3 ft (1 m). Has a short, sturdy stem; spiny, lance-shaped leaves; and succulent reddish-yellow fruit.

Habitat & cultivation Pineapple is native to South America. It is cultivated throughout the tropics for its fruit and, to a lesser extent, its leaf fiber.

Parts used Fruit, leaves.

Constituents Pineapple fruit contains bromelain, a protein-splitting enzyme that aids digestion. It has significant levels of vitamins A and C.

Medicinal actions & uses The sour, unripe fruit improves digestion, increases appetite, and relieves dyspepsia. In Indian herbal medicine, it is thought to act as a uterine tonic. The ripe fruit cools and soothes, and is used to settle gas and reduce excessive gastric acid. Its significant fiber content makes it useful in relieving constipation. The juice of the ripe fruit is both a digestive tonic and a diuretic. The leaves are considered to be useful in encouraging the onset of menstrual periods and easing painful ones.

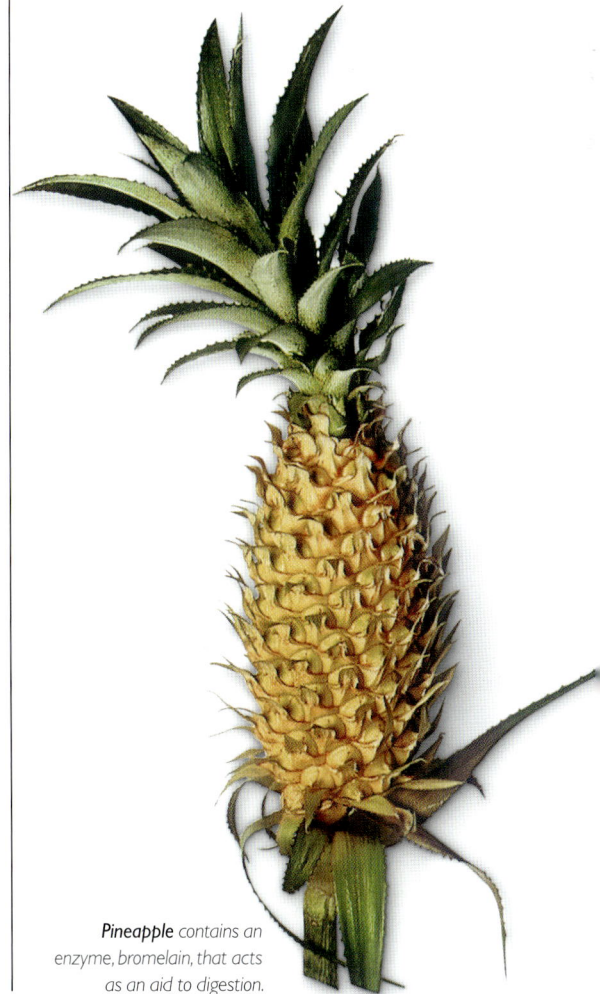

Pineapple contains an enzyme, bromelain, that acts as an aid to digestion.

Anemarrhena asphodeloides (Liliaceae)

Zhi mu

Description Perennial herb with a thick rhizome, thin leaves up to 28 in (70 cm) long, and clusters of small white or light purple flowers.

Habitat & cultivation Native to northern China, Korea, and Mongolia, *zhi mu* grows wild on exposed slopes and hills. It is cultivated in the northern and northeastern China.

Part used Rhizome.

Constituents Contains steroidal saponins, lignans, phenolic compounds, and xanthones.

History & folklore *Zhi mu* is first mentioned in the 1st-century CE herbal, the *Divine Husbandman's Classic (Shen'nong Bencaojing)*.

Medicinal actions & uses *Zhi mu* has a bitter taste and a "cold" temperament and is used in Chinese herbal medicine for "excess heat"—fever, night sweats, and coughs. It has been shown to have significant antibacterial activity and is commonly used to treat sores, mouth ulcers, and coughs, as well as in the treatment of diabetes.

Anemone pulsatilla syn. *Pulsatilla vulgaris* (Ranunculaceae)

Pulsatilla

Description Hairy perennial growing to 6 in (15 cm). Has feathery leaves, and large, purple-blue, bell-shaped flowers, with bright yellow anthers.

Habitat & cultivation Native to Europe, this herb thrives in dry grassland in central and northern parts of the continent, preferring chalky soil. The aerial parts are harvested when it flowers in spring.

Parts used Dried aerial parts.

Constituents Pulsatilla contains the lactone protoanemonin (which on drying forms anemonin), triterpenoid saponins, tannins, and volatile oil.

History & folklore In Greek mythology, the goddess Flora was jealous of her husband's attentions to the nymph Anemone and so transformed her into a flower, at the mercy of the North Wind. Anemone literally means "daughter of the wind" in Greek. The alternate name "pasqueflower" derives from the French name for Easter, when the plant is often in flower.

Medicinal actions & uses Pulsatilla is less commonly used now in herbal medicine than in the past, though it is still considered a valuable remedy for cramping pain, menstrual problems, and emotional distress. It is considered a specific treatment for spasmodic pain of the reproductive system, both male and female, and is given quite frequently for premenstrual syndrome and period pain, especially when these are accompanied by nervous exhaustion. In France, it has traditionally been used for treating coughs and as a sedative for sleep difficulties. Pulsatilla is also used to treat eye problems such as cataracts. The fresh plant is not used because it is strongly irritant. Pulsatilla is one of the most commonly used of all homeopathic remedies.

Related species The meadow anemone (*A. pratensis*) is used interchangeably with pasqueflower; wood anemone (*A. nemorosa*) is now rarely used in herbal medicine.

Cautions Take only under professional supervision. Do not take during pregnancy. Do not take the fresh plant, which is toxic.

Anethum graveolens syn. *Peucedanum graveolens* (Apiaceae)

Dill

Description Aromatic annual that grows to a height of 30 in (75 cm). Has an erect hollow stem, feathery leaves, and numerous yellow flowers in umbels. Fruit is very lightweight and pungent.

Habitat & cultivation Dill is native to southern Europe and central and southern Asia, growing wild on waste ground. It is also widely cultivated, notably in England, Germany, and North America. The leaves are picked as a culinary herb. The seeds are harvested in late summer.

Parts used Seeds, essential oil, leaves.

Constituents Dill seeds contain up to 5% volatile oil (about half of which is alpha-phellandrene), flavonoids, coumarins, xanthones, and triterpenes.

History & folklore An ancient Egyptian remedy in the Ebers papyrus (c.1500 BCE) recommends dill as one of the ingredients in a pain-killing mixture. The ancient Greeks are believed to have covered their eyes with fronds of the herb to induce sleep. Dill was commonly used as a charm against witchcraft in the Middle Ages, when it was burned to clear thunderclouds. Its name comes from the Norse *dylla*—meaning "to soothe."

Medicinal actions & uses Dill has always been considered a remedy for the stomach, relieving gas and calming digestion. Dill's essential oil relieves intestinal spasms and cramps and helps to settle colic, hence it is often used in gripe water mixtures. Chewing the seeds improves bad breath. Dill makes a useful addition to cough, cold, and flu remedies, and is a mild diuretic. Like caraway (*Carum carvi*, p. 187), it can be used with antispasmodics, such as cramp bark (*Viburnum opulus*, p. 154), to relieve period pain. Dill increases milk production, and when taken regularly

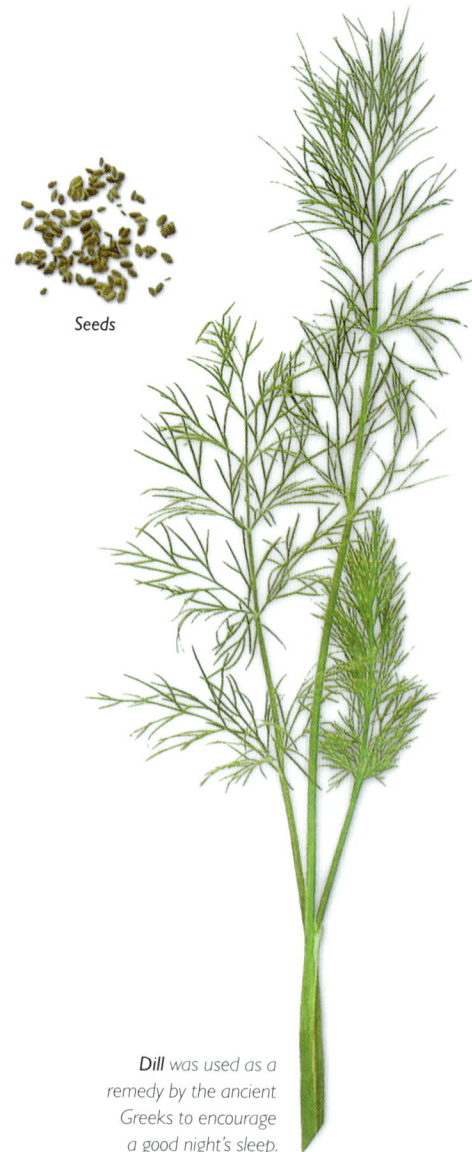

Seeds

Dill was used as a remedy by the ancient Greeks to encourage a good night's sleep.

by nursing mothers, helps to prevent colic in their babies.

Caution Take the essential oil internally only under professional supervision.

Angelica archangelica (Apiaceae)

Angelica

Description Aromatic biennial herb growing to 6½ ft (2 m). Has ridged upright hollow stems, large bright green leaves, and greenish-white flowers in umbels.

Habitat & cultivation Angelica grows in temperate regions in western Europe, Siberia, and the Himalayas. It prefers damp sites and is often found near running water. Leaves and stems are harvested in early summer, seeds as they ripen in late summer, and roots in late fall after one year's growth.

Parts used Root, leaves, stems, seeds.

Constituents Angelica root contains a volatile oil (consisting mainly of beta-phellandrene), lactones, and coumarins. An extract of the root has been shown to be anti-inflammatory.

History & folklore The *British Flora Medica* (1877) reports that "the Laplanders considered this plant as one of the most important productions of the soil …They are subject to a severe kind of colic, against which the root of angelica is one of their chief remedies." The stems are candied for culinary use.

Medicinal actions & uses Angelica is a warming and tonic remedy, having a role to play in a wide range of illnesses. All parts of the plant will help relieve indigestion, gas, and colic. Angelica can also be useful in cases of poor circulation, as it improves blood flow to the peripheral parts of the body. It is considered a specific treatment for Buerger's disease, a condition that narrows the arteries of the hands and feet. By improving blood flow and stimulating the coughing up of phlegm, angelica's warm, tonic properties bring relief from bronchitis and debilitating conditions affecting the chest. For respiratory conditions, the roots are most commonly used, but the stems and seeds may be employed as well. A proprietary extract of Angelica root is used to treat urinary frequency, especially at night.

Caution Do not take as a medicine during pregnancy. Do not confuse with Chinese Angelica.

Self-help use Stomach spasm, p. 315.

Angelica dahurica (Apiaceae)

Bai zhi

Description Aromatic perennial growing to 8 ft (2.5 m). Has a hollow stem, large 3-branched leaves, and umbels bearing many white flower heads.

Habitat & cultivation Grows wild in thickets in China, Japan, Korea, and Russia. Cultivated mainly in central and eastern regions of China.

Part used Root.

Constituents *Bai zhi* contains a volatile oil and the coumarins imperatorin, marmesin, and phellopterin.

History & folklore *Bai zhi* is first mentioned in Chinese herbal medicine in the *Divine Husbandman's Classic* (*Shen'nong Bencaojing*) of the 1st century CE. The famous military physician Zhang Congzheng (1150–1228) classified *bai zhi* as a sweat-inducing herb able to counter harmful external influences on the skin, such as cold, heat, dampness, and dryness.

Medicinal actions & uses The pungent, bitter *bai zhi* is used for headaches and aching eyes, nasal congestion, and toothache. Like its cousins angelica (*A. archangelica, see preceding entry*) and dong quai (*A. sinensis*, p. 67), it is warming and tonic. It is still

given for problems attributed to "damp and cold" conditions, such as sores, boils, and ulcers affecting the skin. *Bai zhi* also appears to be valuable in treating the facial pain of trigeminal neuralgia.

Caution Do not take during pregnancy.

Annona squamosa (Annonaceae)

Sugar apple

Description Tree growing to 33 ft (10 m). Has oblong- to lance-shaped leaves, greenish flowers, and segmented green fruit.

Habitat & cultivation Native to the tropical Americas and the Caribbean, this herb is cultivated throughout the tropics.

Parts used Leaves, bark, fruit, seeds.

Constituents Sugar Apple contains acetogenins, diterpenes, and alkaloids.

Medicinal actions & uses In the Caribbean, the young shoots are used with peppermint (*Mentha × piperita*, p. 118) to relieve colds and chills. In Cuban medicine, the leaves are taken to reduce uric acid levels. The leaves, bark, and unripe fruit are all strongly astringent and are used to treat diarrhea and dysentery. The crushed seeds are mixed with an inert powder and employed as an insecticide.

Research Sugar apple has been shown to have antiprotozoal and anthelmintic (worm-repelling) activity.

Anthemis cotula (Lamiaceae)

Mayweed,
Stinking mayweed

Description Annual or perennial resembling German chamomile (*Chamomilla recutita*, p. 82). Has slightly hairy stems and large solitary daisy-type flowers. As the name stinking mayweed suggests, this plant has an unpleasant smell and taste.

Habitat & cultivation This herb commonly grows wild in Europe, the Americas, Australia, New Zealand, and Siberia. The flowers and leaves are gathered in summer.

Parts used Flowers, leaves.

Constituents Mayweed contains sesquiterpene lactones (including anthecotulide) and polyacetylenes.

History & folklore In his *Irish Herbal* of 1735, the herbalist K'Eogh states that mayweed is "good for women with the falling down of the womb, if they but wash their feet with a decoction of it."

Medicinal actions & uses Although it looks similar to German chamomile, mayweed is far less

effective as a medicine. It has been used as an antispasmodic and to induce menstruation, and was traditionally employed for supposedly hysterical conditions relating to the uterus.

Cautions The whole plant can cause blistering if applied fresh to the skin. Do not take during pregnancy or if breastfeeding.

Anthriscus cerefolium (Apiaceae)

Chervil

Description Annual herb growing to 2 ft (60 cm). Has finely grooved stems, opposite leaves, and many small, white flowers arranged in compound umbels.

Habitat & cultivation Native to Europe, Asia Minor, Iran, and the Caucasus, chervil grows freely on waste grounds. It is cultivated throughout the world. The herb is gathered when in flower in summer.

Parts used Aerial parts.

Constituents Chervil contains a volatile oil, coumarins, and flavonoids.

History & folklore A basket of chervil seeds was one of the items found in Tutankhamen's tomb. The herb is traditionally used as a "spring tonic" in central Europe. Chervil is aromatic and is used extensively in cooking.

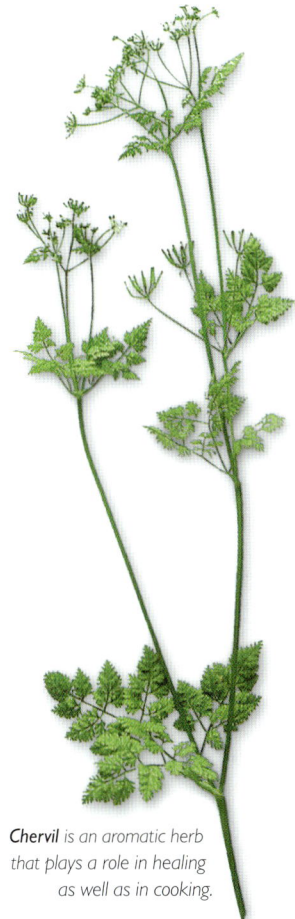

Chervil is an aromatic herb that plays a role in healing as well as in cooking.

Medicinal actions & uses Chervil is a good remedy for settling the digestion. It is also used to "purify the blood" and to help lower blood pressure, as well as being considered a diuretic. Juice from the fresh plant is applied to various skin conditions, including wounds, eczema, and abscesses.

Aphanes arvensis (Rosaceae)

Parsley piert

Description Prostrate, hairy annual growing to 4 in (10 cm). Has small wedge-shaped leaves and tiny green flowers in tufts.

Habitat & cultivation Parsley piert is native to Europe, North Africa, and North America. It grows at an altitude of up to 1,600 ft (500 m), thriving in dry sites, including the top of walls. The herb is harvested when in flower in summer.

Parts used Aerial parts.

Constituents Parsley piert contains tannins.

Medicinal actions & uses Astringent, diuretic, and demulcent, parsley piert is used to treat kidney and bladder problems, especially kidney stones. It is also frequently used in the treatment of bladder stones (gravel), which cause pain and irritation and obstruct urine flow. Best taken in an infusion, the herb is also a useful remedy for cystitis and recurrent urinary infections.

Aralia racemosa (Araliaceae)

American spikenard

Description Aromatic perennial bush growing to 6½ ft (2 m). Has thick fleshy roots, large leathery leaves, small greenish-white flowers, and red or purple berries.

Habitat & cultivation American spikenard is native to North America. The root is unearthed in summer or fall.

Part Used Root.

Constituents American spikenard contains tannins, flavonoids, a volatile oil, saponins, and triterpenes.

History & folklore The Cherokee people made a tea for backache from American spikenard, and the cure was later adopted by Europeans. The Shawnee people used it for flatulence, coughs, asthma, and breast pain; the Menominee people as a cure for blood poisoning. The plant was included in the *US National Formulary* from 1916 to 1965.

Medicinal actions & uses Many of American

spikenard's current uses come directly from Indigenous peoples. The herb encourages sweating, is stimulant, and detoxifying. It is taken for rheumatism, asthma, and coughs. Applied externally as a poultice, the herb is used to treat a number of different skin conditions, including eczema.

Related species Wild sarsaparilla (*A. nudicaulis*) is a North American relative used medicinally in much the same way as American spikenard. The leaves and stalks of two East Asian *Aralia*, *A. chinensis* and *A. cordata*, are eaten as vegetables.

Cautions Do not take during pregnancy.

Arbutus unedo (Ericaceae)

Strawberry tree

Description Evergreen shrub growing to 20 ft (6 m). Has an upright trunk with reddish bark, leathery serrated leaves, white or pink bell-shaped flowers, and round warty red fruit resembling strawberries.

Habitat & cultivation Native to Mediterranean coasts, strawberry tree also grows in western Ireland, Australia, and Africa. The leaves are gathered in late summer and the fruit in the fall.

Parts used Leaves, fruit.

Constituents Strawberry tree contains up to 2.7% arbutin, methylarbutin, and other hydroquinones, a

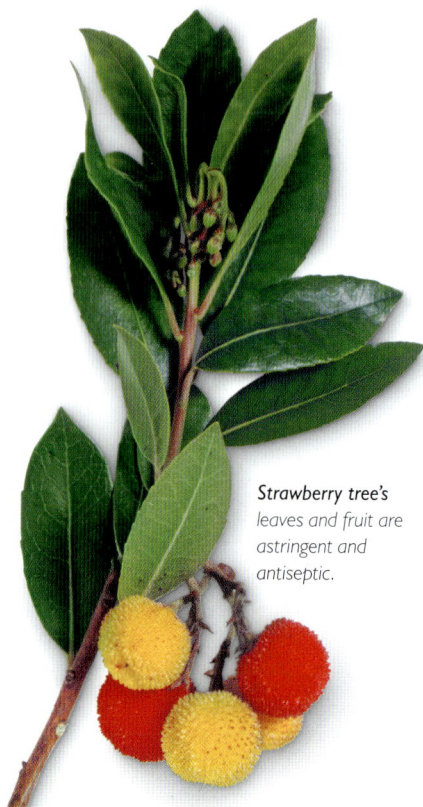

Strawberry tree's leaves and fruit are astringent and antiseptic.

bitter principle, and tannins. Arbutin is powerfully antiseptic in the urinary system.

History & folklore The fruit of strawberry tree is used in preserves, but it is not palatable fresh. The Latin *unedo* comes from *un ede,* meaning "[only] one I eat."

Medicinal actions & uses Strawberry tree is valued as an astringent and antiseptic herb. Its antiseptic action within the urinary tract makes it a useful remedy for treating cystitis and urethritis. Strawberry tree's astringent effect has been put to use in the treatment of diarrhea and dysentery.

Cautions Do not take during pregnancy or if suffering from kidney disease.

Arctostaphylos uva-ursi (Ericaceae)

Uva-ursi,
Bearberry

Description Low-lying evergreen shrub growing to 20 in (50 cm). Has long trailing stems, dark green leaves that are glossy on the upper side, bell-shaped pink flowers, and small glossy red berries.

Habitat & cultivation Uva-ursi is native to Europe, and naturalized throughout the northern hemisphere up to the Arctic. It grows in damp conditions in undergrowth, heathland, and grassland. The leaves are gathered in the fall.

Parts used Leaves, berries.

Constituents The leaves of uva-ursi contain hydroquinones (mainly arbutin, up to 17%), tannins (up to 15%), phenolic glycosides, and flavonoids. Arbutin and other hydroquinones have an antiseptic effect in the urinary tract.

History & folklore The name uva-ursi means "bear's grape" in Latin. Bears are fond of the fruit. The plant is first documented in *The Physicians of Myddfai,* a 13th-century Welsh herbal text.

Medicinal actions & uses Uva-ursi is one of the best natural urinary antiseptics. It has been used extensively in herbal medicine to disinfect and astringe the urinary tract in cases of acute and chronic cystitis and urethritis. However, it is not a suitable remedy if there is a simultaneous infection of the kidneys.

Research Experiments have shown that uva-ursi extracts have an antibacterial effect. This action is thought to be stronger in alkaline urine—thus the efficacy of uva-ursi is likely to increase if it is taken in combination with a vegetable-based diet.

Cautions Do not take during pregnancy or with kidney disease. Unsuitable for children under 12. It is generally advisable to take uva-ursi for no more than 7–10 days at a time.

Arenaria rubra (Carophyllaceae)

Sandwort, Sand spurrey

Description Herbaceous, low-growing, sticky, and hairy annual. Has small thin leaves and pale pink flowers growing to ¼ in (6 mm) across.

Habitat & cultivation Found in the wild throughout Europe, Asia, and Australia, sandwort thrives in sandy and gravelly places, especially close to the sea.

Parts used Aerial parts.

Medicinal actions & uses Sandwort is a diuretic herb that is thought to relax the muscle walls of the urinary tubules and bladder. Sandwort is most commonly taken in the form of an infusion to treat kidney stones, acute and chronic cystitis, and other conditions of the bladder.

Related species Seabeach sandwort (*A. peploides*), a closely related northern plant, is eaten by the Inuit of Alaska as a fresh, pickled, or oil-preserved vegetable. In Iceland, this plant is fermented and eaten in the same way as sauerkraut. Rupturewort (*Herniaria glabra*, p. 224), which is a European plant, has medicinal properties that are similar to those of sandwort.

Argemone mexicana (Papaveraceae)

Mexican poppy, Chicalote

Description Prickly annual growing to 3 ft (1 m). Has spiny white-veined leaves and large yellow flowers with delicate petals.

Habitat & cultivation Mexican poppy grows in tropical regions from the southernmost US to South America. It favors dry soil and is often found in tobacco fields.

Parts used Aerial parts, latex, seeds.

Constituents Mexican poppy contains a wide range of alkaloids, in particular isoquinoline alkaloids, including berberine, as well terpenoids, steroids, and flavonoids.

History & folklore Like most poppies, this plant exudes a milky latex, which was traditionally used in Ecuador to treat cataracts.

Medicinal actions & uses Commonly used through much of Latin America, the whole plant acts as a mild painkiller and sedative, and is taken to relieve muscle ache, toothache, and neuralgic pain. It is also used for a range of more serious health problems, such as bacterial infections, malaria, jaundice, and asthma. The yellow fresh latex contains protein-dissolving properties and is traditionally applied to warts and cold sores. The flowers and

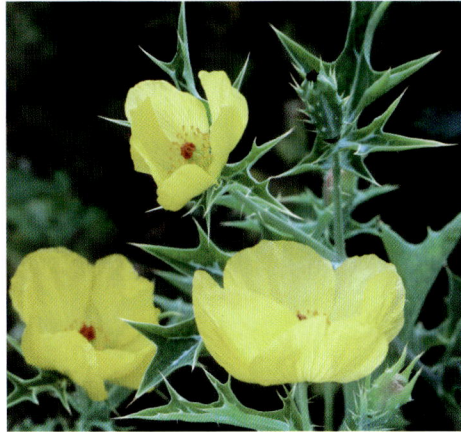

Mexican poppy flowers have expectorant properties and are useful for treating coughs.

seeds are mildly expectorant and can be used to treat irritable coughs and asthma.

Related species In Hawai'i, the latex of *A. glauca* is also used to treat warts.

Cautions Excessive use can cause glaucoma. Use only under professional supervision.

Aristolochia spp. (Aristolochiaceae)

Birthwort

Description Unpleasant-smelling perennial with heart-shaped leaves and tubular yellow flowers with flattened lips.

Habitat & cultivation Native to central and southern Europe, birthwort is also found in southwestern Asia. The root is unearthed in spring or fall.

Parts used Root, aerial parts.

Constituents Birthwort contains aristolochic acids, a volatile oil, and tannins. While stimulating white blood cell activity, aristolochic acid is carcinogenic and toxic to the kidneys (*see Research*).

History & folklore *Aristolochia* means "excellent birth," and refers to the traditional use of the fresh juice to induce labor. Theophrastus (c.372–286 BCE) records that the plant was used to treat disorders of the uterus, reptile bites, and sores on the head.

Medicinal actions & uses No longer in use today and banned in Europe and North America, birthwort was formerly used to treat wounds, sores, and snake bite. It has been taken after childbirth to prevent infection and is also a potent menstruation-inducing herb and a (very dangerous) abortifacient. A decoction was taken to encourage healing of ulcers. Birthwort has also been used for asthma and bronchitis.

Research Birthwort illustrates the fact that though a plant is natural, this has no bearing on its safety.

Aristolochic acid (present within birthwort) is a kidney toxin that induces kidney failure and cancer within the kidneys and urinary tract. However, the slow rate of development of symptoms has meant that in the past no connection was made between these kidney symptoms and the herb. These toxic effects apply to birthwort and all *Aristolochia* species that contain aristolochic acid. Kidney failure and death from aristolochic acid is relatively rare in the West but is "reaching potentially epidemic proportions in the East," according to research published in Taiwan in 2013. Many species of *Aristolochia* continue to be used in Eastern herbal medicine in countries such as China and Japan. All species of *Aristolochia* are banned in most Western countries. More recent research suggests that aristolochic acid may also induce liver cancer.

Cautions Under no circumstance use birthwort or any *Aristolochia* species as medicines.

Armoracia rusticana syn. *Cochlearia armoracia* (Brassicaceae)

Horseradish

Description Perennial with a deep tap root, leaves up to 20 in (50 cm) long, and clusters of 4-petaled white flowers.

Habitat & cultivation Native to Europe and western Asia, this herb is widely cultivated for its root, unearthed in the fall.

Parts used Root, leaves.

Constituents Horseradish root contains glucosilinates (mainly sinigrin), flavonoids, asparagine, resin, and vitamin C. On being crushed, sinigrin produces allyl isothiocyanate, an antibiotic substance.

History & folklore Pliny (23–79 CE) probably had horseradish in mind when describing a plant that warded off scorpions, but for most of its long history, horseradish has been used mainly as a diuretic herb. It is a popular condiment, particularly in Britain and central Europe.

Medicinal actions & uses Now undervalued as a medicinal herb, horseradish has many healing properties. It strongly stimulates digestion, increasing gastric secretions and appetite. It is a good diuretic and promotes perspiration, making it useful in fevers, colds, and flu. It is also expectorant and mildly antibiotic, and can be of use in both respiratory and urinary tract infections. A sandwich of freshly grated root is a home remedy for hay fever. Externally, a poultice of the root can soothe chilblains.

Cautions Over-consumption of horseradish may irritate the gastrointestinal tract. The plant should be avoided by those with low thyroid function. A horseradish poultice may cause blistering.

Arnica montana (Asteraceae)

Arnica

Description Aromatic perennial growing to 1 ft (30 cm). Has downy egg-shaped leaves and bright yellow daisylike flowers.

Habitat & cultivation Arnica grows in mountain woods and pastures in central Europe, the Pyrenees, Siberia, Canada, and the northwestern US. Its flowers are harvested when in full bloom; the rhizomes after the plant has died back in the fall.

Parts used Flowers, rhizome.

Constituents Arnica contains sesquiterpene lactones, flavonoids, a volatile oil that includes thymol, mucilage, and polysaccharides.

History & folklore Arnica has been used extensively in European folk medicine. Johann Wolfgang von Goethe (1749–1832), the German philosopher and poet, drank arnica tea to ease his angina in old age.

Medicinal actions & uses Best known as an effective ointment and compress for bruises, sprains, and muscle pain, arnica improves the local blood supply and accelerates healing. It is anti-inflammatory and increases the rate of reabsorption of internal bleeding. Generally the plant is now taken internally only at a homeopathic dilution, principally for shock, injury, and pain. If taken as a decoction or tincture, it stimulates the circulation and is valuable in the treatment of angina and a weak or failing heart, but it can be toxic even at low dosage and thus is rarely used in this way.

Related species In North America *A. fulgens* is used.

Cautions Do not take internally. Do not apply arnica preparations to broken skin. External use may cause dermatitis. Arnica is subject to legal restrictions in some countries.

Self-help uses Bruises, p. 314; Sprains, p. 322; Tired & aching muscles, p. 322.

Artemisia abrotanum (Asteraceae)

Southernwood

Description Strongly aromatic, shrubby perennial, growing to 3 ft (1 m). Has woody stems, feathery silver-green leaves, and yellow flowers.

Habitat & cultivation Native to southern Europe, this herb is rare in the wild but is cultivated for the perfume industry and, to a lesser extent, for herbal medicine. The aerial parts are harvested in late summer.

Parts used Aerial parts.

Constituents Southernwood contains an essential

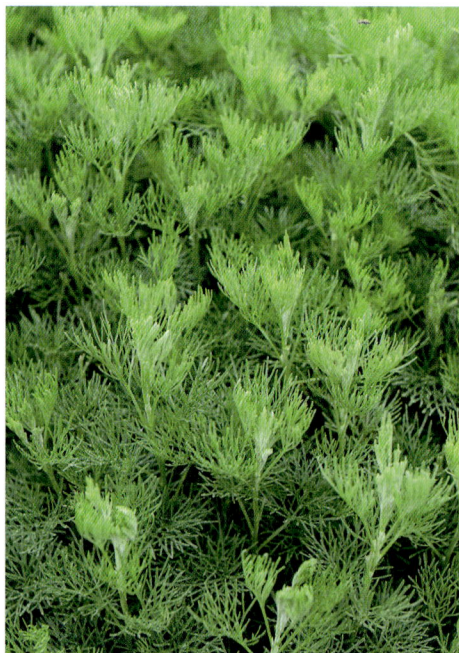

Southernwood leaves were traditionally placed among clothing to repel moths.

oil—mainly composed of borneol and camphor, coumarins, phenolic acids, and flavonoids.

History & folklore Much prized during the Middle Ages and the Renaissance, southernwood is now used infrequently in herbal medicine. The closely related wormwood (*A. absinthium*, p. 70) is considered superior. Like wormwood, southernwood contains a strong volatile oil that repels insects, and the leaves are placed among clothes to repel moths. Mrs. Grieve (*A Modern Herbal*, 1931) reports that in England "even in the early part of the last century a bunch of southernwood and rue [*Ruta graveolens*, p. 273] was placed next to the prisoner in the dock as a preventive from the contagion of jail fever."

Medicinal actions & uses Southernwood is a bitter tonic. It strengthens and supports digestive function by increasing secretions in the stomach and intestines. An infusion of southernwood has been given to children as a treatment for worms, but this is not recommended without professional supervision. Like other *Artemisias*, southernwood stimulates menstruation and is commonly taken to encourage the onset of irregular or absent periods.

Research Recent scientific investigation has shown that southernwood has wide-ranging medicinal benefits. Southernwood, and its essential oil, are reported to have antibacterial, antifungal, antioxidant, anticancer, and anti-allergic properties.

Cautions Do not take during pregnancy. Not suitable for children under 12 unless prescribed professionally.

Artemisia capillaris (Asteraceae)

Yin chen hao

Description Medium-size perennial herb with an erect stem, thin feathery leaves, and clusters of small composite flowers.

Habitat & cultivation Native to Southeast Asia, *yin chen hao* is cultivated in China and other Eastern countries. The young plants are gathered in spring.

Parts used Aerial parts.

Constituents *Yin chen hao* contains a volatile oil, mostly capillene and terpinene, and coumarins.

History & folklore *Yin chen hao* has been used in Chinese herbal medicine for more than 2,000 years. Its medicinal properties were first listed in *Divine Husbandman's Classic* (*Shen'nong Bencaojing*), written in the 1st century CE.

Medicinal actions & uses *Yin chen hao* is an effective remedy for liver problems, being specifically helpful for treating hepatitis with jaundice. Traditional Chinese medicine (see pp. 44–47) holds that it is bitter and cooling, clearing "damp heat" from the liver and gall ducts and relieving fevers. *Yin chen hao* is also anti-inflammatory and diuretic. It was formerly applied in the form of a plaster to treat headaches.

Research Though poorly researched, laboratory studies indicate that *Yin chen hao* has potential value in the treatment of liver disease, including hepatitis B.

Cautions Do not take during pregnancy. Unsuitable for children under 12 unless prescribed professionally.

Artemisia cina (Asteraceae)

Levant wormwood

Description Shrubby perennial with long thin leaves and tiny round tufts of flowers.

Habitat & cultivation This herb is native to the region stretching from the eastern Mediterranean to Siberia. The unopened flower heads are gathered from wild and cultivated plants.

Parts used Flower heads.

Constituents Levant wormwood contains santonin (a sesquiterpene lactone), artemisin, and a volatile oil (with up to 80% cineole). Santonin is directly toxic to roundworms and, to a lesser extent, threadworms.

History & folklore Levant wormwood was known to the classical Greek world as a remedy for intestinal worms, and it has been used for this purpose ever since. Its active constituent, santonin, was first isolated in 1830, and is now more commonly employed than the plant itself.

Medicinal actions & uses Used almost exclusively to expel worms, Levant wormwood is strongly bitter and aromatic and has a tonic and stimulant effect on digestion. The dried flower heads are occasionally mixed with honey to disguise their bitterness.

Cautions Do not take during pregnancy. Use only under professional supervision, especially in the case of children under 12.

Artemisia dracunculus (Asteraceae)

Tarragon

Description Aromatic perennial growing to 3 ft (1 m). Has narrow lance-shaped leaves and small greenish flower heads in long drooping clusters.

Habitat & cultivation Native to Russia, western Asia, and the Himalayas, tarragon is now cultivated as a culinary herb in gardens around the world. The aerial parts are picked in summer.

Parts used Aerial parts, root.

Constituents Tarragon contains tannins, coumarins, and flavonoids, and up to 0.8% volatile oil, consisting of up to 70% methylchervicol, which is toxic and potentially carcinogenic.

History & folklore Tarragon is widely used as an herb in cooking. In French, it is sometimes known as *herbe au dragon*, because of its reputed ability to cure serpent bites.

Medicinal actions & uses While tarragon stimulates digestion, it is reputed to be a mild sedative and has been taken to aid sleep. With its mild menstruation-inducing properties, it is taken if periods are delayed. The root has traditionally been applied to aching teeth.

Cautions Do not take during pregnancy. Do not exceed the standard dose, and do not take for longer than 4 weeks at a time.

Artemisia vulgaris (Asteraceae)

Mugwort

Description Shrubby perennial growing to about 3 ft (1 m). Has dark green deeply indented leaves and numerous clusters of small reddish or yellow flower heads.

Habitat & cultivation Mugwort is found in temperate regions of the northern hemisphere. It flourishes on waste ground and along roads, and is gathered in late summer just before flowering.

Parts used Leaves, root.

Constituents Mugwort contains a volatile oil (mainly caryophyllene), a sesquiterpene lactone, flavonoids, coumarin derivatives, and triterpenes.

History & folklore Known as *Mater Herbarum* (mother of herbs), mugwort was used from the earliest times in Europe and Asia. Roman centurions reputedly placed it in their sandals to keep the soles of their feet in good shape. The Greek physician Dioscorides (1st century CE) recounts that the goddess Artemis (who inspired the plant's genus name) was believed to give succor to women in childbirth. The 13th-century Welsh herbal *The Physicians of Myddfai* recommends: "If a woman be unable to give birth to her child let the mugwort be bound to her left thigh. Let it be instantly removed when she has been delivered, lest there should be hemorrhage." An 18th-century Spanish herbalist, Diego de Torres, recommends the application of a mugwort plaster below the navel as an effective method of inducing labor. In the Isle of Man (UK), sprigs of mugwort are worn at the annual open-air parliamentary assembly, held on Tynwald Hill. In China, mugwort has been valued for millennia. It is the principal ingredient of *moxa* and is used in moxibustion, a process in which heat from a burning, cigar-shaped roll of chopped leaves is applied to acupuncture points.

Medicinal actions & uses A digestive and tonic herb, mugwort has a wide variety of traditional uses. Milder in action than most other *Artemisia* species, it can be taken over the long term at a low dose to improve appetite, digestive function, and absorption of nutrients. In addition, it can be taken to encourage the elimination of worms. Mugwort also increases bile flow and mildly induces the onset of menstruation. The European conception of mugwort as a uterine stimulant is contradicted by Chinese usage, in which it is prescribed to prevent miscarriage and to reduce or stop menstrual bleeding. Mugwort is also antiseptic, and has been used in the treatment of malaria.

Caution Do not take mugwort during pregnancy.

Asclepias tuberosa (Asclepiadaceae)

Pleurisy root

Description Perennial, upright herb growing to 3 ft (1 m). Has narrow lance-shaped leaves and spikes of numerous 5-petaled orange or yellow flowers.

Habitat & cultivation This herb is native to the southern US. The root is unearthed in spring.

Part used Root.

Constituents Pleurisy root contains cardenolides and flavonoids. It is estrogenic.

History & folklore In North American herbal medicine, pleurisy root was considered a cure-all. It was used to treat conditions as diverse as pleurisy, typhoid, pneumonia, congestion, dysentery, colic, eczema, and hysteria. The Omaha people ate the raw root for bronchitis and other chest conditions. Many tribes thought pleurisy root was a good remedy for hot dry fevers.

Medicinal actions & uses Though its most specific usage is relieving the pain and inflammation of pleurisy, pleurisy root has other applications. It is useful for hot, dry, and tight conditions in the chest. It promotes the coughing up of phlegm, reduces inflammation, and, in addition, helps reduce fevers by stimulating perspiration. The root is also taken for the treatment of chronic diarrhea and dysentery.

Related species *A. incarnata* and *A. syriaca* have both been used in North American Indigenous herbal medicine to treat asthma.

Cautions Do not take during pregnancy. Excessive doses may cause vomiting.

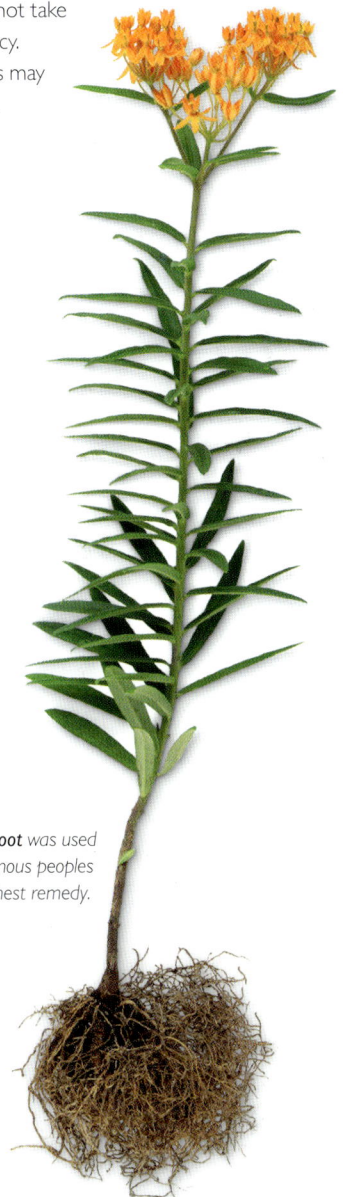

Pleurisy root was used by Indigenous peoples as a chest remedy.

Aspalathus linearis (Fabaceae)

Rooibos, Red bush

Description Variable shrub growing to 6½ ft (2 m) in height, with green, needlelike leaves, yellow, pealike flowers, and small seed pods.

Habitat & cultivation Native to southern South Africa, rooibos is now widely cultivated as a commercial crop, particularly in the Cedarberg mountain area. The seed is hard to germinate and must first be scarified. The young leaves are harvested once a year, chopped, and left to "sweat" or ferment before being dried.

Parts used Young leaves.

Constituents Rooibos contains polyphenols, including flavonoids, with a low tannin content.

History & folklore Rooibos was first used as an appetizing tea by the Khoisan people, indigenous to the Cedarberg region, but also as a sleep aid and for headaches.

Medicinal actions & uses Drunk mostly as a pleasant tasting, caffeine-free drink, rooibos, like green tea, has significant antioxidant activity. There is evidence to suggest that the fermented leaves exert a protective effect on the heart and circulation. In view of the herb's traditional use, it might also prove helpful as a nighttime drink to promote sound sleep.

Asparagus officinalis (Liliaceae)

Asparagus

Description Slender-stemmed perennial growing to 6½ ft (2 m). Has long fronds of delicate needlelike leaves and bell-shaped yellow-green flowers that produce small bright red berries.

Habitat & cultivation Native to temperate regions in Europe, North Africa, and Asia, asparagus is cultivated worldwide as a vegetable. The shoots grow into tender green (and, if sheltered from sunlight, white) stems in spring. The root is gathered after the shoots have been cut.

Parts used Root, shoots.

Constituents Asparagus contains steroidal glycosides (asparagosides), bitter glycosides, asparagine, and flavonoids. Asparagine is a strong diuretic.

History & folklore To judge from ancient Egyptian tomb drawings, asparagus was cultivated as long ago as 4000 BCE. In the 1st century CE, the Greek physician Dioscorides recommended a decoction of asparagus root to improve urine flow and to treat kidney problems, jaundice, and sciatica.

Medicinal actions & uses Asparagus is a strong diuretic that is useful for a variety of urinary

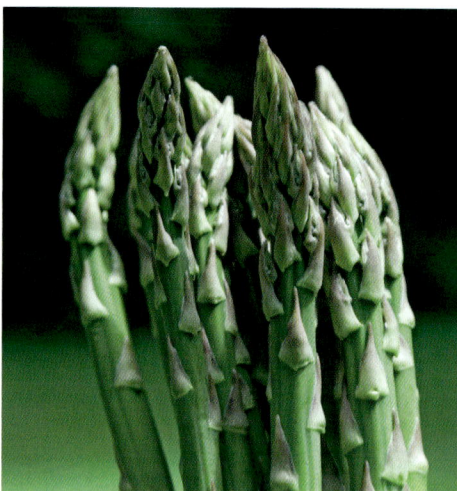

Asparagus is used to treat a range of urinary problems.

problems, including cystitis. It is also useful for rheumatic conditions, helping to "flush" waste products accumulated in the joints out of the body in the urine. Asparagus is also bitter, mildly laxative, and sedative.

Caution Do not take if you suffer from kidney disease.

Asparagus racemosus (Liliaceae)

Shatavari, Indian asparagus

Description Slender perennial fern growing to 23 ft (7 m) in height. Shatavari has fronds of needlelike leaves, tiny white flowers, and purple-black berries.

Habitat & cultivation Native to the Himalayas and the Indian subcontinent, *shatavari* grows wild in gravelly soils up to 3,900 ft (1,200 m) above sea level. It is also found in western China.

Part Used Root.

Constituents *Shatavari* contains steroidal saponins, alkaloids, and mucilage.

History & folklore *Shatavari* is known as the "Queen of herbs" in Ayurvedic medicine. Its name literally means "100 spouses," signifying the herb's ability to act as a sexual tonic and promote fertility.

Medicinal actions & uses A key Ayurvedic remedy, *shatavari* is first and foremost a women's herb, aiding fertility and promoting conception, and acting as a general reproductive and sexual tonic. *Shatavari* can prove particularly helpful in easing menopausal symptoms, such as hot flashes and poor stamina. It appears to improve fertility in both men and women, and may also be taken to treat

impotence. A tonic, strengthening herb, *shatavari* supports immune function and has a place in the treatment of immunosuppressed conditions.

Related species Asparagus (*A. officinalis, see preceding entry*) is a relative.

Asperula odorata syn. *galium odoratum* (Rubiaceae)

Sweet woodruff

Description Perennial growing to 18 in (45 cm). Has a square stem, whorls of narrow elliptical leaves, and small white flowers.

Habitat & cultivation Sweet woodruff is native to Europe, and is also found in Asia and North Africa. It grows in woodlands and shaded places. The herb is gathered when in flower in late spring.

Parts used Aerial parts.

Constituents Sweet woodruff contains iridoids, coumarins (0.6%), tannins, anthraquinones, and flavonoids. The flavonoids act on the circulation and are diuretic.

History & folklore When it dries, sweet woodruff takes on the scent of newly cut grass, and it has often been placed between clothes to impart its aroma. In his *Irish Herbal* of 1735, K'Eogh records that "It is good in healing wounds if bruised and then applied, and also in curing boils and inflammations." In Germany *Maiwein*, made of sweet woodruff steeped in white wine, is drunk to celebrate May Day.

Medicinal actions & uses Sweet woodruff is considered tonic, with significant diuretic and anti-inflammatory effects. Its coumarin and flavonoid constituents make it helpful for varicose veins and phlebitis. It has been used as an antispasmodic, and it is given to children and adults for insomnia.

Cautions In excessive doses, sweet woodruff can cause internal bleeding. Do not use if taking conventional medication for circulatory problems, or during pregnancy.

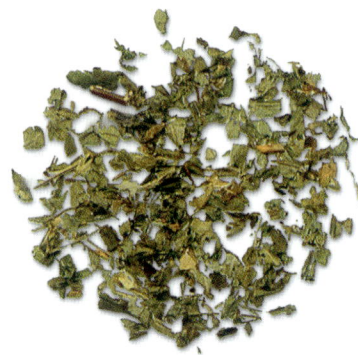

Sweet woodruff aerial parts are dried for medicinal use.

Aspidosperma quebracho-blanco
(Apocynaceae)

White quebracho

Description Tree growing to 100 ft (30 m). Has thick corky bark, leathery leaves, and tubular white flowers.

Habitat & cultivation Quebracho is found in the southern half of South America. The bark and timber are used commercially.

Part used Bark.

Constituents Quebracho contains indole alkaloids (including yohimbine) and tannins.

History & folklore The name quebracho comes from the Spanish *quebrar* (to break) and *hacha* (ax), an allusion to the hardness of this tree's wood.

Medicinal actions & uses With its antispasmodic effect on the bronchial tubes, quebracho is used therapeutically to treat asthma and emphysema. It is also a tonic and reduces fever. Extracts of white quebracho are prescribed to treat erectile dysfunction. It also has tonic properties.

Related species Many other species of *Aspidosperma* are grown for tanning and timber in South America. Some are also considered fever remedies. One, *A. excelsum*, is used to relieve gas, stomach problems, and indigestion.

Cautions Take only under professional supervision. Quebracho is toxic in excessive doses. It is subject to legal restrictions in some countries.

Atractylodes macrocephala (Asteraceae)

Bai zhu

Description Erect perennial herb growing to 2 ft (60 cm). Has alternate oval- to lance-shaped leaves and purple flowers.

Habitat & cultivation *Bai zhu* is rare in the wild. It is cultivated in China, Japan, and Korea. The rhizome is unearthed in late fall or winter.

Part Used Rhizome.

Constituents *Bai zhu* contains a volatile oil (0.35–1.35%), which includes atractylol, and the lactones atractylenolide II and III. Atractylol has a liver-protective activity. It also contains polysaccharides and polyacetylenes.

History & folklore The first record of the use of *bai zhu* is in the *Tang Materia Medica*, written in China in 659 CE. Later, it was one of the 4 herbs that made up the "decoction of the 4 rulers," a mixture prescribed by Wang Ji (1463–1539) as a treatment for syphilis.

Medicinal actions & uses *Bai zhu* has traditionally been used as a tonic, building *qi*

(see p. 44) and strengthening the spleen. The rhizome has a sweet, pungent taste, and is used to relieve fluid retention, excessive sweating, and digestive problems such as diarrhea and vomiting. Combined with Baikal skullcap (*Scutellaria baicalensis*, p. 138), it is employed to prevent miscarriage.

Avena sativa (Poaceae)

Oats

Description Annual grass growing to 3 ft (1 m). Has straight hollow stems, bladelike leaves, and small spikes holding seeds (grain).

Habitat & cultivation Native to northern Europe, oats are now grown in temperate regions worldwide as a cereal crop. They are harvested in late summer.

Parts used Seeds, straw (dried stems).

Constituents Oats contain saponins, alkaloids, sterols, flavonoids, silicic acid, starch, proteins (including gluten), vitamins (especially B vitamins), and minerals (especially calcium).

History & folklore Formerly, oat straw was used to fill mattresses, proving beneficial to those suffering from rheumatism. In *The English Physitian* (1652) Nicholas Culpeper states that "a poultice made of meal of oats and some oil of bay helpeth the itch and the leprosy." Earlier, in 1597, John Gerard was less enthusiastic: "Oatmeal is good to make a fair and well-coloured maid to look like a cake of tallow."

Medicinal actions & uses Oats are best known as a nutritious grain, but they benefit health in many other ways. Oat bran lowers cholesterol, and an oat-based diet may improve stamina (see *Research*). Oats, and oat straw in particular, are tonic when taken medicinally. Oat straw is prescribed by medical herbalists to treat general debility and a wide variety of nervous conditions. The grains and straw are mildly antidepressant, gently raising energy levels and supporting an overstressed nervous system. Oats are used to treat depression and nervous debility, and insomnia in those suffering from nervous exhaustion. Oats are one of the principal herbal aids to convalescence after a long illness. Externally, the grain is emollient and cleansing, and a decoction strained into a bath can help soothe itchiness and eczema.

Research In research undertaken in Australia, athletes who were placed on an oat-based diet for 3 weeks showed a 4% increase in stamina. Oats are thought to help maintain muscle function during training and exercise.

Self-help uses Depression & decreased vitality, p. 326; Eczema, p. 310; Nervous exhaustion & stress, p. 329; Poor sleep & nervous exhaustion, p. 319.

Bacopa monnieri (Scrophulariaceae)

Water hyssop,
Brahmi (Hindi)

Description Creeping succulent perennial growing to 20 in (50 cm). Has spatula-shaped fleshy leaves and pale blue or white flowers on long, slender stalks.

Habitat & cultivation Water hyssop grows in warmer temperate and tropical climates, especially in southern Asia. It thrives in marshland, developing into dense mats on mudflats and at the edges of mangrove swamps.

Parts used Aerial parts.

Constituents Water hyssop contains triterpenoid saponins, including bacosides.

Medicinal actions & uses In India, water hyssop is used principally for disorders of the nervous system, such as neuralgia, epilepsy, and mental illness, but it is also employed for a wide range of other disorders, including indigestion, ulcers, gas and constipation, asthma and bronchitis, and infertility. In China, it is taken as a *yang* tonic for impotence, premature ejaculation, infertility, and rheumatic conditions. In Indonesia, the plant is a remedy for filariasis (a tropical disease caused by worms). In Cuba, water hyssop is used as a purgative, and a decoction of the whole plant is taken as a diuretic and laxative. The expressed juice is mixed with oil and applied as a rub for arthritic pain.

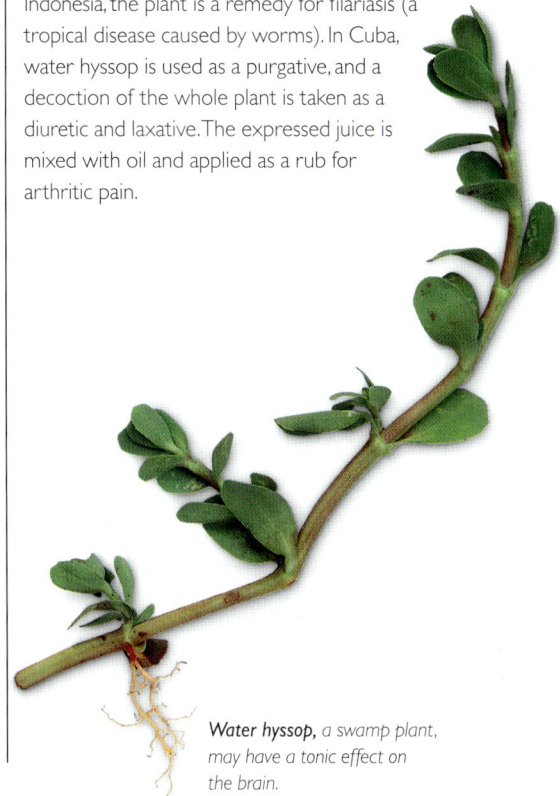

Water hyssop, a swamp plant, may have a tonic effect on the brain.

Research Ongoing research indicates that water hyssop supports healthy cognitive function, including memory and recall, and that it exerts a protective activity in neurological conditions such as epilepsy and dementia.

Ballota nigra (Lamiaceae)

Black horehound

Description Straggling perennial growing to 2 ft (50 cm). Has oval, toothed leaves and pink-purple flowers in whorls at the base of the upper leaves.

Habitat & cultivation This herb is found throughout much of Europe, in North America, and in Asia. It thrives on waste ground, in pavement cracks, and by roadsides, mostly near human habitation. It is harvested when in flower in summer.

Parts used Aerial parts.

Constituents Black horehound contains diterpenoids, including marrubiin, flavonoids, tannins, saponins, and a volatile oil.

History & folklore The Greek physician Dioscorides, writing in the 1st century CE, recommends a plaster of black horehound leaves and salt for dog bites. He also advocates a balm, made from the dried leaves and honey, to purify infected wounds and ulcers.

Medicinal actions & uses Though long considered a remedy for convulsions, low spirits, and menopausal problems, black horehound is rarely used today. Authorities differ over whether there is any substance to claims for its earlier applications. The herb is currently used by Anglo-American herbalists as an antiemetic—preventing or reducing nausea or vomiting. It is perhaps most useful when nausea arises from disorders of the inner ear (such as Ménière's disease) as opposed to those of the digestive system. Black horehound is thought to be mildly sedative and antispasmodic, and is occasionally taken for arthritis and gout.

Black horehound was an ancient Greek remedy for dog bites.

Bambusa arundinaceae (Poaceae)

Spiny bamboo

Description Perennial tree, up to 100 ft (30 m), with multiple stems from its base. Has narrow pointed leaves and long loose clusters of yellow to yellowish-green flowers.

Habitat & cultivation Found throughout tropical Asia, especially in India and China, spiny bamboo thrives up to 6,900 ft (2,100 m) above sea level.

Parts used Root, leaves, sprouts.

Constituents Spiny bamboo juice contains high levels of silica.

History & folklore Spiny bamboo is arguably the most useful plant on earth, being used to make scaffolding, rafts, furniture, paper, and dozens of other items. It also has an important role to play in herbal medicine.

Medicinal actions & uses Various parts of spiny bamboo are used in Indian and Ayurvedic medicine. The root is considered astringent and cooling, and is used to treat joint pain and general debility. The leaves are used to stimulate menstruation, and, being antispasmodic, to help relieve period pain. They are also taken to tone and strengthen stomach function and to expel worms. They are reputed to be aphrodisiac. The young sprouts are eaten to relieve nausea, indigestion, and gas, and a poultice of the sprouts is applied to help drain wounds that have become infected. The juice is rich in silica, and aids in the strengthening of cartilage in conditions such as osteoarthritis and osteoporosis.

Related species In Chinese herbal medicine, the juice and shavings of the black bamboo (*B. breviflora*) are prescribed to counter "excess heat," coughs, and a congested chest. Its roots are used as a diuretic and to treat fevers.

Banisteriopsis caapi (Malpighiaceae)

Ayahuasca

Description Woody vine growing to 100 ft (30 m). Has smooth bark, oval leaves, and bunches of small red or yellow flowers.

Habitat & cultivation Ayahuasca is native to jungles of the Amazon basin. It is cultivated by Indigenous peoples, but the wild herb is preferred for medicinal use.

Part Used Bark.

Constituents Ayahuasca contains beta-carboline alkaloids (including harmine, harmaline, and delta-tetrahydroharmine), which stimulate hallucinations.

History & folklore In the Quechua language, widely spoken in Peru and neighboring countries, *ayahuasca* means "spirit of the dead," indicating the awesome powers traditionally attributed to this plant. Another name used by the Quechua people is *nixi honi xuma*, meaning "vine from which the vision extract is made." Ayahuasca bark, which is often used in combination with members of the *Datura* genus, is the primary hallucinogen among many Amazonian tribes, being prepared as part of complex ritual ceremonies.

Medicinal actions & uses Though known as a powerful hallucinogen, ayahuasca is also a medicine, being used as a remedy to cure a range of diagnosed conditions. However, ayahuasca is usually taken by the healer rather than by the patient. In the shamanistic societies of the Amazon, ayahuasca allows the healer to communicate with the spirit world where illness arises, interceding on behalf of the ill person and the community to restore health and harmony to all—quite unlike the individualized approach of Western medicine. Beyond its ability to affect mood, the bark is emetic and purgative. At low doses it is used as a mild detoxifier.

Caution Ayahuasca is taken traditionally as part of a rich, complex ritual which affects the experience produced. Medicinal use of this plant is not advised.

Baptisia tinctoria (Fabaceae)

Wild indigo

Description Herbaceous perennial growing to 3 ft (1 m). Has a smooth stem, cloverlike leaves, and purplish-blue flowers in small terminal clusters.

Habitat & cultivation Native to eastern parts of North America, wild indigo grows from North Carolina to southern Canada in dry, hilly woods.

Parts used Root, leaves.

Constituents Wild indigo contains isoflavones, flavonoids, alkaloids, coumarins, and polysaccharides.

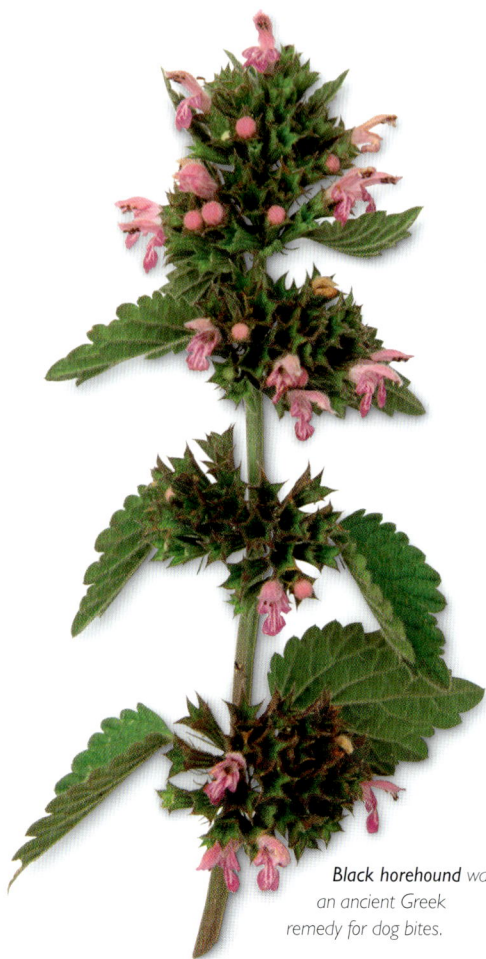

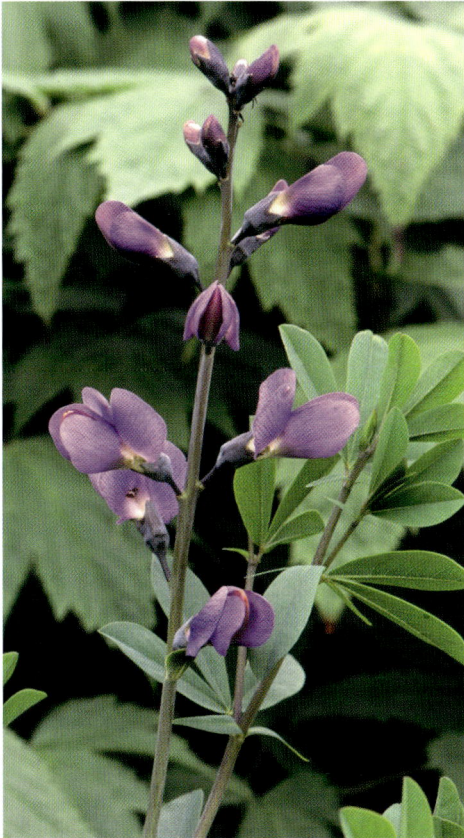

Wild indigo, a North American plant, was used by the Penobscot to treat wounds.

The isoflavones are estrogenic, while the polysaccharides are immunostimulant.

History & folklore Wild indigo was commonly used as a poultice by Indigenous peoples and colonizers to treat snake bite. The Mohican people used a decoction of the root to bathe cuts and heal wounds.

Medicinal actions & uses Wild indigo is a strong antiseptic and immunostimulant, though at more than moderate doses it can produce nausea and vomiting. It is considered particularly effective for upper respiratory infections such as tonsillitis and pharyngitis, and is also valuable in treating infections of the chest, gastrointestinal tract, and skin. Its antimicrobial and immunostimulant properties combat lymphatic problems—when used with detoxifying herbs such as burdock (*Arctium lappa,* p. 69), it helps to reduce enlarged lymph nodes. Wild indigo is frequently prescribed along with echinacea (*Echinacea* spp., p. 96) for chronic viral conditions or chronic fatigue syndrome. A decoction of the root soothes sore or infected nipples and infected skin conditions. When used as a gargle or mouthwash, the decoction treats canker sores, gum infections, and sore throats.

Caution Best taken on professional advice.

Benincasa hispida syn. *B. cerifa* (Cucurbitaceae)

Wax gourd

Description Hairy annual climber. Has 3-lobed leaves, tendrils, and large yellow flowers. Produces rounded fruit (gourds) about 16 in (40 cm) long.

Habitat & cultivation Native to tropical Asia and Africa, this herb is cultivated in India and China as a vegetable. The fruit is harvested in late summer.

Parts used Fruit rind, fruit, seeds.

Constituents Wax gourd contains saponins and guaridine.

History & folklore Wax gourd has been used as a food and medicine for thousands of years. It was first documented in the *Tang Materia Medica,* written in 659 CE.

Medicinal actions & uses In Chinese herbal medicine, a decoction of wax gourd seeds is used to "drain dampness" and "clear heat." It is given for chest conditions and vaginal discharge. In combination with Chinese rhubarb (*Rheum palmatum,* p. 130), it is prescribed for intestinal abscesses. In Ayurvedic medicine, the seeds are used to treat coughs, fever, and excessive thirst, and to expel tapeworms. In an ancient Indian recipe, the fruit juice is mixed with lime juice (*Citrus aurantiifolia*) to prevent or stop bleeding.

Research A 2021 Bangladeshi research paper found that wax gourd, in common with other members of the melon family, has significant cancer protective activity.

Berberis vulgaris (Berberidaceae)

Barberry

Description Thorny deciduous shrub growing to 10 ft (3 m), with leathery leaves, yellow flowers, and red berries in the fall.

Habitat & cultivation Native to Europe, barberry is naturalized in North America. It is cultivated as a garden plant and medicinal herb. The bark is gathered in spring or fall, and the berries in the fall.

Parts used Stem bark, root bark, berries.

Constituents Barberry contains isoquinoline alkaloids, including berberine and berbamine. Berberine is strongly antibacterial and amoebicidal, and stimulates bile secretion. Berbamine is strongly antibacterial. Many of the alkaloids are thought to be cancer-inhibiting.

History & folklore In ancient Egypt, *Berberis* berries were macerated with fennel seed (*Foeniculum vulgare,* p. 217 to make a drink for fevers. The berries are extremely sour but have been used in the past to make preserves—the French *confiture d'épine vinette* is one example.

Medicinal actions & uses Barberry acts on the gallbladder to improve bile flow and ameliorate conditions such as gallbladder pain, gallstones, and jaundice. Its strongly antiseptic property helps amoebic dysentery, cholera, and other similar gastrointestinal infections. The bark is astringent, antidiarrheal, and healing to the intestinal wall—in short, barberry has a strong, highly beneficial effect on the digestive system as a whole. Like Oregon grape (*B. aquifolium, preceding entry*) and goldenseal (*Hydrastis canadensis,* p. 109), barberry helps chronic skin conditions such as eczema and psoriasis. The decoction makes a gentle and effective wash for the eyes, although it must be diluted sufficiently before use.

Research Berberine has been shown to have antibiotic activity against cholera, giardia, shigella, salmonella, and *E. coli.*

Cautions Take only under professional supervision. Do not take during pregnancy.

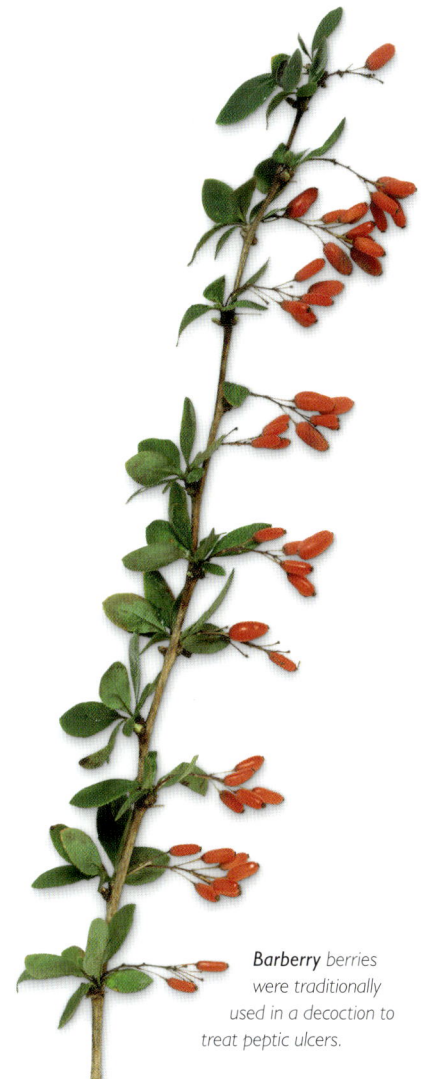

Barberry berries were traditionally used in a decoction to treat peptic ulcers.

Beta vulgaris (Chenopodiaceae)

Red beet, White beet

Description Perennial with swollen edible red or white root, upright shoots, large deep green leaves tinged with red, and spikes of green-petaled flowers.

Habitat & cultivation Sea beet (the wild subspecies) is native to coastal regions of Europe, North Africa, and Asia from Turkey to the East Indies. Red beet is widely cultivated as a vegetable, white beet as a vegetable and source of sugar.

Part used Root.

Constituents White beet contains betaine, which promotes liver regeneration and fat metabolism. Red beet contains betanin (also found in red wine), which is partly responsible for its immune-enhancing effect, and inorganic nitrate, which increases nitric oxide levels within the body and thus lowers blood pressure.

History & folklore *The Materia Medica*, written by Dioscorides in the 1st century CE, recommends the following prescription for clearing the head and relieving earache—mix beet juice with honey and sniff it up the nose.

Medicinal actions & uses White beet acts to support the liver, bile ducts, and gallbladder, influencing fat metabolism and helping to lower blood fat levels. Several clinical trials have shown that red beet juice (due to its high nitrate content) relaxes the arteries and lowers blood pressure in people with high blood pressure. A glass a day of juice will help to support lower blood pressure. Red beet juice is also thought to support immune function and is prescribed by herbalists as part of a cancer-treatment regime—though large quantities must be taken (up to 1 quart a day) to be effective.

Betula pendula syn. *B. verrucosa* (Betulaceae)

Silver birch

Description Handsome slender deciduous tree growing to a height of 100 ft (30 m). Has pale gray papery bark, toothed leaves, and catkins in spring.

Habitat & cultivation Silver birch is common in Europe, in temperate regions of Asia, and in North America. It flourishes in woods and thickets, and is also planted as a garden ornamental. The leaves are gathered in late spring.

Parts used Leaves, bark, sap.

Constituents Silver birch contains saponins, flavonoids, tannin, and a volatile oil that includes methyl salicylate.

History & folklore Silver birch has been used as a medicinal herb in northern Europe and Asia since the earliest times. Its name is thought to derive from the Sanskrit word *bhurga*, meaning "tree whose bark is used for writing on." In the highlands of Scotland, silver birch sap—tapped in the spring—was drunk as a treatment for bladder and kidney complaints.

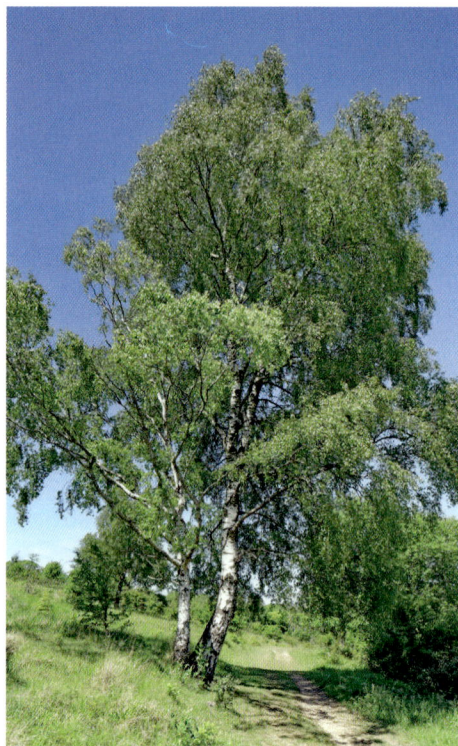

Silver birch is widespread in temperate regions throughout the northern hemisphere. Its leaf oil is used to improve eczema and psoriasis.

Medicinal actions & uses An infusion made with silver birch leaves hastens the removal of waste products in the urine, and is beneficial for kidney stones and bladder stones (gravel), rheumatic conditions, and gout. The leaves are also used, in combination with diuretic herbs, to reduce fluid retention and swelling. Silver birch sap is a mild diuretic. The oil distilled from the leaves is antiseptic and is commonly used in preparations to treat eczema and psoriasis. A decoction of silver birch bark can be used as a lotion for chronic skin problems. The bark can also be macerated in oil and applied to joints for the relief of rheumatism.

Related species The Himalayan silver birch (*B. utilis*), a close relative, is used to treat convulsions, dysentery, hemorrhages, and skin diseases.

Bidens tripartita (Asteraceae)

Bur marigold

Description Annual growing to a height of 2 ft (60 cm). Has toothed lance-shaped leaves, yellow button-like flower heads, and burrlike fruit.

Habitat & cultivation Bur marigold grows throughout Europe and in other temperate regions, including Australia and New Zealand. It is found in damp places and near fresh water.

Parts used Aerial parts.

Constituents Bur marigold contains flavonoids, polyacetylenes, chalcones, coumarins, small amounts of vitamin C, carotenoids, and a volatile oil.

History & folklore The herbalist Nicholas Culpeper, writing in 1652, extolled bur marigold: "It helps the cachexia or evil disposition of the body, the dropsy and yellow jaundice, it opens obstructions of the liver, and mollifies the hardness of the spleen being applied outwardly."

Medicinal actions & uses Little used in medicine today, bur marigold is astringent and diuretic, and employed to treat bladder and kidney problems. It has a longstanding reputation for staunching blood flow, and can be used for uterine hemorrhage and conditions causing blood in the urine. In Uzbekistan a bur marigold lotion is used to treat allergic itching in children.

Bixa orellana (Bixaceae)

Annatto

Description Evergreen tree growing to 26 ft (8 m). Has large leaves, pink or white flowers, and red fruit capsules containing red seeds.

Habitat & cultivation Native to tropical forests in the Americas and the Caribbean, annatto is widely cultivated in similar climatic zones, notably in India. Seeds are collected as the fruit splits open.

Parts used Seeds, leaves, root.

Constituents Annatto seed pulp (not the husk) contains very high levels of carotenoids, notably bixin, and B-carotene. These are bright yellow pigments responsible for the coloring action of the seeds. Carotenoids are generally beneficial for eyesight.

History & folklore In tropical South America, the brilliant red pigment in the seed pulp has traditionally been used in body painting. Annatto dye is also used as a colorant for margarine and cheese.

Medicinal actions & uses In the Caribbean, annatto leaves and roots are used to make an astringent infusion that is taken to treat fever, epilepsy, and dysentery. The infusion is also taken as an aphrodisiac. The leaves alone make an infusion that is used as a gargle. The seed pulp reduces the severity of blistering when applied immediately to burns. Taken internally, the seed pulp acts as a general antidote for poisoning.

Borago officinalis (Boraginaceae)

Borage

Description Hairy annual growing to 2 ft (60 cm). Has a pulpy stem, large basal leaves, and attractive blue flowers in summer.

Habitat & cultivation Borage is a common Mediterranean weed thought to originate from southern Spain and Morocco. Often grown as a garden herb, it is also extensively cultivated for its seed oil.

Parts used Aerial parts, flowers, seed oil.

Constituents Borage contains mucilage, tannins, and pyrrolizidine alkaloids, which in isolation are toxic to the liver. The seeds contain up to 24% gamma-linolenic acid.

History & folklore The herbalist John Gerard, writing in 1597, extols borage's virtues, "A syrup made of the flowers of borage comforteth the heart, purgeth melancholy, and quieteth the phreneticke or lunaticke person." Gerard also quotes the old saying, "I, Borage, bring always courage."

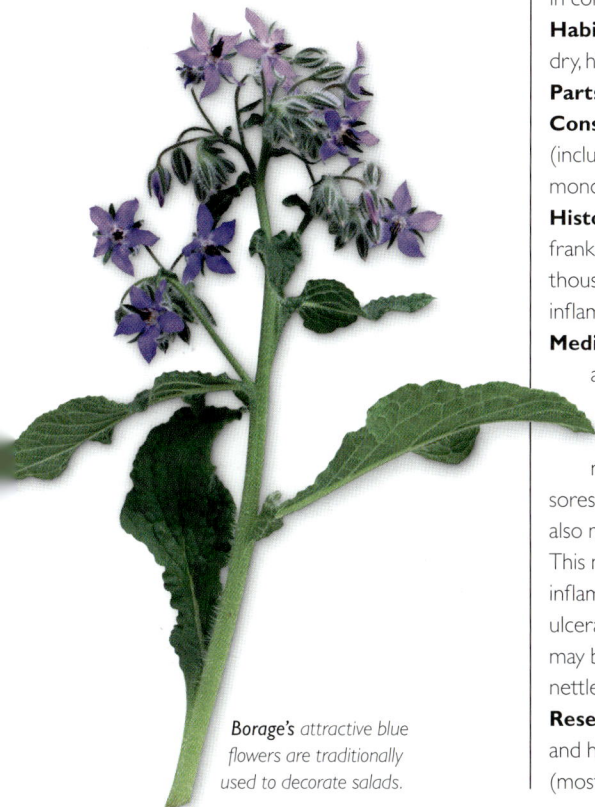

Borage's attractive blue flowers are traditionally used to decorate salads.

Medicinal actions & uses With its high mucilage content, borage is a demulcent herb traditionally used to soothe respiratory problems. Its emollient qualities make it helpful for sore and inflamed skin—prepared either as freshly squeezed juice, in a poultice, or as an infusion. The flowers encourage sweating and the leaves are diuretic. The seed oil is particularly rich in polyunsaturated fats, and is superior in this respect to evening primrose oil (*Oenothera biennis*, p. 241). Borage seed oil is used to treat premenstrual complaints, rheumatic problems, eczema, and other chronic skin conditions.

Cautions Due to the presence of toxic pyrrolizidine alkaloids, there is uncertainty over borage's safety as a medicine. It is subject to legal restrictions in some countries and should not be taken internally. These restrictions and cautions do not apply to borage seed oil.

Boswellia serrata (Burseraceae)

Boswellia,
Indian olibanum, *sallaki* (Sanskrit)

Description Deciduous tree, growing to about 49 ft (15 m), with pale papery bark, compound leaves, and clusters of small white flowers. The gum resin exudes from the bark and is transparent gold in color.

Habitat & cultivation Boswellia grows in dry, hilly regions of central and northern India.

Parts used Gum resin, bark.

Constituents Boswellia contains triterpene acids (including beta-boswellic acid), essential oil, terpenols, monosaccharides, uronic acids, sterols, and tannins.

History & folklore Boswellia, a close relative of frankincense (*B. sacra*), has been used for many thousands of years as an astringent and anti-inflammatory.

Medicinal actions & uses Boswellia makes an effective mouthwash and gargle, the antiseptic and astringent resin helping to heal and tighten inflamed mucous membranes. Sore throat, laryngitis, canker sores, and gum disease will all benefit. Boswellia is also markedly anti-inflammatory and anti-arthritic. This makes it potentially useful in chronic inflammatory diseases such as rheumatoid arthritis, ulcerative colitis, and psoriasis. Other conditions that may benefit include gout, asthma, hay fever, and nettle rash.

Research Research into Boswellia is ongoing and has expanded in recent years. Clinical trials (mostly in India and Germany) indicate that

Boswellia counteracts inflammation in conditions such as arthritis and inflammatory bowel disease. The majority of trials noted that symptoms such as pain, stiffness, and poor grip strength all improved. There is increasing evidence that Boswellia has marked pain-relieving activity, and that it promotes stable blood glucose levels in people with type 2 diabetes.

Brassica oleracea var. *capitata* (Brassicaceae)

Cabbage

Description Biennial or perennial herb growing to 8 ft (2.5 m). Has a thick stem, gray leaves, and 4-petaled yellow flowers. Within the first year, it produces a greatly enlarged terminal bud that develops into the familiar cabbage head in late summer.

Habitat & cultivation Wild cabbage is native to coasts of the English Channel and the Mediterranean. Cultivated varieties are produced worldwide as a vegetable.

Parts used Leaves.

Constituents Cabbage contains glucosinolates, polyphenols, and a range of vitamins. It has anticancer, antioxidant, anti-inflammatory and cardioprotective effects.

History & folklore The wholesome cabbage is one of the oldest vegetables. According to Greek myth, the plant sprang into existence from the perspiration of Zeus. In a Greek ritual, cabbage was given to expectant mothers shortly before birth in order to establish good breast-milk production. The Romans used cabbage as an antidote, especially to alcohol, believing it countered intoxication and prevented or reduced a hangover. They also used cabbage leaves to cleanse infected wounds. It is thought to have been cultivated in Britain from around 500 CE. One traditional method of making a cabbage poultice, still used today, is to cut out the thick midrib of a leaf and iron it, placing it while still hot on the area to be treated.

Medicinal actions & uses Cabbage's best-known medicinal use is as a poultice—the leaves of the wild or cultivated plant are blanched, crushed, or chopped, and applied to swellings, tumors, and painful joints. Wild cabbage leaves eaten raw or cooked aid digestion and the breakdown of toxins in the liver—so the Romans' eating it to ease a hangover was in fact quite justified. Cabbage is also detoxifying and helpful in the long-term treatment of arthritis. The high vitamin C content of cabbage has made it useful in the prevention of scurvy.

Caution A cabbage poultice may cause blisters if left on for several hours.

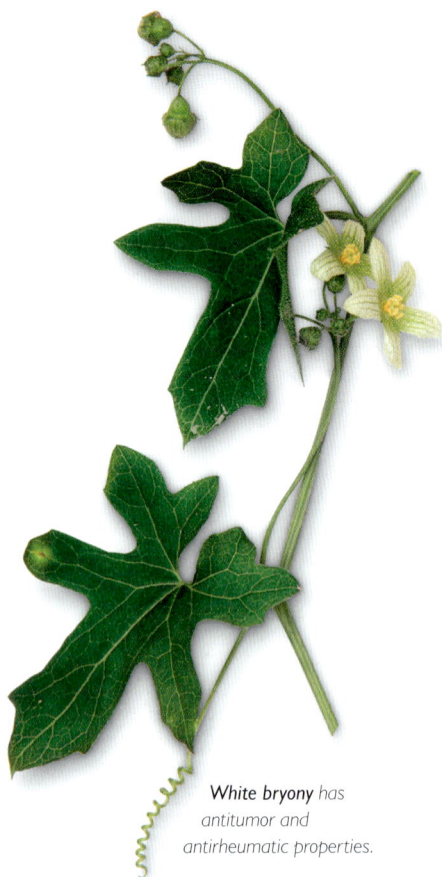

White bryony has antitumor and antirheumatic properties.

Bryonia dioica syn. *b. cretica* subsp. *dioica* (Cucurbitaceae)

White bryony

Description Perennial climbing vine with fleshy taproot up to 6 in (15 cm) thick. Straggling stem with tendrils, greenish flowers, and red berries.

Habitat & cultivation White bryony is native to southern England and parts of Europe. The root is dug up in the fall.

Part Used Root.

Constituents White bryony contains cucurbitacins, glycosides, volatile oil, and tannins. The cucurbitacins kill cells and so act on tumors.

History & folklore From prehistory to the Middle Ages, the thick roots of white bryony were cut into a human shape as a substitute (or a counterfeit) for mandrake root (*Mandragora officinarum*, p. 238), which was believed to afford magical protection. The Greek physician Dioscorides (1st century CE) reports that the leaves, fruit, and root of white bryony were applied to gangrenous wounds. In medieval England, the plant was used to treat leprosy.

Medicinal actions & uses A powerful cathartic and purgative, bryony is used with great caution in herbal medicine today. It is principally prescribed for painful rheumatic conditions. It may be taken internally, or applied as a counterirritant, causing swelling and increased blood flow to the area. White bryony is also given for other inflammatory conditions such as duodenal ulcers, asthma, bronchitis, and pleurisy, and may be used to reduce high blood pressure. The whole herb has antiviral activity and research is now suggesting that it acts as an adaptogen—helping the body to adapt more effectively to stress and strain.

Related species *B. alba* is used in homeopathic medicine. Black bryony (*Tamus communis*) is an unrelated plant with approximately similar uses.

Cautions Bryony is a toxic plant. Use only under professional supervision. Do not take during pregnancy.

Butea monosperma (Fabaceae)

Palas,
Flame of the forest, bengal kino

Description Deciduous tree growing to 49 ft (15 m). Has 3-lobed leaves and large orange-red flowers in clusters.

Habitat & cultivation *Palas* is native to India and Southeast Asia. It grows in forests and in open areas to altitudes of 3,900 ft (1,200 m).

Parts used Bark, flowers, leaves, gum, and seeds.

Constituents All parts of the tree except the seeds contain tannins.

Medicinal actions & uses The gum that oozes from incisions made in *palas* bark is known as Bengal kino. Mildly astringent, it is used as a substitute for the kino derived from bastard teak (*Pterocarpus marsupium*). Bengal kino is taken as a decoction or a tincture for acid indigestion, diarrhea, and dysentery, and used as a gargle for sore throats and as a douche for vaginitis. Early research suggests that the leaves and bark have the potential to treat diabetes, and that the leaves exert a beneficial action on diarrhea.

Caution Do not take during pregnancy.

Caesalpinia bonduc (Caesalpiniaceae)

Nicker nut

Description Thorny bush growing to 30 ft (9 m), with spiny compound leaves, yellow flowers in dense clusters, and prickly pods containing yellow seeds (nuts).

Habitat & cultivation Nicker nut is pan-tropical, common in both tropical Asia and Africa. Its seeds are gathered when ripe.

Parts used Seeds.

Constituents The seeds contain isoflavonoids, diterpenes, a bitter principle, and a fixed oil (20%) rich in linoleic acid (68%).

Medicinal actions & uses Nicker seeds are used to treat fevers and are taken as a tonic and aphrodisiac. In India, they are often mixed with black pepper (*Piper nigrum*, p. 258) for medicinal use. The seeds are also taken for inflammatory conditions such as arthritis. Roasted nicker seeds are used in the treatment of diabetes.

Related species A decoction of the bark of the Caribbean *C. bahamensis* is used for liver and kidney infections, and a decoction of the wood is used for diabetes. An infusion of the leaves of *C. pulcherrima* (native to Asia and Africa) is taken for liver problems and mouth ulcers.

Calluna vulgaris (Ericaceae)

Heather, Ling

Description Small, branched shrub growing to 2 ft (60 cm). Has tiny leaves and white or pink to pale-purple flowers growing on spikes.

Habitat & cultivation Heather grows in temperate regions of the northern hemisphere.

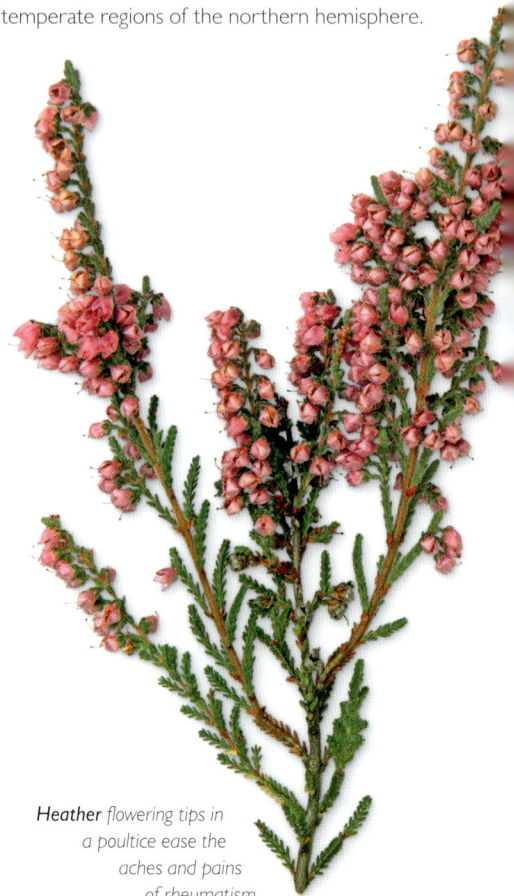

Heather flowering tips in a poultice ease the aches and pains of rheumatism.

It is found on heaths, moors, bogs, and in open woods. The herb is gathered when in flower in late summer.

Parts used Flowering tips.

Constituents Heather contains phenolic compounds, including chlorogenic acid, the hydroquinone, arbutin, flavonoids such as rutin, and tannins.

History & folklore If the "*erica*" that Dioscorides discusses in his 1st century CE *Materia Medica* is indeed heather, as has been surmised, then the flowering tips were used in classical times to treat snake bite. Galen (131–200 CE) wrote of the plant's ability to induce sweating. The rootstock of heather is made into musical pipes, the foliage provides mattress stuffing, and the flowers produce a delicate honey. White heather is considered very lucky, especially in Scotland.

Medicinal actions & uses Heather is a good urinary antiseptic and diuretic, disinfecting the urinary tract and mildly increasing urine production. Besides its role in treating cystitis and inflammatory bladder conditions, heather has been used to treat kidney and bladder stones. Cleansing and detoxifying, it is helpful for rheumatism, arthritis, and gout. A hot poultice of heather tips is a traditional remedy for chilblains and rheumatism.

Research A 2020 scientific paper on heather concluded that the herb "had anti-inflammatory, antimicrobial, anxiolytic, stress-protective, anti-anxiety and antidepressant effects."

Camellia sinensis syn. *Thea sinensis* (Theaceae)

Tea

Description Evergreen shrub clipped to 5 ft (1.5 m) in cultivation, with leathery, dark green leaves and fragrant white flowers.

Habitat & cultivation Cultivated principally in India, Sri Lanka, and China, tea has been grown since the earliest times.

Parts used Leaves, buds.

Constituents Tea contains xanthines, caffeine (1–5%), theobromine, tannins including polyphenols, flavonoids, fats, and vitamin C. Green tea contains significant levels of catechins, a polyphenol compound; black tea has lower levels, due to polymerization during the fermentation process.

History & folklore In China and Japan many rituals have developed around tea drinking. Significantly it is mostly green tea that is drunk in this way.

Medicinal actions & uses Due to its astringency, tea is useful in digestive infections, helping to tighten up the mucous membranes of the gut and reduce looseness. A strong brew of tea may be used to

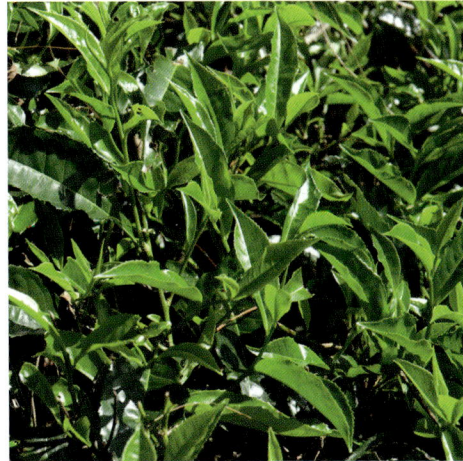

Tea leaves are picked throughout the year and used both as a beverage and medicinally.

soothe irritated eyelids, insect stings, swellings, and sunburn, and in an emergency, if nothing better is on hand, tea makes a serviceable treatment for minor burns. In Ayurvedic medicine tea is considered astringent and a nerve tonic. The caffeine in tea may help to relieve headaches, though less effectively than coffee (*Coffea arabica*, p. 196). In light of research, green tea is recognized as being a much healthier drink than black tea.

Research Green tea's strong antioxidant activity is due to polyphenols, which give the leaf potential as a cancer preventative. The high intake of green tea in China and Japan is thought to be partly responsible for the low incidence of cancer in these countries. Clinical trials indicate that green tea may help to promote weight loss and treat hepatitis, and there is the suggestion that it helps to prevent tooth decay. A recent clinical trial indicated that green tea has a genoprotective action, helping to prevent degenerative changes within the body, and potentially slowing the aging process. A 2013 clinical trial found that green tea extract taken by women for 4 months successfully shrank uterine fibroids.

Cananga odorata syn. *Canangium odoratum* (Annonaceae)

Ylang-ylang

Description Evergreen tree growing to 80 ft (25 m). Has lance-shaped leaves and strongly scented yellow-green flowers.

Habitat & cultivation Native to Indonesia and the Philippines, *ylang-ylang* is cultivated in tropical Asia and Africa.

Parts used Flowers, essential oil.

Constituents The essential oil contains linalool (11–30%), safrole, eugenol, geraniol, and sesquiterpenes (including 15–25% germacrene).

History & folklore The flowers are a traditional adornment in the East. Their scent is thought to have aphrodisiac qualities.

Medicinal actions & uses The flowers and essential oil are sedative, antimicrobial, and antioxidant. The oil has a soothing effect, and its main therapeutic uses are to slow an excessively fast heart rate and to lower blood pressure. With its reputation as an aphrodisiac, *ylang-ylang* may be helpful in treating impotence.

Caution Do not take the essential oil internally without professional supervision.

Canella winterana syn. *C. alba* (Canellaceae)

Canella,
Wild cinnamon

Description White-barked tree growing to 49 ft (15 m). Has elliptical leaves, red flowers, and purple-black berries.

Habitat & cultivation Native to the Caribbean and Florida, canella is found in coastal swamps and scrubland. The bark is collected by gently beating the branches.

Part used Bark.

Constituents Canella contains about 1% volatile oil (including eugenol, alpha-pinene, and caryophyllene), alpha-aldehydes (including canellal), resin, and mannitol.

History & folklore Canella has for a long time been used as a flavoring for tobacco (*Nicotiana tabacum*, p. 247).

Medicinal actions & uses Canella is cytotoxic (kills cells), antifungal, and repels insects. It is also aromatic, stimulant, and antiseptic. Canella is often used in the West Indies and Latin America as a substitute for cinnamon (*Cinnamomum* spp., p. 85). The infusion is drunk for its pleasant flavor and tonic effect (the bark is considered a sexual stimulant). Canella is also used for stomach problems and indigestion.

Capparis spinosa (Capparaceae)

Caper

Description Shrub growing to 3 ft (1 m), with spiny trailing stems, fleshy oval leaves, green buds, large white flowers, and red berries in the fall.

Habitat & cultivation Native to the Mediterranean region, caper thrives in open areas, often growing on stony terrain. The buds are harvested before the flowers open and are pickled for culinary use.

Parts used Root bark, bark, flower buds.

Constituents Caper contains a wide range of active compounds including glucosilinates, phenolics, flavonoids, triterpenoids steroids, and a volatile oil (chiefly docosane).

History & folklore Though much favored as a piquant food by the ancient Greeks, capers were said to disagree with the stomach. They remain a popular condiment to this day.

Medicinal actions & uses The unopened flower buds are laxative and, if prepared correctly with vinegar, are thought to ease stomach pain. The bark is bitter and diuretic and can be taken immediately before meals to increase the appetite. The root bark is purifying and stops internal bleeding. It is used to treat skin conditions, capillary weakness, and easy bruising, and is also used in cosmetic preparations. A decoction of the plant is used to treat yeast and vaginal infections such as candidiasis.

Related species A decoction of the North American *C. cynophallophora* is taken to encourage the onset of menstruation, and is used as a gargle for throat infections.

Cautions Do not take during pregnancy, or if you have kidney stones.

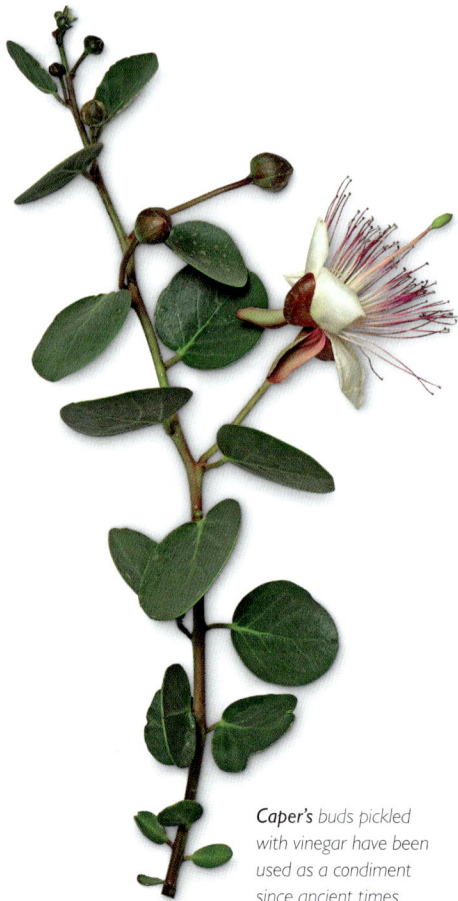

Caper's buds pickled with vinegar have been used as a condiment since ancient times.

Capsella bursa-pastoris syn. *Thlaspi bursa-pastoris* (Brassicaceae)

Shepherd's purse

Description Annual or biennial with an erect stem, rosette of basal leaves, 4-petaled white flowers, and heart-shaped seed pods.

Habitat & cultivation Thought to be native to Europe and Asia, shepherd's purse is now found throughout most temperate regions, and grows profusely as a weed. It is harvested throughout the year.

Parts used Aerial parts.

Constituents Contains flavonoids, polypeptides, choline, acetylcholine, histamine, and tyramine.

History & folklore This herb's name derives from the appearance of the seed pods, which resemble heart-shaped purses. During the World War I, when the standard herbal medicines for staunching blood—goldenseal (*Hydrastis canadensis*, p. 109) and ergot (*Claviceps purpurea*)—were unobtainable in Britain, shepherd's purse was used as an alternative.

Medicinal actions & uses One of the best remedies for preventing or arresting hemorrhage, shepherd's purse has long been a specific treatment for heavy uterine bleeding. While weaker-acting in this respect than ergot, shepherd's purse has none of ergot's toxicity and is better tolerated by the body. It may be used for bleeding of all kinds—from nosebleeds to blood in the urine. An astringent herb, it disinfects the urinary tract in cases of cystitis, and is taken for diarrhea. It is used in Chinese medicine to treat dysentery and eye problems.

Research Reports suggest that the plant is anti-inflammatory and reduces fever.

Caution Do not take during pregnancy.

Self-help use Heavy menstrual bleeding, p. 325.

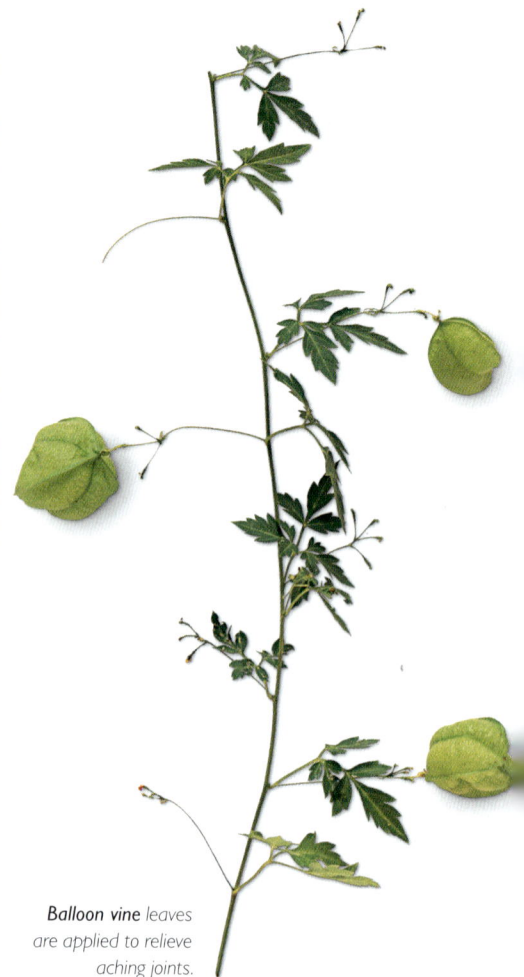

Cardiospermum sp. (Sapindaceae)

Balloon vine

Description Deciduous perennial climbers growing to 10 ft (3 m), with compound leaves, small white flowers, and black seeds.

Habitat & cultivation Balloon vine is found growing in tropical regions around the world.

Parts used Root, leaves, seeds.

Constituents Most *Cardiospermum* species contain cyanogenic glycosides.

History & folklore Indigenous Amazonians string balloon vine seeds into armbands that are worn to ward off snakes.

Medicinal actions & uses In Indian herbal medicine, balloon vine root is used to bring on

Balloon vine leaves are applied to relieve aching joints.

---

delayed menstruation and to relieve backache and arthritis. The leaves stimulate local circulation and are applied to painful joints to help speed the clearing of toxins. The seeds are also thought to help in the treatment of arthritis. The plant as a whole has sedative properties.

Caution Do not take during pregnancy.

Carica papaya (Caricaceae)

Papaya

Description Herbaceous tree growing very rapidly to 26 ft (8 m). Has segmented leaves, yellow flowers, and large, black-seeded yellow to orange fruits weighing up to 11 lb (5 kg).

Habitat & cultivation Native to the tropical Americas, papaya is now cultivated in tropical regions throughout the world.

Parts used Fruit, latex, leaves, flowers, seeds.

Constituents The fruit contains proteolytic enzymes (papain and chymopapain), and traces of an alkaloid, carpaine. Papain, which is found in the milky white latex that flows from incisions in the unripe fruit, is a protein-dissolving enzyme that aids digestion.

History & folklore Papaya juice, shoots, and latex were used in Mayan herbal medicine. In tropical Latin America, the leaves are used as a meat tenderizer.

Medicinal actions & uses Papaya's main medicinal use is as a digestive agent. The leaves and the fruit can both be used (the unripe fruit is especially effective). The latex from the trunk of the tree is applied externally to speed the healing of wounds, ulcers, boils, warts, and cancerous tumors. The seeds are used as a gentle purgative for worms. The latex has a similar but more violent effect. The flowers may be taken in an infusion to induce menstruation, and a decoction of the ripe fruit is helpful for treating persistent diarrhea and dysentery in children. The ripe fruit is mildly laxative and the leaves are used to dress wounds.

Carthamus tinctorius (Asteraceae)

Safflower, *Hong hua* (Chinese)

Description Annual herb growing to 3 ft (90 cm). Has long spiny leaves with 6 oblong-oval leaflets, and groups of yellow flowers arising from the leaf axils.

Habitat & cultivation Thought to be native to Iran and northwestern India, this herb is also found in North America and the Far East. It grows on waste ground and is gathered in summer.

Parts used Flowers, seeds, seed oil.

Constituents Safflower contains lignans, polysaccharides and a volatile oil. The seeds contain a fixed oil, up to 80% linoleic acid.

History & folklore In 19th century North American herbal medicine, safflower was used to induce sweating, to promote the onset of a menstrual period, and as a treatment for measles. Safflower flowers are falsely sold as saffron (*Crocus sativus*, p. 93).

Medicinal actions & uses In Chinese herbal medicine, the flowers are given to stimulate menstruation and to relieve abdominal pain. The flowers are also used to cleanse and heal wounds and sores and to treat measles. In the Anglo-American herbal tradition, the flowers are given as a treatment for fever and skin rashes. The unpurified seed oil is purgative.

Research Chinese research indicates that safflower flowers can reduce coronary artery disease, and lower cholesterol levels. Safflower contains a polysaccharide that has been shown to stimulate immune function in mice. Safflower oil also lowers cholesterol levels.

Caution Do not take the flowers or seeds during pregnancy (seed oil is safe).

Carum carvi (Apiaceae)

Caraway

Description Aromatic annual growing to 2 ft (60 cm). Has ridged stem, feathery leaves, and umbels of white flowers in midsummer. Exploding capsules each contain 2 small narrow seeds.

Habitat & cultivation Caraway grows wild in Europe, North Africa, and Asia. It prefers sunny sites up to 6,600 ft (2,000 m) above sea level. It is cultivated in Europe, Russia, North Africa, and the US, and the seeds are harvested ripe in late summer.

Parts used Seeds, essential oil.

Constituents Caraway contains a volatile oil high in carvone (about 50%) and limonene. It also contains a fixed oil, flavonoids, polysaccharides, proteins, and furanocoumarins.

History & folklore Caraway seed is "conducive to all the cold griefs of the head and stomach … and has a moderate quality whereby it breaketh wind, and provoketh urine" (Nicholas Culpeper, *The*

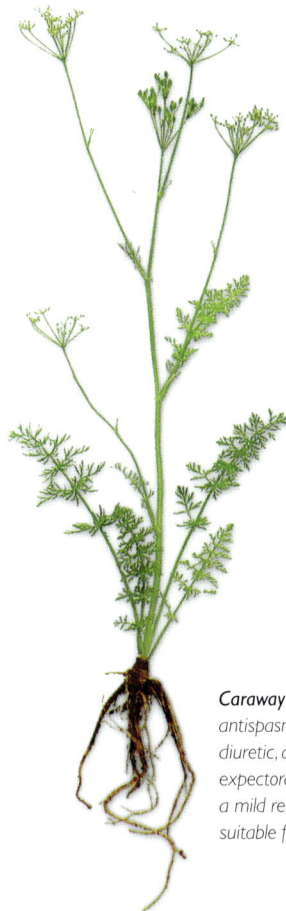

Caraway is antispasmodic, diuretic, and expectorant. It is a mild remedy, suitable for children.

English Physitian, 1652). The seeds are commonly used in cooking.

Medicinal actions & uses Caraway is similar in action to anise (*Pimpinella anisum*, p. 256) and fennel (*Foeniculum vulgare*, p. 212). Being antispasmodic, the seeds soothe the digestive tract, acting directly on the intestinal muscles to relieve colic and cramps as well as bloating and flatulence. They sweeten the breath, improve appetite, counter heart irregularity caused by excess digestive gas, and ease cramping period pain. In addition, the seeds are expectorant and tonic and are frequently used in bronchitis and cough remedies, especially those for children. Caraway has a reputation for increasing breast-milk production. The diluted essential oil is useful for scabies.

Research In a German clinical trial (1999), patients with dyspepsia were given a combination of peppermint and caraway essential oils. Overall, patients experienced a significant reduction in symptoms.

Caution Do not use the essential oil internally except under professional supervision.

Castanea sativa (Fagaceae)

Sweet chestnut

Description Deciduous tree growing to a height of 100 ft (30 m). Has smooth silver-gray bark, lance-shaped dark green leaves, male and female catkins, and spiny yellow-green seed cases containing 2–3 glossy brown nuts.

Habitat & cultivation Native to the Mediterranean, Asia Minor, and the Caucasus, sweet chestnut grows freely across Europe, including Britain. It is cultivated for its timber and for its nuts, which are collected in the fall.

Parts used Leaves, bark.

Constituents Sweet chestnut contains tannins, plastoquinones, and mucilage.

History & folklore Tradition has it that the sweet chestnut tree was carried from Turkey to Sardinia and from there it subsequently spread through Europe, arriving in Britain with the Romans. The nuts are a nutritious foodstuff that can be roasted, candied, or made into a flour. The flowers are sometimes added to blends of aromatic tobaccos.

Medicinal actions & uses An infusion of sweet chestnut leaves is taken to treat whooping cough, bronchitis and bronchial congestion. The preparation tightens the mucous membranes and inhibits racking coughs. A decoction of leaves or bark is also valuable as a gargle for sore throats, and may be taken for diarrhea. The leaves are used in the treatment of rheumatic conditions, to ease lower back pain and also to relieve stiff joints or muscles.

Research Recent laboratory research using a sweet chestnut bark extract suggests that the bark has significant anti-inflammatory and cardioprotective properties.

Related species The Mohican people in North America used an infusion obtained from American chestnut leaves (*C. dentata*) to treat whooping cough. In his *Natural History of North Carolina* (1737), John Brickell reports that the "leaves or bark of the tree boiled in wine are good against the bloody flux [excessive bleeding caused by amoebic dysentery]."

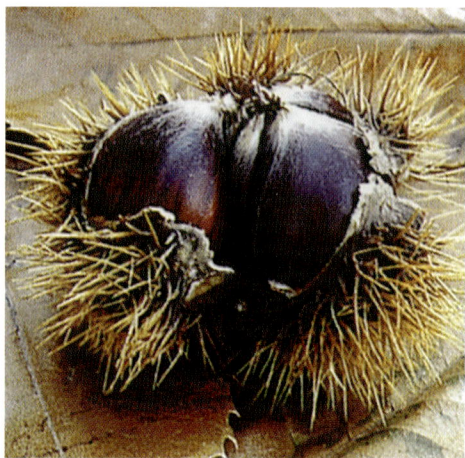

Sweet chestnut nuts are a nutritious food and the leaves are useful for treating coughs.

Catalpa bignonioides (Bignoniaceae)

Indian bean tree, Catalpa

Description Deciduous tree growing to 65 ft (20 m). Has large oval leaves in whorls of 3, white flowers in conical clusters, and long thin fruits (bean pods).

Habitat & cultivation Native to the southeastern US, this tree is often planted in gardens in southern and western Europe.

Parts used Bark, fruit.

Constituents The bark contains catalpin and protocatechuic acids.

History & folklore Indian bean tree bark was formerly used as a substitute for quinine in the treatment of malaria.

Medicinal actions & uses The mildly sedative and narcotic bark is used to treat asthma, whooping cough and other spasmodic coughs in children. The distilled water of the fruit, in combination with herbs commonly used to treat eye problems, such as eyebright (*Euphrasia officinalis*, p. 209) and rue (*Ruta*

graveolens, p. 265), makes an effective eyewash for conjunctivitis and other eye infections.

Caution Never use the roots in any form as they are highly poisonous.

Catha edulis (Celastraceae)

Khat, Catha

Description Tree growing to 49 ft (15 m). Has reddish twigs, oval leathery leaves, and small yellow or white flowers.

Habitat & cultivation Native to the Middle East and the Horn of Africa, khat prefers grassland and arid conditions. It is cultivated in Ethiopia, Somalia, East Africa, and the Arabian peninsula.

Parts used Leaves, twigs.

Constituents Khat contains alkaloids similar to those in *Ephedra* species—norpseudoephedrine (up to 1%) and ephedrine, tannins, and a volatile oil. Ephedrine-type alkaloids strongly stimulate the central nervous system, are anti-allergenic, and suppress the appetite.

History & folklore Khat is taken in some African and Middle Eastern countries as a stimulant, tonic, and appetite suppressant. Infused, smoked, or chewed, khat produces an effect somewhat similar to that of coca leaves (*Erythroxylum coca*, p. 211). Whether khat is addictive is unclear, but withdrawal can produce lethargy.

Medicinal actions & uses Mainly used as a social drug, khat is also chewed fresh or taken in an infusion to treat ailments such as malaria. In Africa, it is taken in old age, stimulating and improving mental function. Khat is used in Germany to counter obesity.

Cautions Khat may cause headaches, raised blood pressure, and general overstimulation if used more than a few weeks at a time. Do not take during pregnancy or while breastfeeding.

Caulophyllum thalictroides (Berberidaceae)

Blue cohosh

Description Upright perennial growing to 3 ft (1 m) with large, 3-lobed leaves, yellow to purple flowers, and striking blue berries.

Habitat & cultivation Blue Cohosh grows wild in much of eastern North America from Manitoba to Alabama, preferring woodland valleys and damp, north-facing slopes. It is mainly wild-harvested but is also cultivated commercially.

Parts used The root and rhizome.

Constituents Blue cohosh contains alkaloids, steroidal saponins, and sterols.

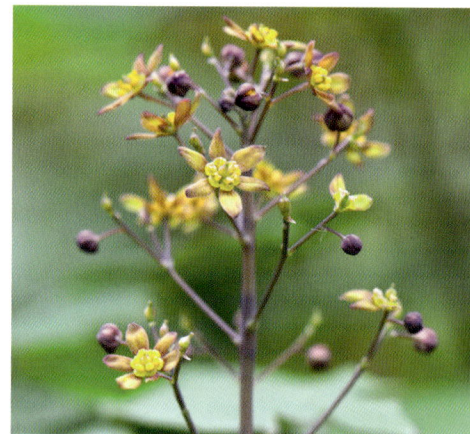

Blue cohosh is mainly wild-harvested but is also cultivated commercially.

History & folklore "Cohosh" is an Algonquin name, and blue cohosh was a popular herb with many Indigenous peoples. Though it was taken by both sexes to treat genitourinary problems, it was primarily considered a women's herb.

Medicinal actions & uses Current medicinal uses of blue cohosh are not that different from the past—the root is still valued as a women's remedy. It is often prescribed as a uterine tonic, bringing relief from uterine and ovarian pain, while regulating to improve menstrual blood flow. The herb also has anti-inflammatory activity and may be used in treatments for arthritic and rheumatic conditions.

Cautions Only take under professional supervision. Do not take during pregnancy or while breastfeeding. The plant can cause contact dermatitis.

Cedrus sp. (Pinaceae)

Cedar

Description Cedar of Lebanon (*C. libani*) is a majestic flat-topped tree growing to 130 ft (40 m). It has dark green needlelike leaves and oval cones. African cedar (*C. atlantica*) grows to 115 ft (35 m).

Habitat & cultivation Cedar of Lebanon is native to mountain forests of Lebanon, Israel, and southwest Turkey (Türkiye). Atlas cedar is native to the Atlas Mountains of Morocco, growing from 4,600–7,200 ft (1,400–2,200 m) above sea level.

Parts used Leaves, wood, essential oil.

Constituents The essential oil of Atlas cedar wood contains mainly alpha-pinene (up to 79%).

History & folklore Cedar of Lebanon is thought to have been used in building Solomon's Temple and the Hanging Gardens of Babylon. The oil has been used for thousands of years in incense, perfumes, and embalming.

Medicinal actions & uses Cedar of Lebanon is antiseptic and expectorant, acting to disinfect the respiratory tract. Cedarwood essential oil has been used for thousands of years for perfumes and for embalming. It is most commonly distilled from Atlas cedar and eastern red cedar (*Juniperus virginicus*). The oil is strongly antiseptic, astringent, diuretic, expectorant, and sedative. Diluted and massaged into the skin, it treats congestion, chest infections, and cystitis. It is used to treat skin wounds and ulcers.

Caution Do not take essential oil of cedar internally except under professional supervision.

Celtis australis (Ulmaceae)

European nettle tree

Description Dome-shaped deciduous tree growing to 80 ft (25 m). Has lance-shaped leaves, green flowers, and small round purple-black fruits.

Habitat & cultivation Native to the Mediterranean region and southwestern Asia, European nettle tree is also planted as a border tree in Italy and France.

Parts used Leaves, fruit.

Constituents European nettle tree contains tannins and mucilage.

Medicinal actions & uses Due to their astringent properties, both the leaves and the fruit of European nettle tree may be taken as a decoction to reduce heavy menstrual and intermenstrual uterine bleeding. The fruit and leaves may be used to astringe the mucous membranes of the gut in peptic ulcers, diarrhea, and dysentery.

Centaurea cyanus (Asteraceae)

Cornflower

Description Annual or biennial plant growing to 3 ft (90 cm). Has a multi-branched stem, a basal rosette of leaves, and sky-blue flowers in summer.

Habitat & cultivation Native to the East, cornflower grows wild in all temperate regions, often in cornfields. The flowers are gathered just after they open.

Parts used Flowers, seeds, leaves.

Constituents Cornflower contains flavonoids, including anthocyanins, sesquiterpene lactones (including cnicin), acetylenes, and coumarins. Cnicin is slightly antibiotic.

History & folklore Cornflower's medicinal properties were first mentioned in the 12th-century writings of Hildegard of Bingen. Later, the doctor Pierandrea Mattioli (1501–1577) recommended it on the basis of the Doctrine of Signatures, which held that a plant's appearance indicated the ailments it would cure. Cornflower's deep blue color symbolized healthy eyes, and for this reason it became a treatment for eye ailments. (In France, the plant is called *casse-lunette*, or "break glasses.")

Medicinal actions & uses Cornflower is still used in French herbal medicine as a remedy for the eyes (the strained infusion is used as an eyewash, and the petals applied as a poultice), but opinion differs as to its efficacy. The petals are also taken as a bitter tonic and stimulant, improving digestion and possibly supporting the liver as well as improving resistance to infection. The seeds have been used as a mild laxative for children. A decoction of the leaves is used to treat rheumatic complaints.

Research A Romanian research paper (2021) compared levels of anthocyanins—the active constituents most responsible for the cornflower's healing effects—in blue-colored and in red colored flowers. Surprisingly, the red flowers had 4–5 times more anthocyanins than the blue flowers. Contrary to traditional use, the paper concluded that the red flowers had greater therapeutic activity.

Related species Greater knapweed (*C. scabiosa*) formed part of the medieval *salve*, an ointment applied to heal wounds and to treat skin infections.

Self-help use Conjunctivitis, p. 320.

Cephaelis ipecacuanha (Rubiaceae)

Ipecac

Description Small shrub with a slender stem growing to 1 ft (30 cm). Has a few oblong leaves, small white flowers, and purple-black berries.

Habitat & cultivation This herb grows mainly in Brazil. Cultivation has been attempted in Southeast Asia with limited success. The root of 3-year-old plants is unearthed when the plant is in flower.

Parts used Root, rhizome.

Constituents Ipecac contains isoquinoline alkaloids, tannins, and glycosides. The alkaloids are expectorant and, at a larger dose, cause vomiting and diarrhea. They are also strongly amoebicidal.

History & folklore Ipecac came to Europe in 1672, and achieved fame as a cure for dysentery. But the cure was not without controversy. It appeared to work well in some cases but to have no effect in others. Now it is possible to see why. There are two types of dysentery—amoebic and bacillary. While the herb is strongly amoebicidal, it has little effect against bacilli.

Medicinal actions & uses Though a highly effective emetic (even moderate doses of ipecac will stimulate vomiting until the contents of the stomach are cleared), it is now rarely used in conventional medicine as safer substitutes have been developed. Ipecac continues to be a common ingredient in patent over-the-counter cough medicines, as its strong expectorant action helps to clear phlegm and ease irritable coughs. It is used in the treatment of bronchitis and whooping cough. Ipecac is also still used for gastroenteritis and amoebic dysentery.

Cautions Do not use the root or rhizome. Take formulations containing ipecac carefully and only as instructed on the label. Several deaths have resulted from overdose.

Ceratonia siliqua (Fabaceae)

Carob

Description Evergreen tree growing to a height of 30 ft (10 m). Has compound leaves, green flowers, and large violet-brown fruit (bean pods).

Habitat & cultivation Native to southeastern Europe, western Asia, and North Africa, carob flourishes in poor soil in warm temperate climates; it is said to "want sight of the sea." It is cultivated for its fruit, and harvested in late summer or fall.

Parts used Fruit, bark.

Constituents The fruit contains up to 70% sugars, fats, starch, proteins, vitamins, and tannins.

History & folklore In ancient Egypt, carob pods were combined with porridge, honey, and wax as a remedy for diarrhea. They also featured in recipes for expelling worms, and treating poor eyesight and eye infections. In the ancient Mediterranean world, carob seeds were used to measure gold, silver, and jewels. The word "carat" comes originally from the ancient Greek for carob seed.

Medicinal actions & uses Carob pods are nutritious and, due to their high sugar content, sweet-tasting and mildly laxative. A decoction of the pulp can be used as an antidiarrheal, gently helping to cleanse and relieve irritation within the gut.

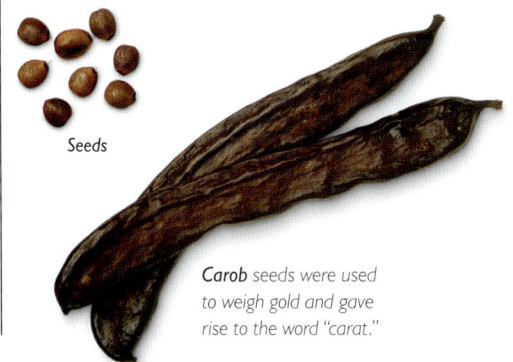

Seeds

Carob seeds were used to weigh gold and gave rise to the word "carat."

Cetraria islandica (Parmeliaceae)

Iceland moss

Description Yellow-green lichen growing in undulating, leathery tufts up to 3 in (8 cm) across.

Habitat & cultivation Iceland moss is native to northern and alpine areas of Europe. It flourishes in sub-Arctic and mountainous regions on rocks and on the bark of trees, especially conifers. It is harvested throughout the year.

Part used Whole plant.

Constituents Iceland moss contains lichen acids (including usnic acid) and about 50% polysaccharides. Usnic acid and the other lichen acids are powerfully antibiotic. The polysaccharides are antiviral.

History & folklore Iceland moss has been used since ancient times as a cough remedy, and has also been used in European folk medicine as a cancer treatment.

Medicinal actions & uses Strongly demulcent, Iceland moss soothes the mucous membranes of the chest, counters congestion, and calms dry and paroxysmal coughs, being particularly helpful as a treatment for elderly people. Iceland moss is also very bitter and, within the gut, has both a demulcent and bitter tonic effect—a combination almost unique in medicinal herbs. It is thus of value in all kinds of chronic digestive problems, for instance irritable bowel syndrome.

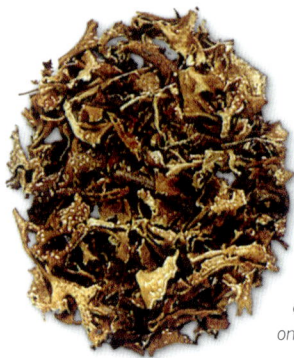

Iceland moss is used to ease coughs and treat congestion. It also has a soothing and bitter tonic effect on the digestive tract.

Chamaelirium lutea (Liliaceae)

Helonias,
False unicorn root

Description Herbaceous perennial growing to 3 ft (1 m) with large, green leaves forming a basal rosette from which emerges a tall spike of green-white flowers.

Habitat & cultivation Native to North America, helonias grows in low, moist, well-drained ground

Helonias root was chewed by Indigenous women to prevent miscarriage.

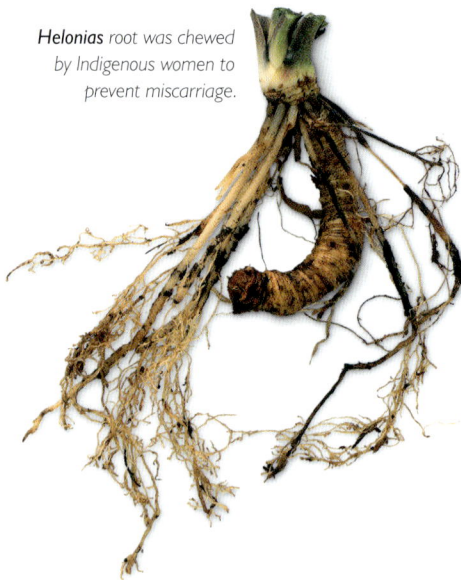

east of the Mississippi river. In view of its rarity in the wild, it is best to use alternative herbs such as black cohosh (*Cimicifuga racemosa*, p. 61) and wild yam (*Dioscorea villosa*, p. 95).

Parts used Rhizome (lifted in the fall).

Constituents Root contains steroidial saponins (up to 9%), including chamaelirin and diosgenin.

History & folklore A traditional Indigenous medicine in North America, Helonias was prized as a woman's herb and used to treat a range of gynecological problems. There is some confusion about its precise use since several herbs share the same (or similar) name.

Medicinal actions & uses In Western herbal medicine, helonias has been valued as a key remedy for conditions affecting the uterus and ovaries. It is thought to have a "normalizing" effect on the female reproductive system. It is thought to regulate the release of hormones by the ovaries and encourage a regular menstrual cycle. It has also been used to treat conditions such as endometriosis, ovarian cysts, and menopausal problems. As it is now an endangered species, other herbs (notably black cohosh) are routinely used in its place.

Caution Do not take during pregnancy.

Chamaemelum nobile syn. *Anthemis nobilis* (Asteraceae)

Roman chamomile

Description Aromatic perennial growing to 20 in (50 cm). Has feathery leaves and daisylike flower heads.

Habitat & cultivation Native to western Europe, Roman chamomile is now cultivated across Europe, and also in other temperate regions. The flowers are harvested as they open in summer.

Parts used Flowers, essential oil.

Constituents Roman chamomile contains up to 1.75% essential oil (including tiglic and angelic acid esters, chamazulene and other sesquiterpene lactones), flavonoids, coumarins, and phenolic acids.

History & folklore Though called Roman chamomile, this herb was not cultivated in Rome until the 16th century, probably arriving there from Britain.

Medicinal actions & uses A remedy for the digestive system, Roman chamomile is often used interchangeably with German chamomile (*Chamomilla recutita*, p. 82). However, an infusion of Roman chamomile has a more pronounced bitter action than its German namesake. It is an excellent treatment for nausea, vomiting, indigestion, and loss of appetite. It is also sedative, antispasmodic, and mildly analgesic, and will relieve colic, cramps, and other cramping pains. By stimulating digestive secretions and relaxing the muscles of the gut, it helps normalize digestive function. Roman chamomile may also be taken for headaches and migraine, even by children. Its marked anti-inflammatory and anti-allergenic properties make it helpful when applied to irritated skin.

Cautions Do not use the essential oil internally except under professional supervision. The essential oil is subject to legal restrictions in some countries.

Chamaenerion angustifolia syn. *Epilobium angustifolium* (Onagraceae)

Rosebay willowherb

Description Perennial growing to 6½ ft (2 m). Has an erect stem, narrow leaves, and long spikes of pink-purple flowers.

Habitat & cultivation This herb is found in Europe and western Asia, and grows in clearings, along roads, and on waste ground. It is picked when in flower in late summer.

Parts used Aerial parts.

Constituents Rosebay willowherb contains flavones and tannins.

History & folklore In Siberia, an alcoholic drink has been made from this herb and the fly agaric mushroom (*Amanita muscaria*).

Medicinal actions & uses Demulcent and astringent, rosebay willowherb treats diarrhea, mucous colitis, and irritable bowel syndrome. It has also been made into an ointment to soothe skin problems in children. Rosebay willowherb is used to treat prostate problems though its close relative the small-flowered willow herb (*Epilobium parviflorum*, p. xxx) is generally considered more beneficial for prostate health.

Cheiranthus cheiri (Brassicaceae)

Wallflower

Description Evergreen perennial growing to 18 in (45 cm). Has lance-shaped leaves and yellow-orange flowers appearing in spring.

Habitat & cultivation Native to southern Europe, wallflower is now found throughout the continent. It grows on cliffs and old walls, and is a common garden plant.

Parts used Leaves, flowers.

Constituents The herb contains cheiranthin and other cardioactive glycosides.

History & folklore In 1735, the Irish herbalist K'Eogh described wallflower thus: "It provokes urination and menstruation and expels a stillborn child, and the afterbirth if a decoction of the dried flowers or a little seed is drunk in wine."

Medicinal actions & uses Although wallflower was formerly used as a diuretic, there was no understanding of its powerful effect on the heart. In small doses it is cardiotonic, supporting a failing heart in a manner similar to foxglove (*Digitalis purpurea*, p. 207). In more than small doses it is toxic, and is

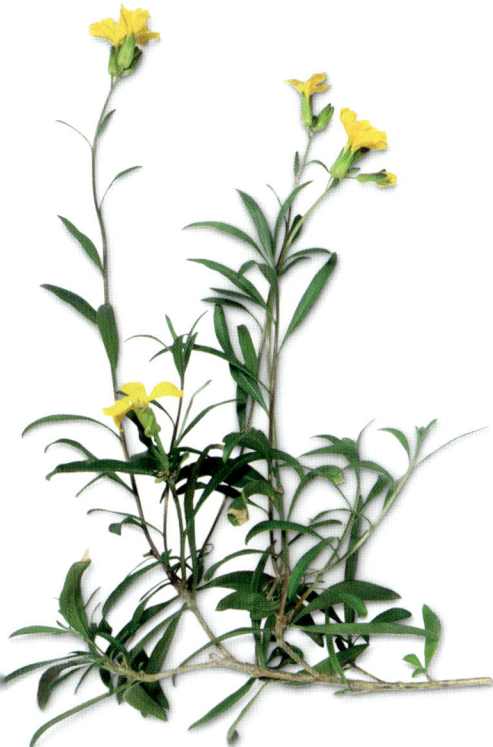

*The Greek physician Dioscorides (1st century CE) used **wallflower** roots to treat gout.*

---

therefore rarely used in herbal medicine.

Cautions Use only under professional supervision. Do not take during pregnancy.

Chelidonium majus (Papaveraceae)

Greater celandine

Description Thin-stemmed perennial herb growing to a height of 3 ft (90 cm). Has indented yellow-green leaflets and 4-petaled flowers, which appear in clusters in late spring.

Habitat & cultivation Native to Europe, western Asia, and North Africa, greater celandine flourishes close to human habitation, preferring open areas, the banks of roadsides, and damp places. The aerial parts of the herb are collected in late spring or early summer.

Parts used Aerial parts, latex.

Constituents Greater celandine contains isoquinoline alkaloids, including allocryptopine, berberine, chelidonine and sparteine. Several of these alkaloids are analgesic. Chelidonine is antispasmodic and also lowers blood pressure. Sparteine, by contrast, raises it.

History & folklore In folk medicine, greater celandine has often been viewed as a cure-all. It has also been used for thousands of years to treat and clear the eyesight, especially cataracts. According to Pliny and Dioscorides (both writing in the 1st century CE), swallows used the latex that flows from cuts in the stems or leaves as a means to sharpen their eyesight. In 1598, Gerard recommended the herb for eye disorders "for it clenseth and consumeth awaie slimie things that cleave about the ball of the eie."

Medicinal actions & uses Greater celandine acts as a mild sedative, relaxing the muscles of the bronchial tubes, intestines, and other organs. In both Western and Chinese herbal traditions, it has been used to treat bronchitis, whooping cough, and asthma. The herb's antispasmodic effect extends to the gallbladder, where it helps to improve bile flow. This would partly account for its use in treating jaundice, gallstones, and gallbladder pain, as well as its longstanding reputation as a detoxifying herb. Greater celandine's sedative action does not, however, extend to the uterus—it causes the muscles of this organ to contract. The herb is applied externally to soothe and encourage the healing of skin conditions such as eczema. The yellow latex of greater celandine is applied to warts, ringworm, and malignant skin tumors, which are slowly broken down by the effect of its protein-dissolving enzymes.

Cautions Use only under professional supervision. Can cause liver damage in rare cases. It is subject to legal restrictions in some countries.

Chelone glabra (Scrophulariaceae)

Balmony

Description Perennial herb growing to 2 ft (60 cm). Has narrow leaves and short spikes of creamy-white to purple double-lipped flowers.

Habitat & cultivation Balmony is native to eastern North America and thrives in habitats such as marshland, wet woodland, and riverbanks. It is harvested when in flower during summer or fall.

Parts used Aerial parts.

Constituents Contains resins and bitters.

History & folklore Balmony's genus name, *Chelone*, means "tortoise" in Greek, referring to the flower head's supposed resemblance to the head of the tortoise.

Medicinal actions & uses A strongly bitter remedy, balmony is principally used to treat gallstones and other gallbladder problems. It stimulates bile flow and has a mildly laxative action. It can be taken to relieve nausea, vomiting, and intestinal colic, and to expel worms. It may also be antidepressant. Balmony is a suitable remedy for children.

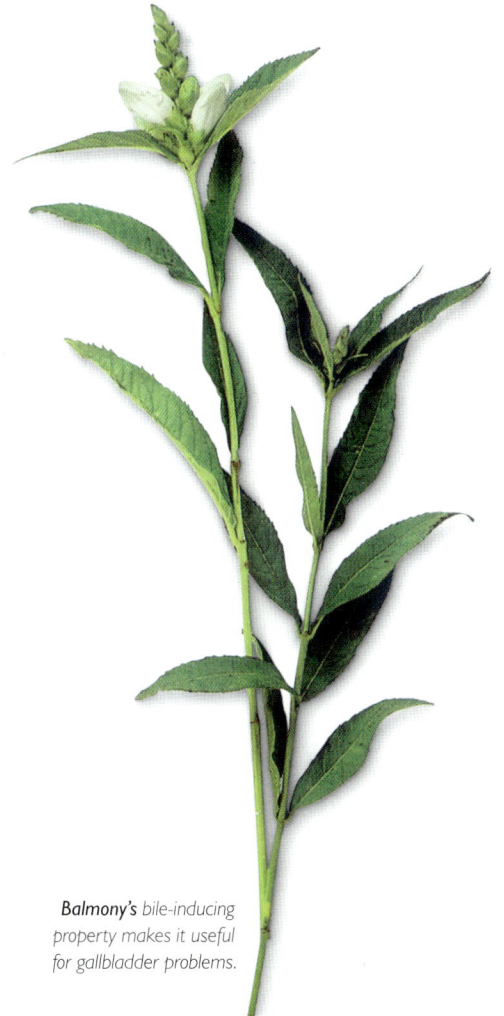

***Balmony's** bile-inducing property makes it useful for gallbladder problems.*

Chenopodium ambrosioides (Chenopodiaceae)

Wormseed

Description Annual herb growing to 3 ft (1 m) with toothed lance-shaped leaves. Yellow-green flowers in round clusters bloom in summer, producing small black seeds in the fall.

Habitat & cultivation Wormseed is native to Central and South America and the Caribbean. It has been extensively cultivated in Maryland, and in China.

Parts used Aerial parts, flowering tops.

Constituents Wormseed contains a volatile oil (up to 90% ascaridol, plus geraniol and methyl salicylate), and triterpenoid saponins. Ascaridol is a powerful worm expellant.

History & folklore An herbal remedy that has been used for centuries, wormseed was used by the Maya in Central America to expel worms. In the eastern US, the herb was similarly employed in the treatment of worms, especially in children. The Catawba people made a poultice from the plant, which they used to detoxify snake bite and other poisonings.

Medicinal actions & uses Wormseed is principally known for its ability to expel worms, especially roundworm and hookworm. It is also used in the Americas as a digestive remedy, the leaves being taken to settle colic and stomach pains. Wormseed's muscle-relaxing action has led to its use in the treatment of spasmodic coughs and asthma. Externally, juice expressed from the whole herb is applied as a wash for hemorrhoids.

Related species Many species of *Chenopodium* are used as foods, and some medicinally. The seeds of *C. rhadinostachyum* are used as food by Aboriginal people in central Australia. Good King Henry (*C. bonus-henricus*), a species that is native to Europe, is both eaten as a vegetable and used medicinally to treat anemia.

Cautions Use only under professional supervision. Wormseed is toxic when taken in overdose. Do not take during pregnancy. The herb is subject to legal restrictions in some countries.

Chenopodium quinoa (Amaranthaceae)

Quinoa

Description An annual herb growing to 10 ft (3 m), with a thick upright stem and lanceolate to triangular leaves. The multiple small green flowers (often petalless), and the seeds, emerge from the main stem.

Habitat and cultivation Native to the Andes, and growing up to 13,000 ft (4,000 m) above sea level, quinoa is thought to originate close to Lake Titicaca on the borders of Bolivia and Peru. A very hardy plant, quinoa prefers a sandy soil and is resistant to cold, salt, and drought. Due to its high food value, it is now cultivated in over 50 countries worldwide, including England, France, Italy, the Netherlands, India, and the US. The seeds are harvested when the leaves have fallen. The seeds contain a bitter tasting saponin which needs to be washed or polished off prior to sale/consumption.

Parts used Seeds

Constituents Quinoa contains 15% protein once dried. As a protein-rich food, it is considered the equivalent of dairy produce, and is a "complete" protein source, containing all 9 essential amino acids. The seeds additionally contain essential fatty acids, polyphenols, sterols, flavonoids, and fiber. The seeds vary in color from white to red, green, and black.

History and folklore Cultivated in the Andes for at least 4,000 years, quinoa was a staple food of the Incas, and its cultivation spread along the Andes into Chile, Ecuador, and Colombia. On his travels in Colombia in 1802, the natural scientist Alexander von Humboldt noted that quinoa was to ancient Andean societies what "wine was to the Greeks, wheat to the Romans, cotton to the Arabs."

Medicinal actions and uses Quinoa is first and foremost a nutritious food crop that contains no gluten, and can be used in place of grains such as rice and wheat. It is mucilaginous, acts as a probiotic, will help soothe acidic digestive symptoms, and may be used as part of a regime to treat gastric ulcers. The seeds slow the absorption of fats and therefore help in maintaining balanced blood cholesterol levels.

Related species Many species of *Chenopodium* are edible. Good King Henry (*Chenopodium bonus-henricus*), a native European plant, can be eaten in much the same way as quinoa. See also Amaranth (*Amaranthus hypochondriacus* p. 170).

Caution Commercially produced quinoa is processed to remove the potentially toxic saponin shell surrounding the seed.

Chimaphila umbellata (Pyrolaceae)

Pipsissewa

Description Evergreen plant with several stems, growing to 8 in (20 cm). Has shiny wedge-shaped leaves and small flat-topped clusters of white flowers tinged with red.

Habitat & cultivation Native to North America, Europe, and Asia, pipsissewa grows in woods and shady places, in sandy soils. The leaves are gathered in summer.

Part used Leaves.

Constituents Pipsissewa contains hydroquinones (including arbutin), flavonoids, triterpenes, methyl salicylate, and tannins. The hydroquinones have a pronounced disinfectant effect within the urinary tract.

History & folklore Pipsissewa was much used by Indigenous North Americans to induce sweating and treat fevers, including typhus. European colonizers used the herb for rheumatism and for urinary and kidney problems. It was listed in the *Pharmacopoeia of the United States* from 1820 to 1916.

Medicinal actions & uses Astringent, tonic, and diuretic, pipsissewa is mainly used in an infusion for urinary tract problems such as cystitis and urethritis. It has also been prescribed for more serious conditions such as gonorrhea and kidney stones. By increasing urine flow, it stimulates the removal of waste products from the body, and is therefore of benefit in the treatment of rheumatism and gout. The fresh leaves of pipsissewa may be applied externally to rheumatic joints or muscles, as well as to blisters, sores, and swellings.

Research Early stage laboratory research suggests that pipsissewa might have potential use in treating breast cancer.

Chionanthus virginicus (Oleaceae)

Fringe tree

Description Deciduous shrub or tree growing to a height of 33 ft (10 m). Has elliptical dark green leaves and long flowering stems with spikes of white flowers. Produces dark blue oval fruits.

Habitat & cultivation Native to the US, fringe tree grows from Pennsylvania south to Florida and Texas. It is also now found in eastern Asia, and thrives on riverbanks and in damp shrubby areas. The root is unearthed in spring or fall, mostly in Virginia and North Carolina.

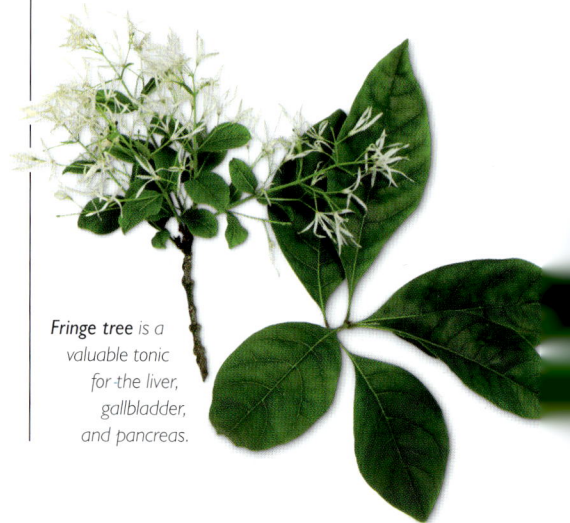

Fringe tree is a valuable tonic for the liver, gallbladder, and pancreas.

Parts used Traditionally root bark, but stem bark is now preferred.

Constituents Fringe tree contains secoiridoids, including oleuropein, and lignans including phyllirin.

History & folklore Fringe tree was commonly used by Indigenous North Americans and European colonizers to treat inflammations of the eye, canker sores, and spongy gums. The Choctaw people of Louisiana applied the mashed bark to cuts and bruises. Indigenous peoples in Alabama used the bark as a treatment for toothache. In the 19th-century Anglo-American Physiomedicalist tradition, fringe tree was valued as a bitter tonic, and the bark was often used to aid recovery from long-term illness.

Medicinal actions & uses The root bark is a liver tonic, stimulates bile flow, and acts as a mild laxative. It is prescribed mainly for gallbladder pain, gallstones, jaundice, and chronic weakness. While it appears to be of benefit to liver and gallbladder function, there is as yet no research to substantiate its effects. The root bark also appears to strengthen function in the pancreas and spleen. Anecdotal evidence indicates that it may substantially reduce sugar levels in the urine. Fringe tree also stimulates the appetite and digestion and is an excellent remedy for chronic illness, especially where the liver has been affected. For external use, the crushed bark may be made into a poultice for treating sores and wounds.

Chondrodendron tomentosum (Menispermaceae)

Pareira

Description Vine climbing to a great height in tropical rainforests. Reaches 100 ft (30 m). Has large leaves up to 1 ft (30 cm) long and trailing clusters of flowers.

Habitat & cultivation Pareira grows wild in rainforests in the upper Amazon region and in Panama. It is collected from the wild as available.

Parts used Root, stem.

Constituents Pareira contains alkaloids, including delta-tubocurarine and L-curarine. Tubocurarine is a potent muscle relaxant.

History & folklore Pareira and similar species are famous for being the source of curare, the paralyzing arrow poison used by Amazonian and other Indigenous South Americans to catch their prey. A dart or spear tipped with curare causes instantaneous paralysis on entering the bloodstream of the animal. Traditional recipes for toxins usually involve blending 10 or more different plants, but pareira or a plant with similar action is always present in the mix.

Medicinal actions & uses Pareira's notoriety as a poison hinges on the effect of its toxic derivative entering directly into the bloodstream. Provided there are no cuts or sores in the mouth, the plant is reasonably safe taken orally as a medicinal remedy. The bitter and slightly sweet-tasting roots and stems are mildly laxative, tonic, and diuretic, and also act to induce menstruation. The plant is chiefly used to relieve chronic inflammation of the urinary tubules. In Brazil, it is also used for snake bite.

Research Pareira's powerful ability to paralyze has led to its being extensively researched. Tubocurarine—one of the many alkaloids within the plant—is now used (as tubocurarine chloride) as an anesthetic to paralyze the muscles during operations.

Related species At least four other closely related species of *Chondrodendron* are used to produce the traditional poison known as curare.

Cautions Use only under professional supervision. Pareira and/or curare are subject to legal restrictions in some countries.

Chondrus crispus (Gigartinaceae)

Irish Moss,
Carragheen

Description Reddish-brown seaweed growing to 10 in (25 cm). Plant body is flat and forked, with a fan-shaped outline.

Habitat & cultivation Irish moss is found on the Atlantic coasts of Europe and North America. It grows just below the waterline, attached to rocks and stones. In summer in North America, and in the fall in Ireland, it is pulled up by hand or with a rake at low tide and dried in the sun.

Part used Whole herb.

Constituents Irish moss contains large amounts of polysaccharides, proteins (up to 10%), amino acids, iodine, and bromine, plus many other minerals. The polysaccharides become jellylike and demulcent when the plant is immersed in water.

History & folklore Irish moss is used extensively in the food and pharmaceutical industries as an emulsifying and binding agent, for example in toothpastes.

Medicinal actions & uses A useful demulcent and emollient, Irish moss is mainly taken for coughs and bronchitis. Its expectorant effect encourages the coughing up of phlegm, and it soothes dry and irritated mucous membranes. It is of value for acid indigestion, gastritis, and urinary infections such as cystitis. For these conditions it is normally combined with other appropriate herbs. Mucilaginous in texture and slightly salty in taste, Irish moss makes a

valuable nutrient in convalescence. Applied externally, this emollient herb soothes inflamed skin. Irish moss also acts to thin the blood.

Caution Due to its blood-thinning property, Irish moss should not be used by people taking anticoagulant medicines.

Cichorium intybus (Asteraceae)

Chicory

Description Deep-rooted perennial growing to 5 ft (1.5 m). Has a hairy stem, oblong leaves, and blue flowers.

Habitat & cultivation Native to Europe, chicory also grows in North Africa and western Asia. It flourishes along paths and roadsides, and in banks and dry fields. The root is unearthed in spring or fall.

Parts used Root, leaves, flowers.

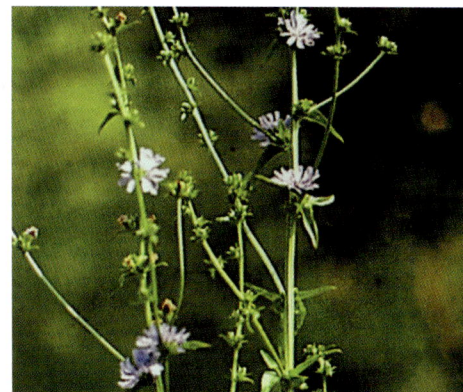

Chicory leaves make a settling digestive tea..

Constituents The root contains up to 58% inulin, caffeic acids, coumarins, flavonoids, polyynes, an essential oil including sesquiterpene lactones, and vitamins and minerals. There is now significant evidence to show that chicory root protects the liver from damage.

History & folklore According to Pliny (23–79 CE), chicory juice was mixed with rose oil and vinegar as a remedy for headaches. The roasted root is commonly used as a coffee substitute. The young root can be boiled and eaten like parsnips.

Medicinal actions & uses Chicory is an excellent mild bitter tonic for the liver and digestive tract. The root is therapeutically similar to dandelion root (*Taraxacum officinale*, p. 145), supporting the action of the stomach and liver and cleansing the urinary tract. Like dandelion, chicory root is a useful remedy in preventing and controlling diabetes. The root is also taken for rheumatic conditions and gout, and as a mild laxative, one particularly appropriate for children. An infusion of the leaves and flowers also aids digestion.

Related species The endive (*C. endiva*) has similar though milder effects.

Cinnamomum camphora syn. *Laurus camphora* (Lauraceae)

Camphor

Description Evergreen tree growing to 100 ft (30 m). Produces red leaves that turn dark green as they mature, small fragrant yellowish flowers, and oval red berries.

Habitat & cultivation Native to China and Japan, this tree is cultivated in tropical and subtropical regions for its wood, from which camphor oil is derived

Parts used Stems, root, wood, leaves, twigs, volatile oil.

Constituents The plant contains a volatile oil comprising camphor, safrole, eugenol, and terpineol. It also contains lignans. Camphor is irritant and antiseptic; safrole is thought to be carcinogenic. A white crystalline substance derived from the stems, root, and other parts of the tree, also called camphor, has powerful antiseptic, stimulant, and antispasmodic properties.

History & folklore In the 13th century, Marco Polo noted that camphor oil was highly valued by the Chinese as a medicine, scent, and embalming fluid.

Medicinal actions & uses Camphor is most commonly applied externally as a counterirritant and analgesic liniment to relieve arthritic and rheumatic pains, neuralgia, and back pain. It may be applied to skin problems, such as cold sores and chilblains, and used as a chest rub for bronchitis and other chest infections. Though the oil has been taken for various complaints, internal use is not advised.

Related species See also cinnamon (*Cinnamomum* spp., p. 85).

Cautions Do not take internally. Camphor oil is subject to legal restrictions in some countries.

Citrullus vulgaris (Cucurbitaceae)

Watermelon

Description Annual vine with hairy, 3–5 lobed leaves, yellow flowers, and green fruit typically growing to 10 in (25 cm) across.

Habitat & cultivation Native to tropical Africa, watermelon is grown throughout warm temperate to tropical regions. The fruit is gathered when ripe.

Parts used Fruit, seeds.

Constituents Watermelon contains polyphenols, notably citrulline, arginine, and lycopene. All three support cardiovascular health, while lycopene is well known for its positive effects on prostate health.

History & folklore Watermelon species have been used in Egypt for more than 4,000 years, figuring in wall paintings dating to the Old Kingdom (2686–2181 BCE). They appear to have been a component in remedies for trembling fingers, constipation, and expelling disease brought on by demons. Egyptian myth recounts that the watermelon originated from the semen of the god Seth.

Medicinal actions & uses Watermelon is best known as a thirst-quenching fruit that comes into season when temperatures are at their hottest. In traditional Chinese medicine it is used precisely to counter "summer heat" patterns—characterized by excessive sweating, thirst, raised temperature, scanty urine, diarrhea, and irritability or anger. Watermelon fruit and juice soothe these symptoms, increasing urine flow and cleansing the kidneys. The fruit's refreshing properties extend to the digestive system, where it clears gas. Watermelon may also be used in the treatment of hepatitis, and as an aid to weight loss. In hot, stifling weather it is helpful for those suffering from bronchitis or asthma. The cooling fruit pulp may be applied to hot and inflamed skin and to soothe sunburn. The seeds can be mashed and used to expel worms.

Related species The watermelons of Egypt (*C. lanata* and *C. colocynthoides*) are very similar species. The colocynth (*C. colocynthus*), native to dry areas of Africa and Asia, is extremely bitter and contains a cucurbitacin glycoside with antitumor properties.

Citrus aurantium (Rutaceae)

Bitter orange

Description Evergreen tree growing to 30 ft (10 m). Has leathery, dark green leaves, delicately perfumed white flowers, and orange fruit.

Habitat & cultivation Native to tropical Asia, this tree is now grown throughout the tropics and subtropics. Orchards of bitter orange are found along the Mediterranean coast, especially in Spain.

Parts used Fruit, peel, leaves, flowers, seeds, essential oil.

Constituents Bitter orange peel contains a volatile oil with limonene (around 90%), flavonoids, coumarins, triterpenes, vitamin C, carotene, and pectin. The flavonoids are anti-inflammatory, antibacterial, and antifungal. The composition of the volatile oils in the leaves, flowers and peel varies significantly. Linalyl acetate (50%) is the main constituent in oil from the leaves (petitgrain) and linalool (35%) in oil from the flowers (neroli). The unripe fruit of the bitter orange contains cirantin, which reportedly is contraceptive.

History & folklore The bitter orange has provided food and medicine for thousands of years. It yields neroli oil from its flowers, and the oil known as petitgrain from its leaves and young shoots. Both distillates are used extensively in perfumery. Orange flower water is a byproduct of distillation and is used in perfumery and to flavor candies and cookies, as well as being used medicinally.

Medicinal actions & uses The strongly acidic fruit of the bitter orange stimulates digestion and relieves flatulence. An infusion of the fruit is thought to soothe headaches, calm palpitations, and lower fevers. The juice helps the body eliminate waste products and, being rich in vitamin C, helps the immune system ward off infection. If taken to excess, however, its acid content can exacerbate arthritis. In Chinese herbal medicine, the unripe fruit, known as *zhi shi,* is thought to "regulate the *qi*," helping to relieve flatulence and abdominal bloating, and to open the bowels. The essential oils of bitter orange, especially neroli, are sedative. In Western medicine, these oils are used to reduce heart rate and palpitations, to encourage sleep, and to soothe the digestive tract. Diluted neroli is applied as a relaxing massage oil. The distilled flower water is antispasmodic and sedative.

Related species The lime (*C. aurantiifolia*) and lemon (*C. limon*, p. 86) have nutritional properties

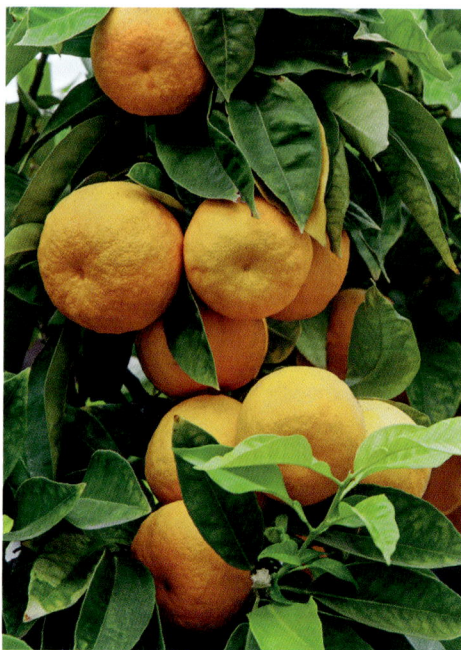

Bitter orange *has a wide range of medicinal uses.*

that are similar to those of bitter orange. See also bergamot (*C. bergamia, following entry*)

Caution Do not take the essential oils internally except under professional supervision.

Citrus bergamia syn. *C. aurantium* var. *bergamia* (Rutaceae)

Bergamot

Description Evergreen tree growing to 30 ft (10 m). Has pointed oval leaves, scented white flowers, and fruit with aromatic peel.

Habitat & cultivation Native to tropical Asia, bergamot is cultivated in subtropical regions, especially in southern Italy.

Part used Essential oil.

Constituents Bergamot contains a volatile oil including linalyl acetate (30–60%), limonene (26–42%), and linalool (11–22%), bergapten, and a diterpene.

History & folklore Bergamot oil, expressed from the peel, provides the distinctive flavor of Earl Grey tea. The oil (or constituents of it) is sometimes added to suntanning oils.

Medicinal actions & uses Bergamot is little used in herbal medicine, but it can be used to relieve tension, relax muscle spasms, and improve digestion.

Caution Do not take bergamot essential oil internally.

Clerodendrum trichotomum (Verbenaceae)

Chou wu tong

Description Upright, deciduous shrub growing to 10 ft (3 m). Has large leaves, clusters of white flowers, and blue berries.

Habitat & cultivation This herb grows in central and southern China. The leaves are harvested just before it flowers.

Parts used Leaves.

Constituents *Chou wu tong* contains clerodendrin, acacetin, and mesoinositol.

History & folklore *Chou wu tong* was first documented in the *Illustrated Classic of the Materia Medica* (1061 CE).

Medicinal actions & uses In Chinese herbal medicine, *chou wu tong* is prescribed for joint pain, numbness, and paralysis, and occasionally for eczema. Traditionally regarded as a plant that "dispels wind-dampness," it is now also being used to help lower blood pressure. The plant is mildly analgesic and, when used with the herb *Siegesbeckia pubescens*, is anti-inflammatory.

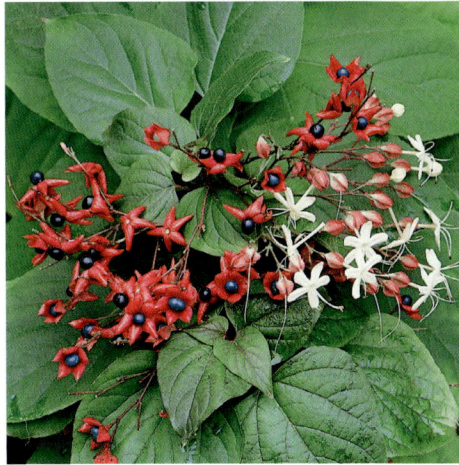

Chou wu tong has been shown by research to lower high blood pressure.

Research In a Chinese trial, 171 people with high blood pressure were given *chou wu tong*. In 81% of those tested, blood pressure levels dropped significantly. This effect was reversed when the treatment was stopped.

Related species *C. serratum* is commonly used in Ayurvedic medicine for respiratory conditions.

Clinopodium menthifolium syn. *Calamintha ascendens* (Lamiaceae)

Calamint

Description Mint-scented perennial growing to 2 ft (60 cm). Has hairy oval leaves, and purple flowers in late summer.

Habitat & cultivation Calamint grows wild in Europe and Asia from the British Isles eastward to Iran, especially in the Mediterranean region. It flourishes along roads and in dry places.

Parts used Aerial parts.

Constituents Calamint contains a volatile oil (about 0.35%) consisting mainly of pulegone.

History & folklore In classical legend, calamint had the power to drive away the Basilisk, a serpent credited with the ability to kill with its gaze or breath.

Medicinal actions & uses Calamint stimulates sweating, and hence helps lower fevers. It also settles gas and indigestion. It is expectorant, and is a good cough and cold remedy. This range of applications makes it a good medicinal herb for mild respiratory infections. It should preferably be mixed with other herbs such as yarrow (*Achillea millefolium*, p. 60) and thyme (*Thymus vulgaris*, p. 147).

Caution Do not take during pregnancy.

Cnicus benedictus syn. *Carbenia benedicta, Carduus benedictus* (Asteraceae)

Holy thistle

Description Erect, red-stemmed annual growing to 26 in (65 cm). Has spiny leathery leaves, a spiny stem, and yellow flowers in summer and fall.

Habitat & cultivation This Mediterranean plant flourishes on dry stony ground and in open areas. The leaves and flowering tops are collected in summer.

Parts used Leaves, flowering tops.

Constituents Holy thistle contains lignans, sesquiterpene lactones (including cnicin), volatile oil, polyacetylenes, flavonoids, triterpenes, phytosterols, and tannins. Cnicin is bitter and anti-inflammatory; the volatile oil is thought to have antibiotic properties.

History & folklore In the Middle Ages, holy thistle was thought to cure the plague. In his herbal of 1568, Nicholas Turner wrote: "There is nothing better for the canker [ulcerous sore] and old rotten and festering sores than the leaves, juice, broth, powder, and water of holy thistle."

Medicinal actions & uses Holy thistle is a good bitter tonic, stimulating secretions within the salivary glands, stomach, gallbladder, and intestines, and thereby improving digestion. It is taken, generally as a tincture, for minor digestive complaints. It has also been a treatment for intermittent fevers. Holy thistle is mildly expectorant and antibiotic. It makes a healing balm for wounds and sores.

Cautions In excessive doses, holy thistle may cause vomiting. It is subject to legal restrictions in some countries.

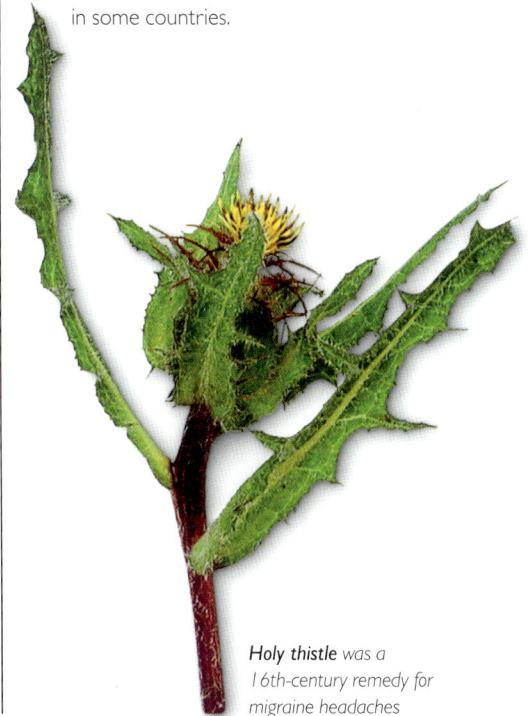

Holy thistle was a 16th-century remedy for migraine headaches

Cochlearia officinalis (Cruciferae)

Scurvy grass

Description Low-growing perennial with fleshy heart-shaped leaves, dense clusters of white 4-petaled flowers, and rounded swollen seed pods.

Habitat & cultivation Native to Europe and temperate regions of Asia and North America, but now rare, scurvy grass thrives in the salty soil of coastal areas and salt marshes. It is occasionally cultivated.

Parts used Leaves, aerial parts.

Constituents Scurvy grass contains glucosilinates, a volatile oil, a bitter principle, tannin, vitamin C, and minerals.

History & folklore As the common name suggests, this plant has long been used for its high vitamin C content. It was used by sailors and others to prevent the onset of scurvy, a potentially fatal vitamin C deficiency marked by bleeding of the gums.

Medicinal actions & uses Besides having a high vitamin C content, scurvy grass has antiseptic and mild laxative actions. The young plant, which has a general detoxicant effect and contains a wide range of minerals, is taken as a spring tonic. Like watercress (*Nasturtium officinale*, p. 246), it has diuretic properties and is useful for any condition in which poor nutrition is a factor. It can be used in the form of a juice as an antiseptic mouthwash for canker sores, and can also be applied externally to spots and pimples.

Cocos nucifera (Arecaceae)

Coconut,
Coconut palm

Description Too familiar to need description, the coconut is a large palm reaching up to 100 ft (30 m) in height with a single, smooth trunk and long-ribbed leaves up to 20 ft (6 m) in length.

Habitat & cultivation Thought to have originated in Southeast Asia, coconut has been described as "the most naturally widespread fruit plant on Earth," and is found throughout the tropics. It thrives in sandy, salty soils (typically coastal) and requires abundant sun and rain. Propagated by seed, the one-seeded nut grows out through one of the three germinating pores at its base. In 2020, coconut was grown commercially in 95 countries, with a total production of 67.8 million tons (61.5 million metric tons). A coconut palm can produce up to 10,000 nuts during its lifetime.

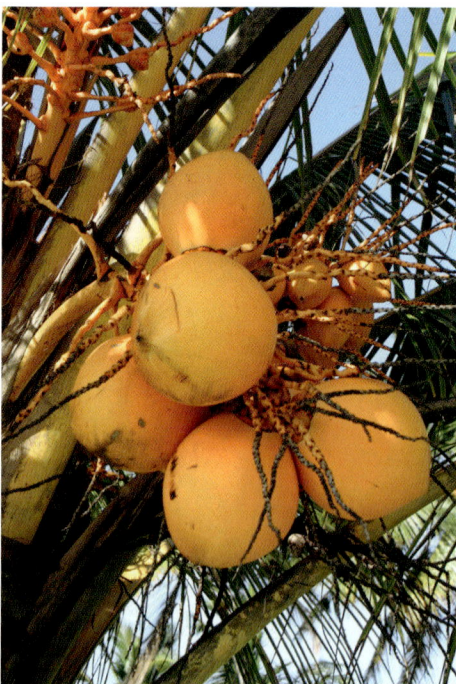

Coconut palms have spread across the tropical regions of the globe. The oil has antimicrobial properties.

Parts used Kernel (fresh or dried), water. Every part of coconut is useful.

Constituents Coconut oil is about 90% saturated fat, mostly medium-chain fatty acids (lauric, myristic, caprylic, and capric acids). Coconut water contains significant levels of minerals, notably potassium. Virgin coconut oil is entirely nontoxic.

History & folklore The coconut palm is described as "Kalpavriksha" (meaning "the all-giving tree") in ancient Indian texts.

Medicinal actions & uses Coconut oil and cream have established antimicrobial and immunostimulant activity. With antibacterial, antifungal, and antiviral properties, the oil and cream can be used to counter many commonly occurring infections, such as influenza, cold sores, shingles, and fungal problems. Coconut has a beneficial action on the gut flora and can prove useful (alongside other treatment) in clearing intestinal worms and parasites. Coconut oil and cream aid digestion and the absorption of nutrients (notably calcium and magnesium), and may be taken as part of a regimen to prevent or treat osteoporosis. Coconut water is reported to lower blood pressure, in part due to its high potassium content, while the oil helps prevent arteriosclerosis. It is also thought to lower cholesterol levels, aid weight loss, and lower blood glucose levels. Coconut oil helps keep skin and hair healthy and is a common ingredient in skin creams and shampoos. Coconut merits its name of "all-giving tree."

Coffea arabica (Rubiaceae)

Coffee

Description Evergreen shrub or small tree growing to 30 ft (9 m). Has dark green, shiny oval leaves and white star-shaped flowers. Produces small red fruit, each containing 2 seeds (beans).

Habitat & cultivation Coffee is native to tropical East Africa, and is now cultivated in tropical areas worldwide. The best-quality beans are produced by fermenting, sun-drying, and roasting the seeds.

Part used Seeds.

Constituents Coffee contains chlorogenic acids, tannins, and xanthines–caffeine (0.6–0.32%), theobromine, and theophylline. Caffeine is a strong stimulant. Theophylline is a stimulant and smooth muscle relaxant. Chlorogenic acids are anti-inflammatory.

History & folklore Native to the plateaus of central Ethiopia, where it is thought to have originated, coffee spread to Yemen in the 6th century CE and then on into the Arabian peninsula. The Arabian physician Rhazes first recorded coffee's use in the 10th century CE. While coffee drinking formed part of Sufi prayer rituals, being taken to enable longer, more ecstatic prayer through the night, coffee gradually became the popular stimulant

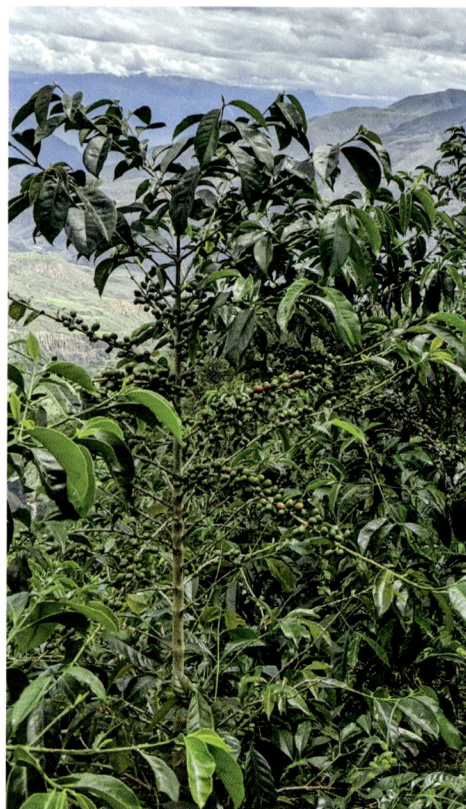

Coffee, native to East Africa, can be used to relieve headaches.

drink that we know today, spreading to Europe in the 17th century. By 2020, the annual export trade in coffee exceeded $20 billion.

Medicinal actions & uses Coffee is an effective and much-loved stimulant of central nervous function, aiding mental alertness and perception. Coffee (and extracts) increase physical performance and heart output, stimulate digestive juices, and act as a powerful diuretic. It can be taken to counter drowsiness and to relieve headaches and migraines. It is nonaddictive, although excess intake or sudden withdrawal from coffee may cause headaches. Many natural medicine practitioners consider overuse of coffee to be unhealthy as it is associated with nervous and endocrine exhaustion. Decaffeinated green coffee bean extract is taken to promote weight loss.

Research Regular coffee drinking is associated with a significantly decreased risk of colon cancer. Coffee may have a protective effect against Alzheimer's and Parkinson's diseases.

Cautions Percolated or boiled coffee is thought to have potentially harmful effects on the heart and circulation and to raise cholesterol levels. Caffeine can increase premenstrual symptoms and period pains.

Cola acuminata (Sterculiaceae)

Kola nut,
Cola nut

Description Evergreen tree growing to 65 ft (20 m) with dark green leaves and yellowish-white flowers. Large woody seed pods contain 5–10 white or red seeds (nuts).

Habitat & cultivation Native to West Africa, kola nut is cultivated widely in the tropics, especially in Nigeria, Brazil, and the Caribbean. The seeds are harvested when ripe and dried in the sun.

Part used Seeds.

Constituents Kola nut contains up to 2.5% caffeine (generally higher than coffee), theobromine, tannins, phlobaphene, and an anthocyanin.

History & folklore Chewed for their digestive, tonic, and aphrodisiac properties, kola nuts have been an integral part of western and central African life for thousands of years. Kola nuts are used in huge quantities today to flavor soft drinks.

Medicinal actions & uses Kola nut stimulates the central nervous system and the body as a whole. It increases alertness and muscular strength, counters lethargy, and has been used extensively both in western African and Anglo-American herbal medicine as an antidepressant, particularly during recovery from chronic illness. Like coffee (*Coffea arabica*, preceding entry), kola is used to treat headaches and migraine. It is diuretic and astringent, and may be taken for diarrhea and dysentery.

Related species *C. nitida*, which grows in Africa, Brazil, and the West Indies, is used in the same fashion.

Cautions Do not take if suffering from high blood pressure, peptic ulcers, or palpitations.

Colchicum autumnale (Liliaceae)

Meadow saffron

Description Attractive perennial growing from a bulblike corm to 4 in (10 cm). Has pointed lance-shaped leaves and tubular 6-petaled pink flowers in the fall.

Habitat & cultivation Common in Europe and North Africa, meadow saffron grows wild in woods and damp meadows. It is also cultivated. The corm is gathered in early summer, the seeds in late summer.

Parts used Corm, seeds.

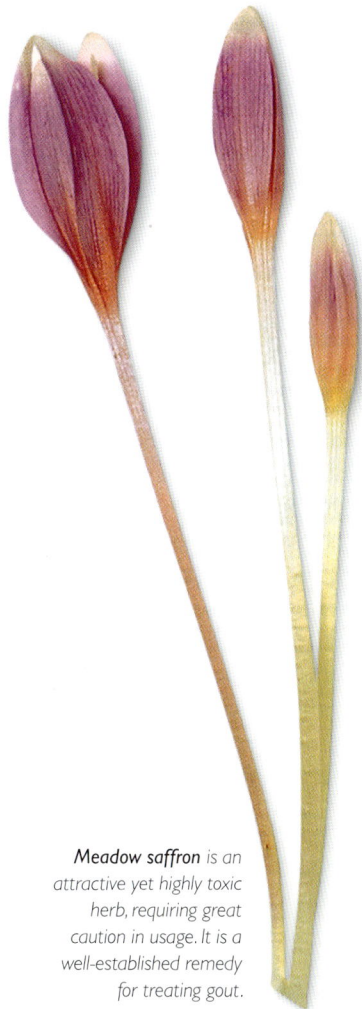

Meadow saffron is an attractive yet highly toxic herb, requiring great caution in usage. It is a well-established remedy for treating gout.

Constituents Meadow saffron contains alkaloids (including colchicine) and flavonoids. Colchicine is anti-inflammatory and is used in conventional medicine for acute attacks of gout. As it affects cell division it can cause fetal abnormality. It has been used in the laboratory to create new genetic strains.

History & folklore Meadow saffron was not used in classical times due to its poisonous nature. Arabian physicians used it in the Middle Ages to treat joint pain and gout, but otherwise herbalists disregarded the plant until the 19th century.

Medicinal actions & uses Despite its toxicity, meadow saffron is considered one of the best remedies for acute gout pain. Leukemia has been successfully treated with meadow saffron, and the plant has also been used with some success to treat Behcet's syndrome, a chronic disease marked by recurring ulcers and leukemia. Taken internally, the herb has significant side effects even at low dosage. Externally, it is applied to relieve neuralgia and itchiness.

Cautions This herb is highly toxic. Use only under professional supervision. Do not use during pregnancy. Meadow saffron is subject to legal restrictions in some countries.

Collinsonia canadensis (Lamiaceae)

Stone root

Description Perennial herb growing to 3 ft (1 m). Has a square stem, oval leaves, and clusters of greenish-yellow flowers.

Habitat & cultivation This herb is native to moist woodlands of eastern North America. The root is dug up in the fall.

Parts used Root, leaves.

Constituents Stone root contains a volatile oil, tannins, and saponins.

History & folklore The *British Medical Journal* of 1887 describes stone root as "highly esteemed as a domestic remedy for gravel and urinary affections."

Medicinal actions & uses Stone root has diuretic and tonic properties, and is chiefly employed in the treatment of kidney stones. It is also prescribed to counteract fluid retention. It has been used to reduce back pressure in the veins, which in turn helps prevent the formation or worsening of hemorrhoids and varicose veins. As an astringent, stone root contracts the inner lining of the intestines, and can be helpful in treating disorders of the digestive system such as irritable bowel syndrome and mucous colitis. The fresh leaves or roots of stone root are applied as a poultice to bruises and sores.

Commiphora mukul (Burseraceae)

Guggul

Description Spiny shrub or tree, growing to 6½ ft (2 m), with oval, serrated leaves, brownish-red flowers, and red fruits. Guggul, the gum resin obtained from the bark, forms pale yellow to brown "tears" on the stems.

Habitat & cultivation Guggul thrives in dry, semiarid and desert environments across much of the Indian subcontinent and the Middle East.

Part used Gum resin.

Constituents Guggul is an oleo-gum resin, its main active constituents being fat-soluble steroids (guggulipids), in particular guggulsterones E and Z.

History & folklore Early Ayurvedic texts describe guggul as being effective in treating obesity. This has led to research into whether the gum resin might be useful for problems associated with fat metabolism, such as raised blood cholesterol levels.

Medicinal actions & uses Guggul has anti-inflammatory, blood-thinning, and cholesterol-lowering activity, and—true to ancient understanding of the herb—can be helpful in treating obesity. In Ayurveda, guggul is principally used to treat arthritic problems, such as osteoarthritis, though it is also considered to have tonic and rejuvenating properties. As a result of research in the 1980s and 1990s, guggul is now most commonly used to lower raised blood cholesterol levels and to improve blood fat profiles in general. It reduces the stickiness of platelets and thins the blood, and may have a protective activity on the heart. Guggul is also useful in the treatment of acne.

Research Extensive research has shown that the guggulipids have anti-inflammatory and anti-arthritic activity and prevent or reverse raised blood cholesterol levels. In several clinical trials, patients showed an average fall in cholesterol levels of about 12%, and in triglycerides of about 14%. The overall blood-fat profile was also shown to improve. Some clinical trials recorded weight loss for patients taking guggulipids.

Related species The closely related myrrh (*Commiphora molmol*) has much similarity with guggul.

Caution Avoid if breastfeeding.

Conium maculatum (Apiaceae)

Hemlock

Description Graceful biennial growing to a height of 8 ft (2.5 m). Has slender, red-speckled stems, finely divided leaves, small clusters of white flowers, and small seeds that have beaded ridges.

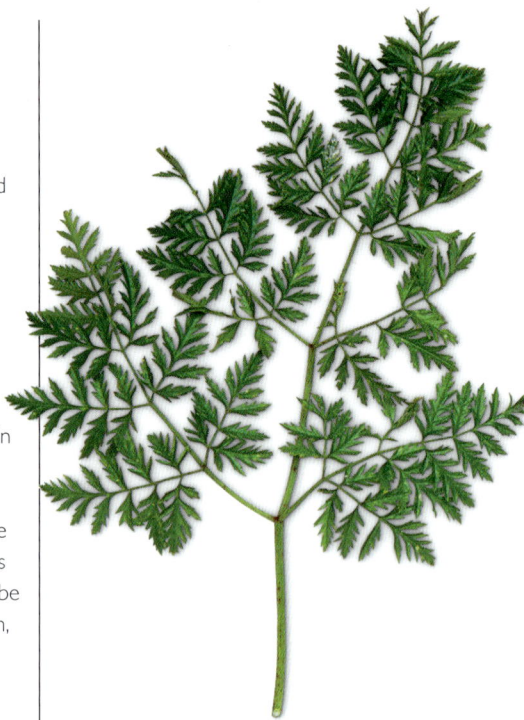

Hemlock is highly poisonous and was used for capital punishment.

Habitat & cultivation Commonly found in Europe, hemlock also grows in temperate regions of Asia and North America. It flourishes in damp meadows, on riverbanks, and on waste ground. The seeds are gathered when almost ripe in summer.

Parts used Leaves, seeds.

Constituents Hemlock contains alkaloids, mainly coniine, and a volatile oil. Coniine is extremely toxic and causes congenital deformities.

History & folklore Hemlock is notorious as the poison administered as a capital punishment in ancient Greece. The Greek philosopher Socrates died in 399 BCE after drinking hemlock juice. According to an old English tradition, the stems took their color in sympathy with the mark placed on Cain's forehead after he murdered Abel. In the 19th century, hemlock was used in conventional medicine as a painkiller.

Medicinal actions & uses In extremely small quantities, hemlock is sedative and analgesic; in larger doses it causes paralysis and death. Rarely used today, it has been prescribed in the past as a treatment for epilepsy, Parkinson's disease, and Sydenham chorea. Hemlock has also been used to treat acute cystitis.

Cautions Do not take internally. Use externally only under professional supervision. Hemlock is subject to legal restrictions in many countries.

Convallaria majalis (Liliaceae)

Lily of the valley

Description Attractive perennial growing to 9 in (23 cm). Has a pair of elliptical leaves, clusters of bell-shaped white flowers on one side of the stem, and red berries.

Habitat & cultivation Native to Europe, this herb is also distributed over North America and northern Asia. It is widely cultivated as a garden plant. The leaves and flowers are gathered in late spring as the plant comes into flower.

Parts used Leaves, flowers.

Constituents Lily of the valley contains cardiac glycosides, including the cardenolides convallatoxin, convalloside, convallatoxol, and others, and flavonoid glycosides. The cardiac glycosides act to strengthen a weakened heart.

History & folklore The herbalist Apuleius, writing in the 2nd century CE, records that Apollo gave lily of the valley as a gift to Asclepius, the god of healing. In the 16th century, the herbalist John Gerard had the following to say about its therapeutic value: "The flowers of the valley lillie distilled with wine, and drunke to the quantitie of a spoonful, restore speech unto those that have the dumb palsie and that are fallen into apoplexy, and are good against the gout, and comfort the heart."

Medicinal actions & uses Lily of the valley is used by European

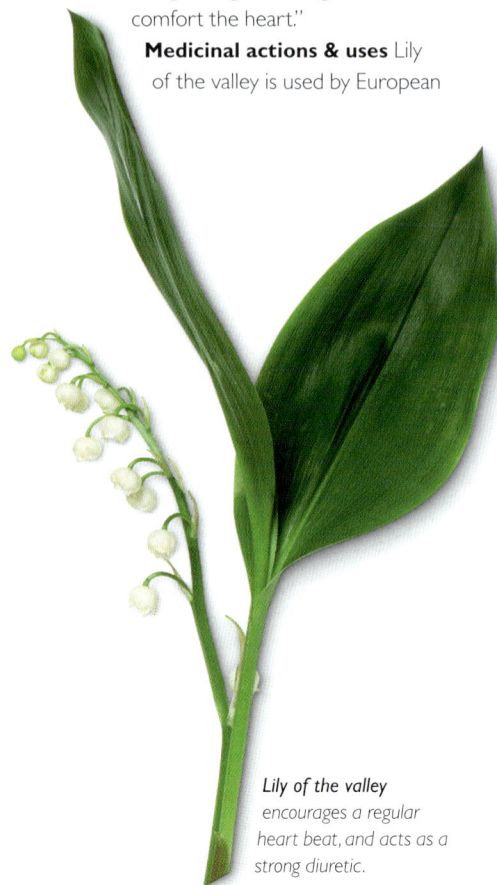

Lily of the valley encourages a regular heart beat, and acts as a strong diuretic.

herbalists in place of common foxglove (*Digitalis purpurea*, p. 207). Both herbs have a profound effect in cases of heart failure, whether due in the long term to a cardiovascular problem, or to a chronic lung problem such as emphysema. Lily of the valley encourages a failing heart to beat more slowly and regularly, and to pump more efficiently, thereby improving blood flow to the heart itself via the coronary arteries. It is also diuretic and lowers blood volume. The herb is better tolerated than foxglove, as it does not accumulate within the body to the same degree. Relatively low doses are required to support heart rate and rhythm, and to increase urine production.

Cautions Use only under professional supervision. Lily of the valley is subject to legal restrictions in some countries.

Conyza canadensis syn. *Erigeron canadensis* (Asteraceae)

Canadian fleabane

Description Erect annual herb growing to 3 ft (1 m). Has narrow, dark green, lance-shaped leaves and clusters of small white flower heads that quickly fade into silky white tufts.

Habitat & cultivation Native to North America, Canadian fleabane is now common in South America and Europe. It thrives on uncultivated and recently cleared land, often invading in large swaths. It is gathered from the wild when in flower.

Parts used Aerial parts.

Constituents Canadian fleabane contains a volatile oil (including limonene, terpineol, and linalool), flavonoids, terpenes, plant acids, and tannins.

History & folklore In traditional North American herbal medicine, Canadian fleabane was boiled to make steam for sweat lodges, taken as a snuff to stimulate sneezing during the course of a cold, and burned to create a smoke that warded off insects—hence its common name.

Medicinal actions & uses An astringent herb, Canadian fleabane is taken for gastrointestinal problems such as diarrhea and dysentery. A decoction of Canadian fleabane is reportedly a very effective treatment for bleeding hemorrhoids. The herb is occasionally used as a diuretic for bladder problems, to clear toxins in rheumatic conditions, and to treat gonorrhea and other genitourinary diseases.

Related species The Philadelphia fleabane (*E. philadelphicus*) was used by the Houma as a treatment for menstrual problems. *E. affinis*, a Mexican relative, is used to make a tooth powder and to treat toothache.

Copaifera spp. (Fabaceae)

Copaiba

Description Evergreen trees growing to 59 ft (18 m). Have compound leaves and small yellow flowers.

Habitat & cultivation Copaiba is native to tropical South America, and also found in southern Africa. Oleoresin, a blend of volatile oil and resin often also referred to as copaiba, is obtained by drilling holes in the trunk.

Part used Oleoresin.

Constituents The oleoresin contains a volatile oil (30–90%), which in turn contains alpha- and beta-caryophyllene, sesquiterpenes, resins, and terpenic acids.

History & folklore Copaiba was used by native Brazilians long before the arrival of Europeans. In 1625, the Portuguese monk Manoel Tristao observed that it was employed to heal wounds and remove scars.

Medicinal actions & uses Antiseptic, diuretic, and stimulant, copaiba is still used extensively in Brazil. Chiefly employed to counter mucus in the chest and genitourinary system, it irritates the mucous membranes and promotes the coughing up of mucus. A solution or tincture of copaiba may be taken for bronchitis, chronic cystitis, diarrhea, and hemorrhoids. Eczema and other skin diseases reportedly benefit from its application.

Related species Several of the 40 *Copaifera* species yield a medicinal oleoresin.

Caution Copaiba is toxic in overdose. Use only under professional supervision.

Coptis chinensis (Ranunculaceae)

Huang lian (Chinese), Chinese goldthread

Description Perennial herb growing to 20 in (50 cm). Has basal leaves and small whitish-green flowers.

Habitat & cultivation This herb is native to the mountains of China, and is most commonly cultivated in Sichuan province. The root is dug up in the fall.

Part used Root.

Constituents *Huang lian* contains isoquiniline alkaloids, including berberine, coptisine, and worenine. Berberine is antibacterial, amoebicidal, and antidiarrheal.

Medicinal actions & uses A bitter-tasting herb, *huang lian* is given in the Chinese herbal tradition as a decoction to "clear heat" and "dry dampness," relieving fever, red and sore eyes, and sore throats. The herb is particularly helpful for diarrhea and dysentery, and has been used to quell vomiting. Skin problems such as acne, boils, abscesses, and burns are also treated with *huang lian*. Like the root of goldthread (*C. trifolia*, see *following entry*), huang lian is taken as a gargle for mouth and tongue ulcers, and for swollen gums and toothache.

Research In a Chinese trial, 30 patients with tuberculosis were given *huang lian*, and all of them showed marked improvement in their symptoms.

Cautions Use only under professional supervision. Do not take during pregnancy.

Coptis trifolia (Ranunculaceae)

Goldthread

Description Perennial growing to 6 in (15 cm). Has a slender golden root, 3-lobed leaves, and single small white flowers.

Habitat & cultivation Native to eastern North America from Labrador to Tennessee, this herb prefers damp sites. The rhizome is dug up in the fall.

Part used Rhizome.

Constituents Goldthread contains isoquiniline alkaloids (including berberine and coptisine)

History & folklore Though little used in herbal medicine today, goldthread was once highly valued. In a book recounting his travels in North America, published in 1779, Jonathan Carver states that the plant "was greatly esteemed both by the Indians [sic] and the colonists as a remedy for any soreness in the mouth." The Montagnais people used a decoction of the root for problems associated with the mouth, lips, and eyes. The Menominee people used the plant as a gargle for children's throat issues and also to treat ulcers and tumors in the mouth.

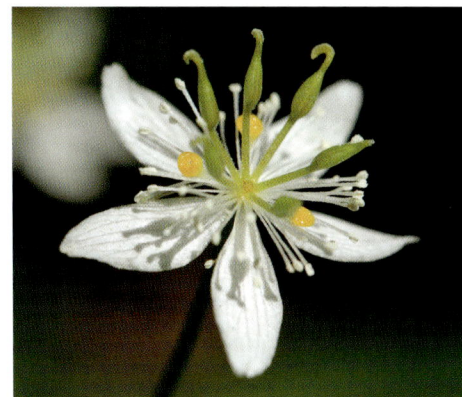

Goldthread is a strongly bitter tonic.

Medicinal actions & uses A strongly bitter tonic, goldthread has been prescribed in the North American tradition principally for indigestion and stomach weakness, though it has also come under consideration as a treatment for peptic ulcers, and has been applied as a wash for vaginal yeast infection. Goldthread has been used as a mouthwash, gargle, or lotion for mouth ulcers, sore lips, and throats. The herb's constituents (and to some degree its actions) are similar to those of goldenseal (*Hydrastis canadensis*, p. 109) and it has been used as a substitute for this herb.

Related species *Huang lian (C. chinensis, preceding entry)* is a close relative that has similar actions.

Cautions Use only under professional supervision. Do not take during pregnancy.

Coriandrum sativum (Apiaceae)

Coriander,
Cilantro

Description Strongly aromatic annual growing to 20 in (50 cm). Has finely cut upper leaves (known as cilantro), small white or pink flowers, and rounded seeds (coriander) in beige seed coats.

Habitat & cultivation Native to southern Europe and western Asia, the herb is cultivated throughout the world. The seeds are gathered ripe in late summer.

Parts used Seeds, essential oil, leaves.

Constituents Coriander contains up to 1.5% volatile oil, consisting mainly of delta-linalool (at around 70%), alpha-pinene and terpinine. It also contains flavonoids, coumarins, phthalides, and phenolic acids.

History & folklore Coriander has been used throughout Asia, northern Africa, and Europe for well over 2,000 years. It is listed in the Ebers papyrus (dating to about 1500 BCE), and apparently was much employed in ancient Egypt. The herb reached China during the Han Dynasty (202 BCE–220 CE). Pliny (23–79 CE) describes its use "for spreading sores … diseased testes, burns, carbuncles, and sore ears, fluxes of the eyes, too, if woman's milk be added".

Medicinal actions & uses Coriander is more often used as a spice than as a medicine. Nevertheless, an infusion of the herb is a gentle remedy for flatulence, bloating, and cramps. It settles spasms within the gut and counters the effects of nervous tension. Cilantro is also chewed to sweeten the breath, especially after consumption of garlic (*Allium sativum*, p. 63). Coriander seed has been used as an expectorant to treat coughs and bronchitis, and in traditional Middle Eastern medicine it is taken to calm anxiety and aid sleep. The ground seed is applied externally as a rub for rheumatic pain. In Europe, it has traditionally been thought to possess aphrodisiac properties.

Caution Do not take coriander essential oil internally.

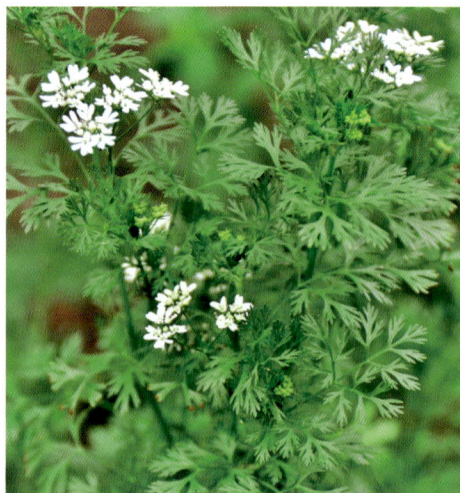

Coriander was used as a digestive aid and a treatment for measles in 6th-century China.

Cornus officinalis (Cornaceae)

Shan zhu yu,
Japanese cornelian cherry

Description Deciduous tree reaching 13 ft (4 m) with glossy elliptical leaves and bright red oval berries.

Habitat & cultivation Native to China, Japan, and Korea, this tree is cultivated in central and eastern China. The fruit is harvested when ripe in the fall.

Part used Fruit.

Constituents *Shan zhu yu* contains an iridoid glycoside (verbenalin), saponins, and tannins. Verbenalin produces a mild tonic effect on the involuntary nervous system, especially that governing the digestive system.

History & folklore Listed in the 1st-century CE *Divine Husbandman's Classic (Shen'nong Bencaojing)*, *shan zhu yu* is one of the constituents of the "Pill of Eight Ingredients," used to "warm up and invigorate the *yang* of the loins."

Medicinal actions & uses As an herb that "stabilizes and binds," *shan zhu yu* is used principally to reduce heavy menstrual bleeding and unusually active secretions, including copious sweating, excessive urine, spermatorrhea (involuntary discharge of semen), and premature ejaculation.

Related species Several *Cornus* species are used medicinally around the world. In Europe, the fruit and bark of the cornelian cherry (*C. mas*) and the bark of common dogwood (*C. sanguinea*) are used as astringents and to relieve fever. The American boxwood (*C. florida*) was used by Indigenous peoples as a fever remedy.

Crithmum maritimum (Apiaceae)

Sea Fennel,
Samphire

Description Maritime herb growing to a height of 2 ft (60 cm). Has long, succulent, bright green leaves and clusters of small yellowish-green flowers.

Habitat & cultivation Sea fennel grows on the Atlantic, Mediterranean, and Black Sea coasts of Europe and Asia Minor. It is found on rocks and cliffs close to the sea, and gathered in early summer.

Parts used Aerial parts.

Constituents Sea fennel contains a volatile oil, pectin, vitamins (especially vitamin C), and minerals.

History & folklore A much-valued herb in the past, sea fennel fell into disfavor but is slowly becoming popular again as a vegetable, either pickled or eaten fresh. The English herbalist John Gerard described it in 1597 as "the pleasantest sauce, most familiar, and best agreeing with man's body, both for the digestion of meates, breaking of stone, and voiding of gravel."

Medicinal actions & uses Though it is currently little used in herbal medicine, sea fennel is a good diuretic, and it has potential as a treatment for obesity. Sea fennel has a high vitamin C and mineral content, and is thought to relieve flatulence and soothe the digestion. In this, the plant resembles its

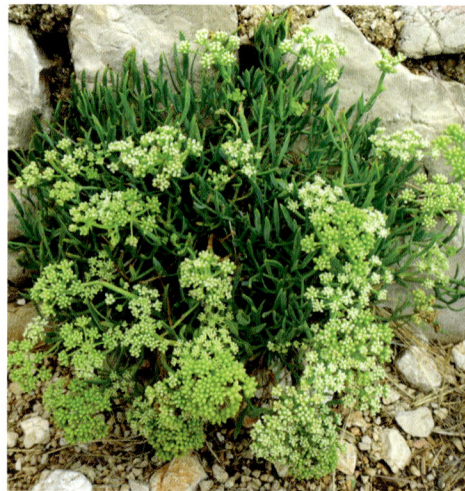

Sea fennel is rich in vitamin C and minerals.

inland namesake, fennel (*Foeniculum vulgare*, p. 217). Glasswort (*Salicornia europaea*), also known as samphire, is an unrelated coastal plant with a high mineral content and is commonly eaten as a vegetable.

Croton spp. (Euphorbiaceae)

Dragon's blood, *Sangre de drago*

Description Fast-growing tree reaching 49 ft (15 m) in height. It has large, heart-shaped leaves and greenish-white flowers.

Habitat & cultivation Dragon's blood is a rainforest tree native to northwestern Amazonia (from Bolivia to Colombia), preferring riverbanks and sites with disturbed soil. It is cultivated by the Indigenous peoples there as an environmentally sustainable crop.

Parts used Latex, sap, resin (fresh or dried), bark.

Constituents Key constituents within dragon's blood include proanthocyanidins, mono- and diterpenes, an alkaloid (taspine), and a lignan (dimethylcedrusine). Many constituents, notably taspine and dimethylcedrusine, have potent anti-inflammatory and wound healing properties. Taspine also has anticancer and antiviral activity.

History & folklore Dragon's blood derives its name from the deep red sap or latex that oozes from the tree when the bark is cut. A prized rainforest medicine, the latex is applied to wounds, fractures, skin infections, and insect bites. Internally, it is taken to treat diarrhea and dysentery, stomach ulcers, viral infections, and as a vaginal bath before and following childbirth. The first written record of its use was in 1653 (Bernabé Cobo, *Historia del Nuevo Mundo*).

Medicinal actions & uses Dragon's blood is a first-rate wound healer and has been described as a "liquid bandage." Tissue healing and repair is strongly stimulated, while the chances of infection developing in open wounds and sores is minimized due to the marked antiseptic action of the latex and its ability to seal off the wound from the open air. The latex (fresh or dried) is a key remedy for herpes, including shingles and genital herpes, and fungal skin infections. Taken internally, it helps to treat and prevent gastrointestinal infection and peptic ulcers, and to control diarrhea in conditions such as ulcerative colitis. A patent US medicine (Crofelemer) derived from dragon's blood is licensed for the treatment of chronic diarrhea, typically in patients with HIV.

Related species *C. lecheri* is most commonly used to make dragon's blood, although similar *Croton* species grow in Central America. *C. flavens* (Yellow balsam), a traditional Mayan and Aztec remedy, is used for fever and infections, and as a wound salve. Dragon trees, such as the Socotra dragon tree (*Dracaena cinnabari*), are desert trees and unrelated to dragon's blood, though some also produce a red latex.

Caution Can permanently stain clothing.

Cucurbita pepo (Cucurbitaceae)

Pumpkin

Description Annual plant with twining stems, lobed leaves, yellow flowers, and large orange fruit.

Habitat & cultivation Probably native to North America, pumpkin is now found worldwide. It is harvested in the fall.

Parts used Seeds, pulp.

Constituents Pumpkin seeds contain a fixed oil (30–50%), which is mostly linoleic acid (43–56%) and oleic acid (24–38%). The oil also contains protein (31–51%), sterols, cucurbitin, vitamin E, beta-carotene, and minerals (4–5%), including significant levels of iron, zinc, and selenium.

History & folklore The pumpkin has been much used as a medicine in Central and North America. The Maya applied the sap of the plant to burns, the Menominee people used the seeds as a diuretic, while Europeans ground up and mixed the seeds with water, milk, or honey as a remedy for worms. This practice became so widespread in homes across North America that the medical profession eventually adopted it as a standard treatment.

Medicinal actions & uses Pumpkin has been used mostly as a safe and effective deworming agent, particularly in children and pregnant women for whom strong-acting and toxic preparations are inappropriate. It is thought most effective in removing tapeworms. The seeds are diuretic and tonic to the bladder, and they have distinct value in treating the early stages of prostate enlargement. The fruit pulp is used as a decoction to relieve intestinal inflammation and is applied as a poultice or plaster for burns.

Research Pumpkin seeds' range of medicinal and nutritional compounds ensures that they have great value as a "natural" food supplement. A good dietary source of zinc, the seeds also contain relatively high levels of selenium, a mineral with important antioxidant and anticancer activity in the body. Cucurbitin repels intestinal worms, and the sterols are anti-inflammatory. Research suggests that pumpkin seed is effective in helping reduce benign enlargement of the prostate gland (BPH), due to both the hormonal influence of the sterols and this anti-inflammatory activity. In one clinical trial pumpkin seeds were combined with saw palmetto (*Serenoa repens*, p. 140) to treat BPH: those taking the herbal extract showed improved urine flow and reduced frequency of urination.

Cuminum cyminum (Apiaceae)

Cumin

Description Small annual growing to 1 ft (30 cm). Has long, narrow segmented leaves, clusters of pink or white flowers, and small oblong ridged fruits.

Habitat & cultivation Cumin is native to Egypt and widely cultivated in southern Europe and Asia. The seeds are gathered when ripe in late summer.

Parts used Seeds.

Constituents Cumin seeds contain 2–5% volatile oil, which consists of 25–35% aldehydes, pinene, and alpha-terpineol. The seeds also contain flavonoids.

History & folklore A popular spice and medicinal herb in ancient Egypt, cumin was used for illnesses of the digestive system, for chest conditions and coughs, as a painkiller, and to treat rotten teeth. The herb is mentioned in the Old Testament and was widely used in the Middle Ages. It has declined in popularity since that time, although it is still frequently used in contemporary Egyptian herbal medicine. In cooking, cumin is an ingredient that is found in many Chinese, Indian, and Middle Eastern recipes, especially curries and pickles.

Medicinal actions & uses Cumin, like its close relatives caraway (*Carum carvi*, p. 187) and anise (*Pimpinella anisum*, p. 256), relieves flatulence and bloating, and stimulates the entire digestive process. It reduces abdominal gases and distension and relaxes the gut. In Indian herbal medicine, cumin is used for insomnia, colds and fevers, and, mixed into a paste with onion juice, has been applied to scorpion stings. The seeds can be taken to improve breast-milk production—a role it shares with fennel seeds (*Foeniculum vulgare*, p. 217). Research indicates that a regular intake of cumin seeds can play a useful role in lowering raised cholesterol levels.

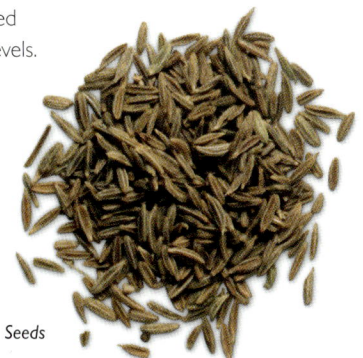

Seeds

Cupressus sempervirens (Cupressaceae)

Cypress

Description Evergreen tree growing to 100 ft (30 m). Has tiny dark green leaves, and male and female cones.

Habitat & cultivation Native to Turkey and cultivated in the Mediterranean, this herb is gathered in spring.

Parts used Cones, branches, essential oil.

Constituents Cypress contains a volatile oil (with pinene, camphene, and cedrol) and tannins.

History & folklore Ancient Greeks took the cones, mashed and steeped in wine, to treat dysentery, the coughing up of blood, asthma, and coughs.

Medicinal actions & uses Applied externally as a lotion or as a diluted essential oil, cypress astringes varicose veins and hemorrhoids, tightening up the blood vessels. A footbath of the cones is used to cleanse the feet and counter excessive sweating. Taken internally, cypress acts as an antispasmodic and general tonic, and is prescribed for whooping cough,

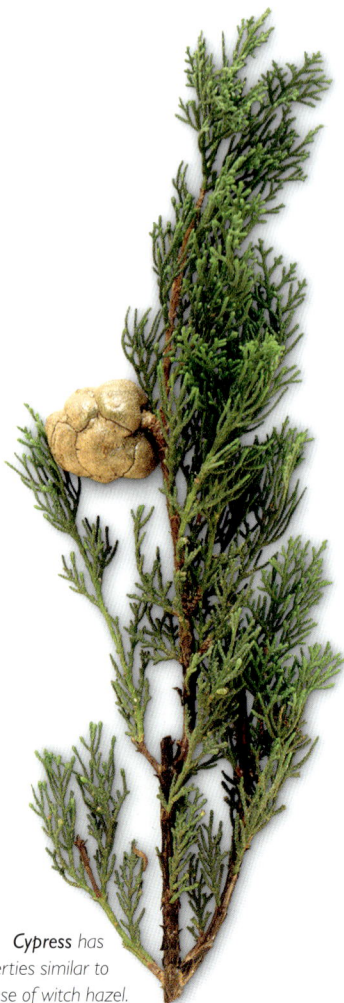

Cypress has properties similar to those of witch hazel.

the spitting up of blood, and spasmodic coughs. Colds, flu, and sore throats, and rheumatic aches and pains, also benefit from this remedy.

Caution Do not take the essential oil internally without professional supervision.

Curcuma zedoaria (Zingiberaceae)

Zedoary

Description Perennial herb with large, tapering, elliptical leaves, pink or yellow flowers, and an aromatic, pale yellow root.

Habitat & cultivation Zedoary is a common Indian and East Asian plant. It is cultivated in India, Bangladesh, Indonesia, China, and Madagascar.

Part used Rhizome.

Constituents Zedoary contains a volatile oil, sesquiterpenes, curcumemone, curcumol, and curdione. Curcumol and curdione have anticancer properties.

Medicinal actions & uses An aromatic, bitter digestive stimulant, zedoary is used in much the same way as ginger (*Zingiber officinale*, p. 159)—to relieve indigestion, nausea, flatulence, and bloating, and generally to improve digestion. The rhizome is used in China to treat certain types of tumors.

Research In trials carried out in China, zedoary was found to reduce cervical cancer, and increase the cancer-killing effects of radiotherapy and chemotherapy.

Related species In Chinese herbal medicine, zedoary is often substituted for turmeric (*C. longa*, p. 94).

Cuscuta epithymum (Convolvulaceae)

Dodder,
Hellweed, Devil's Guts

Description Leafless parasitic plant. Has threadlike stems, which are usually yellow-red in color, and small, scented, pale pink flowers.

Habitat & cultivation Dodder grows throughout Europe, Asia, and southern Africa. It prefers coastal and mountainous regions, and is gathered in summer.

Parts used Aerial parts.

Constituents Dodder contains flavonoids (including kaempferol and quercitin), and hydroxycinnamic acid.

History & folklore Dodder has always been an unpopular country plant. It is also known as hellweed and devil's guts, due to its tendency to overrun and strangle the plant on which it feeds. This host can be thyme (*Thymus vulgaris*, p. 147), gorse (*Ulex*

europaeus), or a crop such as beans. Dodder does, however, have medicinal benefits. In his *Materia Medica*, Dioscorides (1st century CE) notes its use in classical times in combination with honey to purge "black bile" and to lift a melancholy humor. In 1652, the herbalist Nicholas Culpeper similarly recommended it "to purge black or burnt choler." Culpeper further states that dodder plucked off thyme is the most efficacious, making the interesting point that the parasite's medicinal benefits are determined in part by its host.

Medicinal actions & uses In line with its traditional use to purge black bile, dodder is still considered a valuable, though little-used, herb for problems affecting the liver and gallbladder. It is thought to support liver function and is taken for jaundice. Dodder has a mildly laxative effect, and is also taken for urinary problems..

Related species Greater dodder (*C. europaea*) and flax dodder (*C. epilinum*) may be used in the same way as *C. epithymum*. *C. reflexa* is employed in Ayurvedic medicine to treat difficulty in urinating, jaundice, muscle pain, and coughs.

Cyamopsis tetragonoloba (Fabaceae)

Guar gum

Description Erect annual growing to 2 ft (60 cm), with hairy 3-lobed leaves, small purple flowers, and fleshy seed pods.

Habitat & cultivation Native to the Indian subcontinent, guar gum is cultivated extensively in India and Pakistan. The seed pods are harvested when ripe in summer.

Parts used Pods, seeds.

Constituents Guar gum contains about 86% water-soluble mucilage, comprising mainly galactomannan.

History & folklore Guar gum is a viscous substance made from ground guar seed mixed with water. It has been used as a filter in the mining industry, in paper manufacturing, and in cosmetics.

Medicinal actions & uses Guar gum is an effective bulk laxative, similar in action to psyllium (*Plantago ovata*, p. 128). It delays the emptying of the stomach and thus slows down absorption of carbohydrates. As this appears to help stabilize blood-sugar levels, guar gum may prove useful in prediabetic conditions and in the early stages of type 2 diabetes. Research also indicates that guar gum lowers cholesterol levels. In Indian medicine, guar seed is a laxative and a digestive tonic.

Caution Do not exceed the dose. Guar gum can cause flatulence, abdominal distension, and intestinal obstruction.

Cydonia oblonga (Rosaceae)

Quince

Description Deciduous tree growing to 26 ft (8 m). Has green-gray oval leaves, pink or white flowers, and yellow, pear-shaped sweet-smelling fruit.

Habitat & cultivation Native to southwest and central Asia, quince has become naturalized in Europe, especially in the Mediterranean region. It grows in damp, rich soils in hedges and copses. The fruit is harvested when ripe in the fall.

Parts used Fruit, seeds.

Constituents The fruit contains significant levels of antioxidant phenolics and flavonoids, including caffeic acids. The seeds contain a fixed oil, mucilage 20%, amygdalin 0.4%, sterols, triterpenes, tannins, and cyanogenic glycosides.

History & folklore The quince has long been prized as a fruit and medicine in Greece and the eastern Mediterranean. It was used as an astringent in the time of Hippocrates (460–377 BCE). Dioscorides (40–90 CE) records a recipe for quince oil, which was applied to itchy and infected wounds and spreading sores. In northerly climates, quince is often cooked to make a preserve. The English word "marmalade," meaning citrus fruit jam, comes from the Portuguese word for quince, *marmelo*.

Medicinal actions & uses The great astringency of the unripe fruit makes it useful as a remedy for diarrhea, one that is particularly safe for children. The fruit and its juice can also be taken as a mouthwash or gargle to treat canker sores, gum problems, and sore throats. When cooked, much of the fruit's astringency is lost; quince syrup is recommended as a pleasant, mildly astringent, digestive drink. The seeds contain significant quantities of mucilage and are helpful both in treating bronchitis and as a bulk laxative.

Caution Do not use the seeds except under professional supervision.

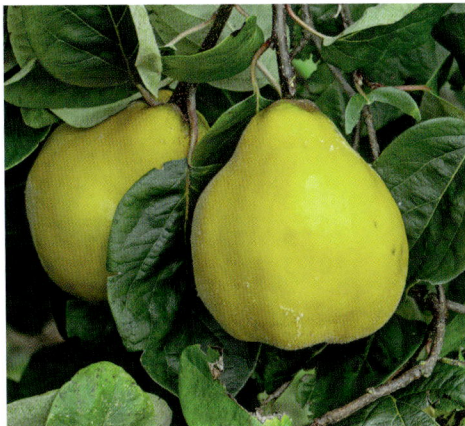

Quince oil was applied to infected wounds and sores.

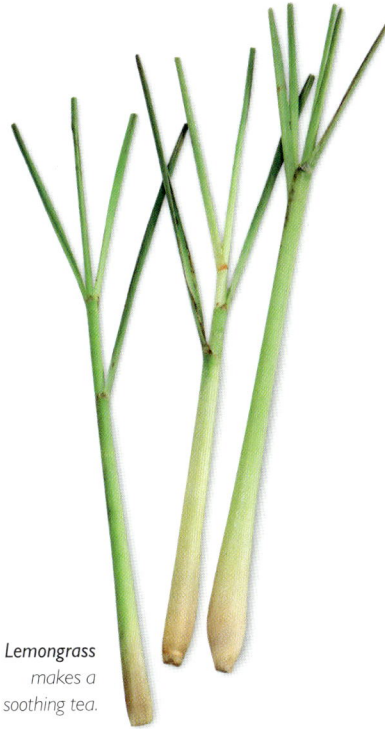

Lemongrass makes a soothing tea.

Cymbopogon citratus (Graminaceae)

Lemongrass

Description Sweetly scented grass growing in large clumps up to 5 ft (1.5 m). Has narrow leaf blades and branched stalks of flowers.

Habitat & cultivation Native to southern India and Sri Lanka, lemongrass is now cultivated in tropical regions around the world.

Parts used Leaves, essential oil.

Constituents Lemongrass contains a volatile oil with citral (about 70%) and citronellal as its main constituents. Both are markedly sedative.

History & folklore Lemongrass is cultivated for its oil, which is used as a culinary flavoring, a scent, and medicinally.

Medicinal actions & uses Lemongrass is principally taken as a tea to remedy digestive problems. It relaxes the muscles of the stomach and gut, relieves cramping pains and flatulence, and is particularly suitable for children. In the Caribbean, lemongrass is primarily regarded as a fever-reducing herb (especially where there is significant congestion). It is applied externally as a poultice or as diluted essential oil to ease pain and arthritis. In India, a paste of the leaves is smeared on patches of ringworm.

Related species *C. martinii* and *C. nardus* yield essential oils that are widely used in soaps and detergents. In Tanzania, traditional healers smoke the flowers of *C. densiflorus* to produce dreams foretelling the future.

Caution Do not take the essential oil internally without professional supervision.

Cynara cardunculus var. *scolymus* (Asteraceae)

Artichoke

Description Perennial herb growing to 5 ft (1.5 m). Has large, thistlelike leaves, gray-green above and woolly white beneath, and very large purple-green flower heads.

Habitat & cultivation Native to the Mediterranean region, artichoke thrives in rich loam in warm temperate climates. Commercially grown plants are renewed after 4 years. The unopened flower heads and leaves are picked in early summer.

Parts used Flower heads, leaves, root.

Constituents All parts of the plant contain the sesquiterpene lactone cynaropicrin (which is strongly bitter) and much inulin. The leaves also contain cynarin, which has liver-protective properties.

History & folklore Artichokes were greatly valued by the ancient Greeks and Romans. Dioscorides (1st century CE) recommended applying the mashed roots to the armpit or elsewhere on the body to sweeten offensive odors.

Medicinal actions & uses Artichoke is a valuable medicinal plant. Like milk thistle (*Silybum marianus*, p. 141), it benefits the liver, protecting against toxins and infection. Though the leaves are particularly effective, all parts of the plant are bitter and stimulate digestive secretions, especially bile. This makes artichoke useful for the treatment of gallbladder problems, nausea, indigestion, and abdominal distension, with the added benefit that

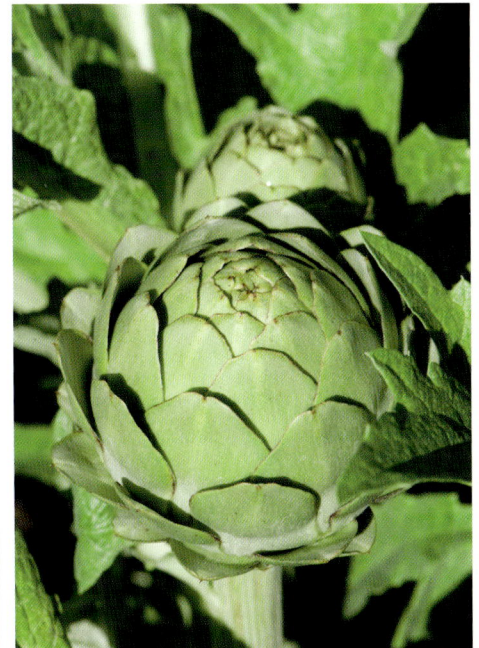

Artichoke *flower heads are nourishing and beneficial for the liver and digestion.*

it lowers blood cholesterol levels. A home recipe from the Mediterranean region uses fresh artichoke leaf juice mixed with wine or water as a liver tonic. Artichoke is also taken during the early stages of type 2 diabetes. It is a good food for diabetics, as it significantly lowers blood sugar. It is also a useful diuretic, and in France it has been used to treat rheumatic conditions.

Research The results of 8 clinical trials show that artichoke leaf extract has a restorative action on the liver. The leaf lowered raised liver enzymes in both fatty-liver disease and in obesity, making it a valuable remedy in metabolic syndrome. The leaf may prove useful in weight loss regimes.

Cyperus esculentus (Cyperaceae)

Chufa, Tiger Nut

Description Erect, grasslike plant growing to 20 in (50 cm). Has cylindrical brown tubers, lance-shaped leaves, and rays of small spikes of green-brown flowers.

Habitat & cultivation Native to the Mediterranean region, chufa was first introduced to Spain and North Africa by the Arabic people. It now grows worldwide, including in India. The tubers (called "nuts") are unearthed in winter and summer.

Parts used Tubers.

Constituents Chufa contains 20–36% fixed oil, known as chufa or tiger nut oil.

History & folklore Chufa nuts have been found in the excavations of the earliest settlements in the Nile Valley, and since ancient times they have remained a popular food in the region. The Greek physician Dioscorides, writing in the 1st century CE, mentions their ability to comfort the stomach.

Medicinal actions & uses Chufa is regarded as a digestive tonic, having a heating and drying effect on the digestive system and alleviating flatulence. It also promotes urine production and menstruation. The juice is taken to heal ulcers of the mouth and gums. Ayurvedic medicine classifies the nuts as digestive, tonic, and aphrodisiac.

Related species Many other species of *Cyperus* are used as foods or medicines. For example, in Chinese herbal medicine *C. rotundus* is used as a liver tonic, to counter indigestion and to promote menstruation. *C. stolonifera*, native to tropical regions of Asia and Australia, is thought to ease stomach pain and act as a heart stimulant. Perhaps the most famous Cyperus species of all is papyrus (*C. papyrus*). This plant provided fiber for the first writing paper, invented by the ancient Egyptians. Papyrus was also chewed like sugar cane, and used medicinally in eye compresses and to bandage wounds.

Cypripedium pubescens (Orchidaceae)

Lady's slipper, American valerian

Description Perennial orchid with several stems sheathed by broad lance-shaped leaves. Has beautiful, complex golden-yellow and purple flowers in late summer.

Habitat & cultivation This herb is native to eastern North America. Its natural habitat is woods and pastures, but due to overharvesting, it is rarely found in the wild. It is cultivated to a limited degree.

Part used Rootstock.

Constituents Lady's slipper is poorly researched, but it is known to contain a volatile oil, resins, glucosides, and tannins.

History & folklore Lady's slipper was held in high regard by Indigenous Americans, who used it as a sedative and antispasmodic. It was commonly taken to ease menstrual and labor pains, and to counter insomnia and nervous conditions. The Cherokee people used one variety to treat worms in children. In the Anglo-American Physiomedicalist tradition, lady's slipper had many uses. Swinburne Clymer (in *Nature's Healing Agents*, 1905) considered the plant "of special value in reflex functional disorders, or chorea, hysteria, nervous headache, insomnia, low fevers, nervous unrest, hypochondria, and nervous depression accompanying stomach disorders."

Medicinal actions & uses Due to its scarcity and cost, lady's slipper is now rarely used. A sedative and relaxing herb, it treats anxiety, stress-related disorders such as palpitations, headaches, muscular tension, panic attacks, and neurotic conditions generally. Like valerian (*Valeriana officinalis*, p. 152), lady's slipper is an effective tranquilizer. It reduces emotional tension and often calms the mind sufficiently to allow sleep. Indeed, its restorative effect appears to be more positive than that of valerian.

Caution In view of its rarity, lady's slipper should no longer be used medicinally.

Cytisus scoparius syn. *Sarothamnus scoparius* (Fabaceae)

Broom

Description Tall deciduous shrub growing to 6½ ft (2 m). Has narrow ridged stems, small trefoil leaves, and bright yellow flowers in leafy terminal spikes.

Habitat & cultivation Native to Europe, broom is commonly found on heaths and verges, and in open woodland. It is naturalized in many temperate regions, including in the US. The flowering tops are picked from spring to fall.

Part used Flowering tops.

Constituents Broom contains quinolizidine alkaloids (particularly sparteine and lupanine), phenethylamines (including tyramine), isoflavones (such as genistein), flavonoids, a volatile oil, caffeic and p-coumaric acids, tannins, and pigments. Sparteine reduces the heart rate and the isoflavones are estrogenic.

History & folklore Both the common and species names of this plant indicate its usefulness as a sweeper ("scopa" means "broom" in Latin). Broom's medicinal value is not mentioned in classical writings, but it does appear in medieval herbals. The 12th-century Welsh Physicians of Myddfai recommend broom as a means to treat suppressed urine: "seek broom seed, and grind into fine powder, mix with drink and let it be drank. Do this till you are quite well." Broom tops have been pickled and used as a condiment similar to capers (*Capparis spinosa*, p. 185)

Medicinal actions & uses Broom is used mainly as a remedy for an irregular, fast heartbeat. The plant acts on the electrical conductivity of the heart, slowing and regulating the transmission of the impulses. Broom is also strongly diuretic, stimulating urine production and thus countering fluid retention. Since broom causes the muscles of the uterus to contract, it has been used to prevent blood loss after childbirth.

Cautions Take broom internally only under professional supervision. Do not take during pregnancy, or if suffering from high blood pressure. The plant is subject to legal restrictions in some countries.

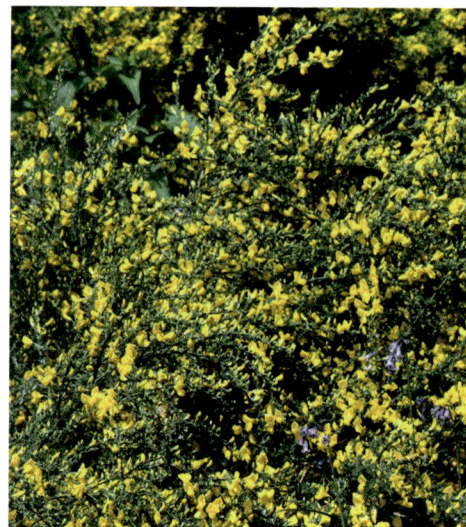

Broom, *taken under professional guidance, helps regulate an overly rapid heartbeat.*

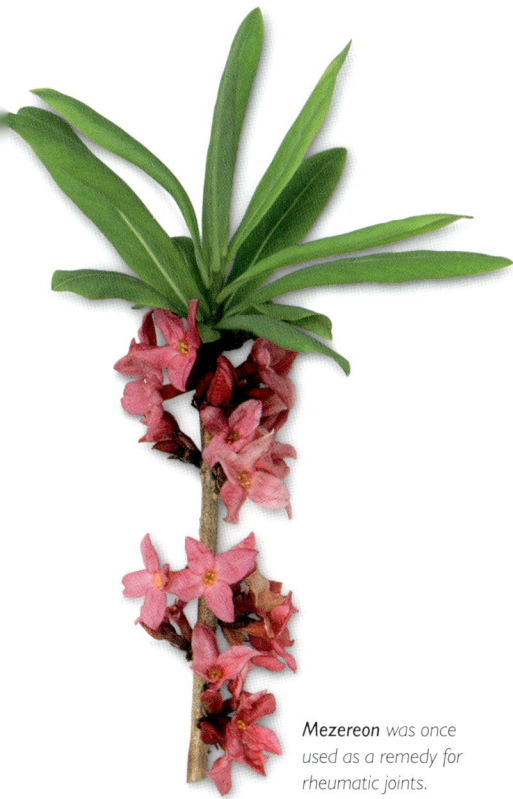

Mezereon was once used as a remedy for rheumatic joints.

Daphne mezereum (Thymelaeaceae)

Mezereon

Description Hardy deciduous shrub growing to 4 ft (1.2 m). Has oval to lance-shaped leaves, clusters of red or pink flowers, and small red berries.

Habitat & cultivation Mezereon is found in Europe, North Africa, and western Asia, in damp mountain woodlands. It is cultivated as a garden plant. The root and bark are gathered in the fall.

Parts used Root, root bark, bark.

Constituents Mezereon contains diterpenes (including daphnetoxin and mezerein), mucilage, and tannins. Though highly toxic, daphnetoxin and mezerein have antileukemic properties and have been used to treat cancer.

History & folklore Mezereon was formerly well used in northern Europe, both internally as a purgative and externally as an ointment for cancerous sores and skin ulcers. The Swedish naturalist Carolus Linnaeus (1707–1778) recorded that the bark was applied to the bites of poisonous reptiles and rabid dogs. People have reportedly died simply from eating birds that have eaten the highly poisonous berries.

Medicinal actions & uses Today, mezereon is considered too poisonous to be ingested. Mezereon is used occasionally as an external counterirritant and is effective on rheumatic joints,

increasing blood flow to the affected area.

Cautions Under no circumstances should mezereon be taken internally. It should only be used externally under professional supervision, and never on open wounds.

Datura stramonium (Solanaceae)

Thornapple

Description Robust annual growing to 3 ft (1 m). Has lobed oval leaves, long white or violet trumpet-shaped flowers, and spiny fruit capsules.

Habitat & cultivation Thornapple grows in the Americas, Europe, Asia, and North Africa. It is cultivated for medicinal use in Hungary, France, and Germany. The leaves and flowering tops are harvested in summer, and the seeds in early fall when the capsules burst.

Parts used Leaves, flowering tops, seeds.

Constituents Thornapple contains 0.2–0.45% tropane alkaloids (especially hyoscyamine and hyoscine), flavonoids, steroidal lactones, withanolides, coumarins, and tannins. The tropane alkaloids are similar to those found in deadly nightshade (*Atropa belladonna*, p. 73), acting to reduce secretions and relax smooth muscle.

History & folklore Thornapple has a long history of medicinal use. If taken in sufficient doses, it causes hallucinations; the Delphic oracle in ancient Greece and the Inca in South America may have used it as an aid to making prophecies. Though it is hallucinogenic, thornapple has traditionally been used to treat insanity.

Medicinal actions & uses At low doses, thornapple is a common remedy for asthma, whooping cough, muscle spasms, and the symptoms of Parkinsonism. It relaxes the muscles of the gastrointestinal, bronchial, and urinary tracts, and reduces digestive and mucous secretions. Like deadly nightshade, thornapple may be applied externally to relieve rheumatic pains and neuralgia.

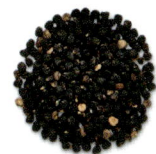

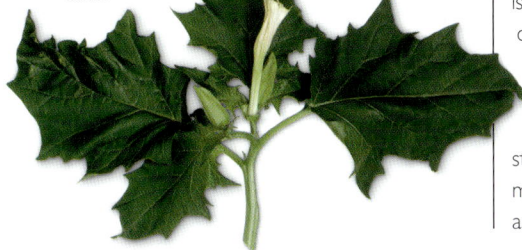

Thornapple seeds and leaves ease asthma, but are hallucinogenic in large doses.

Seeds

Related species *D. metel* and *D. innoxia* are both native to India. These plants are employed in treating asthma, coughs, fevers, and skin conditions.

Cautions Take only under professional supervision. Since it is toxic at more than small doses, thornapple is subject to legal restrictions in most countries.

Daucus carota (Apiaceae)

Carrot

Description Annual (cultivated varieties) or biennial (wild). Has erect stem, which grows to a height of 3 ft (1 m), with feathery leaves, small white flowers, and flat green seeds. Cultivated subspecies have fleshy orange taproots.

Habitat & cultivation Wild carrot is native to Europe, although cultivated subspecies are now grown around the world. The root is harvested in late summer, and the seeds are gathered in late summer or early fall.

Parts used Seeds, root, leaves.

Constituents Wild carrot seeds contain flavonoids, and a volatile oil including asarone, carotol, pinene, and limonene. Cultivated carrot root contains sugars, pectin, carotene, vitamins, minerals, and asparagine. Carrot leaves contain significant amounts of porphyrins, which stimulate the pituitary gland and lead to the release of increased levels of sex hormones.

History & folklore The origins of the familiar garden carrot are a mystery—it was cultivated as a nutritious and cleansing food at least as long ago as ancient Greece and Rome. In the 1st century CE, the physician Dioscorides recommended the seeds to stimulate menstruation, to relieve urinary retention, and to "wake up the genital virtue." The cultivated variety did not reach Britain until the 16th century, when women used its beautiful, finely divided leaves to adorn their hair.

Medicinal actions & uses This common vegetable is also a wonderfully cleansing medicine. It supports the liver, and stimulates urine flow and the removal of waste by the kidneys. The juice of organically grown carrots is a delicious drink and a valuable detoxifier. Carrots are rich in carotene, which is converted to vitamin A by the liver. The raw root, grated or mashed, is a safe treatment for threadworms, especially in children. Wild carrot leaves are a good diuretic. They have been used to counter cystitis and kidney stone formation, and to diminish stones that have already formed. The seeds are also diuretic. They stimulate menstruation and have been used in folk medicine as a treatment for hangovers. Both leaves and seeds relieve flatulence and settle the digestion.

205

Research In a study published in 1995, a carrot extract was shown to protect the liver from toxicity. **Cautions** Do not take carrot seeds during pregnancy. Use only organic carrot juice since the root concentrates artificial fertilizers and insecticides.

Desmodium adscendens (Fabaceae)

Desmodium

Description Perennial, much-branched herb, growing to 20 in (50 cm). Desmodium has light purple flowers, and the leaves each have three small oval leaflets.
Habitat & cultivation A native of West Africa, including Sierra Leone, northern Liberia and Ghana. The aerial parts are harvested as required or after flowering.
Parts used Leaves and stems.
Constituents Contains indole alkaloids, flavonoids, polyphenols, tannins, and saponins.
History & folklore Desmodium has long been used in West African herbal medicine as a treatment for asthma, and also for jaundice.
Medicinal actions & uses Desmodium is chiefly a remedy for asthma and has been used as an anti-asthmatic in Ghanaian hospitals. In France, the herb is taken for liver disorders including viral hepatitis—both A and B—apparently having most effect during the early stages. Desmodium may also be used to relieve headache, backache, and muscle and joint pain—a decoction being taken internally or applied as a lotion.
Research Ghanaian research has shown the herb to have antispasmodic and anti-asthmatic activity. It also appears to increase the resistance of liver cells to inflammation, whether resulting from infection or toxicity. When taken in the early stages of illness, it normalizes liver function.
Caution In rare cases, desmodium can cause nausea or diarrhea.

Dianthus superbus (Caryophyllaceae)

Fringed pink,
Qu mai (Chinese)

Description Upright perennial herb growing to 32 in (80 cm) or more. Has narrow, lance-shaped leaves and large, delicate, fragrant pink or lilac flowers.
Habitat & cultivation Fringed pink is native to Europe and northern Asia (including China and Japan) growing at altitudes of up to 7,900 ft (2,400 m). It grows in clumps on hillsides and crevices, and is cultivated from seed in eastern China. It is only harvested when in flower.
Parts used Aerial parts.
Constituents Fringed pink contains saponins, dianthins, tannins, and flavonoids.
History & folklore Fringed pink is first mentioned in the Chinese herbal known as the *Divine Husbandman's Classic* (*Shen'nong Bencaojing*), which was written in the 1st century CE.
Medicinal actions & uses Although fringed pink is common in Europe, there is little indication that people there have used it as anything other than a vegetable (the young leaves are best boiled or steamed). In Mongolia, it is used to promote contractions and childbirth, and is considered a diuretic, hemostatic, and anti-inflammatory. In Chinese medicine it is widely used for "damp-heat" conditions, and prescribed for kidney stones and urinary tract infections.
Research Research, mostly conducted in Korea and China, indicates that fringed pink has marked anti-inflammatory activity and possible cancer-fighting properties.
Related species The gillyflower (*D. caryophyllus*), of Mediterranean origin, has similar constituents and is traditionally prescribed in European herbal medicine for coronary and nervous disorders.

Dictamnus albus (Rutaceae)

Dittany, Burning bush

Description Strongly aromatic, bushy, and hairy perennial growing to 32 in (80 cm). Has compound leaves and spikes of 5-petaled white or pink flowers

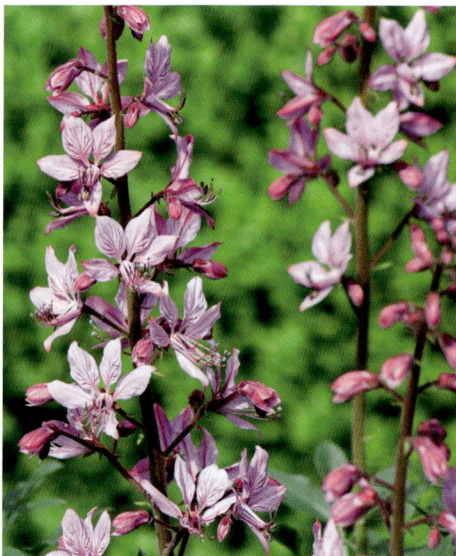

Dittany flowers were formerly used to make a preparation that was sniffed up the nose as a treatment for head colds..

streaked with purple.
Habitat & cultivation This herb grows in southern and central Europe and northern Asia, preferring warm, wooded areas. The flowering tops are gathered in late summer, the root generally in the fall.
Parts used Root, flowering tops.
Constituents Dittany's potent volatile oil contains estragol and anethole, and a toxic alkaloid, dictamnin.
History & folklore Dittany exudes such large amounts of volatile oil that in hot, dry conditions, a match held close will cause the whole plant to burst into flames. The plant has been used to flavor liqueurs and has been brewed as a tea in parts of Siberia. In European folk medicine, dittany was considered an antidote to poison, pestilence, and the bites of all types of venomous animals.
Medicinal actions & uses Very rarely used by herbalists today, dittany has an action similar to that of rue (*Ruta graveolens*, p. 273), in that it strongly stimulates the muscles of the uterus, inducing menstruation and sometimes causing abortion. By contrast, its effect on the gastrointestinal tract is antispasmodic. Dittany relaxes the gut and acts as a mild tonic for the stomach. The plant has also been used as a treatment for nervous conditions.
Cautions This herb is toxic. Take only under professional supervision. Do not take during pregnancy.

Digitalis lutea (Scrophulariaceae)

Yellow foxglove

Description Erect perennial growing to 3 ft (1 m). Has narrow, lance-shaped leaves, and long spikes of yellow, bell-shaped flowers.
Habitat & cultivation Native to western and central Europe, this herb grows in woodland areas, on roadsides, and in mountainous regions. It is cultivated for medicinal use in Russia. The leaves are harvested in the second summer of growth.
Parts used Leaves.
Constituents Yellow foxglove contains cardiac glycosides (including the cardenolides alpha-acetyldigitoxin, acetyldigitoxin, and lanatoside). All act to strengthen the beating of a weakened heart.
History & folklore Unlike the closely related common foxglove (*D. purpurea*, *following entry*), yellow foxglove does not appear to have played a significant role in European herbal medicine.
Medicinal actions & uses Yellow foxglove is little employed in herbal medicine, but in fact it is a less toxic alternative to purple foxglove and woolly foxglove (*D. lanata*). It has similar medicinal actions but its alkaloids are more readily metabolized and flushed out by the body. Like other foxgloves,

this plant supports a weakened or failing heart, increasing the strength of contraction, slowing and steadying the heart rate, and lowering blood pressure by strongly stimulating the production of urine, which reduces overall blood volume

Related species Common foxglove (*following entry*)

Cautions Excessive doses of yellow foxglove can prove fatal. Use only under professional supervision. This plant is subject to legal restrictions in some countries.

Digitalis purpurea (Scrophulariaceae)

Common foxglove, Purple foxglove

Description Perennial growing to 5 ft (1.5 m). Has a single erect stem, broad lance-shaped leaves, and bell-shaped, purple-pink or white flowers in long spikes.

Habitat & cultivation This herb is native to western Europe. Though it is also cultivated, the wild plant is considered superior.

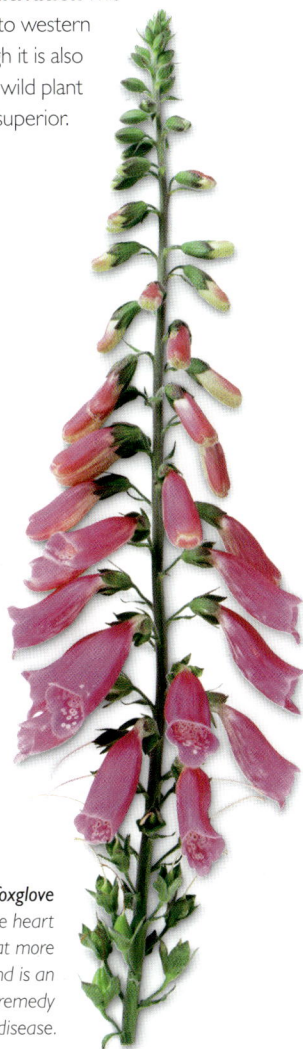

Common foxglove enables the heart to beat more evenly and is an invaluable remedy for heart disease.

The leaves are picked in summer.

Parts used Leaves.

Constituents Foxglove contains cardiac glycosides (including digoxin, digitoxin, and lanatosides), anthraquinones, flavonoids, and saponins. Digitoxin rapidly strengthens the heartbeat, but is excreted very slowly. Digitoxin is therefore preferred as a long-term medication.

History & folklore In medical history, foxglove is best known as the discovery of William Withering, an 18th-century English country doctor. Curious about the formula of a local herbalist, he explored the plant's potential medical uses. His work led to the production of a life-saving medicine.

Medicinal actions & uses Foxglove has a profound tonic effect on a diseased heart. Heart disease worsens when the heart's ability to maintain normal circulation decreases. Foxglove's cardiac glycosides enable the heart to beat more strongly, slowly, and regularly, without requiring more oxygen. At the same time, it stimulates urine production, which lowers the volume of blood, and thus lessens the load on the heart.

Related species Woolly foxglove (*D. lanata*) is today the main source of cardiac glycosides.

Cautions Potentially fatal in overdose. Use only under professional supervision. This plant is subject to legal restrictions.

Dipsacus fullonum (Dipsacaceae)

Teasel

Description Perennial with a spiny ridged stem growing to 6½ ft (2 m), lance-shaped leaves, and lilac-colored flowers blooming from hooked heads.

Habitat & cultivation Common throughout Europe and western Asia, teasel thrives on waste ground, roadsides, and banks. It is cultivated only on a small scale. The root is unearthed in late summer.

Part used Root.

Constituents Teasel contains inulin, bitter substances, and a scabioside.

History & folklore Traditionally, the root was used to treat conditions such as warts, fistulas (abnormal passages opening through the skin), and cancerous sores. The water that collects in the leaf was called "Venus's bath" by early herbalists, and was thought to be very beneficial for the eyes.

Medicinal actions & uses Teasel root is little used medicinally today, and its therapeutic applications are disputed. It is thought to have diuretic, sweat-inducing, and stomach-soothing properties, cleansing the system and improving digestion. Due to its apparent astringency, teasel is considered helpful in diarrhea. It is also thought to increase appetite, to tone the

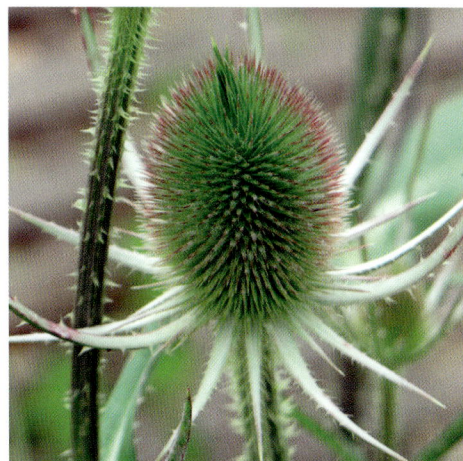

Teasel was traditionally used to treat warts and fistulas.

stomach, and to act on the liver, helping with jaundice and gallbladder problems. A new application of teasel, so far unsubstantiated, is in the treatment of Lyme disease. Research suggests that the root inhibits the breakdown of cholinesterase, making it theoretically useful in the prevention of dementia.

Dorema ammoniacum (Apiaceae)

Ammoniacum

Description Very large perennial herb growing to a height of 10 ft (3 m), with a stout stem, compound leaves, and umbels of white flowers.

Habitat & cultivation Ammoniacum is native to central Asia, Iran, and northern Russia. When pierced, the stem exudes a milky gum, which is pressed into blocks and then ground into a powder.

Part used Oleo-gum-resin.

Constituents Ammoniacum contains a resin (60–70%), gum, volatile oil (including ferulene and linalyl acetate), free salicylic acid, and coumarins.

History & folklore Ammoniacum's medicinal value has been appreciated since ancient times, and is mentioned by Hippocrates (460–377 BCE). The herb's common name reputedly derives from the Temple of Jupiter Ammon in Libya, in an area where it was commonly collected.

Medicinal actions & uses Used in both Western and Indian medicine, ammoniacum is still listed in the *British Pharmacopoeia* as an antispasmodic and as an expectorant that stimulates the coughing up of thick mucus. It is a specific treatment for chronic bronchitis, asthma, and persistent coughs. Ammoniacum is also occasionally used to induce sweating or menstruation.

Other species Ammoniacum is medicinally similar to asafoetida (*Ferula assa-foetida*, p. 215) and galbanum (*Ferula gummosa*, p. 216).

Dorstenia contrajerva (Moraceae)

Contrayerva

Description Stemless perennial herb growing to 1 ft (30 cm). Has palm-shaped leaves and long-stalked greenish flowers.

Habitat & cultivation Native to Central and South America and the Caribbean islands, *contrayerva* is generally gathered from the wild.

Part used Rhizome.

History & folklore *Contrayerva* means "antidote" in Spanish, indicating its traditional use in the treatment of poisoning and venomous bites. The herb was employed in Mayan and Aztec medicine for a variety of purposes, including as a poultice to draw pus.

Medicinal actions & uses *Contrayerva* rhizome is considered aromatic, stimulant, and sweat-inducing. Occasionally used in the early stages of serious fevers such as typhoid, it is also given for gastrointestinal problems such as diarrhea and dysentery. There is no scientific substantiation of its reputation as an antidote.

Related species *D. convexa*, native to Zaire, is used as a wound healer; *D. klainei* is used in tropical Africa as a gargle.

Drosera rotundifolia (Droseraceae)

Sundew

Description Evergreen, insectivorous perennial growing to 6 in (15 cm). Has small white flowers. The hinged, spoon-shaped leaves edged with spines secrete a sticky fluid ("sundew"), which traps insects. They are digested when the leaf closes.

Habitat & cultivation Sundew grows in Europe, Asia, and North America, and is found in marshy ground at altitudes up to 5,900 ft (1,800 m). Formerly it was picked while in flower in summer. As it is now rare, it should not be gathered from the wild.

Parts used Aerial parts.

Constituents Sundew contains flavonoids, naphthoquinones, enzymes, and volatile oil. The naphthoquinones are antimicrobial, antispasmodic, and also cough-suppressing.

History & folklore In the 16th and 17th centuries, sundew was thought to be a remedy for melancholy. In his *Irish Herbal* (1735), K'Eogh advised using sundew to "eat away rotten sores."

Medicinal actions & uses Sundew is of greatest value in the treatment of spasmodic chest conditions such as whooping cough,

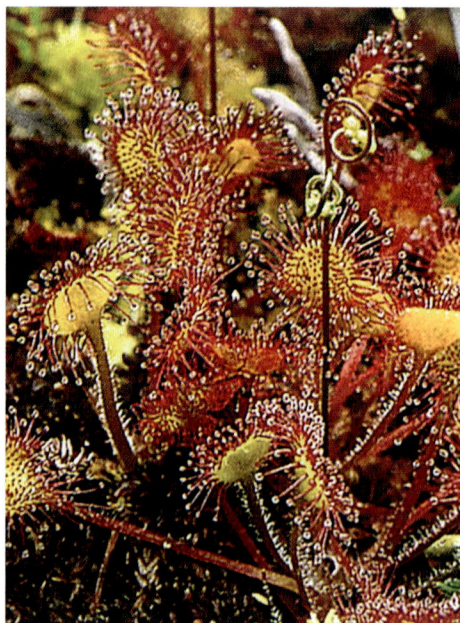

Sundew was once considered a refreshing herb because it maintained its "dew" even in full sun.

bronchial asthma, and asthma. In relaxing the muscles of the respiratory tract, the plant eases breathing, relieves wheezing, and lessens the spasms of whooping cough. Commonly mixed with thyme in a syrup, sundew is a helpful remedy for coughs in children. The herb is also prescribed for gastric problems.

Echium vulgare (Boraginaceae)

Viper's bugloss

Description Abundantly hairy perennial growing up to 3 ft (1 m). Has narrow prickly leaves and pink to violet clusters of flowers in dense spikes.

Habitat & cultivation Native to Europe, viper's bugloss is commonly found on uncultivated land, by roadsides, and in low-lying and coastal regions. The flowering tops are gathered in late summer.

Parts used Flowering tops.

Constituents Viper's bugloss contains pyrrolizidine alkaloids, allantoin, alkannins, and mucilage. In isolation, pyrrolizidine alkaloids are toxic to the liver. The alkannins are antimicrobial and allantoin helps wounds to heal.

History & folklore As its name suggests, viper's bugloss was once considered a preventative and remedy for viper bite. In his 1656 *The Art of Simpling*, herbalist William Coles described the plant: "its stalks all to be speckled like a snake or viper, and is a most singular remedy against poison and the sting of scorpions." Four years earlier, the English herbalist

Nicholas Culpeper had praised its action against "the biting of vipers."

Medicinal actions & uses In many respects, viper's bugloss is similar to borage (*Borago officinalis*, p. 183), in that both herbs have a sweat-inducing and diuretic effect if taken internally. Viper's bugloss has also been taken to treat chest conditions, as its mucilage soothes dry coughs and encourages expectoration. The significant mucilage content in viper's bugloss has also proved helpful in treating skin conditions. Prepared in a poultice or plaster, it is an effective balm for boils and carbuncles. In recent times, this herb has fallen out of use, due partly to lack of interest in its medicinal potential, and partly to its pyrrolizidine alkaloids, which in isolation are toxic. Viper's bugloss may be safely used externally on unbroken skin.

Caution Do not take internally.

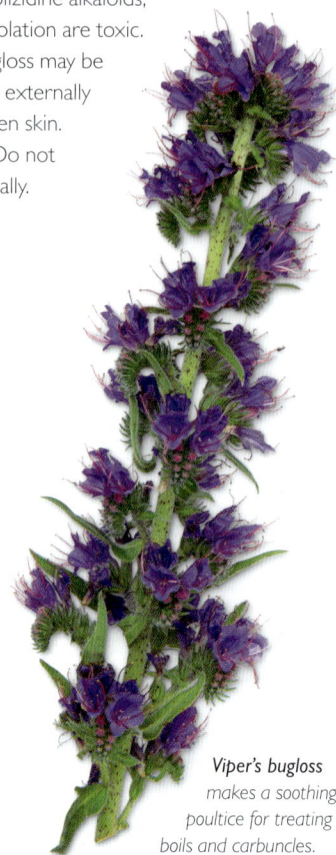

Viper's bugloss makes a soothing poultice for treating boils and carbuncles.

Eclipta prostrata syn. *E. alba* (Asteraceae)

Trailing eclipta

Description Multi-branched annual growing to 2 ft (60 cm). Has lance-shaped leaves and white flowers.

Habitat & cultivation Trailing eclipta is native to Africa, Asia, and Australia. It is now found throughout the tropics, being particularly common in India, China, and Queensland and New South Wales in Australia. It is harvested in early fall.

Parts used Aerial parts.

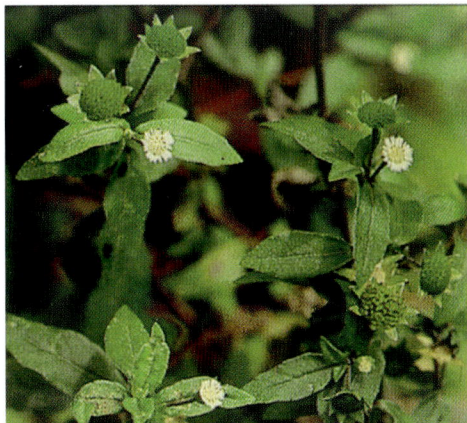

Trailing eclipta is taken in India and China to stop premature graying of the hair..

Constituents Trailing eclipta contains triterpenoid saponins, including ecliptine and alpha-terthienylmethanol, isoflavonoids, and phytosterols.

History & folklore Trailing eclipta is first mentioned in herbal literature in the Chinese *Tang Materia Medica* of 659 CE. The herb contains a black pigment that has been used to color the hair in India, and mothers wash babies' heads in a decoction of the leaves to encourage hair growth. It is also used as an ink for tattooing. The leaves are also eaten as a vegetable.

Medicinal actions & uses Trailing eclipta has remarkably similar uses in Ayurvedic and Chinese herbal medicine. In both of these traditions, a decoction is used to invigorate the liver, to prevent premature graying of the hair, and to staunch bleeding, especially from the uterus. In the Chinese tradition, the herb is considered a *yin* tonic; in Ayurvedic medicine it is thought to prevent aging. In the Caribbean, the juice is sometimes taken for asthma and bronchitis. Trailing eclipta is also used there as a treatment for enlarged glands, as well as for dizziness, vertigo, and blurred vision.

Research Several laboratory experiments have shown that eclipta regulates enzyme levels within the liver and exerts a protective activity on it.

Elymus repens, syn. Agropyron repens

Couch grass

Description Vigorous perennial growing to 32 in (80 cm). Has a long, creeping rhizome, slender leaves, and erect spikes bearing green flowers aligned in two rows.

Habitat & cultivation Found in Europe, the Americas, northern Asia, and Australia, couch grass is an invasive weed. It is harvested throughout the year.

Parts used Rhizome, seeds, root.

Constituents Couch grass contains polysaccharides (such as triticin), a volatile oil (mainly agropyrene), mucilage, and nutrients. Agropyrene has antibiotic properties.

History & folklore In classical times, both Dioscorides (40–90 CE) and Pliny (23–79 CE) recommended couch grass root for poor urine flow and kidney stones. In 1597, the herbalist John Gerard wrote that "Couch-grasse be an unwelcome guest to fields and gardens, yet his physicke virtues do recompense those hurts; for it openeth the stoppings of the liver and reins [ureters] without heat." In times of famine, the root has been roasted and ground as a substitute for coffee and flour.

Medicinal actions & uses A gentle, effective diuretic and demulcent, couch grass is most commonly used for urinary tract infections such as cystitis and urethritis. It both protects the urinary tubules against infection and irritants, and increases the volume of urine, thereby diluting it. It can be taken, usually with other herbs, to help treat kidney stones, reducing the irritation and laceration they cause. Couch grass is also thought to dissolve kidney stones (insofar as this is possible), and in any case will help prevent their further enlargement. Both an enlarged prostate and prostatitis (infection of the prostate gland) will benefit from a couch grass decoction taken over the course of several months. In German herbal medicine, heated couch grass seeds are used in a hot and moist pack that is applied to the abdomen for peptic ulcers. Juice from the roots of couch grass has been advocated for treating jaundice and other liver complaints.

Embelia ribes (Primulaceae)

Embelia

Description Climber with short, elliptical leaves, white or white-green flowers, and round red or black fruits.

Habitat & cultivation Native to India and Southeast Asia, embelia grows in hilly regions. The fruit is harvested when ripe.

Part used Fruit.

Constituents Embelia contains naphthaquinones, including embelin. Embelin stimulates the production of estrogen and progesterone, and it may have a contraceptive effect.

Medicinal actions & uses Embelia has been used in Asia as a home remedy for expelling worms. The herb is also diuretic and relieves flatulence, and is used for indigestion, colic, constipation, and debility.

Cautions Use only under professional supervision. Do not take during pregnancy.

Emblica officinalis (Euphorbiaceae)

Indian gooseberry

Description Deciduous tree with feathery leaves, pale green flowers, and round pale green or yellow fruit. Also known as amla.

Habitat & cultivation Indian gooseberry grows in China, India, and Southeast Asia and is widely cultivated for its fruit.

Part used Fruit.

Constituents Indian gooseberry contains tannins, polyphenols, flavonoids, a fixed oil, and a volatile oil.

History & folklore The Indian gooseberry features in a 7th-century Ayurvedic medical text. The sage Muni Chyawan reputedly restored his vitality with this fruit.

Medicinal actions & uses The astringent Indian gooseberry is given to allay the effects of aging and to restore the organs. In Ayurvedic medicine, the fruit juice is given to strengthen the pancreas of diabetics. It is one of the three herbs in the classic Ayurvedic herbal formula known as "Triphala."

Research Recent research suggests that Indian gooseberry might have a remarkably wide range of potential medicinal benefits. A study in Kerala, India, showed that it may have protective activity against liver cancer. Other studies indicate potential anti-inflammatory and fever-inhibiting effects, and a cholesterol-lowering action. A study undertaken in Bombay concluded that the fruit might prove useful in the treatment of acute pancreatitis.

Entada phaseoloides (Fabaceae)

Matchbox Bean

Description Woody vine with compound leaves and pea-type flowers. Huge, flat brown seed pods, with black seeds grow to 5 ft (1.5 m) in length.

Habitat & cultivation Matchbox bean is native to Australia and tropical regions of Asia and Africa. The seeds are collected when the pods are ripe.

Parts used Seeds.

Constituents Matchbox bean contains high levels of proteins and unsaturated fatty acids, flavonoids, and toxic triterpene saponins.

History & folklore The young leaves and roasted bean are eaten as vegetables, whereas fiber from the stems is made into nets, ropes, and sails. Due to the plant's high saponin content, it is used as a shampoo.

Medicinal actions & uses Australian Aboriginal people use the seeds to treat female sterility and indigestion, and as a painkiller. In the Philippines, juice made from the bark is used to treat conjunctivitis.

Equisetum arvense (Equisetaceae)

Horsetail, Bottlebrush

Description Perennial plant with a yellowish fruiting stem growing to 14 in (35 cm), followed by a sterile segmented and toothed stem growing to 2 ft (60 cm). The latter has whorls of needle-shaped leaves.

Habitat & cultivation Native to Europe, North Africa, northern Asia, and the Americas, horsetail is a common plant, preferring damp soil. The sterile stems are harvested in summer and carefully dried, all discolored parts being discarded.

Parts used Aerial parts.

Constituents Horsetail contains large amounts of silicic acid and silicates (about 15%), flavonoids, phenolic acids, alkaloids (including nicotine), and sterols. Much of the therapeutic effectiveness of this herb is due to its high silica content, a large proportion of which is soluble and can be absorbed. Silica supports the regeneration of connective tissue.

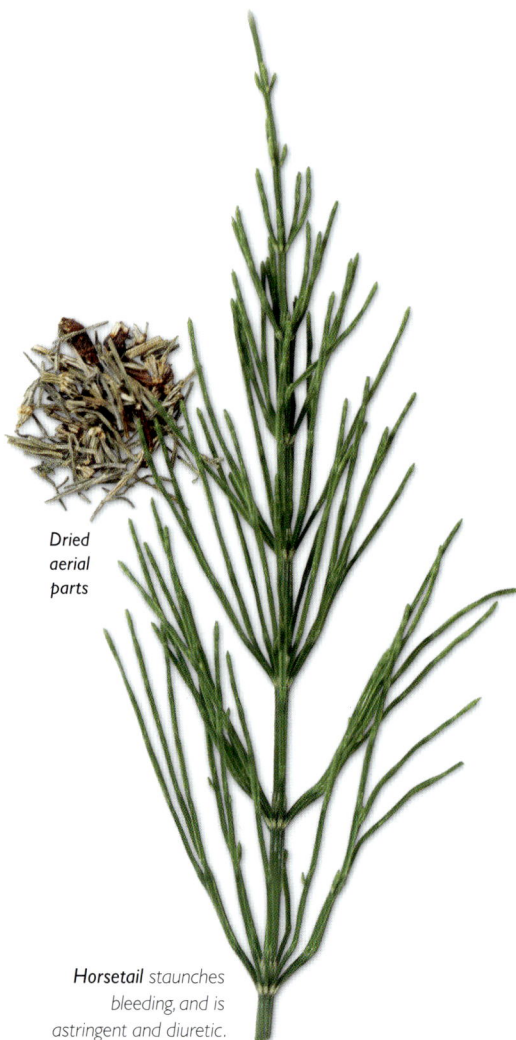

Dried aerial parts

Horsetail staunches bleeding, and is astringent and diuretic.

History & folklore Horsetail is a primitive plant that is descended from huge trees that lived during the Paleozoic era (600–375 million years ago). The herb's high silica content makes it abrasive, and in the past it was used to polish metal and wood. Its common name, bottlebrush, indicates another of its uses. Horsetail was also tied to the tails of livestock to help them ward off flies. It was long considered a wound-healing herb. The English herbalist John Gerard, writing in 1597, recounted: "Dioscorides saith, that the horse-taile being stamped and laid to, doth perfectly cure wounds, yea although the sinues be cut in sunder, as Galen addeth."

Medicinal actions & uses As its traditional usage indicates, horsetail is an excellent clotting agent. It staunches wounds, stops nosebleeds, and reduces the coughing up of blood. In addition, horsetail has an astringent effect on the genitourinary system, proving especially valuable where there is bleeding within the urinary tract, and in cases of cystitis, urethritis, and prostate disease. Horsetail helps speed the repair of damaged connective tissue, improving its strength and elasticity. The herb is also prescribed to treat problems related to rheumatic and arthritic problems, for chest ailments (such as emphysema), for chronic swelling of the legs, and for various other conditions. A decoction of the herb's aerial parts added to a bath benefits slow-healing sprains and fractures, as well as certain irritable skin conditions such as eczema.

Research Several of horsetail's traditional uses have been upheld by clinical research, notably its value as a diuretic and in treating an enlarged prostate.

Cautions Horsetail breaks down vitamin B1 (thiamine) and should generally be taken long term only in tandem with a vitamin B supplement.

Eriodictyon californicum (Boraginaceae)

Yerba santa

Description Sticky evergreen shrub growing to 8 ft (2.5 m). Its narrow lance-shaped leaves are shiny green on the upper side and hairy white underneath. Trumpet-shaped white or blue flowers grow in clusters.

Habitat & cultivation Native to California and Oregon in the US, and northern Mexico, *yerba* santa flourishes on dry mountain slopes. It grows at altitudes of up to 3,900 ft (1,200 m).

Parts used Leaves.

Constituents *Yerba* santa contains a volatile oil, flavonoids (including eriodictyol), and resin.

History & folklore The name yerba santa (holy weed) was given to this plant by Spanish colonists who learned of its medicinal virtues from Indigenous North Americans. Traditionally, the leaves were infused and taken for coughs, colds, sore throats, mucus, and asthma. The infusion was also used as a wash to ease fever, and the mashed leaves were applied as a poultice to treat sores.

Medicinal actions & uses An aromatic herb with a pleasant sweet taste, *yerba santa* is a valuable expectorant that can be used to treat tracheitis, bronchitis, and asthma, and similar respiratory tract ailments.

Eryngium maritimum (Apiaceae)

Sea holly, Eryngo

Description Evergreen perennial growing to 2 ft (60 cm). Has spiny silver leaves, and tiny flowers in summer.

Habitat Sea holly is found in coastal areas of Europe, preferring sandy soils. The root is unearthed in the fall.

Part used Root.

Constituents Sea holly contains saponins, coumarins, flavonoids, and plant acids.

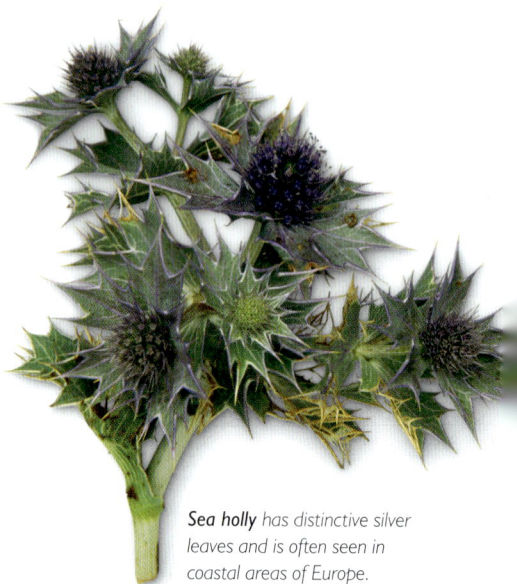

Sea holly has distinctive silver leaves and is often seen in coastal areas of Europe.

History & folklore In 17th-century England, sea holly root was candied and eaten as a sweetmeat. It was also consumed as a means of preventing scurvy. In his *Irish Herbal* (1735), K'Eogh states that the herb "provokes urination and menstruation, encourages flatulence, and removes obstructions of the liver, kidneys, and bladder." In K'Eogh's time, sea holly was a popular medicinal herb, and was considered helpful in the treatment of a wide array of neurological conditions, including paralysis and convulsions.

Medicinal actions & uses In contemporary European herbal medicine, sea holly is used as a diuretic. It is prescribed as a treatment for cystitis and urethritis, and taken as a means to alleviate kidney stones. It is unlikely that the herb actually dissolves established stones, but it probably helps retard their formation. Sea holly is also used to treat enlargement or inflammation of the prostate gland, and may be of benefit in treating chest problems.

Erythraea centaurium (Gentianaceae)
Centaury

Description Biennial herb growing to 9½ in (24 cm) with a basal rosette of leaves and 5-petaled pink flowers in clusters.

Habitat & cultivation Native to Europe and southwestern Asia, centaury is now found in temperate regions throughout the world. The plant is harvested in summer when just about to flower.

Parts used Aerial parts.

Constituents Centaury contains many bitter constituents, including secoiridoids, also found in gentian (*Gentiana lutea*, p. 103).

History & folklore In classical myth, the centaur Chiron used this herb to treat a poisoned arrow wound.

Medicinal actions & uses One of the most useful bitter herbs, centaury has a relatively mild bitter action, stimulating appetite as well as digestive secretions from the salivary glands, stomach, intestines, and gallbladder. With increased digestive juices, food is processed and broken down more effectively, leading to better absorption of nutrients. For best results, centaury should be taken over several weeks. The preparation should be slowly sipped so that the components (detectable at a dilution of up to 1:3,500) can stimulate reflex activity throughout the upper digestive tract.

Self-help uses Weak digestion, p. 316; Gas & bloating, p. 316.

Erythrina variegata (Fabaceae)
Indian coral tree, *Dadap* (Hindi)

Description Deciduous tree growing to 59 ft (18 m). Has prickly stems, leaves with triangular leaflets, and pealike red flowers.

Habitat & cultivation Indian coral tree grows in deciduous forests throughout much of the Indian subcontinent.

Parts used Bark, leaves.

Constituents Indian coral tree contains alkaloids, isoflavonoids, triterpenoids, and lectins. The alkaloids are anti-inflammatory and analgesic, and the isoflavonoids display antibacterial activity.

Medicinal actions & uses In Ayurvedic medicine, Indian coral tree is used to treat inflammatory conditions, period pain, and problems related to eating and digestion, including anorexia, flatulence, colic, and worms. The bark is used to treat skin problems and fever. A paste made from the leaves is applied to heal wounds.

Erythronium americanum (Liliaceae)
Trout lily

Description Perennial growing to 10 in (25 cm) from a small, bulblike corm. Has two oblong leaves mottled with purple and a large, bright yellow lily flower.

Habitat & cultivation Native to North America, trout lily is found mainly in the east, from New Brunswick to Florida. It prefers damp woodland and open ground. The leaves are gathered in summer.

Parts used Leaves.

Constituents Very little is known about the constituents of this plant. It contains alpha-methylenebutyrolactone.

History & folklore Trout lily was little used by Indigenous North American peoples. European colonizers considered its medicinal properties to be similar to those of meadow saffron (*Colchicum autumnale*, p. 197). Trout lily was listed in the *Pharmacopoeia of the United States* from 1820 to 1863 as a treatment for gout.

Medicinal actions & uses An infusion of the leaves is taken for skin problems such as ulcers and tumors, and for enlarged glands. The leaves (or the whole plant) may also be applied as a poultice for skin conditions. The fresh leaves are strongly emetic.

Caution Take trout lily only under professional supervision.

Erythroxylum coca (Erythroxylaceae)
Coca

Description Evergreen shrub growing to 10 ft (3 m). Has alternate oval leaves, small white flowers, and small red berries that each contain a single seed.

Habitat & cultivation Native to Peru and Bolivia, coca grows in high-rainfall areas of the eastern Andes to altitudes of 4,900 ft (1,500 m). It is mostly cultivated for the illegal market. The leaves are picked when they begin to curl.

Parts used Leaves.

Constituents Coca contains cocaine and various

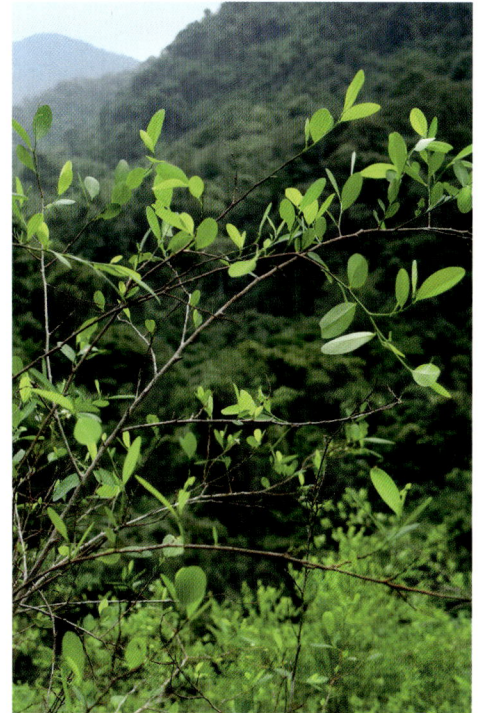

Coca is cultivated in the Andes and chewed as a tonic to help counter the effects of cold.

other alkaloids, a volatile oil, flavonoids, vitamins A and B$_2$, and minerals. The plant's stimulant and anesthetic action is due largely to cocaine.

History & folklore The Indigenous peoples of the Andes carry pouches containing coca leaves and lime, which they chew throughout the day. Early European travelers noted that individuals chewing coca never had tooth or gum problems, and local folk medicine traditionally considered the plant a treatment for toothache. Coca leaf extract is still used as a flavoring for cola drinks—but cocaine has long been banned from the formulas.

Medicinal actions & uses In Bolivia and Peru, coca leaves play an important part in the culture and herbal medicine of the Indigenous Aymara and Quechua peoples. High altitudes, cold, and an impoverished diet place great physical demands on the population. Coca leaves, chewed with lime or ashes, release small amounts of the active constituents, which act as a tonic and help block the effects of cold, exhaustion, and poor nutrition. Coca leaves are also used in South American herbal medicine to treat nausea, vomiting, and asthma, and have been used to speed convalescence. Cocaine extracted from coca leaves is used legally in conventional medicine as a local anesthetic. It is also taken illegally as a narcotic, stimulant drug. As an isolated chemical, cocaine is extremely addictive.

Cautions Take only under professional supervision. Coca is subject to legal restrictions in most countries.

Eschscholzia californica (Papaveraceae)

California poppy

Description Annual or perennial growing to 2 ft (60 cm). California poppy has finely cut leaves and bright orange, yellow, pink, or red flowers.

Habitat & cultivation California poppy is native to western North America. Widely cultivated as a garden plant, it prefers sandy soils.

Parts used Aerial parts.

Constituents California poppy contains isoquinoline alkaloids (including protopine, cryptopine, and chelidonine) and flavone glycosides.

History & folklore Indigenous North American peoples used the sap of California poppy for its pain-killing properties, particularly for toothaches. The leaves were also eaten as a vegetable. Early colonizers used California poppy for sleep issues, especially in children, and for whooping cough. It is California's state flower.

Medicinal actions & uses Though the California poppy is a close relation of the opium poppy (*Papaver somniferum*, p. 251), it has a significantly different effect on the central nervous system. California poppy is not a narcotic. In fact, rather than disorienting the user, it actually tends to normalize psychological function. California poppy's gently antispasmodic, sedative, and analgesic effects make it a valuable herbal medicine for treating physical and psychological problems in children. The herb may prove beneficial in attempts to overcome nervous tension and anxiety, bed-wetting, and difficulty in sleeping.

Research A French study confirmed the traditional usage of California poppy by showing that extracts were sedative, reduced anxiety levels, and were nontoxic.

California poppy contains a latex that has sedative, pain-killing, and antispasmodic properties. It is a gentle remedy, suitable for children.

Eucalyptus smithii (Myrtaceae)

Gully gum

Description Aromatic evergreen tree growing to 165 ft (50 m).

Habitat & cultivation Native to Australia, eucalyptus now grows in temperate and subtropical zones around the globe. It prefers moist soil, and so is found in swamps, gullies, and at the foot of slopes.

Part used Essential oil.

Constituents The volatile oil contains about 70% eucalyptol (1,8-cineole), as well as pinene, limonene, alpha-terpineol, and linalool. While it is similar to the oils of related species, this oil appears to be better tolerated by the skin.

Medicinal actions & uses *Eucalyptus smithii* oil is an antiseptic and decongestant, and is used for inhalations as well as aromatherapy massages. See eucalyptus (*Eucalyptus globulus*, p. 100) for further details.

Cautions Though less toxic than the oils of other eucalyptus species, *E. smithii* essential oil should be used with care. Follow the label instructions, or take on professional advice.

Eucommia ulmoides (Eucommiaceae)

Eucommia bark,
Du zhong (Chinese)

Description Deciduous tree growing to 65 ft (20 m). Has elliptical leaves, with male flowers in loose clusters and solitary female flowers in the leaf axils.

Habitat & cultivation Eucommia bark grows in temperate zones in China. It is cultivated, but only in small amounts.

Part used Bark.

Constituents Eucommia bark contains gutta-percha, alkaloids, flavonoids, iridoids and other glycosides, and phenolic compounds.

History & folklore The herb is mentioned in the Chinese herbal, the *Divine Husbandman's Classic* (*Shen'nong Bencaojing*), which was written in the 1st century CE.

Medicinal actions & uses Eucommia bark is considered an excellent tonic for the liver and kidneys. Eucommia bark is said to "tonify the *yang*," to improve the circulation, and also to prevent miscarriage in women who are weak or suffering from back pain.

Research Much interest has been aroused by eucommia bark's ability to reduce high blood pressure, which it is thought to do by increasing nitric oxide levels within the arteries. In a clinical trial in China involving 119 people, 46% of those treated with the herb showed a significant blood pressure reduction. However, eucommia bark appears to have little effect in cases of severe hypertension. Recent studies indicate that eucommia bark is an antioxidant and may help to prevent the onset of type 2 diabetes. A small clinical trial in Japan published in 1996 concluded that an infusion of eucommia bark reduced the body's exposure to mutagen-forming compounds naturally present within the diet.

Euonymus atropurpureus (Celastraceae)

Wahoo bark

Description Deciduous tree growing to 26 ft (8 m). Has smooth branches, serrated elliptical leaves, clusters of purple flowers, and 4-lobed scarlet fruit.

Habitat & cultivation Native to eastern North America, wahoo bark thrives in damp woods and close to water. The bark is gathered in the fall.

Parts used Stem bark, root bark.

Constituents Wahoo bark contains cardenolides (cardiac glycosides) similar to digitoxin, asparagine, sterols, and tannins.

History & folklore The Sioux, Cree, and other Indigenous North American peoples used wahoo bark in various ways—as an eye lotion, as a poultice for facial sores, and for gynecological conditions. Indigenous peoples introduced the plant to early European colonizers, and it became very popular in North America as well as in Britain in the 19th century.

Medicinal actions & uses Wahoo bark is considered a gallbladder remedy with laxative and diuretic properties. It is prescribed for biliousness and liver problems, as well as for skin conditions such as eczema (which may result from poor liver and gallbladder function) and for constipation. In the past, it was often used in combination with herbs such as gentian (*Gentiana lutea*, p. 103) as a fever remedy, especially if the liver was under stress. Following the discovery that it contains cardiac glycosides, wahoo bark has been given for heart conditions.

Cautions Wahoo bark is toxic. Use only under professional supervision. Do not take during pregnancy or while breastfeeding.

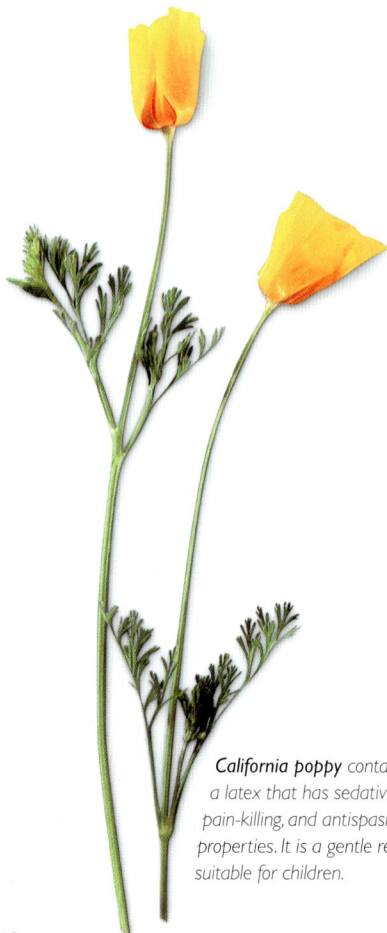

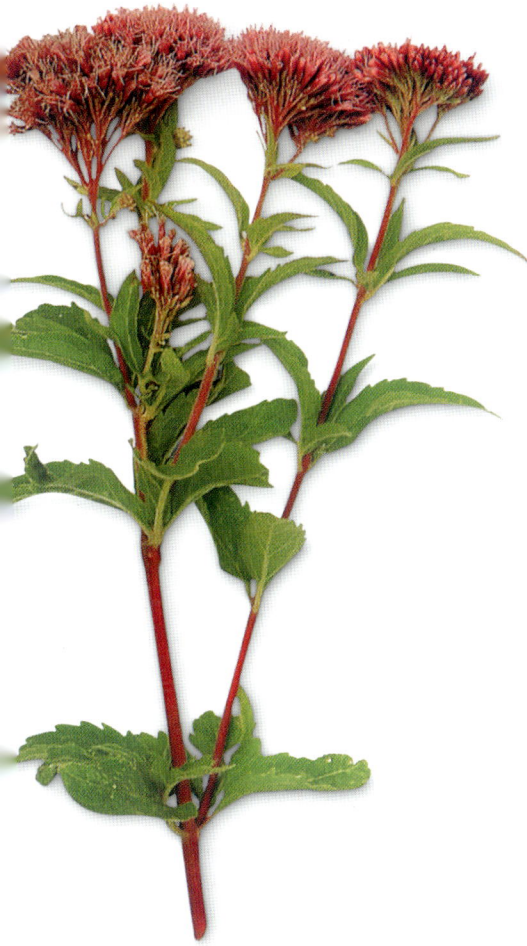

Hemp agrimony was formerly taken as a spring tonic in Holland.

Eupatorium cannabinum (Asteraceae)

Hemp agrimony

Description Perennial growing to a height of 5 ft (1.5 m). Has a red stem, downy leaves, and dense bunches of pink to mauve florets.

Habitat & cultivation Native to Europe, hemp agrimony is now also found in western Asia and North Africa. It grows in damp woods, ditches, marshes, and on waste ground, and is gathered when in flower in summer.

Parts used Aerial parts, root.

Constituents Hemp agrimony contains a volatile oil (with alpha-terpinene, p-cymene, thymol, and an azulene), sesquiterpene lactones (especially eupatoriopicrin), flavonoids, pyrrolizidine alkaloids, and polysaccharides. P-cymene is antiviral, while eupatoriopicrin has anticancer properties and inhibits cellular growth. The polysaccharides stimulate the immune system. In isolation, the pyrrolizidine alkaloids are toxic to the liver.

History & folklore Hemp agrimony was known to Ibn Sina (980–1037 CE) and other practitioners of Arabian medicine in the early Middle Ages.

Medicinal actions & uses Hemp agrimony has been employed chiefly as a detoxifying herb for fever, colds, flu, and other acute viral conditions. The root is laxative and diuretic, and the whole herb is considered to be tonic. Recently, hemp agrimony has found use as an immunostimulant, helping to maintain resistance to acute viral and other infections.

Related species See also boneset (*E. perfoliatum*, following entry) and gravel root (*E. purpureum*, subsequent entry).

Caution In view of hemp agrimony's pyrrolizidine alkaloid content, take only under professional supervision.

Eupatorium perfoliatum (Asteraceae)

Boneset

Description Erect perennial growing to 5 ft (1.5 m). Has tapering lance-shaped leaves and many white or purple florets.

Habitat & cultivation Native to eastern North America, boneset is found in meadows and marshland. It is gathered when in flower in summer.

Parts used Aerial parts.

Constituents Boneset contains sesquiterpene lactones (including eupafolin), polysaccharides, flavonoids, diterpenes, sterols, and volatile oil. The sesquiterpene lactones and polysaccharides are significant immunostimulants. Boneset also contains pyrrolizidine alkaloids (see Cautions below).

History & folklore Indigenous North American peoples used boneset to make an infusion for treating colds, fever, and arthritic and rheumatic pain. European colonizers learned of the plant's benefits, and by the 18th and 19th centuries it was regarded as a virtual cure-all. Boneset's common name derives from its ability to treat "break-bone fever." Commonly used to treat malaria, constituents within boneset are now known to have antiprotozoal activity.

Medicinal actions & uses A hot infusion of boneset will bring relief to symptoms of the common cold. The plant stimulates resistance to viral and bacterial infections, and reduces fever by encouraging sweating. Boneset also loosens phlegm and promotes its removal through coughing, and it has a tonic and laxative effect. It has been taken for rheumatic illness, skin conditions, and worms.

Cautions The pyrrolizidine alkaloids that occur in this plant are likely to be hepatotoxic—toxic to the liver. Use only under professional supervision.

Self-help uses Allergic rhinitis with mucus, p. 310; Colds, flu, & fevers, p. 321; High fever, p. 321.

Euphorbia hirta syn. *E. pilulifera* (Euphorbiaceae)

Pill-bearing Spurge, Asthma Plant

Description Erect annual or perennial plant growing to 20 in (50 cm), with pointed oval leaves and clusters of small flowers.

Habitat & cultivation Native to India and Australia, pill-bearing spurge is now widespread throughout the tropics. The aerial parts of the plant are gathered when it is in flower.

Parts used Aerial parts.

Constituents Pill-bearing spurge contains flavonoids, terpenoids, alkanes, phenolic acids, shikimic acid, and choline. The latter two constituents may be partly responsible for the antispasmodic action of this plant.

History & folklore As its name suggests, this plant was traditionally used in Asia to treat asthma.

Medicinal actions & uses A specific treatment for bronchial asthma, pill-bearing spurge relaxes the bronchial tubes and eases breathing. Mildly sedative and expectorant, it is also taken for bronchitis and other respiratory tract conditions. It is most often used along with other anti-asthmatic herbs, notably gumplant (*Grindelia camporum*, p. 222) and lobelia (*Lobelia inflata*, p. 114). In the Anglo-American tradition, pill-bearing spurge is taken to treat intestinal amebiasis.

Related species The Cherokee people used *E. maculata* to treat sore nipples and skin disorders. Many other North American *Euphorbia* species were used for constipation. A decoction of *E. lancifolia*, native to the West Indies, is used to stimulate breast-milk production. *E. atoto* is used in Malaysia and Indochina to induce a delayed period and as an abortifacient. Many species of *Euphorbia* are used as arrow poisons.

Caution Take only under professional supervision.

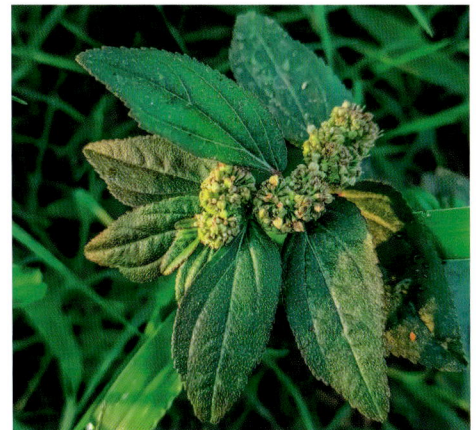

Pill-bearing spurge is recommended as a treatment for asthma.

Euphrasia spp. (Scrophulariaceae)
Eyebright

Description Creeping semiparasitic annual growing to 20 in (50 cm). Has tiny oval leaves and small scallop-edged white flowers with yellow spots and a black center, somewhat resembling an eye.

Habitat & cultivation Common in Europe, eyebright thrives in meadows and open grassland. It is gathered in summer when in flower.

Parts used Aerial parts.

Constituents Eyebright contains iridoid glycosides (including aucubin), flavonoids, tannins, lignans, and phenolic acids. Aucubin has antibacterial, anti-inflammatory, and antispasmodic activity.

History & folklore Eyebright's use for eye problems was due in part to the Doctrine of Signatures, an ancient belief that the way that a plant looks—its "sign"—indicates the ailments for which it should be used as a medicine.

Medicinal actions & uses Eyebright relieves inflammation and tightens mucous membranes and finds specific use in the treatment of conjunctivitis and blepharitis. Its ability to counter mucus means that it is often used for infectious and allergic conditions affecting the eyes, middle ear, sinuses, and nasal passages. Eyebright counters liquid mucus, but it should be used guardedly for dry and stuffy congestion, which tends to be made worse by the plant's astringency.

Self-help uses Allergic rhinitis with mucus, p. 310; **Conjunctivitis**, p. 320; **Prevention of nosebleeds**, p. 320.

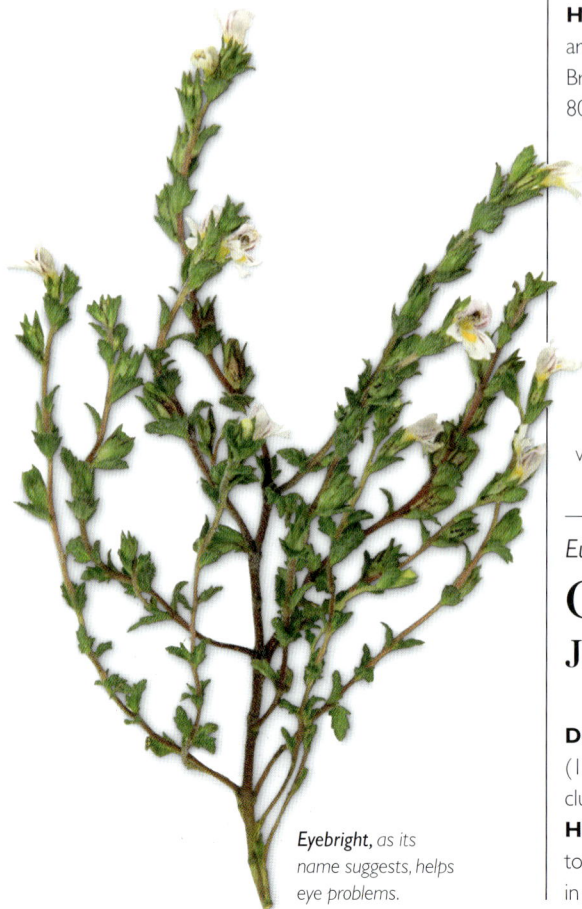

Eyebright, as its name suggests, helps eye problems.

Euterpe oleracea (Arecaceae)
Acai

Description A rainforest palm reaching 80 ft (25 m), with 4–8 slender trunks and pinnate leaves up to 10 ft (3 m) long. The berries (about the size of a grape) hang down in large bunches.

Habitat & cultivation Found throughout much of Central America and northern South America, the acai palm is widely grown for its berries and palm hearts.

Parts used Drupe (the "berries"), seed, root, palm heart.

Constituents The berries contain high levels of polyphenols, especially anthocyanins and proanthocyanidins (as found in other dark purple berries, such as blueberry). They are strong antioxidants and anti-inflammatories.

History & folklore Acai berries and their juice are a nutritious part of many Brazilians' diet. In Brazil and Peru, the crushed seeds (which make up 80% of the berry) are used to treat fever.

Traditionally, the essence of the root is extracted to treat conditions such as hepatitis and enlarged prostate.

Medicinal actions & uses Less a medicine than a nourishing addition to the diet, acai supports vitality and a healthy heart and circulation. Acai juice has much in common with blueberry and pomegranate (*Punica granatum*, p. 267) juices—all helping to sustain good health. The Acai palm is the main source of palm hearts, which are eaten worldwide as a vegetable.

Eutrochium purpureum (Asteraceae)
Gravel Root,
Joe Pye weed

Description Erect perennial growing to 5 ft (1.5 m). Has whorls of pointed oblong leaves and clusters of purple-pink florets.

Habitat & cultivation Gravel root is native to eastern North America. The root is unearthed in the fall.

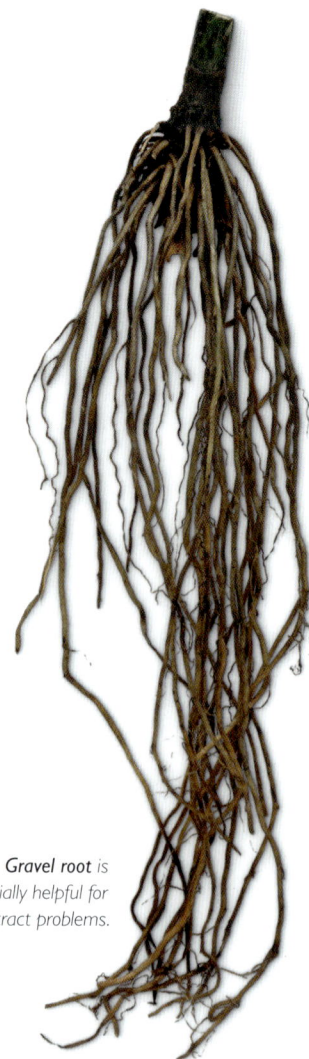

Gravel root is especially helpful for urinary tract problems.

Part used Root.

Constituents Gravel root contains a volatile oil, flavonoids, and resin.

History & folklore The plant's alternative name, Joe Pye weed, is in honor of the Indigenous North American said to have used it to cure New Englanders of typhus. Indigenous peoples used the herb as a diuretic and as a remedy for genitourinary conditions. The root was listed in the *Pharmacopoeia* of the *United States* from 1820 to 1842.

Medicinal actions & uses As its common name indicates, gravel root is a valuable herb for urinary tract problems. It helps prevent the formation of kidney and bladder stones and may diminish existing stones. Gravel root is also useful for cystitis, urethritis, prostate enlargement (and other forms of obstruction), and for rheumatism and gout. The root is thought to help the latter two conditions by increasing the removal of waste by the kidneys.

Cautions The pyrrolizidine alkaloids that occur in this plant are likely to be hepatotoxic—toxic to the liver. Use only under professional supervision.

Evodia rutaecarpa (Rutaceae)

Evodia,
Wu zhu yu (Chinese)

Description Deciduous tree growing to 33 ft (10 m). Has compound leaves, clusters of white flowers, and greenish-red fruit.

Habitat & cultivation Native to China, and the eastern Himalayas, evodia is cultivated in China. The partially ripe fruit is gathered in late summer.

Part used Fruit.

Constituents Evodia contains the alkaloids evodine, evodiamine, and rutaecarpine.

History & folklore Evodia is listed in the *Divine Husbandman's Classic* (*Shen'nong Bencaojing*) of the 1st century CE.

Medicinal actions & uses Evodia has a marked warming effect on the body, helping relieve headaches and a wide range of digestive problems. In Chinese herbal medicine, evodia is used mainly for abdominal pains, vomiting, diarrhea, headaches, and a weak pulse.

Research Chinese studies indicate that evodia is analgesic and reduces blood pressure.

Caution Use evodia only under professional supervision.

Fagopyrum esculentum (Polygonaceae)

Buckwheat

Description Annual growing to about 20 in (50 cm). Has arrow-shaped leaves and clusters of white or pink 5-petaled flowers.

Habitat & cultivation Buckwheat is native to central and northern Asia, and is cultivated extensively in temperate regions, especially the US. It is harvested in summer.

Parts used Leaves, flowers.

Constituents Buckwheat contains bioflavonoids, especially rutin, which is strongly antioxidant. Rutin strengthens the inner lining of blood vessels.

History & folklore Buckwheat's French name, *blé Sarrasin*, alludes to its ancient Middle Eastern origins. The grain was either introduced to Europe during the Crusades (11th and 12th centuries), or it was brought to Spain by the Arabic people several centuries earlier.

Medicinal actions & uses Used for a wide range of circulatory problems, buckwheat is best taken as a tea or tablet, accompanied by vitamin C or lemon juice (*Citrus limon*, p. 86) to aid absorption. Buckwheat is used particularly to treat fragile capillaries (seen as small bruises with no apparent cause), but also helps strengthen varicose veins and heal chilblains. Often combined with linden flowers (*Tilia spp.*, p. 286),

buckwheat is a specific treatment for hemorrhage into the retina. Buckwheat is also commonly taken in combination with other herbs for high blood pressure.

Related species Recent research has shown that the Chinese *F. dibotrys* and *F. cymosum* are immunostimulant. They are prescribed for chronic bronchitis, inflamed gallbladder, and pulmonary abscesses.

Cautions Interacts with blood-thinning medication. Do not take as a medicine if taking prescribed anticoagulants.

Self-help uses High blood pressure & arteriosclerosis, p. 311; Poor circulation & high blood pressure, p. 329.

Feronia limonia (Rutaceae)

Wood Apple

Description A spiny tree growing to 30 ft (9 m), it has feathery leaves, red flowers, and round whitish fruit the size of oranges.

Habitat & cultivation Native to southern India, wood apple is cultivated in tropical Asia.

Parts used Fruit, leaves.

Constituents The fruit contains fruit acids, vitamins, and minerals. The leaves contain tannins and a volatile oil.

Medicinal actions & uses Wood apple fruit is used mainly to stimulate the digestive system. In India, the fruit forms part of a paste applied to tone the breasts. The astringent leaves are used to treat

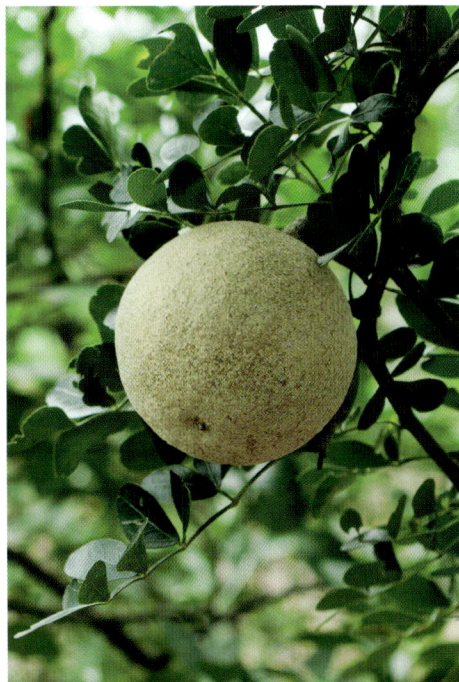

Wood apple is native to southern India and mainly used to stimulate the digestive system.

indigestion, flatulence, diarrhea, dysentery (particularly in children), and hemorrhoids. It is traditionally thought to act as a male contraceptive, although there is limited research to support this.

Ferula assa-foetida (Apiaceae)

Asafoetida,
Devil's dung

Description Perennial plant growing to about 6½ ft (2 m). Has a fleshy taproot, hollow stem, compound leaves, and many white flowers in umbels.

Habitat & cultivation Native to Iran, Afghanistan, and Pakistan, asafoetida produces a gum obtained in summer from 4-year-old plants. The stems are cut off and successive slices are made through the roots. The gum wells up and is collected after it has hardened.

Part used Oleo-gum-resin.

Constituents Asafoetida exudate contains 6–17% volatile oil, as well as resin and gum. The volatile oil contains disulfides (about 58%), which have an expectorant action. The oil also settles the digestion. Asafoetida resin contains sesquiterpenoid coumarins, including foetidin.

History & folklore In the 4th century BCE, *Charaka Samhita*, a Hindu medical treatise, proclaimed asafoetida the best remedy for clearing gas and bloating. The name devil's dung notwithstanding, the plant is thought to have been the most popular spice in ancient Rome. Asafoetida is as persistent in aroma as garlic (*Allium sativum*, p. 63), and is still used as a flavoring.

Medicinal actions & uses In Middle Eastern and Indian herbal medicine, asafoetida is used for simple digestive problems such as gas, bloating, indigestion, and constipation. Asafoetida's volatile oil, like that of garlic, has components that leave the body via the respiratory system and aid the coughing up of congested mucus. Asafoetida is taken (usually in tablet form) for bronchitis, bronchial asthma, whooping cough, and other chest problems. Asafoetida also lowers blood pressure and thins the blood. The herb has a reputation for helping in neurotic states.

Related species *F. silphion* was used in ancient Rome as a contraceptive. It was overharvested and died out in about 300 CE. *F. persica* is used in the Middle East for rheumatic problems and backache. The central Asian *F. sumbul* is used as a nerve tonic. *F. jaeschkeana* has recently been investigated as a potential contraceptive. See also *F. gummosa* (*following entry*)

Caution While safe in adults, asafoetida may be harmful to young babies.

Ferula gummosa syn. *F. galbaniflua* (Apiaceae)

Galbanum

Description Perennial with a smooth, hollow stem, finely toothed compound leaves, and umbels of small white flowers.

Habitat & cultivation Native to central Asia, galbanum produces a gum that is obtained when stems are cut off and successive slices are made through the roots. Gum wells to the surface and is collected after it has hardened.

Part used Oleo-gum-resin.

Constituents Galbanum exudate contains a volatile oil, resins, gums, as well as a coumarin (umbelliferone).

History & folklore Galbanum has been used medicinally for centuries.

Medicinal actions & uses Galbanum is a digestive stimulant and antispasmodic, reducing flatulence, cramps, and colic. It is also expectorant. Applied as an ointment, the gum may help heal wounds.

Related species See asafoetida (*F. assa-foetida*, preceding entry).

Self-help use Acidity & indigestion, p. 317.

Ficus benghalensis (Moraceae)

Banyan tree

Description Tree growing to 65 ft (20 m) with oval leaves, fig-type fruit, and roots that grow into the ground from branches.

Habitat & cultivation Growing wild in India and Pakistan, the banyan tree is also cultivated across the Indian subcontinent.

Parts used Fruit, bark, leaves, latex, aerial roots.

Constituents Banyan tree contains ketones, sterols, ficusin, and bergaptin.

History & folklore The banyan tree is sacred to Hindus and is frequently found in the proximity of Hindu temples. The god Shiva is often shown sitting peacefully in the shade of a banyan tree. The banyan tree is the national tree of India.

Medicinal actions & uses The astringent leaves and bark of the tree are employed to relieve diarrhea and dysentery and to reduce bleeding. As with other *Ficus* species, the latex is applied to hemorrhoids, warts, and aching joints. The fruit is laxative and the roots are chewed to prevent gum disease. The bark is used in Ayurvedic medicine for diabetes.

Research In laboratory studies an extract of the leaves was shown to counter diarrhea. Glycosides in banyan have been shown to

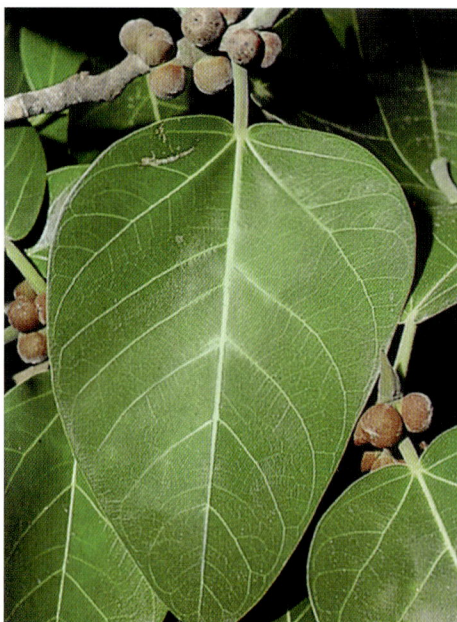

Banyan tree leaves are astringent and are used to tighten mucous membranes.

have an antidiabetic activity, lowering blood-sugar levels.

Related species See fig (*F. carica*, following entry).

Caution The latex is toxic and should not be taken internally.

Ficus carica (Moraceae)

Fig

Description Deciduous tree growing to 13 ft (4 m). Has large leaves and fleshy receptacles that ripen into purple-brown, pear-shaped fruit.

Habitat & cultivation Native to western Asia, fig now grows wild and is cultivated in many temperate and subtropical regions. Fruit is harvested in summer.

Parts used Fruit, latex.

Constituents Figs contain around 50% fruit sugars (mainly glucose), flavonoids, vitamins, and enzymes.

History & folklore The fig leaf was used by Adam and Eve to hide their nakedness in the Garden of Eden. There are many other references to the plant in the Old Testament, mainly to the sweetness of the fruit and to its use as a medicine. Spartan athletes in Ancient Greece were said to eat figs in order to improve their performance.

Medicinal actions & uses The fruit sugars within the fig (especially the dried fruit) have a pronounced but gentle laxative effect; syrup of figs is still a remedy for mild constipation. The fruit's emollient pulp helps relieve pain and inflammation, and it has been used to treat tumors, swellings, and gum abscesses—the fruit often being roasted before application. Figs are also mildly expectorant and, when used with herbs such as elecampane (*Inula helenium*, p. 111), are helpful in treating dry and irritable coughs and bronchitis. The milky latex from leaves and stems is reputed to be analgesic, and has long been used to treat warts, insect bites, and stings.

Related species Research published in 1999 showed that an extract of leaves of *F. racemosa*, a native of northern India, had a marked protective activity on the liver in rats. The juice and powdered bark of the Central American *F. cotinifolia* are applied to wounds and bruises. *F. indica* is used in Ayurvedic medicine as a tonic, diuretic, and treatment for gonorrhea. *F. lacor* is used in Chinese herbal medicine to induce sweating, while *F. retusa*, which is native to China, Indonesia, and Australia, is used in the Chinese tradition to treat toothache and tooth decay. See also banyan tree (*F. benghalensis*, preceding entry) and peepal (*F. religiosa*, following entry).

Cautions The latex is toxic and should not be used internally. Applied to the skin, it may cause an allergic reaction to sunlight.

Ficus religiosa (Moraceae)

Peepal

Description Tree growing to around 26 ft (8 m) with large, leathery, heart-shaped leaves and purple fruit growing in pairs.

Habitat & cultivation Peepal grows in northern and central India, in forests, and alongside water. It is also widely cultivated throughout the subcontinent and southern Asia. The fruit is gathered when ripe.

Parts used Fruit, leaves, bark, latex.

Constituents The fruit contains fruit sugars, flavonoids, and enzymes.

History & folklore Sacred to Hindus and Buddhists, the peepal is the tree under which the Buddha attained enlightenment. It is a long-living tree; a peepal in Sri Lanka is thought to be over 2,000 years old.

Medicinal actions & uses Peepal's uses are similar to those of the banyan (*F. benghalensis*, p. 216). Its astringent bark and leaves are taken for diarrhea and dysentery, whereas the leaves alone are used for constipation. The leaves are applied with ghee (clarified butter) as a poultice to boils and to swollen salivary glands in mumps. The powdered fruit may be taken for asthma and the latex is used to treat warts.

Related species See preceding entries, fig (*F. carica*) and banyan tree (*F. benghalensis*).

Foeniculum vulgare (Apiaceae)

Fennel

Description Aromatic perennial growing to about 5 ft (1.5 m). Has dark green, feathery leaves, umbels of yellow flowers, and small, ridged, oval-shaped seeds.

Habitat & cultivation Native to the Mediterranean region, fennel is now cultivated in temperate regions around the world. The seeds are gathered in the fall.

Parts used Seeds, essential oil.

Constituents "Sweet" fennel seeds contain about 8% volatile oil (about 80% anethole, plus fenchone and methylchavicol), flavonoids, coumarins (including bergapten), and sterols. The volatile oil relieves gas and is antispasmodic. "Bitter" fennel seeds contain significantly higher levels of fenchone.

History & folklore Dioscorides, in the 1st century CE, states that "the juice, when put into the eye, aids vision, and into the ear, kills the worms (i.e. bacteria) that develop there."

Medicinal actions & uses The primary use of fennel seeds is to relieve bloating, but they also settle stomach pain, stimulate the appetite, and are diuretic and anti-inflammatory. Like anise (*Pimpinella anisum*, p. 256) and caraway (*Carum carvi*, p. 187), the seeds make an excellent infusion for settling digestion and reducing abdominal distension. The seeds help in the treatment of kidney stones, and, combined with urinary antiseptics such as uva-ursi (*Arctostaphylos uva-ursi*, p. 174), make an effective treatment for cystitis. An infusion of the seeds may be taken as a gargle for sore throats and as a mild expectorant. Fennel is safe for children when taken at a low dose and, as an infusion or syrup, can be given for colic and painful teething in babies. Fennel increases breast milk production and the herb is still used as an eyewash for sore eyes and conjunctivitis. The seeds have a longstanding reputation as an aid to weight loss and to longevity. Essential oil from the sweet variety is used for its digestive and relaxing properties. It also has estrogenic activity and may prove helpful in relieving menopausal symptoms.

Cautions Fennel seeds are potentially toxic; do not exceed the recommended dose. Do not take the essential oil internally.

Self-help uses Acidity & indigestion, p. 317; Morning sickness & nausea, p. 327; Stomach spasm, p. 315; Gas & bloating, p. 316.

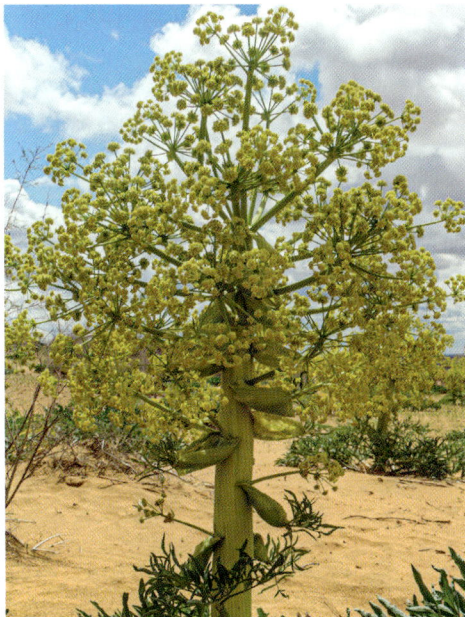

Fennel has a long history of use as a remedy for ailments of the digestive tract.

Forsythia suspensa (Oleaceae)

Weeping forsythia, *Lian qiao* (Chinese)

Description Deciduous shrub growing to 16 ft (5 m). Has toothed leaves, bright yellow flowers, and woody fruit.

Habitat & cultivation Native to China and Japan, weeping forsythia is grown for its bright yellow blossoms in temperate gardens all over the world. The fruit is harvested in the fall, just before it is fully ripe.

Part used Fruit.

Constituents The fruit contains flavonoids, including rutin, lignans, glycosides, and forsythin. Research suggests that forsythin is antimicrobial, antiemetic, and anti-inflammatory.

History & folklore Weeping forsythia was first listed in the *Divine Husbandman's Classic (Shen'nong Bencaojing)*, written in the 1st century CE. Weeping forsythia features in a remedy for infections devised in the 18th century.

Medicinal actions & uses A bitter-tasting, pungent herb with antiseptic and antiviral activity, weeping forsythia is used to treat infections such as colds, flu, sore throats, and tonsillitis. In traditional Chinese medicine, it is used to treat a range of other conditions (including boils, swollen glands, and skin infections). The American herbal scientist James A. Duke recommends it be taken as a warm tea, combined with honeysuckle (*Lonicera* spp., p. 235) and lemon balm (*Melissa officinalis*, p. 117), at the onset of colds and similar viral infections.

Caution Not advisable in pregnancy.

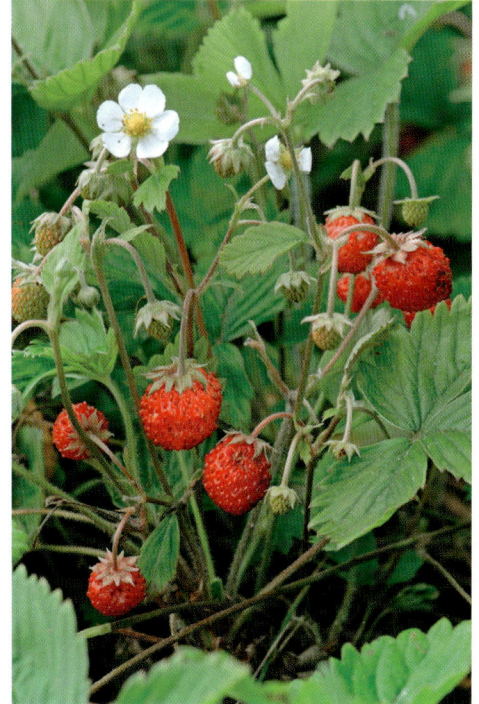

Wild strawberry was said to "comfort fainting spirits."

Fragaria vesca (Rosaceae)

Wild Strawberry

Description Low-growing perennial herb spread by runners. Has 3-lobed leaves, white flowers, and small red berries.

Habitat & cultivation Wild strawberry is native to Europe and temperate regions of Asia. The leaves and fruit are gathered in early summer.

Parts used Leaves, fruit.

Constituents The leaves contain flavonoids, tannins, and a volatile oil. The fruit contains fruit acids and a volatile oil with methyl salicylate and borneol.

History & folklore Wild strawberry appears to have been little used medicinally until the Middle Ages. Writing in 1652, Nicholas Culpeper listed its benefits: "the berries are excellent good to cool the liver, the blood, and the spleen, or a hot cholerick stomach … the leaves and roots thereof [are] also good to fasten loose teeth and to heal spongy foul gums."

Medicinal actions & uses Wild strawberry leaves are mildly astringent and diuretic. The plant is little used medicinally today, but it can be taken to treat diarrhea and dysentery. The leaves were used as a gargle for sore throats, and in a lotion for minor burns and grazes. In Europe, the fruit is considered to have cooling and diuretic properties, and has been prescribed as part of a diet in cases of tuberculosis, gout, arthritis, and rheumatism.

Fraxinus excelsior (Oleaceae)

Ash

Description Deciduous tree growing to 130 ft (40 m). Has pale gray bark, black conical leaf buds, and bright green leaves with 7–13 oval leaflets.

Habitat & cultivation Common in Europe, ash thrives in lowland and moorland. The leaves are gathered in summer, but the bark is gathered in spring.

Parts used Leaves, bark, seeds.

Constituents Ash leaves contain flavonoids, tannins, mucilage, triterpenes, and iridoids.

History & folklore The ash was the "world-tree" of Norse mythology, its roots spreading to the domain of the gods, and its branches extending to the remotest corners of the universe. In Norse myth, the first man was carved from a piece of ash wood. In parts of Europe, ash bark was used as a cost-free substitute for quinine in the home treatment of malaria. Such use probably continued in rural areas into the 20th century.

Medicinal actions & uses Ash bark is tonic and astringent. Little used in herbal medicine today, it is occasionally taken for fever. The leaves are also astringent, and they have a laxative and diuretic effect. They have been used as a mild substitute for senna (*Cassia senna*, p. 80).

Related species The bark of the American white ash (*F. americana*) has been used as a bitter tonic and astringent. Several ash species exude a nutritious sap, called "manna," which is used as a laxative for children. In particular, the manna ash (*F. ornus*), which has antioxidant activity, has been cultivated in southern Europe for its high yield of manna sap.

Fucus vesiculosus (Fucaceae)

Bladder wrack, Kelp

Description Brownish-green alga growing to 3 ft (1 m) in length. Has flat, usually forked, fronds containing air bladders.

Habitat & cultivation Bladder wrack is native to the North Atlantic shores and western Mediterranean, and is harvested all year.

Part used Whole plant.

Constituents Bladder wrack contains polyphenols, polysaccharides, and minerals, especially iodine (up to 0.1%). The polysaccharides are immunostimulant. The iodine may stimulate the thyroid gland.

History & folklore Bladder wrack has been employed as a fuel, as a winter feed for cattle, and as a source of iodine and potash.

Medicinal actions & uses Due to its iodine content, bladder wrack is taken as an antigoiter remedy. The plant appears to raise the metabolic rate by increasing hormone production by the thyroid gland, though this increase may be limited to poorly functioning thyroids. Bladder wrack is reputedly helpful in rheumatic conditions

Research In one clinical trial (Italy 1976), patients taking bladder wrack lost much more weight than the control group. In more recent German research, the polyphenols and polysaccharides appeared to have antiviral and anti-HIV activity.

Cautions Do not take if pregnant or breastfeeding. If suffering from a thyroid illness or taking insulin, take only under professional advice.

Fumaria officinalis (Fumariaceae)

Fumitory

Description Climbing annual growing to 1 ft (30 cm). Has compound leaves and maroon-tipped pink tubular flowers.

Habitat & cultivation Native to Europe and North Africa, fumitory also grows in Asia, North America, and Australia.

Parts used Flowering aerial parts.

Constituents Fumitory contains isoquinoline alkaloids and flavonoids.

Medicinal actions & uses A notably bitter-tasting herb, fumitory has a stimulant and cleansing action on the liver and gallbladder, and is principally used to treat chronic itchy skin problems such as eczema. It is also diuretic and mildly laxative.

Related species Fumitory is related to corydalis

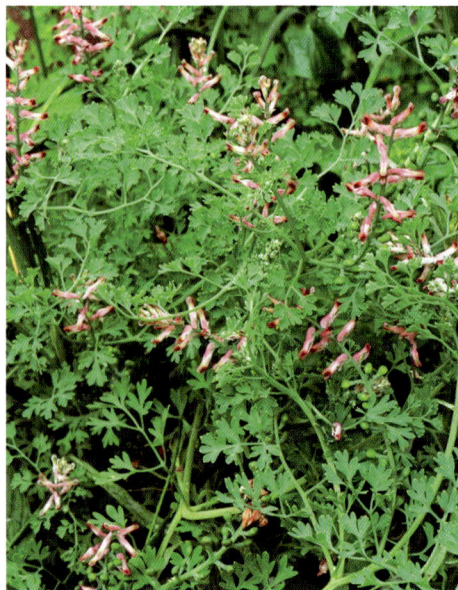

Fumitory may be applied externally as a treatment for eczema.

(*Corydalis yanhusuo*, p. 90), and *F. parviflora* from central Asia. The latter, like fumitory, is used as a detoxifying, laxative, and diuretic herb.

Caution Fumitory is toxic in excessive doses. Use only with professional advice..

Galega officinalis (Fabaceae)

Goat's rue

Description Bushy perennial growing to about 3 ft (1 m) in height. Goat's rue has compound leaves with lance-shaped leaflets and delicate pink pea-type flowers on terminal spikes, and produces red-brown seed pods in the fall.

Habitat & cultivation Native to Asia and continental Europe, and naturalized in Britain, goat's rue grows in damp and low-lying areas. It is harvested in summer.

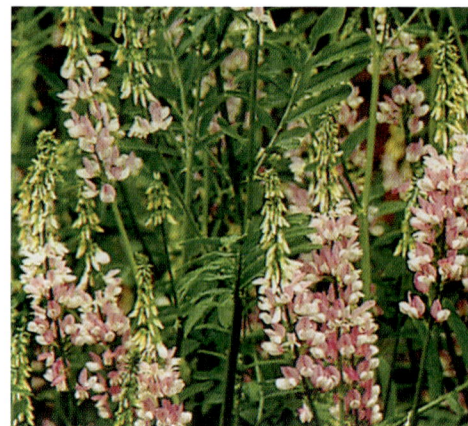

Goat's rue was once taken to treat the plague.

Parts used Aerial parts.

Constituents Goat's rue contains alkaloids (including galegine), lectins, flavonoids, and tannins. Galegine strongly reduces blood-sugar levels.

History & folklore Formerly used as a treatment for the plague, goat's rue has been widely cultivated as a cattle feed.

Medicinal actions & uses Today, goat's rue is chiefly used as an antidiabetic herb, having the ability to reduce blood-sugar levels. It is not a substitute for conventional drugs, but can be valuable in the early stages of type 2 diabetes and is best used as an infusion. The herb may help regenerate cells in the pancreas that secrete insulin, and appears to have immune-protective activity. The herb can be taken to increase breast milk production, and it makes a useful diuretic.

Caution Use as part of the treatment of diabetes only under professional supervision.

Galipea officinalis syn. *G. cusparia* (Rutaceae)

Angostura

Description Evergreen tree growing to 49 ft (15 m) with gray bark, shiny bright green leaflets, and foul-smelling flowers.

Habitat & cultivation Angostura is native to some Caribbean islands and to tropical South America. The bark is gathered throughout the year.

Part used Bark.

Constituents Angostura bark contains bitter principles, quinoline alkaloids including cusparine, and 1–2% volatile oil. The alkaloids have antimicrobial activity against the tuberculosis bacillus.

History & folklore Angostura is a traditional tonic and fever remedy in South America, used chiefly for digestive infections. Indigenous Amazonians use the plant as a fish poison. Angostura has been used as a source of "bitters," although it is unknown whether it is an ingredient of the cocktail flavoring bearing its name as the drink's composition is a trade secret.

Medicinal actions & uses Strong bitter with tonic properties, angostura stimulates the stomach and digestive tract as a whole. It is antispasmodic and is reported to act on the spinal nerves, helping in paralytic conditions. Angostura is typically given for weak digestion, and is considered valuable as a remedy for diarrhea and dysentery. In South America, it is sometimes used as a substitute for cinchona (*Cinchona* spp., p. 84) to control fevers.

Caution Use under professional guidance only.

Galium aparine (Rubiaceae)

Cleavers, Goose grass

Description Straggling, square-stemmed annual growing to a height of 4 ft (1.2 m) with whorls of lance-shaped leaves, clusters of small white flowers, and small, round, green fruit with hooked prickles.

Habitat & cultivation Common throughout Europe and North America, cleavers is found in many other temperate regions, including in Australia. It grows prolifically in gardens and along roadsides, and is gathered when just about to flower in late spring.

Parts used Aerial parts.

Constituents Cleavers contains iridoids (including asperuloside), polyphenolic acids, anthraquinones (only in the root), alkanes, flavonoids, and tannins. Asperuloside is a mild laxative.

History & folklore The name cleavers refers to the plant's ability to cling (or cleave) to fur or clothing. Dioscorides, a Greek physician of the 1st century CE, considered it useful for countering weariness, and

described how shepherds used the stems to make sieves for straining milk.

Medicinal actions & uses A valuable diuretic, cleavers is often taken for skin diseases such as seborrhea, eczema, and psoriasis; for swollen lymph glands; and as a general detoxifying agent in serious illnesses such as cancer. The plant is commonly prepared in the form of an infusion, but for conditions such as cancer, it is best taken as a juice, which is strongly diuretic. The juice and the infusion are also taken for kidney stones and other urinary problems.

Research According to French research (1947), an extract of the plant appears to lower blood pressure.

Related species The Mexican *G. orizabense* is used by the Mazatecs to treat intestinal parasites and to relieve fever. *G. umbrosum* from New Zealand has been used to treat gonorrhea. See also lady's bedstraw (*G. verum*, following entry).

Galium verum (Rubiaceae)

Lady's bedstraw

Description Short, sprawling perennial growing to 32 in (80 cm). Has whorls of narrow dark green leaves and tufts of very small bright yellow flowers.

Habitat & cultivation Found throughout Europe and western Asia, and naturalized in North America, lady's bedstraw thrives in dry meadows, along roadsides, and in wayside places. It is gathered when in flower in summer.

Parts used Aerial parts.

Constituents Lady's bedstraw contains iridoids (including asperuloside), flavonoids, anthraquinones, alkanes, and rennin.

History & folklore The name of this pleasant-scented herb derives from its traditional use as a stuffing for mattresses. In medieval times, it was used as a "strewing" herb on floors. Lady's bedstraw curdles milk and gives a yellow color to cheese produced from the curd. In his *Irish Herbal* (1735), K'Eogh states, "when applied to burns, the crushed flowers alleviate inflammation, and when applied to wounds, they can heal them."

Medicinal actions & uses A slightly bitter-tasting remedy, lady's bedstraw is used mainly as a diuretic and for skin problems. Like its close relative, cleavers (*G. aparine, preceding entry*), the herb is given for kidney stones, bladder stones, and other urinary conditions, including cystitis. It is occasionally used as a means to relieve chronic skin problems such as psoriasis, but, in general, cleavers is preferred as a treatment for this condition. Lady's bedstraw has had a longstanding reputation, especially in

France, of being a valuable remedy for epilepsy, though it is rarely used for this purpose today.

Related species *G. elatum* has also been considered a remedy for epilepsy in France. (*See also G. aparine, preceding entry.*)

Gardenia jasminoides syn. *G. augusta*, *G. florida* (Rubiaceae)

Gardenia, *Zhi zi* (Chinese)

Description Evergreen shrub growing to 6½ ft (2 m). Has green leaves, scented double flowers, and orange-red fruit.

Habitat & cultivation Native to southeastern provinces of China, gardenia prefers humid, tropical climates. The fruit is gathered when it turns reddish-yellow.

Part used Fruit.

Constituents Gardenia fruit contains iridoid glycosides. The flowers are the source of the essential oil

History & folklore Gardenia has been used in Chinese medicine for at least 2,000 years. It provides an important essential oil used to flavor teas. The oil is also used to make perfumes. Gardenia perfumes often blend gardenia, jasmine, and tuberose.

Medicinal actions & uses In the Chinese herbal tradition (pp. 44–47), gardenia is a "bitter, cold" herb

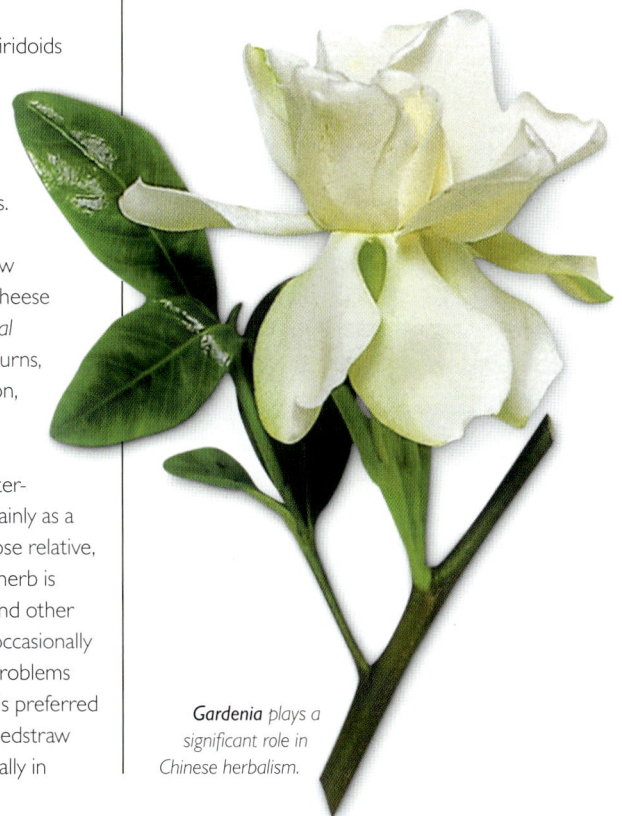

Gardenia plays a significant role in Chinese herbalism.

used mostly to relieve symptoms associated with heat. These include fever, irritability, restlessness, insomnia, cystitis, painful urination, and jaundice. The fruit staunches bleeding and is taken for nosebleeds, and urinary and rectal bleeding. The essential oil is an antiseptic and has a reputation for being an aphrodisiac.

Related species The fruit of the northern Indian *G. campanulata* is cathartic and used to expel worms. *G. gummifera*, from eastern India, is antiseptic and digestive. The Pacific region *G. taitensis* relieves headaches. The African *G. thunbergia* is used to relieve constipation.

Cautions Avoid in diarrhea. Do not take if taking prescribed medication for high blood pressure.

Gaultheria procumbens (Ericaceae)

Wintergreen

Description Aromatic low-lying shrub growing to 6 in (15 cm). Has leathery, oval leaves, small white or pale pink bell-shaped flowers, and brilliant red fruit.

Habitat & cultivation Native to North America, wintergreen is found in woodland and exposed mountainous areas. The leaves and fruit are gathered in summer.

Parts used Leaves, fruit, essential oil.

Constituents Wintergreen contains phenols (including gaultherin and salicylic acid), 0.8% volatile oil (up to 98% methyl salicylate), mucilage, resin, and tannins.

History & folklore Wintergreen was popular with Indigenous North American peoples who used it for treating back pain, rheumatism, fever, headaches, sore throats, and many other conditions. Samuel Thomson, founder of the 19th-century Physiomedicalist movement, combined it with hemlock (*Conium maculatum*, p. 198) to treat severe fluid retention. The leaves have been used as a substitute for tea (*Camellia sinensis*, p. 185), for example during the American Revolution (1776–1784).

Medicinal actions & uses Wintergreen is strongly anti-inflammatory, antiseptic, and soothing to the digestive system. It is an effective remedy for rheumatic and arthritic problems, and taken as a tea it relieves flatulence and colic. The essential oil, in the form of a liniment or ointment, brings relief to inflamed, swollen, or sore muscles, ligaments, and joints, and can also prove valuable in treating neurological conditions such as sciatica (pain resulting from pressure on a nerve in the lower spine) and trigeminal neuralgia (pain affecting a facial nerve). The oil is sometimes used to treat cellulitis, a bacterial infection causing the skin to become inflamed.

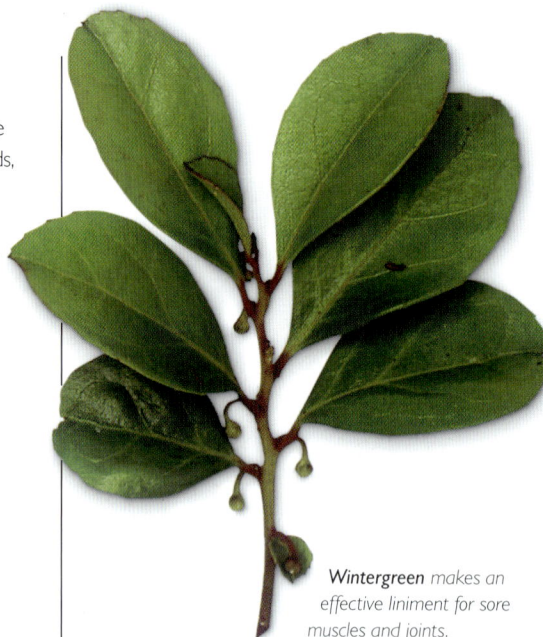

Wintergreen makes an effective liniment for sore muscles and joints.

Cautions People who are sensitive to aspirin should not take wintergreen internally. Oil of wintergreen should never be taken internally, nor applied (even well diluted) to the skin of children under the age of 12 unless with professional supervision.

Gelidium amansii (Rhodophyceae)

Agar

Description Seaweed with red-brown, translucent, multi-branched ribbons and fronds growing to about 3 ft (1 m) in length. It has spherical fruit that appears in late fall and winter.

Habitat & cultivation Agar is native to the Pacific coasts of China and Japan and the coast of South Africa. It grows to a depth of 100 ft (30 m) below sea level. Commercial harvesters rake plants off banks and rocks. The cleaned seaweed, after being boiled with sulfuric acid for 6 hours, yields agar, which sets to form a jelly. Around 6,500 tons of processed agar are produced each year.

Part used Seaweed extract (agar).

Constituents Agar contains polysaccharides, mainly agarose and agaropectin (up to 90%), which are very mucilaginous.

History & folklore Agar is commonly used as a thickening agent in food preparation, but its most widespread application is in scientific research, where it is used as a culture medium for growing microorganisms in petri dishes.

Medicinal actions & uses Like most seaweeds and their derivatives, agar is nutritious and contains large amounts of mucilage. Its chief medicinal use is as a bulk laxative. In the intestines, agar absorbs water

and swells, stimulating bowel activity and the subsequent elimination of feces.

Related species While *G. amansii* is the main agar-producing species, *G. cartilagineum* (found on the Pacific coast of North America) and other closely related species around the world are being used as alternative sources

---

Gelsemium sempervirens (Loganiaceae)

Yellow jasmine, Gelsemium

Description Evergreen woody climber growing to 20 ft (6 m). Has shiny, dark green leaves and clusters of fragrant, trumpet-shaped yellow flowers.

Habitat & cultivation Native to the southern US and Central America, yellow jasmine prefers damp sites. The rootstock is unearthed in the fall.

Part used Rootstock.

Constituents Yellow jasmine contains indole alkaloids (including gelsemine and gelsedine), iridoids, coumarins, and tannins. The alkaloids are toxic and act as a depressant to the central nervous system.

History & folklore It is unclear whether yellow jasmine was used in Indigenous North American medicine. The plant came into regular use only in the middle of the 19th century. It was first employed by followers of the Eclectic herbal movement, and then later became an official medicine, listed in the *Pharmacopoeia* of the *United States* from 1863 to 1926.

Medicinal actions & uses A potent medicinal herb, yellow jasmine is prescribed in small doses as a sedative and antispasmodic, most commonly for neuralgia (pain caused by nerve irritation or damage). Yellow jasmine is often given for nerve pain affecting the face. The herb is also applied externally to treat intercostal neuralgia (nerve pain between the ribs) and sciatica (pain resulting from pressure on a nerve in the lower spine). Yellow jasmine's antispasmodic property is used in treating whooping cough and asthma. The herb is occasionally taken for migraine, insomnia, and bowel problems, and also to reduce blood pressure. Yellow jasmine is also used in homeopathic medicine.

Cautions Yellow jasmine is an extremely toxic plant that should be used only under professional supervision. The plant is subject to legal restrictions in some countries.

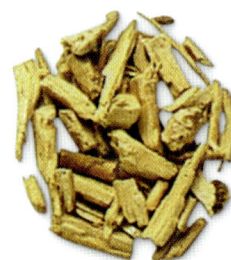

Dried rootstock

Geranium maculatum (Geraniaceae)

Wild geranium

Description Perennial growing to 2 ft (60 cm). Has deeply cleft leaves, pink-purple flowers, and beak-shaped fruit.

Habitat & cultivation Native to woodlands of eastern and central North America, the root is dug up in early spring, and the aerial parts are gathered in summer.

Parts used Root, aerial parts.

Constituents Wild geranium contains up to 30% tannins.

History & folklore Indigenous North American peoples used wild geranium for sore throats, mouth ulcers, infected gums, and oral thrush. The herb was later used by European settlers for diarrhea, internal bleeding, cholera, and venereal diseases.

Medicinal actions & uses An astringent and clotting agent, wild geranium is often prescribed for irritable bowel syndrome and hemorrhoids, and it is used to staunch wounds. It may also be used to treat heavy menstrual bleeding and excessive vaginal discharge.

Related species See herb robert (*G. robertianum, following entry*).

Caution Wild geranium should only be taken for a few weeks at a time.

Geranium robertianum (Geraniaceae)

Herb robert

Description Strong-smelling annual or biennial herb growing to 20 in (50 cm). Has deeply cleft red-green leaves, bright pink flowers, and pointed seed capsules.

Habitat & cultivation Native to Europe and Asia, herb robert is naturalized in North America. It is gathered in summer.

Parts used Aerial parts, root.

Constituents Herb robert contains tannins, notably geraniin, flavonoids, phenolic acids including caffeic and chlorogenic acids, and a trace of volatile oil.

History & folklore Herb robert's unpleasant odor has earned it the name "stinking Bob" in parts of England.

Medicinal actions & uses Herb robert is little used in contemporary European herbal medicine. It is occasionally employed in much the same way as Wild geranium (*G. maculatum, preceding entry*),

as an astringent and wound healer. The herb bears closer investigation as a remedy. According to one authority it is effective against stomach ulcers and inflammation of the uterus, and it holds some potential as a treatment for cancer.

Geum urbanum (Rosaceae)

Avens

Description Downy perennial growing to 60 cm (2 ft). Has wiry stems, compound leaves, small, yellow 5-petaled flowers, and fruit covered with hooks.

Habitat & cultivation Native to Europe and central Asia, avens is a common wayside plant. The root is dug up in spring, and the aerial parts are picked in summer.

Parts used Aerial parts, root.

Constituents Avens contains phenolic glycosides (including eugenol), tannins, a volatile oil, and possibly a sesquiterpene lactone (cnicin).

History & folklore Once known as *herba benedicta* (blessed herb), avens was credited with significant magical powers in the Middle Ages. A German text of 1493 states that if avens root is in the house, the devil is powerless. According to tradition, the root should be unearthed on March 25th.

Medicinal actions & uses Avens is an astringent herb, used principally for problems affecting the mouth, throat, and gastrointestinal tract. The herb tightens up soft gums, heals mouth ulcers, makes a good gargle for infections of the pharynx and larynx, and reduces irritation of the stomach and gut. It may be taken for peptic ulcers, irritable bowel syndrome, diarrhea, and dysentery. Avens has been used in a lotion or ointment as a soothing remedy for hemorrhoids. The herb may also be used as a douche for treating excessive vaginal discharge. Avens reputedly has a mild quinine-type action in lowering fever.

Glechoma hederacea syn. *Nepeta glechoma* (Lamiaceae)

Ground Ivy, Alehoof

Description Creeping perennial herb growing to 6 in (15 cm). Has long rooting runners, notched kidney-shaped leaves, and purple-blue flowers in whorls.

Habitat & cultivation Native to Europe and western Asia, ground ivy is now naturalized in other temperate regions, including North America. It thrives on the outskirts of woods and alongside paths and hedges. It is gathered in summer.

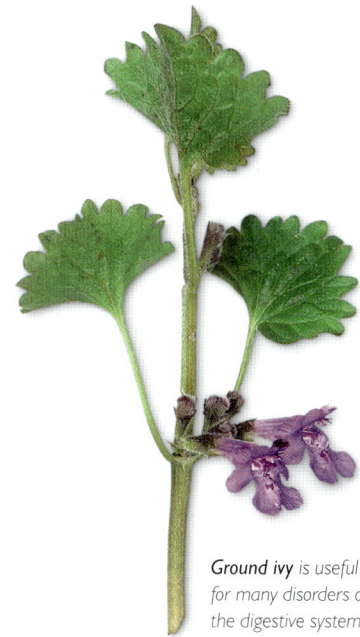

Ground ivy is useful for many disorders of the digestive system.

Parts used Aerial parts.

Constituents Ground ivy contains phenolic acids, flavonoids, lignans, triterpenes, and a lectin.

History & folklore Known in parts of England as "alehoof," ground ivy was used to flavor and clarify ale, the traditional drink of the Anglo-Saxons. In Medieval times, it was recommended for fever, and was a popular treatment for chronic coughs. The 16th-century herbalist John Gerard considered it a valuable remedy for tinnitus.

Medicinal actions & uses Ground ivy is tonic, diuretic, and decongestant, and is used to treat many problems involving the mucous membranes of the ear, nose, throat, and digestive system. A well-tolerated herb, it can be given to children to clear lingering congestion and to treat chronic conditions such as "glue ear" and sinusitis. Throat and chest problems, especially those due to excess mucus, also benefit from this remedy. Ground ivy is also a valuable treatment for gastritis and acid indigestion. Further along the gastrointestinal tract, its binding nature helps to counter diarrhea and to dry up watery and mucoid secretions. Ground ivy has been employed to prevent scurvy and as a spring tonic, and is considered beneficial in kidney disorders.

Glycine max (Fabaceae)

Soy, Soybean

Description Annual growing to 6½ ft (2 m). Has leaves with 3 leaflets, white or purple flowers, and pods with 2–4 beans.

Habitat & cultivation Soy is native to south-western Asia, and is cultivated in warm temperate regions. The pods are gathered when ripe.

Parts used Beans, sprouts.

Constituents Soy contains protein (about 30%), fixed oil (about 17%), including lecithin (2% or more), linoleic acid, and alpha-linolenic acid, isoflavones, coumestrol, sterols, saponins, vitamins, and minerals. Coumestrol and the isoflavones closely mimic estrogen within the body.

History & folklore A staple food in much of Asia, soy has been used in China for at least 5,000 years. Soy was introduced in the United States in 1804 and has become a major crop in the South and Midwest. It is now one of the world's most important food crops.

Medicinal actions & uses Although soybeans and soy produce have little direct medicinal value, they are highly important as foods, providing unusually high levels of protein, lecithin, and essential fatty acids. However, the beans may have a protective role against cancer, notably breast cancer. Their significant estrogenic activity makes them a particularly good medicinal food for women going through menopause, helping to relieve symptoms such as hot flashes, and to protect against osteoporosis. In Chinese medicine, soybean sprouts (also highly nutritious) are thought to help relieve "summer heat" and fever.

Research Soybean is a remarkable nutrient, rich in protein, fats, and estrogenic substances, all of which make it an excellent food. The isoflavones, sterols, saponins, and fiber contribute to soy's protective activity against cancer, and countries such as Japan are thought to have lower levels of cancer because of the great quantity of soy produce eaten there. The isoflavones, coumestrol, and sterols are all phytoestrogens. These appear to inhibit estrogen within the body when estrogen levels are too high (for example, in menstrual disorders), and to compensate when estrogen levels are low (such as during menopause). Unrefined soybean oil contains high levels of lecithin and polyunsaturated essential fatty acids, which support healthy levels of blood fat such as cholesterol.

Gnaphalium uliginosum (Asteraceae)

Marsh cudweed

Description Annual plant growing to 8 in (20 cm). Has narrow silver-gray leaves and tiny yellow flower heads.

Habitat & cultivation Marsh cudweed is native to Europe, the Caucasus, and western Asia, and is naturalized in North America. It prefers damp areas, and is gathered in summer when in flower.

Parts used Aerial parts.

Constituents Marsh cudweed contains sterols, fatty acids, triterpenes, and a volatile oil, mainly a-pinene and estragol.

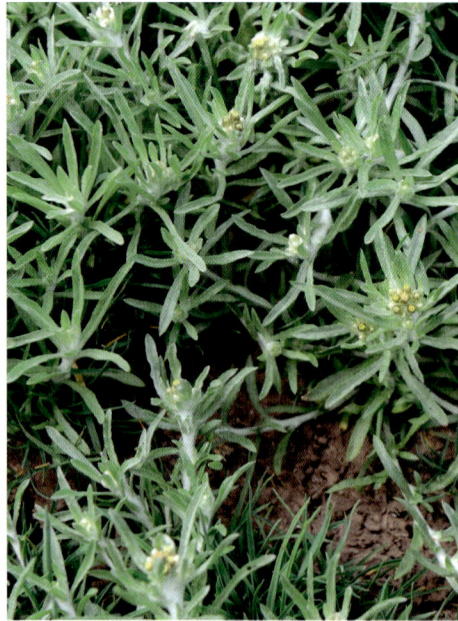

Marsh cudweed is commonly found in damp areas in Europe, North America, and Asia.

Medicinal actions & uses While little used medicinally today, marsh cudweed has astringent, antiseptic, and decongestant properties. In British herbal medicine, it is occasionally taken for tonsillitis, sore throat, and hoarseness, and for mucus in the throat, nasal passages, and sinuses. Marsh cudweed is used in Russia to reduce high blood pressure. It is thought to be antidepressant and aphrodisiac.

Related species A North American relative, *G. polycephalum*, was used to treat respiratory and intestinal congestion, and was applied as a poultice for bruises. *G. keriense*, native to New Zealand, is also considered a remedy for bruises.

Gossypium herbaceum (Malvaceae)

Cotton

Description Biennial or perennial growing to about 8 ft (2.5 m). Has lobed leaves, large white or pink flowers, and seed capsules surrounded by fluffy white tufts.

Habitat & cultivation Native to the Americas, Africa, and Asia, cotton thrives in warm temperate and tropical climates. It is widely cultivated for its fiber. The root and seeds of the plant are harvested in the fall.

Parts used Root bark, seed oil.

Constituents Cotton root bark contains gossypol (a sesquiterpene) and flavonoids. Cotton seed contains a fixed oil, which is about 2% gossypol, and flavonoids. Gossypol causes infertility in men.

History & folklore In India and the Middle East, cotton has been cultivated since the earliest times for its fiber and medicinal properties. The plant was particularly valued for its ability to induce menstruation. Cotton seed oil's contraceptive effect in men was first discovered in China when men became infertile after eating food cooked in the oil.

Medicinal actions & uses Cotton root bark is rarely used medicinally today. It was once employed as a substitute for ergot (*Claviceps purpurea*), the widely used labor-inducing herb. Cotton root bark is both milder-acting and safer in effect, stimulating uterine contractions and hastening a difficult labor. It also promotes abortion or the onset of a period, and reduces menstrual flow. Cotton root bark encourages the blood to clot and the secretion of breast milk. Cotton seed oil is used to treat heavy menstrual bleeding and endometriosis.

Research Cotton seeds and seed oil cause infertility in men, and have been tested as a male contraceptive in China. However, in addition to lowering sperm count, cotton seed oil causes the degeneration of sperm-producing cells.

Related species The American species *G. hirsutum* was used extensively as a medicinal herb by the Maya and Aztecs, and was also cultivated for its fiber. Columbus carried samples of this species back to Europe from his first voyage. Indigenous North American peoples used the bark to ease the pain of childbirth, and by the 19th century it was used as an inducer of menstruation and abortion.

Cautions Cotton root bark and seed oil are potentially toxic and should only be used under professional supervision. Do not use during pregnancy.

Grindelia camporum syn. *G. robusta* var. *rigida* (Asteraceae)

Gumplant

Description Perennial herb growing to 3 ft (1 m). Has triangular leaves and yellow-orange daisy-type flowers.

Habitat & cultivation Native to the southwestern US and Mexico, gumplant grows in arid and saline soil. It is harvested in late summer when in flower.

Parts used Leaves, flowering tops.

Constituents Gumplant contains diterpenes (including grindelic acid), resins, and flavonoids.

History & folklore Gumplant was used by Indigenous North American peoples to treat bronchial problems and skin afflictions. Gumplant was officially recognized in the *Pharmacopoeia* of the United States from 1882 to 1926.

Medicinal actions & uses Gumplant is a valuable remedy for bronchial asthma, and when phlegm in the airways impedes respiration. Both antispasmodic and expectorant, gumplant helps to relax the muscles of the smaller bronchial passages and to clear congested mucus. Additionally, it is thought to desensitize the nerve endings in the bronchial tree and to slow the heart rate, both leading to easier breathing. Gumplant is also taken for bronchitis and emphysema. It has been used in the treatment of whooping cough, hay fever, and cystitis, and externally to help speed the healing of skin irritation and burns.

Related species *G. squarrosa*, a North American species used interchangeably with *G. camporum*, was taken by Indigenous North American peoples to treat respiratory problems such as colds, coughs, and tuberculosis.

Cautions Toxic in excessive doses. Only take under professional supervision. Do not take if suffering from kidney or heart problems.

Guaiacum officinale (Zygophyllaceae)

Lignum vitae,
Guayacan (Spanish)

Description Evergreen tree growing to 33 ft (10 m). Has compound oval leaves, small, deep blue star-shaped flowers, and heart-shaped seed capsules.

Habitat & cultivation Lignum vitae is native to South America and the Caribbean islands. It grows in tropical rainforests. The tree is felled for its timber, and resin is extracted from the heartwood.

Parts used Wood, resin.

Constituents Lignum vitae contains lignans

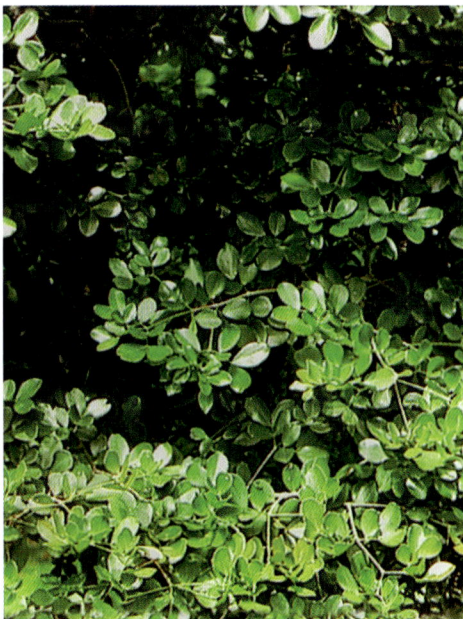

Lignum vitae was once in high demand in Europe as a purported cure for syphilis.

(furoguaiacidin, guaiacin, and others), triterpene saponins, 18–25% resin, and volatile oil.

History & folklore In 1519, Ulrich von Hutten, a German satirist, was said to have cured himself of syphilis after a 40-day regimen involving fasting, profuse sweating, and drinking decoctions of lignum vitae. Furthermore, in 1526, Oviedo, one of the earliest chroniclers of American natural history, wrote that "Caribbean Indians [sic] cure themselves very easily" of venereal disease with this plant. For some years, lignum vitae was in great demand in Europe but it slowly fell into disrepute, its use as a cure for syphilis being seen as a long-lasting hoax. However, it is plausible that the herb would have potent antimicrobial activity against syphilis, if combined with an intense naturopathic sweating regimen.

Medicinal actions & uses Used in Europe, especially in Britain, as a remedy for arthritic and rheumatic conditions, lignum vitae has anti-inflammatory properties that help to reduce joint pain and swelling. It is also diuretic, laxative, and sweat-inducing and speeds the elimination of toxins, which makes it valuable for treating gout. Tincture of lignum vitae is commonly used as a friction rub on rheumatic areas. Absorbent cotton moistened with the resin may be applied to aching teeth. A decoction of the wood chips acts as a local anesthetic, and is used to treat rheumatic joints and herpes blisters.

Related species *G. sanctum*, which grows in Central America and parts of Florida, and *G. coulteri*, native to Mexico, are used in the same manner as lignum vitae.

Caution Lignum vitae is subject to legal restrictions in some countries and is endangered.

Guarea rusbyi syn. *G. guidonia* (Meliaceae)

Cocillana, Guapi bark

Description Evergreen tree growing to 150 ft (45 m) with pale gray bark, compound lance-shaped leaves, and green-white flowers.

Habitat & cultivation Cocillana is native to the eastern Andes. The bark is gathered throughout the year.

Part used Bark.

Constituents Cocillana contains anthraquinones, proanthocyanids, and a volatile oil.

History & folklore Cocillana has been used as an emetic in traditional South American and Caribbean medicine, probably for many centuries. The plant was first introduced to Western medicine by H. H. Rusby, who collected samples in Bolivia in 1886.

Medicinal actions & uses Cocillana is used in

cough mixtures, being an even more powerful expectorant than ipecac (*Cephaelis ipecacuanha*, p. 189). Cocillana is taken as a treatment for coughs, excessive mucus production in the throat and chest, and bronchitis. At a high dosage, the plant induces vomiting.

Related species A gum resin derived from the Caribbean *G. guara* is used as a clotting agent, and a decoction of the leaves is taken as a treatment for internal bleeding.

Caution Use cocillana only under professional supervision.

Gymnema sylvestre (Apocynaceae)

Gymnema,
Gurmar (Hindi)

Description Large, evergreen, twining plant, climbing up through forest trees, sometimes to a considerable height. Has dull green leaves about 2 in (5 cm) long, and umbels of small yellow flowers.

Habitat & cultivation Gymnema is native to forests of central and southern India, Southeast Asia, and as far south as northern Australia. It prefers loamy soil

Parts used Leaves.

Constituents Gymnema contains saponins (gymnemic acids) and a polypeptide (gurmarin).

History & folklore Gymnema has long been used in Indian domestic medicine as a remedy for sugar cravings and diabetes. Its Hindi name means "sugar destroyer."

Medicinal actions & uses Gymnema has real value in treating diabetes, especially in the early stages of type 2 diabetes, which develops in middle to old age. If taken consistently for a year or more, it will help prevent the condition deteriorating. Gymnema may help to regenerate cells in the pancreas that secrete insulin, so it may be possible to control or reverse mild diabetes with diet and gymnema. The plant's remarkable ability to block sweet tastes means that it can reduce sugar cravings and contribute to weight-loss programs.

Research In recent research in India and Japan, gymnema has shown promise as a safe and effective natural treatment for diabetes. In two clinical trials in India, patients with diabetes needed less insulin or other treatments to lower blood-sugar levels. There is an indication that gymnema may encourage repair of the islet cells of the pancreas, responsible for insulin secretion. The leaves have been shown to anesthetize the sweet taste buds of the tongue, and temporarily reduce appetite.

Haronga madagascariensis (Guttiferae)

Haronga

Description Small evergreen tree growing to 26 ft (8 m). Has black-dotted leaves with a dark green upper surface and red-brown hairs underneath, and clusters of creamy-white flowers.

Habitat & cultivation Haronga is native to Madagascar and East Africa, and grows in tropical areas. The leaves and bark are collected throughout the year.

Parts used Leaves, bark.

Constituents Haronga bark contains phenolic pigments, triterpenes, anthraquinones, and tannins. The leaves contain phenolic pigments, the diterpene hypericin, flavonoids, and tannins. Hypericin, which is also found in St. John's wort (*Hypericum perforatum*, p. 110), has antiviral properties.

History & folklore Haronga resin has traditionally been used in Africa to secure arrowheads onto shafts.

Medicinal actions & uses Thought to stimulate bile secretion, haronga is used in European herbal medicine to treat indigestion and poor pancreatic function. In African herbal medicine, haronga is chiefly employed as an astringent and mild laxative, and is also given for digestive system ailments such as diarrhea and dysentery.

Hedera helix (Araliaceae)

Ivy, English ivy

Description A woody climber up to 100 ft (30 m) with leathery, dark green leaves, clusters of greenish-yellow flowers and black or orange berries.

Habitat & cultivation Native to Europe and northern and central Asia, ivy has been introduced, often as a garden climber, in many parts of the world. In the wild, it typically grows on trees and in hedges.

Parts used Leaves, berries.

Constituents Ivy contains saponins, sterols, polyacetylenes, a volatile oil, and flavonoids. The saponins are expectorant, amebicidal, and antifungal, and kill liver flukes.

History & folklore In the classical world, common ivy was dedicated to Dionysus, the god of wine making and intoxication. Ivy was thought to be able to prevent or undo drunkenness. The leaf was traditionally used in England to treat corns and warts—it was soaked in vinegar and bound on as a poultice, or placed inside a sock, overlying the corn.

Medicinal actions & uses Ivy is chiefly used for congestion of the ear, nose, and throat, as well as for bronchitis. It acts as an expectorant,

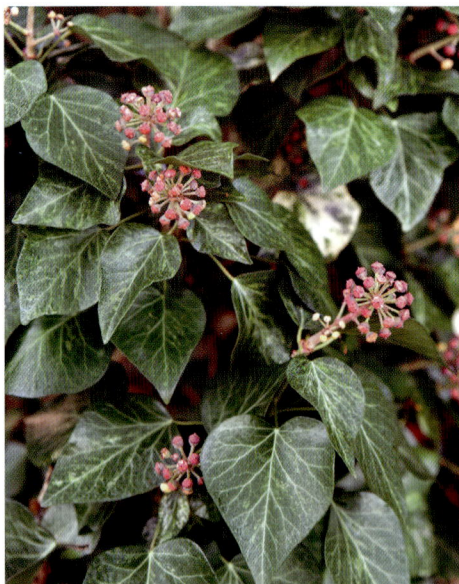

Ivy was thought, in the classical world, to undo drunkenness.

stimulating the coughing up and clearance of phlegm. It has a beneficial effect on mucous membranes and is generally combined with tonic herbs, especially thyme (*Thymus vulgaris*, p. 147). Ivy extracts are common ingredients in cosmetic formulations for cellulite.

Caution Fresh leaves can irritate the skin.

Helichrysum italicum (Asteraceae)

Curry plant, Immortelle

Description A strongly aromatic, small bushy evergreen herb with silver-gray needle shaped leaves and yellow composite flowers on domed clusters, growing to about 20 in (50 cm) in height.

Habitat & cultivation Native to the Mediterranean region, curry plant thrives in poor quality and sandy soils, typically growing close to the sea or on riverbanks, but found inland up to 2,600 ft (800 m) above sea level. The flowering tops are gathered when just opening in June.

Parts used Flowering tops.

Constituents Curry plant contains a volatile oil (0.44%), mostly sesquiterpenes including alpha-cedrene, alpha-curcurmene, and geranyl acetate, phloroglucinols, notably arzanol, phenolic acids, and flavonoids. Arzanol is a potent anti-inflammatory.

History & folklore The plant's botanical name "Helichrysum" comes from the classical Greek meaning "sun—gold." If dried carefully, curry plant flower heads can last for long periods of time, thus

its other name of "Immortelle."

Medicinal actions & uses A neglected, traditional southern European medicinal herb, much used in the past, and now undergoing something of a renaissance. The flowers have longstanding use in treating allergies and upper respiratory infections, and healing wounds and inflammatory skin problems. The essential oil has marked anti-inflammatory and photoprotective (protects against solar radiation) activity supporting its traditional use in enhancing skin health.

Research A 2020 clinical trial found that a night cream containing curry plant essential oil, among other constituents, was effective at reducing the negative impact of environmental factors on the skin and reducing clinical signs of aging.

Herniaria glabra (Caryophyllaceae)

Rupturewort

Description Prostrate annual or perennial with bright green oval leaves and clusters of green flowers.

Habitat & cultivation Rupturewort is found throughout Europe and western Asia. It thrives in barren areas, in lime and sandy soils. It is gathered when in flower.

Parts used Aerial parts.

Constituents Rupturewort contains coumarins (including 3% herniarin and scopoletin), flavonoids, phenolic acids, and saponins.

History & folklore Rupturewort was first documented in European herbals of the 16th century. Its genus name, *Herniaria*, refers to its reputed ability to heal hernias.

Medicinal actions & uses Rupturewort is of value chiefly as a diuretic herb. The fresh plant treats urinary problems such as cystitis, irritable bladder, and kidney stones. It is also astringent, and has been applied as a poultice to speed the healing of ulcers. The whole plant appears to have an antispasmodic effect on the bladder.

Hibiscus sabdariffa (Malvaceae)

Hibiscus, Jamaica

Description Shrub growing to 6½ ft (2 m) in height.

Habitat & cultivation Native to North Africa and Southeast Asia, hibiscus grows in tropical regions around the world. It is primarily cultivated across Africa and in Thailand, China, and Mexico.

Parts used Calyx (the outer base of the flower), flowers, leaves.

Constituents Hibiscus contains polyphenols especially anthocyanins and protocatechuic acid, polysaccharides, and organic acids.

History & folklore "Hibiscus" means "plant that is consecrated to the ibis," a bird held sacred in ancient Egypt.

Medicinal actions & uses Hibiscus makes a refreshing, pleasant-tasting tea that is cooling and mildly sedative, soothing hot and feverish conditions. The calyces are gently tonic and will ease colds, coughs, and chest problems. They also aid digestion and gently stimulate appetite. Both the calyces and flowers act to reduce cholesterol levels. All parts of hibiscus are demulcent, mildly soothing sore or inflamed mucous membranes within the digestive and respiratory tracts.

Research Several clinical trials have shown that hibiscus lowers raised blood pressure and can form part of a natural approach to its treatment. Studies also indicate that it helps to lower raised blood sugar and blood cholesterol levels.

Hieracium pilosella syn. *Pilosella officinarum* (Asteraceae)

Mouse-ear hawkweed

Description Perennial herb growing to a height of 8 in (20 cm) from a rosette of basal leaves. Stems bear single bright yellow flower heads.

Habitat & cultivation Mouse-ear hawkweed is common throughout much of Europe and temperate regions of Asia and North America. Found growing in dry pastures and on sandy soil, it is collected when in flower in summer

Parts used Aerial parts.

Constituents Mouse-ear hawkweed contains a coumarin (umbelliferone), flavonoids, and caffeic acid. It is thought to be mildly antifungal.

History & folklore In his *Irish Herbal* (1735), K'Eogh summarizes mouse-ear hawkweed's medicinal benefits: "good against the spitting of blood, all kinds of flow, coughs, ulcers of the lungs, mouth and eyes, and shingles."

Medicinal actions & uses Mouse-ear hawkweed relaxes the muscles of the bronchial tubes, stimulates the cough reflex, and reduces the production of mucus. This combination of actions makes the herb effective in respiratory problems, including asthma and wheeziness, whooping cough, bronchitis, and other chronic and congested coughs. The herb is used to control heavy menstrual bleeding, and to ease the coughing up of blood. It may be applied as a poultice to heal wounds.

Hippophae rhamnoides (Elaeagnaceae)

Sea buckthorn

Description Thorny deciduous shrub growing to 16 ft (5 m). Has narrow silvery leaves, male or female flowers, and clusters of brownish-orange berries.

Habitat & cultivation Native to Europe and Asia, sea buckthorn grows mainly in sandy coastal areas and in dry riverbeds in mountainous regions. The berries are harvested in the fall.

Parts used Berries.

Constituents The fruit contains flavonoids, flavones, carotenoids, vitamins A, C (present in very high quantities), and E, and high levels of minerals including sulfur, selenium, zinc, and copper. The seeds contain appreciable levels of alpha-linolenic acid.

History & folklore The sour-tasting berries have traditionally been eaten with milk and cheese by Siberians and Tartars, who also used them to make a pleasant-tasting jelly.

Medicinal actions & uses Sea buckthorn berries are very high in vitamin C. They have principally been used to help improve resistance to infection. The berries are mildly astringent, and a decoction of them has been used as a wash to treat skin irritation and eruptions, and to promote healing.

Research Research into sea buckthorn fruit, seed, and seed oil indicates that they have definite therapeutic value. The fruit especially supports heart and circulatory health and is useful in treating conditions such as capillary fragility, arteriosclerosis, and a weak heart. The seed oil nourishes the skin, promotes tissue healing, and will often prove useful in treating eczema.

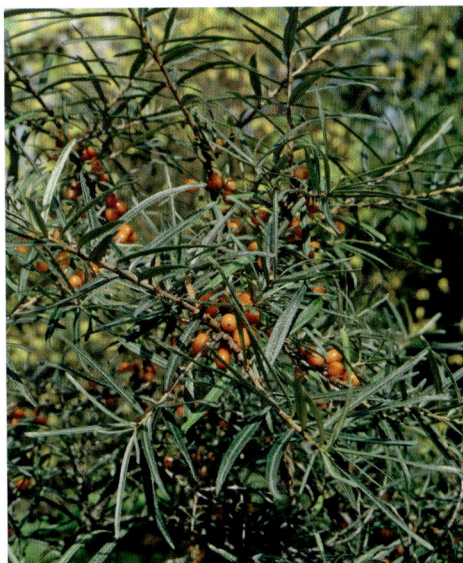

Sea buckthorn is distinguished by its thorny stems and narrow silvery leaves. The berries help improve the body's resistance to infection.

Hoodia gordonii (Apocynaceae)

Hoodia

Description Unusual-looking succulent growing to 3 ft (1 m), hoodia has multiple spiny, gray-green stems and light purple flowers.

Habitat & cultivation Native to the Kalahari desert, hoodia is now extensively cultivated in Namibia and South Africa. The plant is grown from seed or cuttings. Trade in the hoodia plant is legally restricted due to its threatened survival in the wild.

Parts used The peeled stem.

Constituents Hoodia contains steroidal glycosides. It is thought to have a stimulant (sympathomimetic) effect and thus is used as an appetite suppressant.

History & folklore The San people of the Kalahari traditionally used this plant to suppress sensations of thirst and hunger, when on journeys through the desert. Such use was first recorded in 1937.

Medicinal actions & uses Hoodia provides a cautionary tale for herbal medicines and supplements in the 21st century. There is little evidence that taking it leads to weight loss other than the plant's traditional use as an appetite suppressant, while its safety profile is unknown. Despite this, after media coverage by the BBC in 2003, sales of hoodia supplements rocketed, with prices in the *LA Times* reaching $40 per ounce (30 g) in 2006. At such a price, it is not hard to see why hoodia's survival in the wild is severely threatened. It would seem sensible to opt instead for herbs that are endorsed for their use for weight loss by scientific studies and where there is no risk of the herb disappearing from the wild, such as gymnema (*Gymnema sylvestre*, p. 223).

Cautions Seek professional advice before taking hoodia products, especially if taking prescribed blood-thinning medication for conditions such as diabetes or high blood pressure.

Hordeum vulgare (Poaceae)

Barley

Description Annual grass growing to about 3 ft (1 m). Has an erect hollow stem, lance-shaped leaves, and ears bearing twin rows of seeds and long bristles.

Habitat & cultivation Barley is cultivated in temperate regions worldwide. It is harvested when the seeds are mature.

Parts used Seeds.

Constituents Barley contains polysaccharides, proteins, sugars, fats, and vitamins B and E.

The young seedlings also contain the amines tyramine and gramine.

History & folklore Barley has been consumed for many thousands of years. Dioscorides (1st century CE) recommended it "to weaken and restrain all sharp and subtle humours, and sore and ulcerated throats."

Medicinal actions & uses An excellent food for convalescence in the form of porridge or barley water, barley is soothing to the throat and provides easily assimilated nutrients. It can also be taken to clear mucus. Its demulcent quality soothes inflammation of the gut and urinary tract. Barley aids in the digestion of milk and is given to babies to prevent the development of curds within the stomach. It is commonly given to children suffering from minor infections or diarrhea, and it is particularly recommended as a treatment for feverish states. Made into a poultice, barley is an effective remedy for soothing and reducing inflammation in sores and swellings.

Research The fiber in barley, like that in oats, has an established action in reducing fat absorption from the gut, aiding lower cholesterol levels. In common with other fiber foods, it may also help to stabilize blood sugar levels and to prevent bowel cancer.

Wild hydrangea

Hydrangea arborescens (Hydrangeaceae)

Description Woody-stemmed deciduous shrub growing to a height of about 10 ft (3 m). Has oval leaves and clusters of small, creamy-white flowers.

Habitat & cultivation Native to the eastern US from New York to Florida, wild hydrangea grows in woodlands and on riverbanks. The root is dug up in the fall.

Part used Root.

Constituents Hydrangea is thought to contain flavonoids, a cyanogenic glycoside (hydrangein), saponins, and a volatile oil.

History & folklore The Cherokee used hydrangea as a remedy for kidney and bladder stones. The 19th-century Physiomedicalist herbal movement used a formula comprising hydrangea, couch grass (*Agropyron repens*, p. 209), and hollyhock (*Althaea rosea*) to treat serious kidney disorders, including nephritis.

Medicinal actions & uses Western herbal medicine considers the diuretic hydrangea as being particularly helpful in the treatment of kidney and bladder stones. It is thought both to encourage the expulsion of stones and to help dissolve those that remain. The herb is given for many other troubles

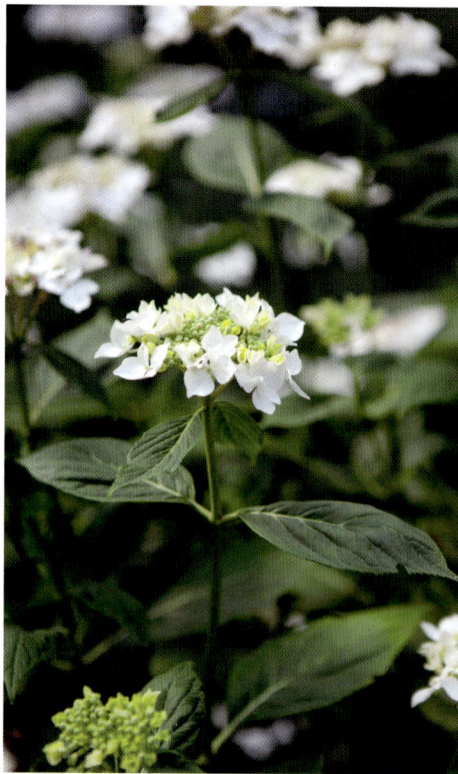

Wild hydrangea is used to treat kidney and bladder stones.

affecting the genitourinary system, including cystitis, urethritis, enlarged prostate, and prostatitis.

Cautions Do not take during pregnancy or while breastfeeding. Wild hydrangea is best taken on professional advice.

Gokulakanta

Hygrophila spinosa (Acanthaceae)

Description Thorny, red-stemmed annual growing to 2 ft (60 cm). Has bright blue flowers and small, flat, dark red seeds.

Habitat & cultivation Native to India, gokulakanta is now widely distributed throughout tropical regions. It is gathered when in flower.

Parts used Aerial parts, root.

Constituents Gokulakanta contains mucilage, fixed and volatile oils, and an alkaloid.

Medicinal actions & uses Commonly used as a remedy in India, gokulakanta is taken chiefly for its reputed aphrodisiac properties. Both the aerial parts and ash of the burned plant are strongly diuretic, and are used to flush water from the body in cases of excess fluid retention.

Related species The South American *H. guayensis* is bactericidal and has been used as a local treatment for the tropical disease, leishmaniasis.

Henbane

Hyoscyamus niger (Solanaceae)

Description Annual or biennial herb growing to 3 ft (1 m). Has delicate, slightly lobed leaves and bell-shaped flowers, pale yellow in color with fine purple veining.

Habitat & cultivation Native to western Asia and southern Europe, henbane is now found across much of western and central Europe, and North and South America. It is cultivated for therapeutic use in parts of Europe, including England, and in North America. The leaves and flowers are picked just after the plant has flowered, in the first year for the annual variety and in the second year for the biennial.

Parts used Leaves, flowering tops.

Constituents Henbane contains 0.045–0.14% tropane alkaloids, especially hyoscyamine and hyoscine, and flavonoids. Hyoscyamine and hyoscine are common to other members of the *Solanaceae* family, but henbane's relatively high hyoscine content gives it a more specifically sedative action than its relatives thornapple (*Datura stramonium*, p. 205) and deadly nightshade (*Atropa belladonna*, p. 73).

History & folklore Henbane has been used as a medicinal herb for thousands of years. Babylonian accounts and the Egyptian *Ebers papyrus* (c. 1500 BCE) record that henbane was smoked to relieve toothache. In Greek myth, the dead were adorned with henbane when they arrived in Hades. Writing in the 1st century CE, Dioscorides recommended henbane for insomnia, coughs, congestion, heavy menstrual bleeding, eye pain, gout, and as a general

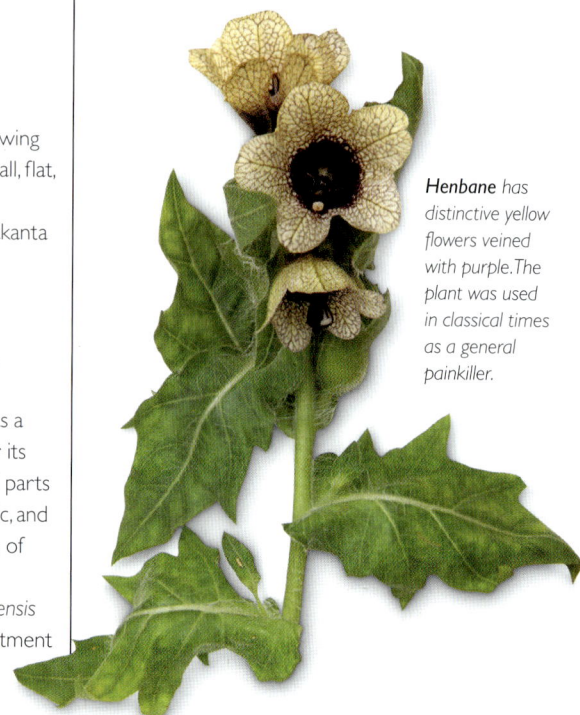

Henbane has distinctive yellow flowers veined with purple. The plant was used in classical times as a general painkiller.

pain reliever, and advised that the herb should be used within a year as it deteriorates quickly. In the Middle Ages, henbane had the Latin name *dentaria*, denoting its use as a remedy against toothaches. Henbane reputedly produces a sensation of lightness, as though one were flying, and it was one of the chief components of witches' "flying ointments."

Medicinal actions & uses Henbane is used extensively in herbal medicine as a sedative and painkiller. Its specific use is for pain affecting the urinary tract, especially pain due to kidney stones, though it is also given for abdominal cramping. Its sedative and antispasmodic effect makes it a valuable treatment for the symptoms of Parkinson's disease, relieving tremor and rigidity during the early stages of the illness. Henbane has also been used to treat asthma and bronchitis, usually as a "burning powder" or in the form of a cigarette. Applied externally as an oil, it can relieve painful conditions such as neuralgia, sciatica, and rheumatism. Henbane reduces mucus secretions, as well as saliva and other digestive juices. Like its cousin deadly nightshade, it dilates the pupils. Hyoscine is commonly employed as a preoperative anesthetic and in motion sickness formulations.

Related species Other *Hyoscyamus* species are used in a similar way. The North African *H. muticus* is traditionally smoked by Bedouins to relieve toothaches. See also deadly nightshade (*Atropa belladonna*, p. 73).

Cautions Use only under professional supervision. Potentially toxic in overdose, henbane is subject to legal restrictions in some countries.

Hyssopus officinalis (Lamiaceae)

Hyssop

Description Semi-evergreen shrub growing to 2 ft (60 cm). Has narrow leaves and clusters of blue double-lipped flowers.

Habitat & cultivation Native to southern Europe, hyssop grows freely in Mediterranean countries, especially in the Balkans and Turkey. It prefers sunny, dry sites and is a common garden herb. The flowering tops are harvested when the plant is in flower in summer

Parts used Flowering tops, essential oil.

Constituents Contains terpenes (including marubiin, a diterpene), a volatile oil (consisting mainly of camphor, pinocamphone, and beta-pinene), flavonoids, tannins, and resin. Marubiin is a strong expectorant. Pinocamphone is toxic, and the volatile oil can cause epileptic seizures.

History & folklore In the past, hyssop was so highly esteemed it was regarded as a virtual cure-all. An old saying went, "Whoever rivals hyssop's virtues, knows too much." In the 1st century CE, Dioscorides recommended a recipe containing a mixture of hyssop, figs (*Ficus carica*, p. 216), rue (*Ruta graveolens*, p. 273), honey, and water for treating a number of conditions, including pleurisy, asthma, tight-chestedness, respiratory congestion, and chronic coughs.

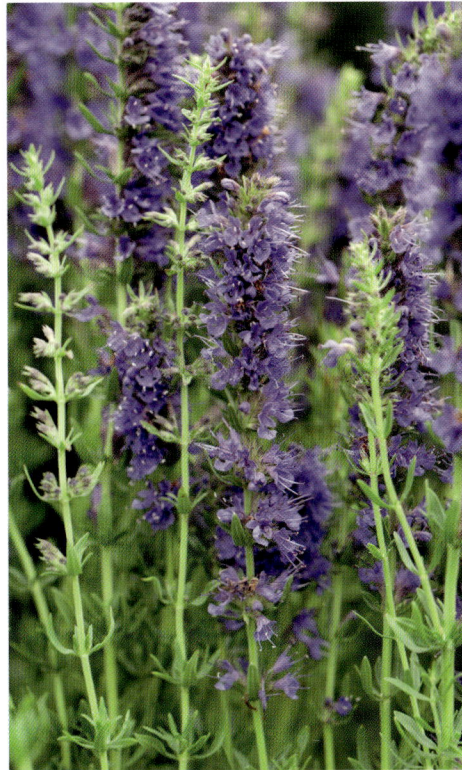

Hyssop has a positive effect on respiratory infections.

Medicinal actions & uses Currently an undervalued medicinal herb, hyssop is potentially useful as it is both calming and tonic. It has a positive effect when used to treat bronchitis and respiratory infections, especially where there is excessive mucus production. Hyssop appears to encourage a more liquid mucus, and at the same time gently stimulates expectoration. This combined action clears thick and congested phlegm. Hyssop can irritate the mucous membranes, so it is best given after an infection has peaked, when the herb's tonic action encourages a general recovery. As a sedative, hyssop is a useful remedy against asthma in both children and adults, especially where the condition is exacerbated by mucus congestion. Like many herbs with a strong volatile oil, it soothes the digestive tract and can be an effective remedy against indigestion, gas, bloating, and colic.

Cautions Hyssop essential oil can induce epileptic seizures. It should only be used under professional supervision. Hyssop essential oil is subject to legal restrictions in some countries.

Ilex paraguariensis syn. *I. paraguensis* (Aquifoliaceae)

Maté

Description Evergreen shrub or small tree growing to 20 ft (6 m). Has large leaves, white flowers, and small reddish fruit.

Habitat & cultivation Maté grows wild in northern Argentina, Paraguay, Uruguay, and southern Brazil, and is widely cultivated in Argentina, Spain, and Portugal. The leaves are picked when the berries are ripe, heated over a wood fire, ground, and then stored in sacks for a year before being sold.

Parts used Leaves.

Constituents Maté contains xanthine derivatives, including about 1.5% caffeine, about 0.2% theobromine, theophylline, and up to 16% tannins. The high tannin content means that maté should not be consumed with meals, as tannins impair the absorption of nutrients.

Medicinal actions & uses Maté is a traditional South American tea that increases short-term physical and mental energy levels. It is taken as a fortifying beverage in much the same way as tea (*Camellia sinensis*, p. 185) is consumed throughout Asia and Europe. Maté has properties similar to those of tea and coffee (*Coffea arabica*, p. 196). It stimulates the nervous system and is mildly analgesic and diuretic. As a medicinal herb, maté is used to treat headaches, migraine, neuralgic and rheumatic pain, fatigue, and mild depression. It has also been used in the treatment of diabetes.

Related species *I. guayusa*, from Ecuador, is used in much the same way as maté but is also employed medicinally to treat malaria, liver pain, and syphilis. It is thought to aid digestion and cleanse the digestive tract.

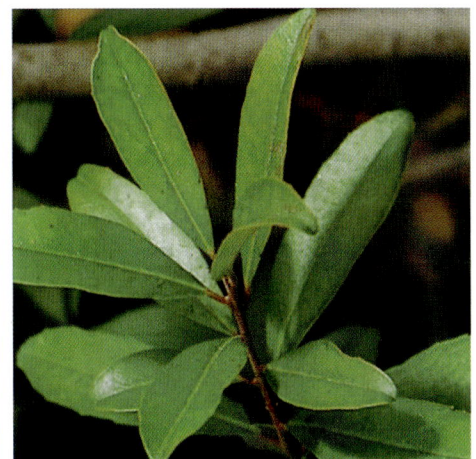

Maté makes a pleasant-tasting tea that has a stimulant, mildly analgesic, and diuretic effect.

Illicium verum (Schisandraceae)

Star anise, *Ba jiao hui xian* (Chinese)

Description Evergreen tree growing to 59 ft (18 m). Has tapering leaves, pale greenish-yellow flowers and star-shaped segmented fruit (seed pods).

Habitat & cultivation Native to China, India and Vietnam, star anise grows in tropical regions across the world. The fruit is harvested when ripe.

Parts used Fruit and seeds.

Constituents Star anise contains a volatile oil (mostly anethole), sesquiterpenoids, and flavonoids, including quercetin. Anethole calms the digestive system and relieves gas. The sesquiterpenoids have analgesic activity. Shikimic acid, found in the seed pods, was until recently used as the main source for the production of Tamiflu, a prescribed antiviral medicine. Star anise has antibacterial, antifungal, antiviral, anti-inflammatory, and insecticidal activity.

History & folklore Due to its high anethole content, star anise has a similar taste to anise (*Pimpinella anisum*, p. 256), and both are used principally as spices. The herb's Chinese name, *ba jiao hui xian*, means "8-horned fennel."

Medicinal actions & uses Used in Chinese herbal medicine as a remedy for rheumatism, back pain, and hernias, star anise has stimulant, diuretic, and digestive properties. It makes an effective remedy for gas and indigestion—especially colic—and can safely be given to children. To treat hernias of the intestine or bladder, star anise is often mixed with fennel (*Foeniculum vulgare*, p. 217). Both herbs help to relax the organ's muscles and relieve spasm. Star anise is also used for toothache.

Caution Japanese star anise (*Illicium anisatum*), which is very similar to star anise, contains a toxic compound and can cause serious side effects.

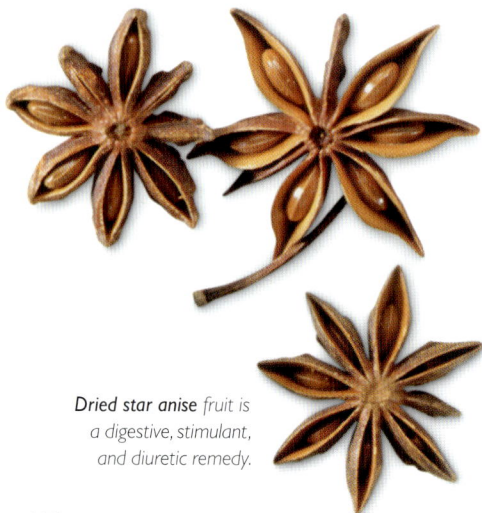

Dried star anise fruit is a digestive, stimulant, and diuretic remedy.

Ipomoea purga syn. *Convolvulus jalapa* (Convolvulaceae)

Jalap

Description Evergreen vine reaching about 13 ft (4 m). Has heart-shaped leaves and trumpetlike purple flowers.

Habitat & cultivation Native to Mexico, jalap is cultivated in Central America, the Caribbean, and Southeast Asia. The root is unearthed in summer.

Part used Root.

Constituents Jalap contains the resin convolvulin.

History & folklore Spanish colonizers learned of jalap's strong purgative effect from Indigenous Mexican peoples. Introduced into Europe in 1565, the herb was used for all types of illnesses until the 19th century.

Medicinal actions & uses Jalap is such a powerful cathartic that its medicinal value is questionable. Even in moderate doses it stimulates the elimination of profuse watery stools, and in larger doses it causes vomiting.

Related species *I. turpethum*, native to Asia and Australia, is also a drastic purgative. Other *Ipomoea* species, such as the sweet potato (*I. batatas*, from South America), are important food plants. The seeds of morning glory (*I. violacea*), native to Mexico, contain compounds similar to LSD, and were taken ritually by the Zapotecs and Aztecs.

Caution Do not take jalap under any circumstances.

Iris versicolor (Iridaceae)

Blue flag, Wild iris

Description Perennial growing to about 3 ft (1 m). Has erect stems and long sword-shaped leaves. Each stem bears 3–5 resplendent blue to violet flowers with white-veined areas on the petals.

Habitat & cultivation Blue flag is native to North America. Preferring damp and marshy areas in the wild, it is also widely cultivated as a garden plant. The rhizome is unearthed in the fall.

Part used Rhizome.

Constituents Blue flag contains triterpenoids, salicylic, and isophthalic acids, a very small amount of volatile oil, starch, resin, an oleoresin, and tannins.

History & folklore Blue flag was one of the medicinal plants most frequently used by Indigenous North American peoples. Different nations made use of it variously as an emetic, cathartic, and diuretic, to treat wounds, and for colds, earache, and cholera. In the Anglo-American Physiomedicalist tradition, blue

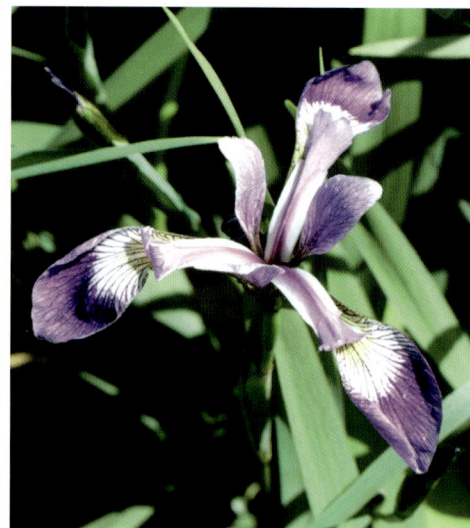

Blue flag was very widely used by Indigenous North American peoples to treat wounds and sores.

flag was used as a glandular and liver remedy. Blue flag is Quebec's provincial flower.

Medicinal actions & uses Blue flag is currently used mainly to detoxify the body. It increases urination and bile production, and has a mild laxative effect. This combination of cleansing actions makes it a useful herb for chronic skin diseases such as acne and eczema, especially where gallbladder problems or constipation contribute to the condition. Blue flag is also given for biliousness and indigestion. However, in large doses blue flag will itself cause vomiting. The traditional use of blue flag for gland problems persists. It is also believed by some to aid weight loss.

Cautions Excessive doses cause vomiting. Do not take this plant during pregnancy.

Jasminum grandiflorum (Oleaceae)

Jasmine

Description Slender evergreen rambler growing to 20 ft (6 m). Has dark green compound leaves and large, sweetly scented tubular white flowers.

Habitat & cultivation Native to northern India, Pakistan, and the northwestern Himalayas, jasmine is now cultivated as a garden plant and for its essential oil.

Parts used Flowers, essential oil.

Constituents Jasmine's volatile oil contains benzyl alcohol, benzyl acetate, linalool, and linalyl acetate.

History & folklore Jasmine was introduced to Europe in the 16th century, and is mainly used as a source of perfume.

Medicinal actions & uses Jasmine flowers make a calming and sedative infusion, taken to relieve tension. The oil is considered antidepressant and relaxing. It is used externally to soothe dry or sensitive skin. Due to frequent adulteration, the oil is rarely used in aromatherapy.

Related species Actually native to Southeast Asia, Arabian jasmine (*J. sambac*) is used as an eyewash, is added to tea (*Camellia sinensis*, p. 185) to produce jasmine tea, and is used in Buddhist ceremonies.

Caution Jasmine essential oil should not be taken internally.

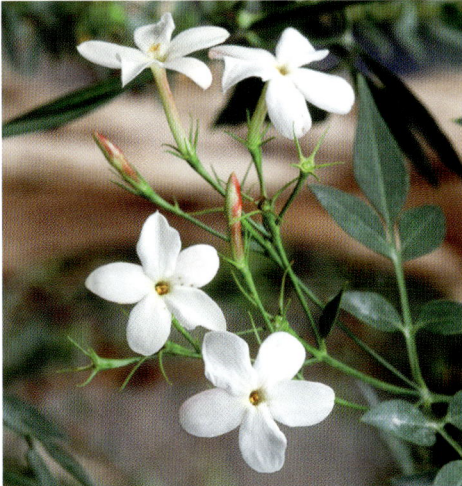

Jasmine flowers are the source of an essential oil that is used to treat stress and depression.

Jateorhiza palmata (Menispermaceae)
Calumba

Description Creeping vine with a perennial rootstock, growing to a great height and often reaching the tops of trees. Has large palm-shaped leaves, small greenish-white flowers, with male and female flowers on separate plants, and round, fleshy fruit.

Habitat & cultivation Native to the rainforests of eastern Africa, especially Mozambique and Madagascar, calumba is also grown in other tropical regions. The roots are dug up in dry weather in March and dried.

Parts used Bark.

Constituents Calumba contains isoquinoline alkaloids (notably palmatine, columbamine, and jatrorrhizine), diterpene bitter principles, mucilage, and volatile oil (about 1%).

Medicinal actions & uses Profoundly bitter, calumba is an extremely good remedy for underactive or weakened digestion, stimulating stomach acid production and increasing appetite. It is a specific for loss of appetite and anorexia, and by making the stomach more acidic (and therefore

hostile to pathogens) helps to prevent digestive infections and improve the breakdown and absorption of foods. It is a useful treatment for chronic intestinal infection such as dysentery.

Research Calumba's bitterness is due both to the bitter principles and the alkaloids. Palmatine and jatrorrhizine reduce blood pressure, palmatine is a uterine stimulant, and jatrorrhizine is sedative and antifungal.

Other species Calumba has much in common with gentian (*Gentiana lutea*, p. 103), although it owes its bitterness to a different range of constituents

Caution Avoid during pregnancy.

Juglans cinerea (Juglandaceae)
Butternut

Description Deciduous tree growing to 100 ft (30 m). Has gray bark, long leaves with many leaflets, male catkins and female flowers, and an oval-shaped fruit containing a hard dark-colored nut.

Habitat & cultivation Native to North American forests, butternut is cultivated for its timber in other temperate regions. The bark is collected in the fall.

Part used Inner bark.

Constituents Contains naphthaquinones (including juglone, juglandin, and juglandic acid), a fixed and a volatile oil, and tannins. The naphthaquinones have an approximately similar laxative effect to the anthraquinones found in plants such as senna (*Cassia senna*, p. 80) and Chinese rhubarb (*Rheum palmatum*, p. 130). Juglone is purgative, antimicrobial, antiparasitic, and has anticancer activity.

History & folklore Butternut bark was employed by Indigenous North American peoples and colonizers as a laxative and tonic remedy. Butternut was used to treat a variety of conditions, including rheumatic and arthritic joints, headaches, dysentery, constipation, and wounds.

Medicinal actions & uses Used to this day as a laxative and tonic, butternut is a valuable remedy for chronic constipation, gently encouraging regular bowel movements. It is especially beneficial if combined with a carminative herb, such as ginger (*Zingiber officinale*, p. 159) or angelica (*Angelica archangelica*, p. 172). Butternut also lowers cholesterol levels, and promotes the clearance of waste products by the liver. It has a positive reputation in treating intestinal worms, and, being antimicrobial and astringent, it has been prescribed as a treatment for dysentery.

Related species Black walnut (*J. nigra*) is used in the same way as butternut. The bark of the walnut tree (*J. regia*) is used as a gentle purgative, and is also

applied to skin afflictions. The nut is used in Chinese herbal medicine as a kidney tonic. The nuts of both varieties are highly nutritious, lower cholesterol levels, and contain significant quantities of alpha-linolenic acid.

Juniperus communis (Cupressaceae)
Juniper

Description Coniferous shrub sometimes growing to 49 ft (15 m). Has slender twigs with whorls of needlelike leaves, yellow male and blue female flowers on separate plants, and spherical blue-black fruit.

Habitat & cultivation Juniper is found in Europe, southwestern Asia up to the Himalayas, and North America, where it grows from southern coastal sites to more northerly moorland and mountainous regions. The ripe fruit (berries) is gathered in the fall.

Parts used Fruit, essential oil.

Constituents Juniper fruit contains 1–2% volatile oil, consisting of over 60 compounds, which include myrcene, sabinene, alpha- and beta-pinene, and cineole. Juniper also contains tannins, flavonoids, diterpenes, and coumarins. The fruit has antimicrobial, anti-inflammatory, diuretic, and pain-relieving activity.

History & folklore Juniper is the main flavoring used in gin. Juniper berries are still mostly gathered

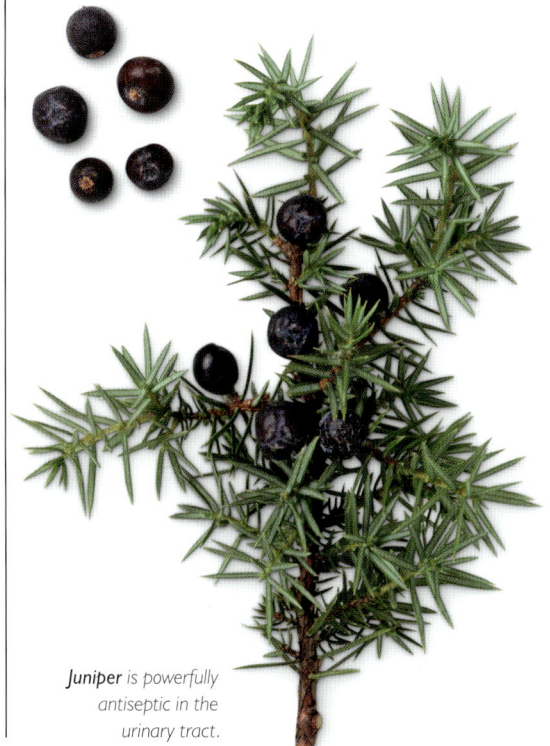

Juniper is powerfully antiseptic in the urinary tract.

from the wild. In former times, sprigs of juniper flung into the fire were thought to protect against evil spirits.

Medicinal actions & uses Juniper is tonic, diuretic, and strongly antiseptic within the urinary tract. It is a valuable remedy for cystitis, and helps relieve fluid retention, but should be avoided in cases of kidney disease. In the digestive system, juniper is warming and settling, easing colic and supporting the function of the stomach. Taken internally or applied externally, juniper is helpful in the treatment of chronic arthritis, gout, and rheumatic conditions. Applied externally as a diluted essential oil, it has a slightly warming effect on the skin and is thought to promote the removal of waste products from underlying tissues. Juniper also stimulates menstruation and tends to increase menstrual bleeding.

Research Laboratory research suggests juniper may have neuroprotective activity, possibly protecting against Parkinson's disease. It also appears to help lower blood cholesterol levels.

Related species Oil of Cade is produced from *J. oxycedrus* and is applied to treat skin rashes. Savin (*J. sabina*) is toxic and a powerful abortifacient. The Japanese *J. rigida* is used as a diuretic.

Cautions Do not use juniper during pregnancy or if prone to heavy menstrual bleeding. Do not take if suffering from a kidney infection or kidney disease. Do not take the essential oil internally except under professional supervision.

Self-help use Urinary infections, p. 324.

Kigelia pinnata syn. *K. africana* (Bignoniaceae)

Kigelia,
African sausage tree

Description Semi-deciduous tree growing to 80 ft (25 m) with smooth, gray-brown bark and brown-purple flowers. The tree gets its name from the spectacular sausage-shaped fruit, up to 3 ft (1 m) in length, which hangs from a ropelike stalk and weighs up to 22 lb (10 kg).

Habitat & cultivation Kigelia grows throughout Africa south of the Sahara but is native to the eastern half from Tanzania to South Africa. The tree is cultivated from seed or cuttings and flowers after 6 years. The fruit is harvested when ripe.

Parts used Fruit pulp, leaves, bark, roots.

Constituents Kigelia fruit contains norviburtinal, coumarins, iridoids, flavonoids, fatty acids, sterols, glycosides, and napthaquinones. Norviburtinal has tumor-reducing activity, the iridoids and sterols are anti-inflammatory, the flavonoids are antifungal, and

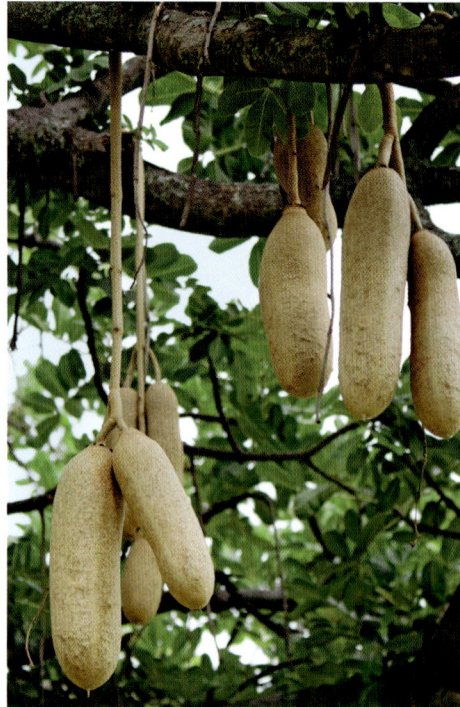

Kigelia is a key remedy for treating skin problems.

the napthaquinones are thought to be cytotoxic.

History & folklore Prized by traditional healers throughout Africa south of the Sahara, kigelia has been put to many uses. The Shona of southern Africa use the bark or root to treat skin infections and ulcers, toothache, backache, and pneumonia. In Central Africa, the unripe fruit is used as a dressing for wounds, hemorrhoids, and rheumatism. In West Africa, the leaves are given for stomach and kidney problems, and the fruit is used as a purgative and applied as a paste to sores. Kigelia is commonly included in traditional herbal formulations for malaria.

Medicinal actions & uses Thanks to the knowledge and experience of African traditional healers, kigelia is now understood to be a valuable remedy for skin problems, particularly sores and ulcers, produced by bacterial and fungal infection. Kigelia has been described as a "natural antibacterial." Given its marked anti-inflammatory and wound healing properties, kigelia is also being investigated as a skin toner and restorer, as well as potential treatment for skin disorders such as eczema, psoriasis, and solar keratosis (a precancerous skin problem caused by overexposure to sunlight). Various patents exist for kigelia products, and over time kigelia may become widely known as a key herbal resource for the skin.

Cautions Take kigelia internally only under professional guidance. Do not take during pregnancy or while breast-feeding.

Krameria triandra (Krameriaceae)

Rhatany

Description Dense evergreen shrub growing to 3 ft (90 cm). Has a deep root, oblong leaves, and large red flowers.

Habitat & cultivation Rhatany is found in Ecuador, Peru, and Bolivia on western slopes of the Andes at altitudes of 3,000–9,800 ft (900–3,000 m). The root is unearthed throughout the year.

Part used Root.

Constituents Rhatany contains 10–20% tannins, including phlobaphene, benzofurans, and n-methyltyrosine.

History & folklore A traditional South American remedy, rhatany was used by Indigenous peoples as an astringent and a tooth preservative. Its Spanish name, *raiz para los dientes* (root for the teeth), points to this traditional usage.

Medicinal actions & uses Rhatany is astringent and antimicrobial. It is a useful remedy taken principally for problems affecting the gastrointestinal tract. It is most commonly used for diarrhea and dysentery. In addition, rhatany makes a good mouthwash and gargle for bleeding and infected gums, mouth ulcers, and sore throats. The plant's astringency makes it useful in the form of an ointment, suppository, or wash for treating hemorrhoids. Rhatany may also be applied to wounds to help staunch blood flow, to varicose veins, and over areas of capillary fragility that may be prone to easy bruising.

Related species The Mexican *K. cystisoides* is an astringent remedy used in much the same way as rhatany. Another species native to North and Central America, *K. parvifolia*, was used by the Papago people as an eyewash.

Lactuca virosa (Lamiaceae)

Wild lettuce

Description Hollow-stemmed biennial growing to about 4 ft (1.2 m). Has broad spiny leaves and clusters of pale yellow composite flowers. All parts of the plant exude a white milky latex.

Habitat & cultivation Common throughout Europe, wild lettuce grows on waste ground, along roadsides, and in hedges. It is gathered when in flower in late summer.

Parts used Leaves, latex, seeds.

Constituents The latex contains sesquiterpene lactones (including lactucopicrin and lactucerin); the leaves also contain flavonoids and coumarins. The sesquiterpene lactones have a sedative effect.

History & folklore In Assyrian herbal medicine, lettuce seeds were reportedly used with cumin (*Cuminum cyminum*, p. 201) as a poultice for the eyes. Dioscorides (1st century CE) wrote that the plant's effect resembled that of the opium poppy (**Papaver somniferum**, p. 251).

Medicinal actions & uses Wild lettuce is a safe sedative that can be given to adults and children to encourage a sound night's sleep or to calm overactivity or overstimulation. Most commonly, it is recommended for excitability in children. It is also taken to treat coughs, often in combination with herbs such as licorice (*Glycyrrhiza glabra*, p. 105). Wild lettuce is thought to lower the libido. It may also be used to relieve pain.

Research A 2011 Egyptian clinical trial found that lettuce seed oil improved sleep in people suffering from insomnia. Lettuce seed oil has traditionally been used in Egypt for sleep problems.

Related species Garden lettuce (*L. sativa*) may be used like wild lettuce, but has a much weaker therapeutic action.

Lamium album (Lamiaceae)
White deadnettle

Description Perennial growing to 2 ft (60 cm). Has a square stem, toothed oval leaves, and clusters of white double-lipped flowers.

Habitat & cultivation White deadnettle is native to and widespread in Europe and central and northern Asia. It thrives in fields and on waste ground. It is gathered when in flower in summer.

Parts used Flowering tops.

Constituents White deadnettle flowering tops contain hydroxycinnamic acids, iridoids, secoiridoids, flavonoids, anthocyanins, steroids, benzoxazinoids, and betaine.

History & folklore Deadnettle is so called because it resembles true nettle (*Urtica dioica*, p. 150), without the stinging hairs. It was also known as archangel, a plant "to make the heart merry, to make a good colour in the face, and to refresh the vital spirits" (John Gerard, *The Herball*, 1597).

Medicinal actions & uses White deadnettle is astringent and demulcent. It is chiefly used as a uterine tonic, to arrest intermenstrual bleeding, and to reduce excessive menstrual flow. It is also a traditional treatment for abnormal vaginal discharge. The herb is sometimes taken to relieve painful periods. Its astringency helps treat diarrhea, and, used externally, it can relieve hemorrhoids and varicose veins.

Research Laboratory studies into white deadnettle show that its constituents to some degree have antimicrobial, antiviral, anti-inflammatory, pain-relieving, and cell protective activity. However, such results need to be put in context. In a 2009 clinical study investigating the anti-inflammatory activity of fresh nettle leaves (*Urtica dioica* p. 150), white deadnettle leaves—which look very similar —were used by way of comparison (as a placebo). Those taking part had arthritis of the thumb and applied either fresh nettle leaves or white deadnettle leaves to the affected area each day. Within a week, those applying the nettle leaves noted a significant reduction in symptoms, while those applying the white deadnettle leaves saw no such improvement —indicating that nettle has significantly stronger anti-inflammatory activity than white deadnettle.

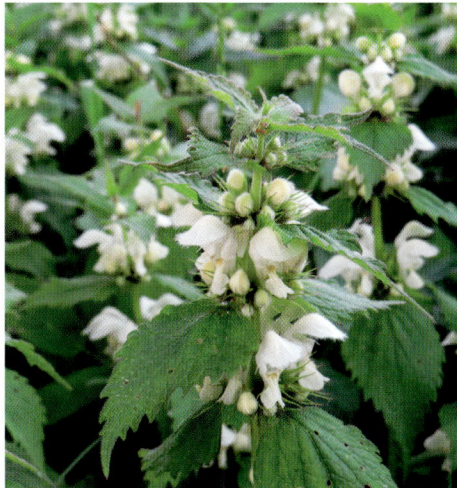

White deadnettle is used to treat gynecological conditions.

Larix decidua syn. *L. europaea* (Pinaceae)
European larch

Description Deciduous conifer growing to 165 ft (50 m). Has clusters of needlelike leaves, male and female flowers, and small, light brown cones.

Habitat & cultivation Native to the Alps and the Carpathian mountains of eastern Europe, larch grows to altitudes of 6,600 ft (2,000 m). It is widely cultivated for its timber. The resin is tapped in autumn; the bark is collected when the tree is felled.

Parts used Inner bark, resin.

Constituents Larch contains lignans, resins, and volatile oil (consisting mainly of alpha- and beta-pinene and limonene).

Medicinal actions & uses Larch has astringent, diuretic, and antiseptic properties. The bark may be used to treat bladder and urinary tubule infections such as cystitis and urethritis, and respiratory problems, including bronchitis. The resin is applied to wounds, where it protects and counters infection. A decoction of the bark is used to soothe eczema and psoriasis.

Caution Do not take if suffering from kidney disease.

Larrea tridentata (Zygophyllaceae)
Chaparral,
Creosote bush

Description Thorny shrub growing to 6 1/2 ft (2 m), with small finely divided leaves.

Habitat & cultivation Chaparral is found in large numbers in the deserts of the southwestern US and Mexico.

Parts used Aerial parts.

Constituents Chaparral contains about 12% resin and lignans, including nordihydroguaiaretic acid. The latter is reportedly harmful to the lymph glands and kidneys, though recent research shows that it has beneficial antidiabetic properties. US research published in 1996 demonstrated that other lignans have antiviral activity against HIV.

History & folklore Widely used by Indigenous North American peoples, chaparral was taken in the form of a decoction to treat stomach troubles and diarrhea. Young twigs were used for toothache. The leaves were applied as a poultice for respiratory problems and as a wash for skin problems.

Medicinal actions & uses Until the 1960s, chaparral remained in wide use in the US, with an average of 10 tons (9.07 metric tons) consumed each year. It was thought to be a beneficial remedy for rheumatic disease, venereal infections, urinary infections, and certain types of cancer, especially leukemia. Chaparral was also taken internally for skin afflictions such as acne and eczema, and applied as a lotion to sores, wounds, and rashes. In the early 1990s, sales of chaparral were banned in the US and Britain due to concern over its potential toxic effect on the liver. It now seems likely that this is another herb that can, in rare cases, cause liver damage, as with some conventional medicines. In view of the uncertainty about its safety, any potential benefit from taking the herb must be weighed against the risks.

Related species The North American *L. divaricata*, a close relative of chaparral, contains lignans, which have been shown to inhibit lymphoid tumor growth with no apparent harmful effect on normal lymphatic tissue.

Cautions Only take chaparral on professional advice. People with a history of liver disease should never take chaparral.

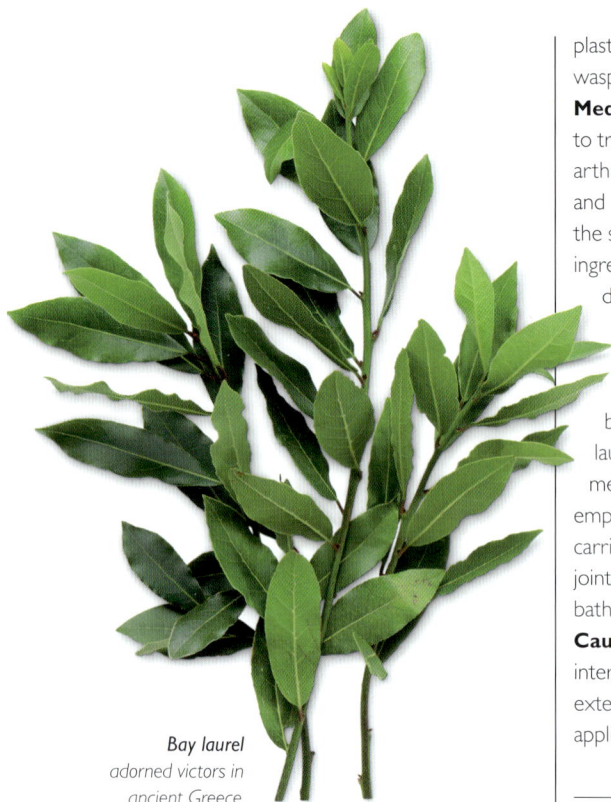

Bay laurel
adorned victors in
ancient Greece.

Laurus nobilis (Lauraceae)

Bay laurel

Description Aromatic evergreen shrub or tree growing to 65 ft (20 m). Has leathery, dark green leaves, small yellow male and female flowers, and shiny black berries.

Habitat & cultivation Native to Mediterranean countries, bay laurel prefers damp and shady sites. It is also a popular garden herb, cultivated largely for culinary use. The leaves are picked year round.

Parts used Leaves, essential oil.

Constituents Bay laurel contains up to 3% volatile oil (including 30–50% cineole, linalool, alpha-pinene, alpha-terpineol acetate, mucilage, tannin, and resin). The essential oil has significant antibacterial and antifungal activity.

History & folklore In ancient Greece, bay laurel was used in divination by the Delphic Oracle. From ancient Rome comes the tradition that the sudden withering of a bay laurel tree bodes disaster for the household. In ancient Rome, bay laurel leaves were used as a medicine, a spice, and a decorative garland during the December festival of Saturnalia. Bay laurel was sacred to the gods Apollo and Asclepius, who together oversaw healing and medicine. The herb was thought to be greatly protective and healing. An infusion of the leaves was taken for its warming and tonic effect on the stomach and bladder, and a plaster made from the leaves was used to relieve wasp and bee stings.

Medicinal actions & uses Bay laurel is used mainly to treat upper digestive tract disorders and to ease arthritic aches and pains. It is settling to the stomach and has a tonic effect, stimulating the appetite and the secretion of digestive juices. When used as an ingredient in cooking, bay laurel leaves promote the digestion and absorption of food. The leaves have much the same kind of positive effect as spearmint (Mentha spicata) and rosemary (Rosmarinus officinalis, p. 132) in assisting the breakdown of heavy food, especially meat. Bay laurel has also been used to promote the onset of menstrual periods. The essential oil is chiefly employed as a friction rub, being well diluted in a carrier oil and massaged into aching muscles and joints. A decoction of the leaves may be added to a bath to ease aching limbs.

Cautions Never take bay laurel essential oil internally. An allergic reaction may result from external use, therefore the oil should only be applied in very dilute (2%) concentrations.

Lawsonia inermis syn. *L. alba* (Lythraceae)

Henna

Description Heavily scented evergreen shrub or tree growing to 20 ft (6 m). Has narrow pointed leaves, clusters of small white or pink flowers, and blue-black berries.

Habitat & cultivation Native to the Middle East, North Africa, and the Indian subcontinent, henna grows in sunny areas and is widely cultivated for use as a hair restorative and dye. The leaves are picked during the growing season.

Parts used Leaves, bark.

Constituents Henna contains coumarins, naphthaquinones (including lawsone), flavonoids, sterols and tannins.

History & folklore Henna has been used for thousands of years in North Africa and Asia as a red dye and as a scent. Mummies were wrapped in henna-dyed cloth in ancient Egypt. In the Middle East and India, the leaves have traditionally been used to make a pigment for dyeing intricate linear patterns on the fingers, palms, and feet. The leaves have also been used to dye not only human hair but the manes and tails of horses. Before meeting Antony, Cleopatra reputedly soaked the sails of her barge in heady henna flower oil.

Medicinal actions & uses Used mainly within Ayurvedic and Unani medicine, henna leaves are commonly taken as a gargle for sore throats, and as an infusion or decoction for diarrhea and dysentery. The leaves are astringent, prevent hemorrhaging, and strongly promote menstrual flow. A decoction of the bark is used to treat liver problems. Applied in the form of a plaster, henna treats fungal infections, acne, and boils.

Leonurus cardiaca (Lamiaceae)

Motherwort

Description Perennial herb growing to 5 ft (1.5 m). Has toothed, palm-shaped leaves and double-lipped pink flowers blossoming in clusters.

Habitat & cultivation Native to central Asia, motherwort is now naturalized in much of Europe and North America. It grows wild in woodlands, on waste ground, and along roadsides. It is also cultivated as a garden plant. Motherwort is harvested when it comes into flower in summer.

Parts used Aerial parts.

Constituents Motherwort contains alkaloids (including L-stachydrine), an iridoid (leonurine), diterpenes, flavonoids, caffeic acid, and tannins.

History & folklore As its species name *cardiaca* indicates, motherwort has long been considered a heart remedy. The herbalist Nicholas Culpeper stated that "there is no better herb to drive away melancholy vapours from the heart, to strengthen it and make the mind cheerful" (1652). The Italian physician and herbalist Pierandrea Mattioli held it "useful for palpitations and a pounding heart, spasms and paralysis … [it] thins thick and viscid humours [and] stimulates urine and menstrual bleeding" (1548).

Medicinal actions & uses A remedy for the heart and nerves and often prescribed for palpitations, motherwort strengthens heart function, especially where it is weak. Antispasmodic and sedative, the herb soothes anxiety and promotes

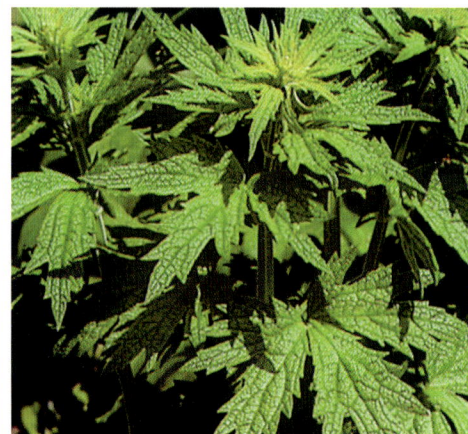

Motherwort has been used to treat palpitations since at least the 16th century.

relaxation. However, motherwort stimulates the muscles of the uterus, and is particularly suitable for delayed periods, period pain, and premenstrual syndrome (especially if shock or distress is a factor). It should not be used if menstrual bleeding is heavy.

Related species Two East Asian species, *L. heterophyllus* (from China) and *L. sibiricus* (from Siberia), are both used therapeutically for the same purposes as motherwort. *L. heterophyllus* appears to lower blood pressure and to induce menstruation.

Cautions Do not take motherwort during pregnancy. It should also be avoided where there is heavy menstrual bleeding.

Self-help uses Menstrual problems— irregular cycle, p. 325; Panic attacks, p. 312.

Lepidium meyenii (Brassicaceae)

Maca root

Description Maca is a perennial plant growing between 11,000–15,000 ft (3,500–4,500 m) above sea level. Between 12–20 leaves form a basal rosette, from which the main stem emerges up to 8 in (20 cm) in height. Its white flowers are about 3/16 in (5 mm) long. The tuberous roots, similar to turnips, grow to around 3 in (8 cm) in diameter, varying in color from white to red to yellow to purple.

Habitat & cultivation A plant of the high Andes in Bolivia and Peru, Maca has been cultivated as a staple food and tonic medicine for over 3,500 years. It is grown from seed, 2½ acres (1 hectare) producing roughly 5½ tons (5 metric tons) of dried root. Mostly grown in its native Andes, the root is now being cultivated in the Himalayas.

Parts used Tuberous roots

Constituents Maca root contains polyunsaturated fatty acids, including macaenes and macamides, alkaloids, glucosinolates, sterols, and polysaccharides.

History & folklore Maca root is taken as a juice, or cooked as a "porridge" or paste as a nourishing food. It has longstanding use as a restorative tonic and aid to fertility in both men and women. In the 1800s, the Indigenous people of the Junin area made annual payments to Spanish colonizers of 9 tons of maca root, which was given to horses as a tonic feed.

Medicinal actions & uses Maca is another plant that blurs the boundary between food and medicine. A nourishing vegetable, ideally suited to aid survival in the high Andean plateau, maca root is also an adaptogen that promotes nonspecific resistance to stresses of all kinds. As such it has a wide range of potential uses, including improving fertility and the chances of conception, anemia, menopausal symptoms, chronic fatigue, and failure to thrive. It can equally be taken to promote and maintain good

health—children in Peru are given maca to improve school performance.

Research A 2010 review investigating maca's effect on human sexual function noted that two clinical trials showed a significant positive effect of maca on sexual dysfunction or sexual desire in healthy menopausal women, and in healthy adult men. It is thought that maca can also prove helpful with erectile dysfunction and an enlarged prostate.

Lepidium virginicum (Brassicaceae)

Virginia peppergrass

Description Annual herb growing to about 2 ft (60 cm). Has slender lance-shaped leaves and small white flowers.

Habitat & cultivation Virginia peppergrass is native to eastern North America and the Caribbean, and is naturalized in Australia. The leaves are gathered in spring and are consumed as food. The seedpods can serve as a substitute for black pepper.

Parts used Leaves, root.

Constituents Virginia peppergrass contains high levels of vitamin C.

History & folklore The Menominee people of eastern North America applied a lotion of Virginia peppergrass (or a bruised fresh plant) to poison ivy eruptions.

Medicinal actions & uses Virginia peppergrass is nutritious and generally detoxifying. It has been used to treat vitamin C deficiency and diabetes, and to expel intestinal worms. The herb is also diuretic and of benefit in easing rheumatic pain. The root is taken to treat excess phlegm within the respiratory tract.

Related species Maca (*L. meyenii*) is a low-growing Andean perennial. The root is valued as a staple food and medicine by Andean peoples, notably to support immune function and for hormonal disorders including sterility. Maca is now commonly available in supplement stores and has acquired a reputation as a tonic, hormone balancer, and aphrodisiac.

Leptandra virginica syn. *Veronicastrum virginicum* (Scrophulariaceae)

Black root

Description Perennial herb growing to 3 ft (1 m). Has an erect stem, lance-shaped leaves, and white flowers.

Habitat & cultivation Black root grows across

North America in meadows and woodlands. The root is unearthed in the fall.

Part used Dried root.

Constituents Black root contains a volatile oil, saponins, sugars, and tannins.

History & folklore Known to the Indigenous peoples of Missouri and Delaware as a violent purgative, black root was used in moderate doses as a laxative, a detoxifier, and a remedy for liver disorders. In the 19th century Physiomedicalist tradition, black root was taken to stimulate bile production.

Medicinal actions & uses Black root is used in small doses today as a laxative and a remedy for liver and gallbladder disorders. The herb also treats flatulence and bloating, and eases the discomfort of hemorrhoids, chronic constipation, and rectal prolapse.

Root

Cautions Do not use the fresh root. Do not take during pregnancy.

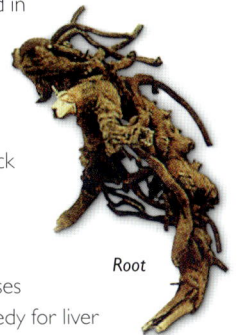

Levisticum officinale syn. *Ligusticum levisticum* (Apiaceae)

Lovage

Description Perennial growing to 6½ ft (2 m). Has glossy, toothed compound leaves, greenish-yellow flowers, and tiny oval seeds.

Habitat & cultivation Lovage is found in southern Europe and southwestern Asia. It thrives on sunny mountain slopes. The leaves are gathered in spring or early summer, the seeds in late summer, the root in the fall.

Parts used Root, seeds, leaves.

Constituents Lovage root contains a volatile oil (about 70% phthalides), coumarins (including bergapten, psoralen, and umbelliferone), alkynes, plant acids, sterols, resins, and gums. The phthalides are sedative and anticonvulsant.

History & folklore The *Trotula* texts, written in Salerno during the 12th century, recommend lovage for skin lightening. The Irish herbalist K'Eogh follows this recommendation: "lovage clears the sight and removes spots, freckles, and redness from the face."

Medicinal actions & uses Lovage is a warming and tonic herb for the digestive and respiratory systems. It treats indigestion, poor appetite, gas and colic, and bronchitis. Lovage is significantly diuretic and antimicrobial and is commonly taken for urinary tract problems. It also promotes menstruation and relieves period pain. Its warming nature improves poor circulation.

Related species The Chinese *chuan xiong* (*Ligusticum chuanxiong*) is used principally as a means to bring on absent menstrual periods and to treat period pain. The Chinese *gao ben* (*Ligusticum sinense*) is also used for pain.

Cautions Do not take during pregnancy. Do not take if you suffer from kidney disease. Can increase sensitivity to sunlight.

Self-help use Heavy menstrual bleeding, p. 325.

Lippia alba (Verbenaceae)

Lippia,
Bushy lippia, *Prontoalivio*

Description Multi-branched, square-stemmed, aromatic shrub growing to 5 ft (1.5 m), with opposite leaves and small white or pink flowers close to the leaf axils.

Habitat & cultivation Lippia grows throughout South and Central America from northern Argentina to the southern US. It is a common garden herb, and may be grown from seed or cuttings, the latter used for commercial cultivation.

Parts used Leaves.

Constituents Lippia leaves contain about 0.15% volatile oil with different plant strains, or chemotypes, producing several essential oils with quite a distinct range of compounds, notably citral and carvone. The citral chemotype oil is thought to have strong anti-*Candida* activity.

History & folklore In many parts of Central and South America, Lippia is valued for its ability to resolve common illnesses, such as stomach upset, nausea, gas and bloating, coughs, colds, sore throat, and headache. Its Colombian name, *prontoalivio* (meaning "quick relief") points to its place in popular Latin American medicine.

Medicinal actions & uses Lippia has pain-relieving, anti-inflammatory, relaxant, and antispasmodic properties, making it useful in many non-severe health problems. In Brazil, where it is regulated as a medicinal herb, the herb is typically used for upper digestive problems, coughs, colds, and bronchitis, as well as for high blood pressure and as a sedative. The herb has been little researched, though a small clinical trial in Brazil found it effective in treating migraine headache. The essential oil is increasingly used in pharmaceutical and cosmetic preparations, for example, within Europe, and has significant antifungal and antibacterial activity on the skin.

Related species The sweet tasting *L. dulcis* has broadly similar medicinal use and is found across Central America and the Caribbean. See also lemon verbena (*Lippia citriodora*, p. 168).

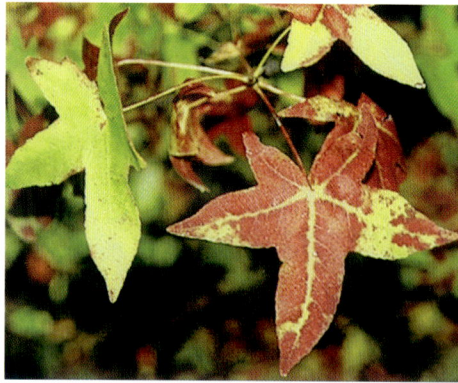

Oriental sweetgum can relieve congestive chest problems.

Liquidambar orientalis (Altingiaceae)

Oriental sweetgum

Description Deciduous tree growing to 100 ft (30 m). Has purplish-gray bark, lobed leaves, and small single yellow-white flowers

Habitat & cultivation Oriental sweetgum is found in southwestern Turkey. Storax balsam, a viscid gray-brown liquid, is extracted from the bark, which is pried off the tree in the fall.

Part used Bark extract.

Constituents Oriental sweetgum contains cinnamic acid, cinnamyl cinnamate, phenylpropyl cinnamate, triterpene acids, and a volatile oil.

History & folklore Oriental sweetgum has been the *Liquidambar* species most commonly used medicinally since the 19th century. Oriental sweetgum is also employed as a fixative for perfumes.

Medicinal actions & uses Storax balsam acts as both an irritant and an expectorant within the respiratory tract, and it is one of the ingredients of Friar's Balsam, an expectorant mixture that is inhaled to stimulate a productive cough. In addition, storax balsam is applied externally to encourage the healing of skin diseases and problems such as scabies, wounds, and ulcers. Mixed with witch hazel (*Hamamelis virginiana*, p. 106) and rosewater (*Rosa species*), Oriental sweetgum makes an astringent face lotion. In China, Oriental sweetgum is used to clear mucus congestion and to relieve pain and constriction in the chest.

Related species American storax (*L. styraciflua*), which grows mainly in Honduras but is also found further north, has been used since the time of the Maya for its healing properties.

Lobaria pulmonaria (Peltigeraceae)

Tree lungwort

Description Gray or light green lichen with forked irregular lobes measuring up to $^5/_8$ in (1.5 cm) across.

Habitat & cultivation Found throughout Europe, tree lungwort grows on trees and rocks in woodland areas. It is gathered year round.

Part used Lichen.

Constituents Tree lungwort contains a variety of plant acids (including stictic and succinic acid), fatty acids, mucilage, and tannins.

History & folklore Tree lungwort has been used since ancient times as a remedy for lung problems. The Italian physician and herbalist Pierandrea Mattioli (1501–1577) recommended it for healing pulmonary ulcers and for treating blood-flecked phlegm. It was also used to treat wounds, heal ulcers, reduce excessive menstrual bleeding, relieve dysentery, and halt "choleric vomiting."

Medicinal actions & uses A beneficial but underused remedy, tree lungwort has expectorant and tonic properties. It aids in clearing congested mucus, reduces phlegm, and helps increase the appetite. In a decoction sweetened with honey, it is appropriate for all conditions that are marked by chronic respiratory infections, especially coughs and bronchitis. The plant also treats asthma, pleurisy, and emphysema. Being astringent and demulcent, tree lungwort makes a useful treatment for pulmonary ulcers as well as for a variety of gastrointestinal problems. It is highly suitable for treating ailments in children.

Lomatium dissectum (Apiaceae)

Lomatium,
Desert parsley

Description Erect perennial, growing to $6^1/_2$ ft (2 m), with a large woody taproot, divided triangular leaves, and flowers in flat-topped umbels.

Habitat & cultivation Native to coastal and inland regions of western North America from California as far north as British Columbia.

Part used Root.

Constituents Lomatium contains flavonoids, coumarins, tetronic acids, and volatile oil.

History & folklore One of the most important medicinal plants of the Pacific Northwest, lomatium was "big medicine" for Indigenous North American peoples and widely used for respiratory infections. In Nevada, lomatium root was combined with yarrow (*Achillea millefolium*, p. 60) to treat sexually transmitted diseases. In Oregon, a decoction of the root was applied to horses to rid them of ticks. During the 1917 influenza epidemic an American doctor, Ernest Krebbs, successfully used lomatium in his own practice, after noting the effective use of the herb by Indigenous peoples.

Medicinal actions & uses Lomatium is today used mostly by botanical practitioners in North America to treat a broad range of viral infections, from chronic fatigue syndrome to influenza and herpes infections. A good tonic herb, it promotes peripheral blood flow and stimulates immune function. It is usually combined with other herbs such as echinacea (*Echinacea* spp., p. 96) or wild indigo root (*Baptisia tinctoria*, p. 180).

Research The tetronic acids have been shown to be markedly antimicrobial and toxic to fish (Indigenous peoples used to place the fresh root in streams or pools in order to stun fish). Preliminary studies in Canada and the US suggest that lomatium has significant antiviral activity.

Cautions A red measles-like rash, which clears on stopping treatment, may develop when taking lomatium. Like other members of the carrot family, lomatium can increase sensitivity to sunlight.

Lonicera spp. (Caprifoliaceae)

Honeysuckle, & *Jin yin hua*

Description A climber growing to 13 ft (4 m) that is deciduous (honeysuckle, *L. caprifolium*) or semi-evergreen (jin yin hua, *L. japonica*). Has paired oval leaves, yellow-orange (honeysuckle) or yellow-white (jin yin hua) tubular flowers, and red (honeysuckle) or black (jin yin hua) berries.

Habitat & cultivation Honeysuckle is native to southern Europe and the Caucasus. Jin yin hua is native to China and Japan. Both plants are commonly found growing on walls, on trees, and in hedges. The flowers and leaves are gathered in summer just before the flowers open.

Parts used Flowers, leaves, bark.

Constituents In Europe, *L. caprifolium* and *L. japonica* are often used interchangeably and contain approximately the same quantity of volatile oil. Nonetheless, Romanian research indicates that the Asian species contains a much wider range of therapeutically active antiseptic compounds.

History & folklore Honeysuckle is one of the Bach Flower Remedies, and in this system of herbal cures it is believed to counter feelings of nostalgia and homesickness. Jin yin hua has long been used in Chinese medicine to "clear heat and relieve toxicity."

Medicinal actions & uses Honeysuckle flowers from both species can be successfully used to treat fever, colds, and upper respiratory tract infections. The leaves are traditionally used as a gargle for sore throats and as a mouthwash. In Chinese herbal medicine, honeysuckle finds frequent use in inflammatory conditions, such as conjunctivitis, mastitis (inflammation of the breasts), and rheumatoid arthritis.

Research Chinese research indicates that the Asian species has significant antimicrobial activity, including against the tuberculosis bacillus. Clinical studies suggest that this species can also help to lower high blood pressure.

Caution Do not eat the berries, which are thought to be toxic.

Lophophora williamsii (Cactaceae)

Peyote

Description Cactus growing to 2 in (5 cm). Has a squat gray-green body with tufted hairs, and pink or white flowers.

Habitat & cultivation Peyote is native to northern Mexico and the southwestern region of the US.

Part used Whole plant.

Constituents Peyote contains alkaloids, principally mescaline, which is a powerful hallucinogen.

History & folklore Peyote has been used by Indigenous peoples of North America in religious ceremonies for over 6,000 years. Its use as a hallucinogen was popularized by Aldous Huxley in his book *The Doors of Perception*.

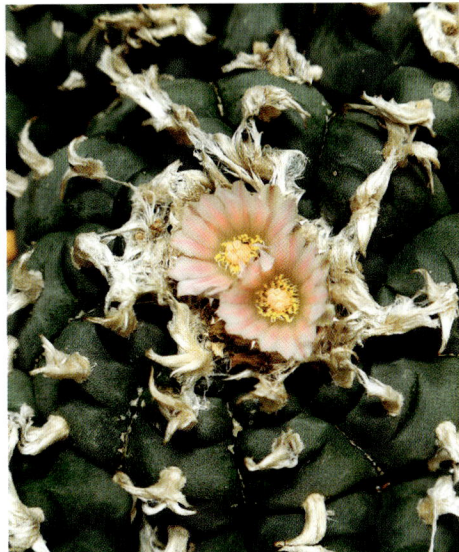

Peyote is a powerful hallucinogen. It is used in ceremonies by Indigenous peoples in North America.

Medicinal actions & uses Peyote is a shamanistic plant, taken in Indigenous North American rituals to deepen spiritual understanding. It plays an important part in the emotional and mental state of the community. It is also used to treat fevers, as a painkiller for rheumatism, and to treat paralysis. It is applied as a poultice for fractures, wounds, and snake bite. Peyote is also used to induce vomiting.

Caution The use of peyote and mescaline is illegal in most countries.

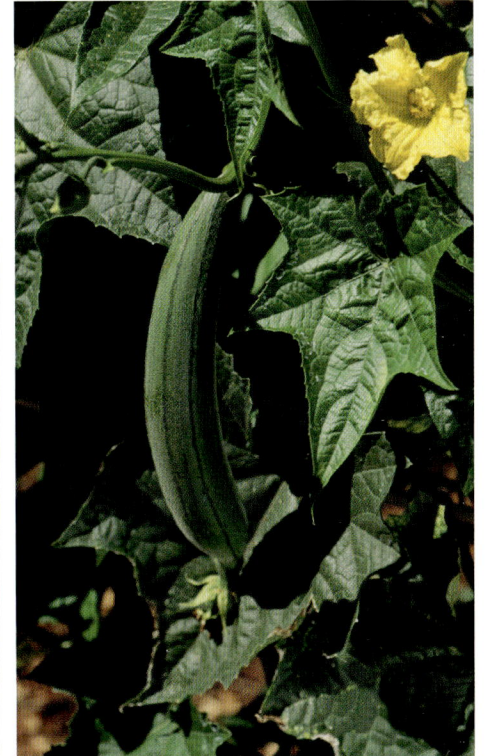

Loofah fruit is dried and used in Chinese medicine to treat muscle and joint pain.

Luffa aegyptiaca syn. *L. cylindrica* (Cucurbitaceae)

Loofah, *Si gua luo* (Chinese)

Description Annual vine climbing to 49 ft (15 m). Has large lobed leaves, tendrils, and yellow female flowers producing long cylindrical squash-like fruit.

Habitat & cultivation Loofah is native to the tropics of Asia and Africa. It is now grown as a fruit in tropical regions around the world. It is harvested when ripe in summer.

Part used Fruit.

Constituents Loofah contains polysaccharides, xylan, xylose, and galactan.

History & folklore Loofah was brought from India to China in the Tang Dynasty (618–907 CE). It is best known in the West as a shower accessory—the fibrous skeleton makes a good skin scrubber.

Medicinal actions & uses In Chinese medicine, the inner skeleton of the dried fruit is used to treat pain in the muscles, joints, chest, and abdomen. It is prescribed for chest infections accompanied by fever and pain, and is used to clear congested mucus. Loofah has also been prescribed to treat painful or swollen breasts.

Research Chinese research indicates that the fresh vine has a stronger expectorant effect than the dried fruit. German research (1999) using a homeopathic preparation of the plant concluded it was effective as a standard nasal spray for relief of hay fever.

Lycopodium clavatum (Lycopodiaceae)

Club moss

Description Creeping evergreen moss growing to 4³/₄ in (12 cm). Has numerous straggling branchlets covered with bright green linear leaves, and scaly spikes bearing yellow spores.

Habitat & cultivation Club moss is found throughout temperate regions of the northern hemisphere. It is common on mountains and in moorland. The plant is gathered in summer.

Parts used Moss, spores.

Constituents Club moss contains about 0.1–0.2% alkaloids (including lycopodine), polyphenols, flavonoids, and triterpenes.

History & folklore Club moss has been used medicinally since at least the Middle Ages. The whole plant was employed as a diuretic to aid in the flushing out of kidney stones. In Wales, club moss was used for certain back problems and for colds and sore throats. Being strongly water-resistant, the spores are still used to coat tablets. The spores ignite explosively and have been used in making fireworks.

Medicinal actions & uses Club moss is diuretic, sedative, and antispasmodic, and is particularly useful for treating chronic urinary issues. The herb may also be taken for indigestion and gastritis. The spores can be applied to the skin to relieve itchiness. Club moss is frequently used in homeopathic medicine, being prescribed for headache, liver problems, and digestive symptoms such as gas and burping.

Caution Club moss is potentially toxic in overdose. This plant should only be used with the supervision of a professional practitioner.

Lycopus virginicus (Lamiaceae)

Bugleweed

Description Perennial herb growing to 2 ft (60 cm). Has a square stem, lance-shaped leaves, and whorls of whitish flowers.

Habitat & cultivation Bugleweed is common throughout most of North America, thriving close to water. It is harvested in summer when in flower

Parts used Aerial parts.

Constituents Bugleweed contains phenolic acids (including derivatives of caffeic, chlorogenic, and ellagic acids).

History & folklore In the 19th-century Physiomedicalist tradition, bugleweed was regarded as astringent and calming to the nerves, and was given for loose coughs, internal bleeding, and urinary incontinence. Herbal practitioners once considered the plant to be a mild narcotic.

Medicinal actions & uses Bugleweed has sedative properties and today the herb is principally prescribed to treat an overactive thyroid gland and the racing heartbeat that often accompanies this condition. Bugleweed is also considered an aromatic and tonic astringent that reduces the production of mucus.

Research Studies indicate that bugleweed and, to some degree, gipsywort (*see Related species, below*) reduce the activity of the thyroid gland.

Related species Gipsywort (*L. europaeus*), a European native, has astringent and cardiotonic properties. It is taken for palpitations and anxiety, and has been used to lower fever.

Cautions Take only under professional supervision. Do not take during pregnancy.

Lysimachia vulgaris (Primulaceae)

Yellow loosestrife

Description Attractive perennial growing to 3 ft (1 m) with whorls of broadly lance-shaped leaves and bright yellow flowers.

Habitat & cultivation Native to Europe, yellow loosestrife commonly grows in damp hedgerows and near water. It is also cultivated as a garden plant. It is gathered when in flower in summer.

Parts used Aerial parts.

Constituents Yellow loosestrife contains a benzoquinone, triterpenoid saponins, flavonoids, and tannins.

History & folklore Pliny (23–79 CE) recorded that lysimachia, the plant's Latin name, was a tribute to King Lysimachus of Sicily, who discovered its medicinal benefits. The name "loosestrife" refers to the plant's reputed power to prevent conflict, particularly between animals, and to repel insects. The Greek physician Dioscorides (40–90 CE) recommended loosestrife to staunch wounds and for nosebleeds, and noted that its smoke would drive away snakes and flies.

Medicinal actions & uses An astringent herb, yellow loosestrife is principally used to treat gastrointestinal conditions such as diarrhea and dysentery, to stop internal and external bleeding, and to cleanse wounds. It makes a workable mouthwash for sore gums and mouth ulcers, and may be used to treat nosebleeds. Yellow loosestrife has also been taken as an expectorant.

Related species The yellow pimpernel (*L. nemorum*), another European native, is astringent and staunches blood. Jin qian cao (*L. christinae*), from China, is a diuretic used to treat urinary pain. A Chinese trial showed that the latter is also effective in treating both kidney stones and gallstones.

Lythrum salicaria (Lythraceae)

Purple loosestrife

Description Attractive perennial growing to about 5 ft (1.5 m). Has straight red stems, pointed lance-shaped leaves, and spikes of brilliant purple flowers.

Habitat & cultivation Purple loosestrife is native to Europe but well-established in the wild in North America. It thrives in marshes and along rivers and streams, to altitudes of 3,300 ft (1,000 m). It is gathered when in flower in summer.

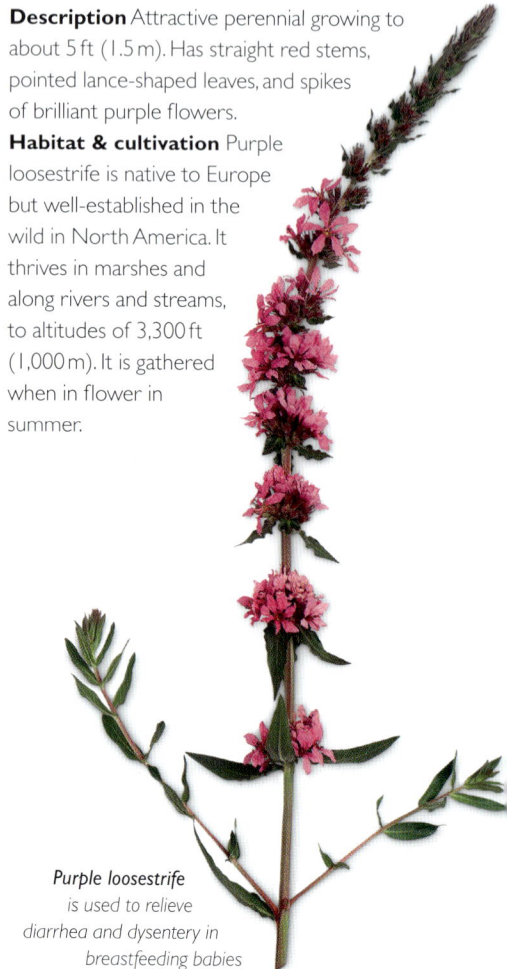

Purple loosestrife
is used to relieve diarrhea and dysentery in breastfeeding babies

Parts used Aerial parts.

Constituents Purple loosestrife contains tannins, flavonoids, anthocyanins, phenolic acids, alkaloids, steroids, and triterpenes.

History & folklore In 1654, the herbalist Nicholas Culpeper praised this herb, writing that "the distilled water is a present remedy for hurts and blows on the eyes, and for blindness … it also cleareth the eyes of dust or any other thing gotten into them, and preserveth the sight." A common plant in Ireland, purple loosestrife was much used there against diarrhea.

Medicinal actions & uses The astringent purple loosestrife is mainly employed as a treatment for diarrhea and dysentery. It can be safely taken by people of all ages; some herbalists recommend it to help arrest diarrhea in breastfeeding babies. The herb may also be used to treat heavy periods and for intermenstrual bleeding. Externally, it is applied as a poultice or lotion to wounds, leg ulcers, and eczema, and used to treat excess vaginal discharge and vaginal itching. Purple loosestrife is now little used to treat eye problems, but, as Culpeper's experience suggests, the herb could be worth further investigation as a remedy for disorders of the eyes and vision.

Research In animal experiments, extracts of the flowers and leaves have been shown to be hypoglycemic—lowering blood sugar levels. The plant is also thought to have antibiotic activity.

Madhuca longifolia (Sapotaceae)

Butter tree

Description Large deciduous tree with spreading crown growing to 16 m (50 ft). Has leathery leaves, clusters of scented white flowers, and greenish fruit.

Habitat & cultivation Madhuca species are native to India, Nepal and Burma growing up to 656 ft (200 m) above sea level. The flowers, leaves and seeds are gathered in summer.

Parts used Flowers, seed oil.

Constituents The leaves contain an alkaloid and a saponin; the seeds a saponin and fixed oil.

History & folklore Butter tree has been a source of food and medicine in India for at least 2,000 years. Its flowers are eaten and are fermented to make alcoholic drinks.

Medicinal actions & uses The expectorant flowers are used to treat chest problems such as bronchitis. They are also taken to increase breast milk production. The leaves are applied as a poultice to eczema. The seed oil is laxative and is taken for constipation and to loosen the stool of hemorrhoid sufferers.

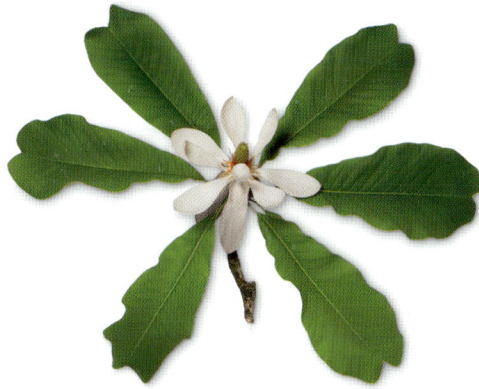

Magnolia is distinguished by its beautiful creamy-white flowers.

Magnolia officinalis (Magnoliaceae)

Magnolia,
Hou po (Chinese)

Description Deciduous tree growing to 80 ft (25 m). Has aromatic bark, large leaves, and fragrant creamy-white flowers.

Habitat & cultivation Native to China, magnolia grows wild in mountainous regions. It is now planted in many parts of the world as an ornamental tree. The bark is stripped in spring.

Part used Bark.

Constituents Magnolia bark contains alkaloids, coumarins, flavonoids, and lignans. The lignan honokiol, found in the bark of several magnolia species appears to have antitumor and anti-anxiety activity. Another lignan, magnolol, has antibacterial and anti-anxiety activity.

Medicinal actions & uses Magnolia bark is aromatic, warming, and pungent. It relieves cramping pain and flatulence, and is taken for abdominal distension, indigestion, loss of appetite, vomiting, and diarrhea. It is now also used to treat anxiety, chronic stress, and lowered mood, and as a neuroprotective remedy that aids memory and mental function.

Research Research suggests that magnolia bark extract is antimicrobial and may have specific use as an oral antiseptic to control bacteria and relieve bad breath (halitosis). Two Italian clinical studies found that magnolia extract helped relieve anxiety and support positive mood in menopausal women. A 2012 Korean study concluded that magnolia may be useful in treating Alzheimer's disease.

Related species North American species, notably *M. grandiflora*, are used in much the same way as magnolia (above), with traditional uses including for fever and rheumatism.

Caution Do not take during pregnancy.

Mahonia aquifolium syn. *Berberis aquifolium*

Oregon grape

Description Evergreen shrub growing to 6½ ft (2 m). Has shiny leaves, clusters of small yellowish-green flowers, and purple berries in the fall.

Habitat & cultivation Native to western North America, Oregon grape grows in the Rocky Mountains up to 6,600 ft (2,000 m), and in woods from Colorado to the Pacific coast. It is abundant in Oregon and northern California.

Part used Root.

Constituents Oregon grape contains isoquinoline alkaloids (including berberine, berbamine, and hydrastine) and other alkaloids of aporphine-type. These alkaloids are strongly antibacterial and are thought to reduce the severity of psoriasis.

History & folklore Indigenous peoples in California took a decoction or tincture of the bitter-tasting root for loss of appetite and debility. In the 19th and early 20th centuries, Oregon grape was an important herb in the Physiomedicalist movement, based on a combination of orthodox and Indigenous North American practices. In this context, it was prescribed as a detoxifier and tonic.

Medicinal actions & uses Oregon grape is chiefly used for gastritis and general digestive weakness, to stimulate gallbladder function, and to reduce congestion problems (mainly of the gut). It also treats eczema, psoriasis, acne, boils, and herpes, and skin conditions linked to poor gallbladder function.

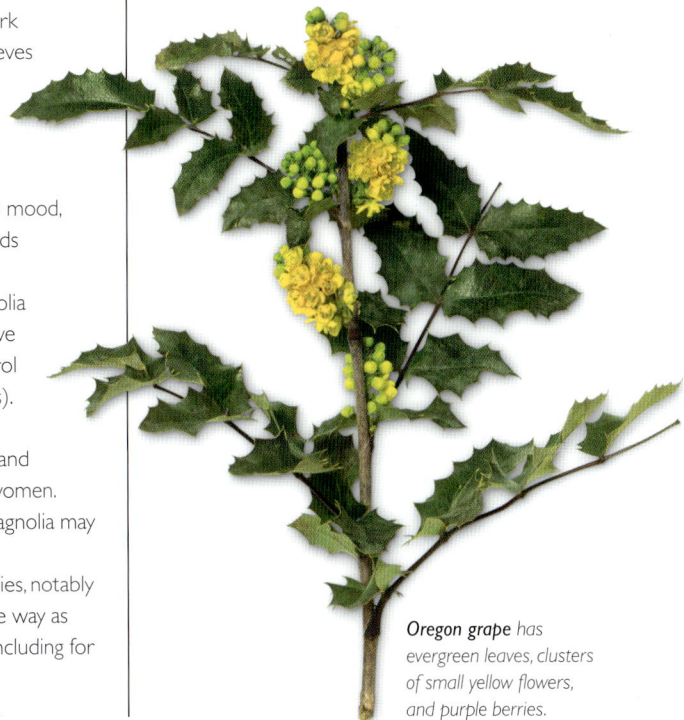

Oregon grape has evergreen leaves, clusters of small yellow flowers, and purple berries.

Research Clinical use of extracts of Oregon grape has been investigated in Germany and there is now evidence that the root can be effective in relieving psoriasis. Extracts can be taken internally and applied locally on the skin. The alkaloid berberine is thought to prevent cell proliferation.

Related species Barberry (*B. vulgaris*, p. 181) is similar to Oregon grape in its overall action, but it is generally stronger in the effect it produces.

Caution Do not take during pregnancy.

Malva sylvestris (Malvaceae)

Common mallow

Description Biennial growing to 5 ft (1.5 m). Has a pulpy taproot, 5-lobed scalloped leaves, and pink to mauve flowers.

Habitat & cultivation Common mallow is native to Europe and Asia. It is naturalized in the Americas and Australasia, growing on waste ground and on hedges and fences. The leaves are gathered in spring, the flowers when in bloom in summer.

Parts used Leaves, flowers, root.

Constituents Common mallow contains flavonol glycosides, mucilage, and tannins. The flowers also contain malvin (an anthocyanin).

History & folklore The young leaves and shoots of this plant have been eaten since at least the 8th century BCE. The plant's many uses gave rise to the Spanish adage, "A kitchen garden and mallow, sufficient medicines for a home."

Medicinal actions & uses Though less useful than marsh mallow (*Althaea officinalis*, p. 169), common mallow is an effective demulcent. The flowers and leaves are emollient and good for sensitive areas of the skin. It is applied as a poultice to reduce swelling and draw out toxins. Taken internally, the leaves reduce gut irritation and have a laxative effect. When common mallow is combined with eucalyptus (*Eucalyptus globulus*, p. 100), it makes a good remedy for coughs and other chest ailments. As with marshmallow, the root may be given to children to ease teething.

Mandragora officinarum (Solanaceae)

Mandrake

Description Perennial growing to 2 in (5 cm). Has a deep branching root, a rosette of broad floppy leaves, funnel-shaped white to purple flowers, and yellow fruit.

Habitat & cultivation Native to the Mediterranean region of Europe, mandrake grows

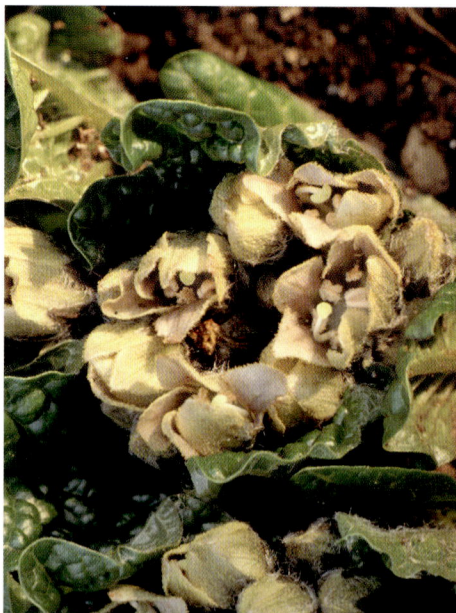

Mandrake's narcotic properties and human-shaped root have inspired much legend and lore.

on dry riverbeds. Its root is unearthed in late summer.

Part used Root.

Constituents Mandrake contains 0.4% tropane alkaloids (hyoscine and hyoscyamine).

History & folklore Legend held that the mandrake, on being uprooted, emitted a scream that was so powerful it could kill the person harvesting the plant. Consequently, reported one classical authority, mandrake was pulled up by dogs that had the stems tied to their tails. The fantastic powers attributed to the plant were partly due to the narcotic-like properties of the root. Also influential was the root's shape, which often vaguely resembles the human form. The roots have been carved and used as talismans for thousands of years, especially to aid fertility in women, and as a charm against misfortune. From Roman times onward, mandrake was used as an anesthetic for surgical operations and to relieve pain. Later Arabian physicians developed a "sleep sponge" applying an extract of mandrake over the mouth and nose to induce unconsciousness in patients about to undergo surgery.

Medicinal actions & uses Mandrake has now largely fallen out of use. The herb is sometimes applied as a poultice or plaster for rheumatic and arthritic pains, or as a decoction, for ulcers and similar kinds of skin disorders.

Cautions Mandrake is toxic. Do not take internally. Use externally only under professional supervision. The plant is subject to legal restrictions in some countries.

Manihot esculenta (Euphorbiaceae)

Cassava, Manioc

Description Shrub growing to 6½ ft (2 m). Has fleshy roots, woody stems, large palm-shaped leaves, and green flowers.

Habitat & cultivation Cassava is native to tropical Central and South America. Possibly the most grown root crop in the world, bitter and sweet varieties are grown commercially throughout the tropics (Nigeria, Thailand, and Brazil being the foremost producers). The plant was first cultivated in Peru around 4,000 years ago. The root is unearthed 8 to 24 months after planting.

Part used Root.

Constituents Cassava contains cyanogenic glycosides (0.02–0.03% in the bitter varieties, 0.007% in the sweet) and starch.

History & folklore Bitter cassava has large quantities of highly toxic glycosides, and must be carefully soaked and cooked before it is safe to eat. (Sweet cassava is safe to eat without such processing.) *Tapioca* is a native Brazilian name for the processed root, which is used in commercial food preparation as a thickening agent. The Witoto of the Colombian Amazon poison fish with the water used to wash bitter cassava. The Makuna use the wash water to treat scabies.

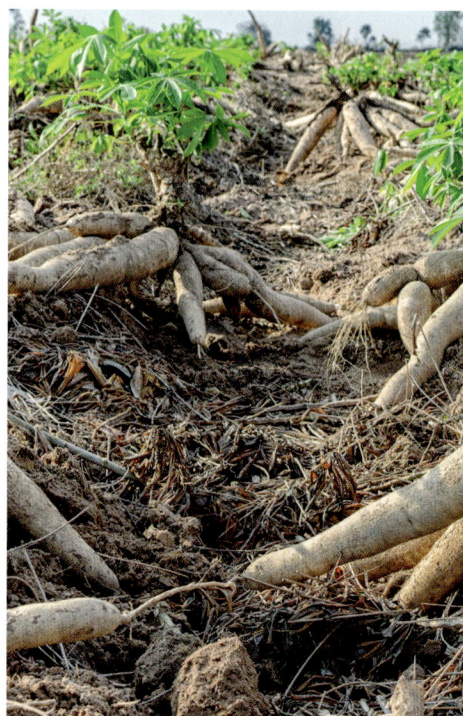

Cassava is a staple food in many tropical regions of the world.

Medicinal actions & uses Cassava root is easily digestible and makes a suitable, if low-protein, food for convalescence. The bitter variety may be used to treat scabies, diarrhea, and dysentery. Cassava flour may be used to help dry weeping skin. In China, a poultice is made of cassava, wheat flour, and ginger (*Zingiber officinale*, p. 159) to draw out pus when infection is present.

Caution Raw bitter cassava is toxic and has caused many deaths. The root must be carefully soaked and cooked before eating.

Maranta arundinacea (Marantaceae)

Arrowroot

Description Perennial growing to 6½ft (2 m). Has a creeping rhizome, many long-stemmed oval leaves, and flowering stems with clusters of creamy-white flowers.

Habitat & cultivation Native to northern South America and the Caribbean islands, arrowroot is cultivated mostly on the island of Saint Vincent. The rhizome is unearthed 10 to 11 months after planting.

Part used Rhizome.

Constituents Arrowroot contains 25–27% neutral starch.

History & folklore In Central America, the Maya made the root into a poultice for smallpox sores, and an infusion for urinary infections. Arrowroot was a staple food of the Arawak people of the Caribbean. The plant reputedly gets its name from its use to treat poisoned arrow wounds—presumably as a drawing poultice.

Medicinal actions & uses Arrowroot is used in herbal medicine in much the same manner as slippery elm (*Ulmus rubra*, p. 149), as a soothing demulcent and a nutrient of benefit in convalescence and for those with weak digestions. It helps to relieve acidity, indigestion, and colic, and is mildly laxative. It may be applied as an ointment or poultice mixed with antiseptic herbs such as myrrh (*Commiphora molmol*, p. 89).

Self-help use Acidity & indigestion, p. 317.

Marrubium vulgare (Lamiaceae)

White horehound

Description Square-stemmed perennial growing to about 20 in (50 cm). Has toothed, downy leaves and double-lipped white flowers.

Habitat & cultivation Native to Europe, white horehound is naturalized in North and South America. It flourishes in dry, bare, or on waste ground, and is gathered in spring.

Parts used Leaves.

Constituents White horehound contains the diterpenes marrubiin (0.3–1.0%) and marrubenol, tannins, phenolic acids, coumarins, and 0.06% volatile oil. Marrubiin is thought to be chiefly responsible for the herb's expectorant and bitter activity. It also acts on the heart to correct an irregular heartbeat.

History & folklore White horehound has been a remedy for chest problems since ancient times, perhaps most frequently taken as a syrup made with honey or sugar. The Greek physician Dioscorides (40–90 CE) recommended a decoction of white horehound as a treatment for tuberculosis, asthma, and coughs.

Medicinal actions & uses White horehound is helpful for wheeziness, bronchitis, bronchiectasis (a damaged air passage within the lung), bronchial asthma, nonproductive coughs, and whooping cough. The herb apparently causes the secretion of a more fluid mucus, which is readily cleared by coughing. As a bitter tonic, white horehound increases the appetite and supports the function of the stomach. It is widely used in Mexico to help control type 2 diabetes. The herb appears to relax arterial muscles and has long traditional use in treating high blood pressure. It is thought to have a beneficial action on the heart, helping to stabilize heart rate and rhythm. Poorly researched, there is clearly more to this herb than is currently known.

Marsdenia condurango syn. *Gonolobus condurango* (Apocynaceae)

Condurango

Description Climbing vine growing to 33 ft (10 m). Has heart-shaped leaves and funnel-shaped, white-green flowers.

Habitat & cultivation Condurango is native to deciduous forests of the Andes in Peru and Ecuador. It generally grows at altitudes between 3,300–6,600 ft (1,000–2,000 m). The bark is collected year round.

Parts used Bark, latex.

Constituents Condurango bark contains glycosides (based on condurangogenins), a volatile oil, and phytosterols.

History & folklore Early in the last century, condurango was erroneously yet widely believed to be a remedy for cancer.

Medicinal actions & uses The bark's main effect is to stimulate stomach secretions. It is often used in South American folk medicine as a potent bitter and digestive tonic. Condurango is a specific treatment for nervous indigestion and anorexia nervosa, since its bitterness slowly increases the appetite as well as the stomach's ability to process more food. The herb is also thought to stimulate the liver and pancreas, and may be taken for liver disorders. Condurango also encourages menstruation. The caustic white latex has been applied topically to remove warts.

Research The condurangogenins in condurango may act to counter tumors. The whole plant, however, does not seem to have cancer preventative activity.

Caution The latex is poisonous and should not be taken internally.

Medicago sativa (Fabaceae)

Alfalfa,
Lucerne

Description Perennial herb growing to 32 in (80 cm). Has 3-lobed leaves, flowers that range in color from yellow to violet-blue, and spiraling seed pods.

Habitat & cultivation Native to Europe, Asia, and North Africa, alfalfa is found in meadows and on waste ground and cultivated areas. Grown as a fodder crop in temperate climates, it is harvested in summer.

Parts used Aerial parts, seeds, sprouting seeds.

Constituents Alfalfa contains isoflavones, coumarins, alkaloids, vitamins, and porphyrins. The isoflavones and coumarins are estrogenic.

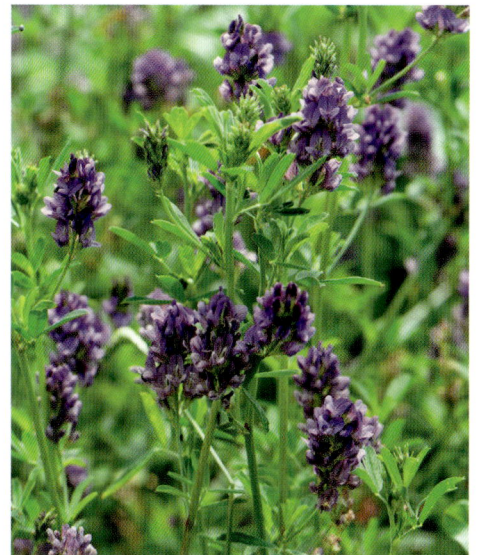

Alfalfa has been cultivated for centuries for its nutritional and medicinal properties.

History & folklore Though mostly used as an animal feed, alfalfa seeds have been consumed as food for thousands of years. Pliny (23–79 CE) records that alfalfa was brought to Greece by Darius, King of Persia (550–486 BCE), during his attempt to conquer Athens.

Medicinal actions & uses Alfalfa is perhaps more therapeutically useful as a food than a medicine, as it is the seeds that are taken to help lower cholesterol levels. In view of alfalfa's estrogenic activity, it can prove useful in treating problems relating to menstruation and menopause.

Cautions Do not take alfalfa alongside the anticoagulant medication warfarin. Avoid sprouted seeds in compromised immune states. Using large amounts is not advisable in pregnancy or in autoimmune diseases.

Melaleuca leucadendron (Myrtaceae)

Cajuput

Description Aromatic, evergreen tree growing to 130 ft (40 m). Has peeling bark, pale green oval leaves, and clusters of small white flowers on long spikes.

Habitat & cultivation Native to Southeast Asia, cajuput is cultivated for its essential oil and timber. The leaves and twigs are gathered throughout the year.

Part used Essential oil.

Constituents The volatile oil contains terpenoids, mainly cineole (50–60%), beta-pinene, alpha-terpineol, and others. Cineole is strongly antiseptic. Early investigations suggest the fruit may have antiviral properties.

Medicinal actions & uses Cajuput is normally combined with other essential oils such as eucalyptus (*Eucalyptus globulus*, p. 100). Its antiseptic properties treat colds, sore throats, coughs, and, especially, chest infections. The diluted oil may either be steam-inhaled or applied to the chest or throat to treat laryngitis, tracheitis, and bronchitis. As cajuput stimulates the circulation and is antispasmodic, it is used as a friction rub for rheumatic joints and neuralgia.

Related species Niaouli (*M. viridiflora*), of New Caledonia, has properties similar to those of cajuput. See also tea tree (*M. alternifolia*, p. 116).

Cautions Take internally only under professional supervision. Do not use during pregnancy. Cajuput essential oil is subject to legal restrictions in some countries

Self-help use Chesty coughs & bronchitis, p. 320.

Melilotus officinalis syn. *M. arvensis* (Fabaceae)

Melilot

Description Biennial herb growing to about 3 ft (1 m). Has 3-lobed leaves, spikes of yellow flowers, and brown seedpods.

Habitat & cultivation Melilot is native to Europe, North Africa, and temperate regions of Asia, and is naturalized in North America. It grows in dry and on waste ground. It is harvested in late spring.

Parts used Aerial parts.

Constituents Melilot contains flavonoids, coumarins, resin, tannins, and volatile oil. If allowed to spoil, the plant produces dicoumarol, a powerful anticoagulant.

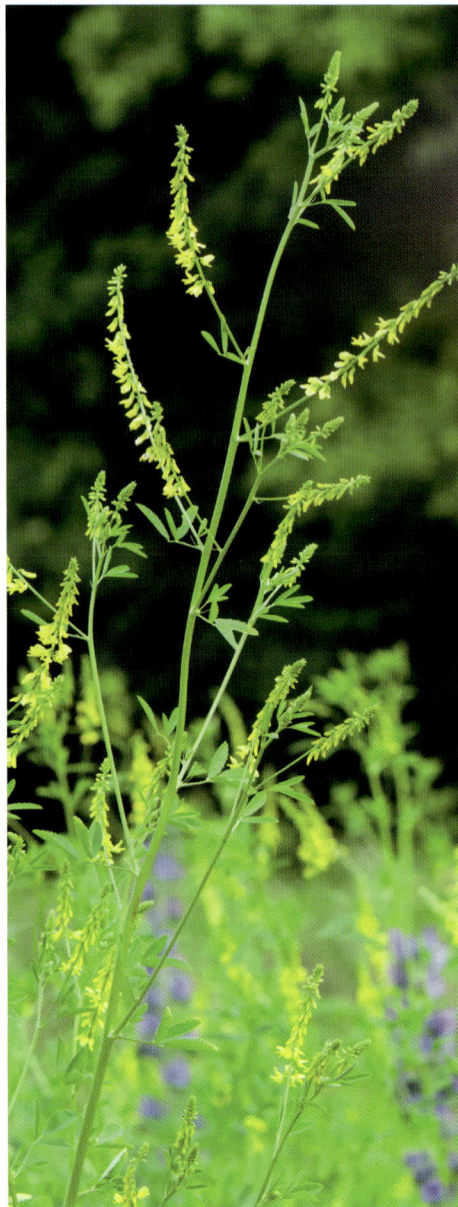

Melilot is an effective remedy for venous disorders.

History & folklore The Irish herbalist K'Eogh reported in 1735, "a gentlewoman of my acquaintance … had a swelling for a year or more on her right side, which was cured by three or four times rubbing the grieved part with an oil made of this herb."

Medicinal actions & uses As with horse chestnut (*Aesculus hippocastanum*, p. 62), long-term use of melilot—internally or externally—can help varicose veins and hemorrhoids. Melilot also helps reduce the risk of phlebitis and thrombosis. The plant is mildly sedative and antispasmodic, and is given for insomnia (especially in children) and anxiety. It has been used to treat flatulence, indigestion, bronchitis, problems associated with menopause, and rheumatic pains.

Cautions Do not take melilot if using anticoagulants. If harvested from the wild, melilot should be dried or used immediately, as the spoiled plant is toxic.

Mentha canadensis syn. *M. haplocalyx*

Bo he (Chinese), American wild mint

Description Perennial herb growing to 2 ft (60 cm). Has a square stem, oval toothed leaves, and whorls of pale lilac flowers growing from the leaf axils.

Habitat & cultivation American wild mint is native to temperate regions of the northern hemisphere, and is widely cultivated in China. Harvested 2–3 times a year, the best crops are in early summer and early fall.

Parts used Aerial parts.

Constituents American wild mint contains a volatile oil comprising mainly menthol (up to 95%) with menthone, menthyl acetate, camphene, limonene, and other terpenoids.

History & folklore American wild mint was first mentioned in *Grandfather Lei's Discussion* of Herb Preparation (c. 470 CE). A 15th-century Chinese prescription recommends *bo he* for dysentery with blood

Medicinal actions & uses In Chinese herbal medicine *bo he* is a popular treatment for colds, sore throats, sore mouth and tongue, and a host of other conditions ranging from toothache to measles. Like peppermint (*M. x piperita*, p. 118), it helps to lower the temperature, has anti-mucus properties, and may be taken for dysentery and diarrhea. The juice has also been used to treat earache. American wild mint is often combined with *ju hua* (*Chrysanthemum* × *morifolium*, p. 83) to treat headaches and bloodshot or sore eyes.

Related species Several varieties of American wild

mint are cultivated as a source of menthol. The closely related spearmint (*M. spicata*) native to Europe and Asia, is used mainly as a flavoring and culinary herb. See also peppermint (*M. x piperita*, p. 118) and pennyroyal (*M. pulegium, following entry*).

Mentha pulegium (Lamiaceae)

Pennyroyal

Description Powerfully aromatic perennial growing to 16 in (40 cm). Has oval, toothed leaves and whorls of lilac flowers.

Habitat & cultivation Pennyroyal is native to Europe and western Asia, and has become naturalized in the Americas. It thrives in damp areas and is gathered when in flower in summer.

Parts used Aerial parts.

Constituents Pennyroyal's volatile oil contains mainly menthone, pulegone, and neomenthone.

History & folklore The Roman natural historian Pliny (23–79 CE) wrote that pennyroyal was considered a better medicinal herb than roses, and that it purified bad water. His contemporary, Dioscorides, stated that pennyroyal "provokes menstruation and labour." In 1597, John Gerard wrote that "a garland of pennie royal made and worne about the head is of great force against the swimming of the head, and the pains and giddiness thereof." The name pulegium derives from the Latin word for flea, referring to pennyroyal's traditional use as a flea-repellent.

Medicinal actions & uses Similar in many respects to peppermint (*M. x piperita*, p. 118), pennyroyal is a good digestive tonic. It increases the secretion of digestive juices, relieves flatulence and colic, and occasionally is used as a treatment for intestinal worms. It makes a good remedy for headaches and for minor respiratory infections, helping to check fever and reduce catarrh. Pennyroyal powerfully stimulates the uterine muscles and encourages menstruation. An infusion of pennyroyal can be used externally to treat itchiness and formication (a sensation of ants crawling over the body) and rheumatic conditions including gout.

Research A 2015 study in Turkey (Türkiye), using wild-harvested pennyroyal, found that extracts of the herb had strong antibacterial activity against *Staphylococcus epidermis*, a bacterium that normally lives in the skin but which occasionally causes moderate to severe illness.

Related species See peppermint (*M. x piperita*, p. 118) and bo he (*M. haplocalyx*, preceding entry). American pennyroyal (*Hedeoma pulegoides*), while only distantly related, has constituents similar to those of pennyroyal. American pennyroyal is traditionally used as a remedy for colds, headaches, and delayed menstrual periods..

Cautions Do not use the essential oil, which is highly toxic. Do not take pennyroyal during pregnancy, or if menstrual periods are heavy.

Self-help uses Digestive headaches & biliousness, p. 319; Nausea with headache, p. 316

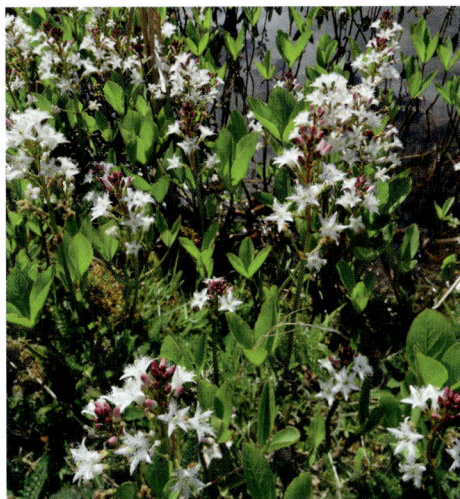

Bogbean leaves are gathered in summer, after the plant has come into flower.

Menyanthes trifoliata (Menyanthaceae)

Bogbean

Description Perennial aquatic plant growing to 9 in (23 cm). Has trefoil leaves and spikes of pink and white flowers with fringed petals.

Habitat & cultivation Bogbean is native to Europe, Asia, and America. It is found in shallow fresh water. The leaves are picked in summer.

Parts used Leaves.

Constituents Bogbean contains iridoid glycosides, flavonol glycosides, coumarins, phenolic acids, sterols, triterpenoids, tannin, and very small amounts of pyrrolizidine alkaloids. The iridoids are strongly bitter and stimulate digestive secretions.

History & folklore Long used as a folk remedy for rheumatism and arthritis, bogbean has also been taken to treat fluid retention, scabies, and fever. In the past, because of the herb's pronounced bitterness, it was used as an adulterant of, or a substitute for, hops (*Humulus lupulus*, p. 108).

Medicinal actions & uses Bogbean is a strongly bitter herb that encourages the appetite and stimulates digestive secretions. It is taken to improve underactive or weak digestion, particularly if there is abdominal discomfort. Bogbean has long traditional use as an anti-inflammatory remedy for kidney disease, such as nephritis. The herb is also thought to be an effective anti-inflammatory treatment for rheumatic disease, especially where this is associated with weakness, weight loss and lack of vitality. For the most part, bogbean is prescribed in combination with other herbs such as celery seed (*Apium graveolens*, p. 68) and white willow (*Salix alba*, p. 133).

Research A 2019 Polish research article concluded that bogbean should be researched in detail in view of its potential anticancer activity.

Cautions Do not take if suffering from diarrhea, dysentery or colitis. Excessive doses may cause vomiting.

Mikania spp. (Asteraceae)

Guaco

Description A shrubby climbing plant growing to about 6½ ft (2 m) in height and up to 16 ft (5 m) in spread. It has distinctive bright green heart-shaped leaves and white to pale yellow flowers.

Habitat & cultivation *Mikania glomerosa* and closely related species are found through much of tropical south and central America.

Parts used Leaves.

Constituents Guaco contains about 10% coumarin, a strong anticoagulant, sesquiterpenes, phenolic acids, and tannins.

History & folklore Guaco has a strong, spicy scent that is thought to be repellent to snakes. In Brazil and Colombia, the leaves have been used both to treat snake bite and to keep snakes away, leaves or a lotion being applied around sleeping areas or onto clothing or skin. In a Colombian tradition, guaco's antivenin effects were learned by observing kites eat guaco leaves and spread sap on their wings, before hunting snakes. Guaco was listed in the first edition of the *Brazilian Pharmacopoeia* (1926).

Medicinal actions & uses Guaco is a commonly used and valued herbal medicine in Brazil, where it is taken, as an infusion or extract, for all manner of health problems affecting the respiratory system. Coughs, colds, flu, sore throat, and bronchitis are the main indications. However, guaco has notable muscle relaxant activity and can also be helpful in asthma. Applied topically, a guaco lotion can soothe itchy skin and insect bites and act as an insect repellent.

Research Brazilian research indicates that guaco has strong anti-inflammatory activity and has a key action in countering the toxic effects of snake bite. The herb also has marked antispasmodic, antibacterial, and antifungal activity.

Mitchella repens (Rubiaceae)

Partridge berry

Description Evergreen herb growing to 1 ft (30 cm) and forming mats on the ground. Has rounded shiny leaves, a flowering stem bearing fragrant white flowers and small, bright red berries.

Habitat & cultivation Partridge berry is native to the eastern and central US. It grows in dry sites in woodlands, and is harvested in late summer.

Parts used Aerial parts, berries.

Constituents Partridge berry is believed to contain tannins, glycosides, and saponins.

History & folklore An infusion of partridge berry was commonly taken by Indigenous North American women to hasten childbirth. It was also occasionally used for a variety of other complaints, including insomnia, rheumatic pain, and fluid retention.

Medicinal actions & uses Partridge berry is still extensively used to aid labor and childbirth, and is considered to have a tonic action on the uterus and the ovaries. It is taken to normalize menstruation and to relieve heavy periods and period pain. This herb has also been recommended for stimulating breast milk production, but other herbs with a similar action, such as fennel (*Foeniculum vulgare*, p. 217), are preferred. The berries, crushed and mixed with tincture of myrrh (*Commiphora molmol*, p. 89), are helpful for sore nipples. An astringent herb, partridge berry has also been prescribed for diarrhea and colitis.

Research A recent laboratory study in the US demonstrated that partridge berry has a strong stimulant activity on muscle contraction in uterine cells, providing some confirmation of the herb's traditional use.

Caution Do not take during the first 6 months of pregnancy.

Momordica charantia (Cucurbitaceae)

Bitter melon, Kerala

Description Annual climber growing to about 6½ ft (2 m). Has deeply lobed leaves, yellow flowers, and orange-yellow fruit.

Habitat & cultivation Native to southern Asia, bitter melon is common throughout tropical regions of the world. It is harvested year round.

Parts used Leaves, fruit, seeds, seed oil.

Constituents Bitter melon contains a fixed oil, an insulin-like peptide, cucurbitacins, glycosides (mormordin and charantin), and an alkaloid (mormordicine). The peptide is known to lower sugar levels in the blood and urine.

History & folklore Bitter melon is traditionally taken in Asia, Africa, and the Caribbean to treat the symptoms of diabetes.

Medicinal actions & uses The unripe fruit is mainly used to treat type 2 diabetes. The ripe fruit is a stomach tonic, and induces menstruation. In Turkey (Türkiye), it is used to treat ulcers. The fruit is much used in the Caribbean for worms, urinary stones, and fever. The fruit juice is taken as a purgative, and is prescribed for colic. A decoction of the leaves is taken for liver problems and colitis, and it may be applied to skin conditions. The seed oil is used to help heal wounds.

Research Bitter melon seeds are androgenic and inhibit sperm production and were tested as a contraceptive in China in the 1980s. In diabetic laboratory animals, bitter melon fruit juice stimulated regeneration of the pancreatic cells, which secrete insulin. A major body of evidence now supports the traditional use of bitter melon fruit juice to treat non-insulin-dependent diabetes.

Related species The seeds of the Asian *M. cochinchinensis* are applied as a poultice to relieve abscesses, hemorrhoids, and scrofula. Recent research indicates that a paste of the seeds may help psoriasis and ringworm.

Cautions While bitter melon is relatively safe at low dosage, do not use for more than 4 weeks. Do not take if prone to low blood-sugar levels.

Monarda punctata (Lamiaceae)

Horsemint

Description Strongly aromatic perennial growing to 3 ft (90 cm). Has downy lance-shaped leaves, and double-lipped, red-spotted yellow flowers growing in whorls from the leaf axils.

Habitat & cultivation Native to the eastern and central US, horsemint is found in dry and sandy areas. It is gathered when in flower in summer and fall.

Parts used Aerial parts.

Constituents Horsemint's volatile oil has thymol as the main constituent.

History & folklore Horsemint's genus name, *Monarda*, was bestowed in honor of Nicolas Monardes, a Spanish physician, whose herbal of 1569 detailed the medicinal uses of a number of New World plants. Horsemint was used by the Winnebago and Dakota peoples as a stimulant and

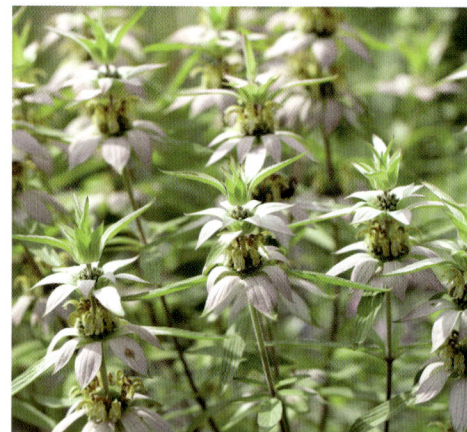

Horsemint strongly encourages sweating and the onset of menstruation.

to treat cholera. Other Indigenous peoples used the herb for a wide variety of problems, including nausea, backache, fluid retention, chills, and headache.

Medicinal actions & uses Having a strong volatile oil, horsemint is primarily used for digestive and upper respiratory problems. It is taken as an infusion to relieve nausea, indigestion, colic, and flatulence. It is also employed to reduce fevers and upper respiratory mucus. The herb has an antiseptic action within the chest. Taken internally or applied externally, horsemint reduces fever by encouraging sweating. It also strongly stimulates menstruation.

Related species In 19th-century America, Oswego tea (*M. didyma*) was considered a tonic for young mothers, and was traditionally given to brides. It is thought to be a mild menstrual regulator and an appetite stimulant.

Caution Do not take during pregnancy.

Monsonia ovata (Geraniaceae)

Monsonia

Description Small herbaceous plant with multi-branched stems, very small oblong leaves and white solitary or paired geranium-like flowers.

Habitat & cultivation Native to South Africa and Namibia, monsonia is found growing in arid conditions. It is gathered when in flower.

Parts used Aerial parts.

History & folklore In Zulu medicine, monsonia is used to treat snake bite.

Medicinal actions & uses Monsonia is used throughout southwestern Africa as a treatment for diarrhea, acute and chronic dysentery, and ulcerative colitis. The plant's astringent properties act to tighten and protect the inner linings of the intestinal tract. Given monsonia's long traditional use for intestinal disorders and infections, it is possible—but as yet unsubstantiated by research—that the plant has a direct antimicrobial effect.

Montia perfoliata (Portulacaceae)

Miner's lettuce

Description Annual growing to 4 in (10 cm) with pointed oval leaves (one pair enveloping the stem), and white 5-petaled flowers.

Habitat & cultivation Miner's lettuce is native to western North America, and has become naturalized in temperate regions around the world, especially in Australia. The plant thrives in acid sandy soils. It is generally gathered from the wild before and during the flowering period. It has also been cultivated as a vegetable.

Parts used Aerial parts.

Constituents Miner's lettuce is rich in vitamin C.

History & folklore Miner's lettuce was a readily available salad vegetable on the West Coast of America. It most probably acquired its name during the California gold rush of 1849. Itinerant miners may have later taken the plant with them to Australia, where it is now common.

Medicinal actions & uses Apart from its value as a vegetable, miner's lettuce, like its relative purslane (*Portulaca oleracea*, p. 263), may also be taken as an invigorating spring tonic and an effective diuretic.

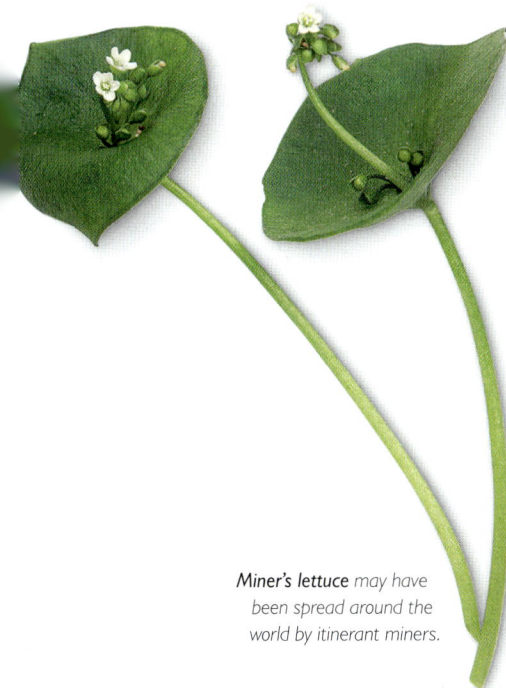

Miner's lettuce may have been spread around the world by itinerant miners.

Morinda citrifolia (Rubiaceae)

Noni,
Indian mulberry

Description Shrub or small tree, growing to 26 ft (8 m), with 4-angled stems, and elliptical to oval leaves to 14 in (35 cm) long. Large creamy-white flowers produce a fruit resembling a breadfruit, about 4$^3/_4$ in (12 cm) long, green turning yellow to white, with a pungent, very unpleasant odor.

Habitat & cultivation Originally native only to Southeast Asia, noni has spread to India in the west and across the Pacific to eastern Polynesia and Hawaii. It prefers volcanic soils in coastal areas and lowland forests up to about 1,300 ft (400 m) above sea level, and until recently was infrequently cultivated. The fruit is gathered when ripe; other parts of the tree are picked as required.

Parts used Fruit and juice, leaves, bark.

Constituents Noni fruit contains polysaccharides, coumarins, iridoids, flavonoids, and alkaloids. No active compounds unique to noni have been identified.

History & folklore Different parts of the plant have been used in Polynesia for at least 2,000 years, chiefly to counter infection and to treat chronic disease. For example, noni leaves are used to treat boils and stomach ulcers and, chewed, are applied as a poultice to relieve inflammation. In Hawaii, traditional healers have long used noni in order to promote recovery from bouts of serious illness.

Medicinal actions & uses Since the late 1990s, word of noni's reputed medicinal benefits has spread and noni is being presented as a medicinal food with an astonishing variety of potential uses. These include treating obesity, diabetes, cancer, pain, lowered immunity, high blood pressure, heart disease, and depression. With lists like this, many people are justifiably skeptical about noni's value as a medicinal food. Nonetheless, noni fruit and juice is highly unlikely to do harm and may well prove useful in treating chronic illness, including pain, inflammatory disorders, heart and circulatory problems, and cancer. Traditionally, juice from the fruit is used as a mouthwash and gargle for infections in the mouth and throat. Noni juice is probably best drunk on an empty stomach.

Research The limited research into noni suggests that it may support immune function and be useful in treating chronic inflammation. A 2012 review of noni research concluded that the fruit "may have a small degree of anticancer activity." One theory advanced is that noni contains appreciable

levels of proxeronine, which the body needs to produce xeronine. This alkaloid appears to enable cells throughout the body to counter inflammation, promote healing, and support cellular regulation. In times of stress or infection, the body's need for xeronine increases, and many people are thought to lack sufficient proxeronine to maintain adequate xeronine levels.

Morinda officinalis (Rubiaceae)

Morinda,
Ba ji tian (Chinese)

Description Deciduous plant with white flowers and a root that yields a yellow dye.

Habitat & cultivation Morinda is native to China. It is cultivated in Guangdong, Guangxi, and Fujian provinces. The root is unearthed in early spring.

Part used Root.

Constituents Morinda contains anthraquinones, terpenoids, and polysaccharides.

History & folklore The earliest written record of morinda's use is in the *Divine Husbandman's Classic* (*Shen'nong Bencaojing*) of the 1st century CE.

Medicinal actions & uses Pungent and sweet-tasting, morinda root is an important tonic herb within traditional Chinese medicine. It has hormonal and antidepressant properties. As a sexual tonic, it is commonly used to treat impotence and premature ejaculation in men, and is taken by both sexes to aid fertility. Morinda is employed in various other conditions, notably in the treatment of menstrual disorders. Researchers are investigating the root for its potential to prevent bone loss and help in treating osteoporosis.

Moringa oleifera (Moringaceae)

Drumstick tree

Description A small, slender deciduous tree growing to 33 ft (10 m), Moringa has an open crown of drooping branches, feathery pale green leaves and fragrant white flowers. The brown hanging pods grow up to 3 ft (1 m) long and contain about 20 seeds.

Habitat & cultivation Native to the foothills of the Himalayas, Moringa is drought-tolerant and is now cultivated in tropical and subtropical regions around the world, especially in arid conditions. It is propagated by branch cuttings.

Parts used Leaves, seed oil (topical use). All parts of

the tree have been used as food and medicine in its native India.

Constituents Moringa leaves contain high levels of protein (25–30% by dry weight), vitamins A, C, E, and B12, and significant amounts of minerals, notably calcium, magnesium, and potassium. Key medicinal constituents include flavonoids such as quercitin, and phenolic acids, including chlorogenic and caffeic acids, as well as alkaloids, glucosilinates, and saponins.

History & folklore The name Moringa comes from the Tamil meaning "drumstick." In India, Moringa trees are planted on graves to keep away hyenas. Moringa has also been used as a charm against witchcraft. Moringa seeds act as a natural water filter, absorbing suspended particles and microorganisms within untreated water.

Medicinal actions & uses Moringa leaves have great medicinal use, benefiting almost every organ in the body. The leaves lower blood pressure and support cardiovascular health, act to strengthen immune resistance, with indications of activity against the Epstein-Barr virus, counter inflammation, exert a neuroprotective activity, stabilize blood glucose and blood fat levels, and protect the liver and kidneys from toxicity. Unsurprisingly, traditional use is wide-ranging. Moringa has been used to treat diabetes; chronic inflammatory diseases, such as rheumatoid arthritis; bacterial, viral, and fungal infections; heart disease; and cancer, among many other conditions.

Research Five clinical studies show that dried moringa leaf acts to normalize blood glucose and blood fat levels. Another clinical study found that moringa seed kernel extract improved lung function in 20 patients with mild to moderate asthma. A 2017 research paper concluded that moringa leaves had value in "protecting against cardiovascular disease, diabetes, non-alcoholic liver disease, Alzheimer's, and hypertension," though to date this list is based only on laboratory research. Preliminary research also indicates that moringa actively supports nerve cell regrowth.

Morus alba (Moraceae)

White mulberry, *Sang ye* (Chinese)

Description Deciduous tree growing to about 49 ft (15 m). Has toothed leaves, flowers in catkins, and white berries.

Habitat & cultivation White mulberry is native to China. It is grown worldwide as a garden

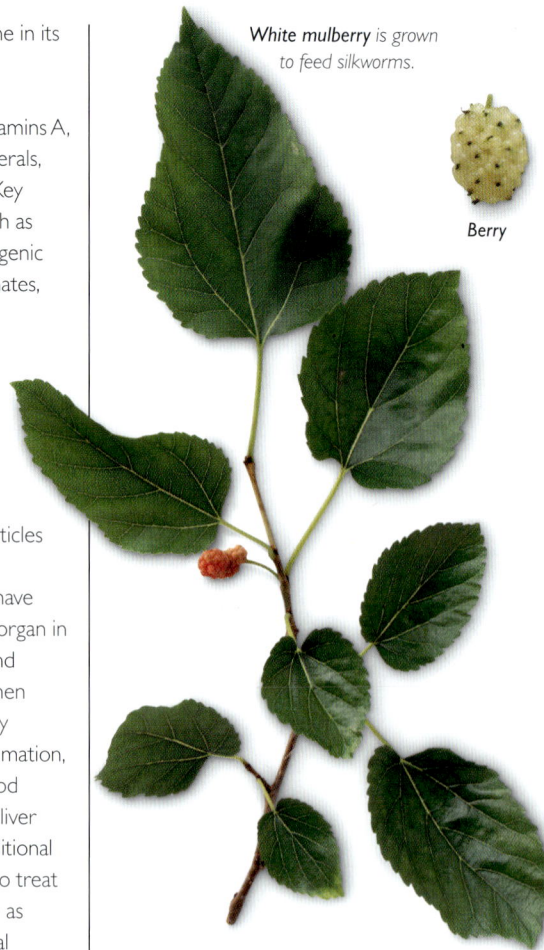

White mulberry is grown to feed silkworms.

Berry

ornamental. The leaves are gathered in late fall, the twigs in early summer, and the berries when ripe in summer. The root is dug up in winter.

Parts used Leaves, twigs, fruit, root bark.

Constituents The leaves contain phenolic acids, flavonoids, anthocyanins, tannins, and chalcones. The fruit contains flavonoids, anthocyanins, alkaloids, and appreciable levels of pro-vitamins A, B_1, B_2 and C.

History & folklore White mulberry has been cultivated for over 5,000 years for its leaves (*sang ye*), the preferred food of the silkworm. The silkworm's feces are used in Chinese medicine to treat vomiting.

Medicinal actions & uses White mulberry leaves are expectorant, encouraging the loosening and coughing up of phlegm, and are prescribed in China as a treatment for coughs. The leaves are also taken to treat fever, sore and inflamed eyes, sore throats, headaches, dizziness, and vertigo. The fruit juice is cleansing and tonic, and has often been used as a gargle and mouthwash. The root bark may be used for toothache, and it is considered laxative. An extract of the leaves has been given by injection for elephantiasis. The twigs are used to combat excess fluid retention and joint pain. The fruit is taken to prevent premature graying of the hair, and to treat

dizziness, ringing in the ears, blurred vision, and insomnia.

Research Several small-scale clinical trials in India and Thailand have investigated the effectiveness of mulberry leaf in supporting a healthy blood fat profile. In one study those taking 3 g of leaf a day for 4 weeks were found to have on average a 12% reduction in cholesterol levels, a 23% reduction in LDL-cholesterol, and an 18% increase in HDL-cholesterol. In another small trial in Thailand, 60 healthy middle-aged and elderly volunteers took mulberry leaf extract for 3 months. The results showed "improved working memory and cognitive enhancement without any toxic effects."

Related species The black mulberry (*M. nigra*), native to Iran, is cultivated for its sweet, deep red, highly nutritious fruit.

Murraya koenigii (Rutaceae)

Curry tree

Description Aromatic deciduous shrub or tree growing to 20 ft (6 m). Has strongly scented leaves, clusters of small, fragrant white flowers, and pink to black berries.

Habitat & cultivation Curry tree is native to subtropical forests in much of southern Asia. It is widely cultivated in India for its leaves.

Parts used Leaves, berries.

Constituents Curry tree contains over 20 alkaloids, a glycoside (koenigin), volatile oil, and tannins.

History & folklore Curry tree is a common flavoring in Indian food.

Medicinal actions & uses Curry tree leaves increase digestive secretions and relieve nausea, indigestion, and vomiting. They are also used to treat diarrhea and dysentery. Curry tree aids healing, for example in gastric ulcers, and the leaves are applied as a poultice on wounds and burns. It helps to stabilize blood-sugar levels and is useful for type 2 diabetes.

Related species The very bitter leaves of cosmetic bark (*M. paniculata*) are taken to treat stomach ache, dysentery, toothache, and bruises.

Musa spp. (Musaceae)

Banana, Plantain

Description Evergreen, palmlike perennials growing to 30 ft (9 m). Have large, shiny green leaves, hanging flowering stems, and bunches of elongated green fruit that turn yellow on ripening.

Habitat & cultivation *Musa* species are native

to India and Southeast Asia, and are extensively cultivated in tropical and subtropical regions. The fruit is generally picked when immature and then allowed to ripen. The leaves are gathered as required

Parts used Fruit, leaves, root.

Constituents The fruit contains flavonoids and is rich in vitamins B, C, and E, potassium, serotonin, and noradrenaline.

History & folklore The delicious and highly nutritious banana fruit is the yield of careful horticulture, which had its origins with wild plants in prehistoric times.

Medicinal actions & uses Ripe banana fruit is gently laxative, while the unripe fruit is astringent and used to treat diarrhea. The fruit stimulates hemoglobin production and can therefore prove useful in preventing or treating anemia. Banana makes a simple addition to diets aimed at lowering high blood pressure. Given the fruit's serotonin content, some practitioners recommend taking three bananas a day to help treat migraines and depression. A syrup made from plantain is taken for coughs and chest conditions such as bronchitis.

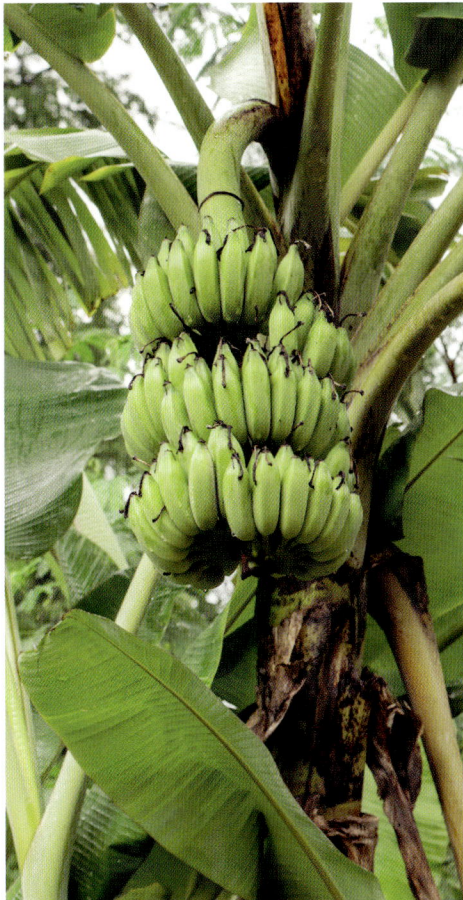

Bananas are picked before they fully ripen. They are a useful remedy for diarrhea.

Myrica cerifera (Myricaceae)
Bayberry

Description Evergreen shrub or small tree growing to 33 ft (10 m). Has narrow leaves, small yellow flowers in catkins, and waxy gray berries.

Habitat & cultivation Bayberry is found in coastal regions of the eastern and southern US, as far west as Texas. The root bark is collected in the fall or spring.

Part used Root bark.

Constituents Bayberry contains triterpenes (including taraxerol, taraxerone, and myricadiol), flavonoids, tannins, phenols, resins, and gums. Myricadiol has a mild effect on potassium and sodium levels.

History & folklore Colonizers in North America extolled the medicinal benefits of bayberry. A 1737 account stated that the plants "expel wind and ease all manner of pains proceeding from cold, therefore are good in colic, palsies, convulsions, epilepsies, and many other disorders." Bayberry was a key herb in the frontier style "Thomsonian" herbal medicine popular in both the US and Great Britain during the 19th and early 20th centuries, its heating and drying effect being particularly valued. The root bark was listed in the *US National Formulary* from 1916 to 1936.

Medicinal actions & uses Bayberry is used to increase circulation, stimulate perspiration, and keep bacterial infections in check. Colds, flu, coughs, and sore throats benefit from treatment with this herb. It helps to strengthen resistance to infection and to tighten and dry mucous membranes. An infusion is helpful for spongy gums, and a gargle is used for sore throats. Bayberry's astringency is beneficial for irritable bowel syndrome and mucous colitis. An infusion can help treat excess vaginal discharge. A paste of the powdered root bark may be used externally on ulcers and sores.

Caution Do not take in pregnancy.

Myrica gale (Myricaceae)
Sweet gale,
Bog myrtle

Description Low-growing, fragrant shrub, growing to 6½ ft (2 m), with lance-shaped leaves. Male plants produce resinous catkins in spring.

Habitat & cultivation Sweet gale thrives in wet and damp heaths and moorlands across northerly regions of the northern hemisphere. The leaves are collected in summer, the catkins in spring.

Parts used Leaves, branches, catkins.

Constituents Sweet gale contains an essential oil (chiefly alpha-pinene and delta-cadinene), flavonoids, and resin.

History & folklore In Scotland, where the plant grows freely, Highlanders slept on flea-proof beds of sweet gale and placed it among linen to repel moths. Enterprising anglers are also reported to have worn sprigs of sweet gale to keep away midges. In Scotland and Sweden, a strong decoction was used to kill insects and intestinal worms.

Medicinal actions & uses Sweet gale is mostly used as an insect repellent and insecticide and offers a safe and ecologically sound way to protect against insect bites. Over-the-counter preparations are available, though a decoction of the plant bathed on exposed areas will also prove effective.

Research Since the 1990s, the essential oil of sweet gale has become recognized as an effective insect repellent (especially of midges), and is now available in blended formulations. In one trial in Scotland, volunteers exposed their arms to midges, with one arm covered in a gel containing essential oil of sweet gale. After 10 minutes, the protected arms averaged 1.6 bites, the unprotected arms 9.4.

Cautions Do not take the essential oil internally. Do not use sweet gale internally in pregnancy or while breastfeeding. The essential oil is thought to be toxic.

Myroxylon pereirae syn. *M. balsamum* var. *pereirae* (Fabaceae)
Peruvian balsam

Description Evergreen tree growing to 115 ft (35 m). Has gray bark, compound leaves dotted with oil glands, white pealike flowers, and yellow seed pods.

Habitat & cultivation Native to Central America, Peruvian balsam grows wild in tropical forests. It is cultivated in Central and South America and India. Oleoresin (balsam) is taken from cuts in the bark.

Part used Oleo-resin.

Constituents The oleoresin contains 50–65% volatile oil (mainly benzyl benzoate and benzyl cinnamate) and resins.

Medicinal actions & uses Peruvian balsam is strongly antiseptic and stimulates repair of damaged tissue. It is most commonly taken internally as an expectorant and anticatarrhal remedy to treat bronchitis, emphysema, and bronchial asthma. It may also be taken to treat sore throats and diarrhea, and applied topically to skin disorders.

Related species The balsam from similar species was used by the Inca to relieve fevers and colds.

Caution Peruvian balsam may cause allergic skin reactions..

Myrtus communis (Myrtaceae)

Myrtle

Description Evergreen shrub growing to a height of 10 ft (3 m). Has dark green leaves, white flowers, and purple-black berries.

Habitat & cultivation Myrtle is native to the Mediterranean region and it is cultivated for its essential oil. The leaves are gathered in spring.

Parts used Leaves, essential oil.

Constituents Myrtle contains tannins, flavonoids, and a volatile oil (mainly alpha-pinene, cineole, and myrtenol).

History & folklore In ancient Greece, myrtle was dedicated to Aphrodite, who was the goddess of love, and brides bedecked themselves with myrtle leaves. A liqueur is made from the berries.

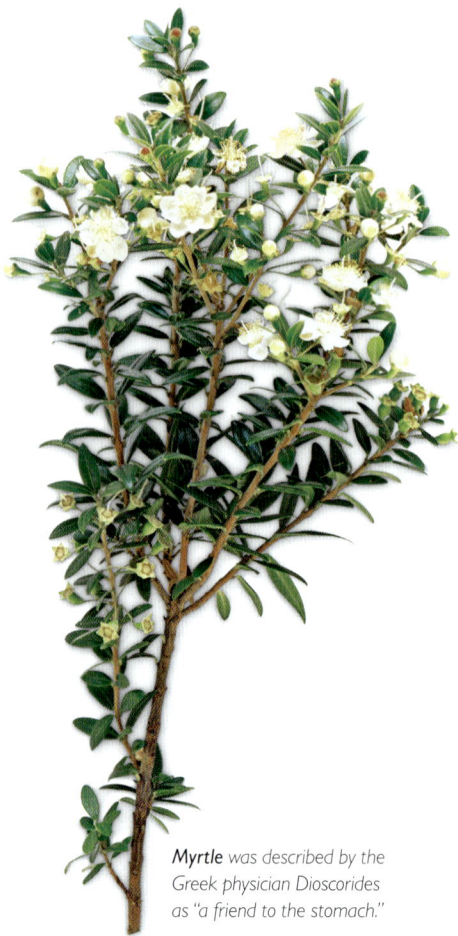

Myrtle was described by the Greek physician Dioscorides as "a friend to the stomach."

Medicinal actions & uses Myrtle leaves are astringent, tonic, and antiseptic. An infusion of the leaves can be used externally to clean and heal wounds and ulcers, or internally to remedy disorders of the digestive and urinary systems. In Ethiopia, both fresh and dried myrtle leaves are used to treat dandruff and fungal infections of the scalp. The essential oil is strongly antiseptic and anticatarrhal. In Spain it is traditionally used to treat bronchial and respiratory infections.

Caution Do not take the essential oil internally except with professional advice.

Nasturtium officinale (Cruciferae)

Watercress

Description Creeping perennial growing to 2 ft (60 cm), with compound leaves, spikes of white 4-petaled flowers, and small sickle-shaped pods.

Habitat & cultivation Found in temperate regions throughout the world, watercress thrives alongside or in fresh running water. While commonly found in the wild, it is also widely cultivated as a salad herb. Watercress is best gathered before it flowers in summer.

Parts used Aerial parts.

Constituents Watercress contains isothiocyanates and is rich in vitamins A, B1, B2, C, and E, and minerals (especially iodine, iron, and phosphorus). Allyl isothiocyanate has broad-spectrum antibiotic activity. Research in the 1960s suggested that watercress might have antitumor activity.

History & folklore Watercress has long been valued as a food and medicinal plant. Xenophon, a Greek general in the 5th century BCE, attributed other virtues to it, recommending the Persians to feed it to their children to build up their strength. In European folk medicine, watercress has primarily been considered a "blood-cleanser," and was used in former times as a spring tonic.

Medicinal actions & uses Watercress provides excellent, easily digested nutrition. Its high mineral and vitamin C content makes it particularly suited for chronic ill health and convalescence. It is thought to stimulate appetite, ease indigestion, and counter mucus. A detoxifying herb and food, watercress cleanses the liver, blood, kidneys, and lungs.

Research Several scientific papers have proposed that diets rich in cruciferous vegetable plants, including watercress, can reduce the risk of lung cancer, colorectal cancer, and prostate cancer.

Nepeta cataria (Lamiaceae)

Catnip

Description Downy, aromatic perennial growing to 3 ft (1 m). Has heart-shaped, gray-green leaves and whorls of white flowers with purple spots.

Habitat & cultivation Catnip is native to Europe and naturalized in North America. It grows in dry wayside places and in mountainous regions up to altitudes of 5,000 ft (1,500 m). Catnip is gathered when in flower in summer and fall.

Parts used Aerial parts.

Constituents Catnip contains iridoids, tannins, and volatile oil (mainly comprising alpha- and beta-nepetalactone, citronellol, and geraniol).

History & folklore Pechey's *Compleat Herbal* (1694) describes catnip: "'Tis hot and dry. 'Tis chiefly used for obstructions of the womb, for barrenness, and to hasten delivery, and to help expectoration. 'Tis used outwardly in baths for the womb, and the itch." Catnip has an excitatory effect on cats.

Medicinal actions & uses Catnip settles the stomach, is sedative and, as it stimulates sweating, reduces fever. The herb's pleasant taste and gentle action make it suitable for colds, flu, and fever in children, especially when mixed with elderflower (*Sambucus nigra*, p. 132) and sweetened with honey. Catnip is markedly antiflatulent, helping to settle indigestion and colic. The herb is also useful in treating headaches related to digestive problems. A tincture is beneficial as a friction rub for rheumatism and arthritis.

Self-help use Digestive infections, p. 315.

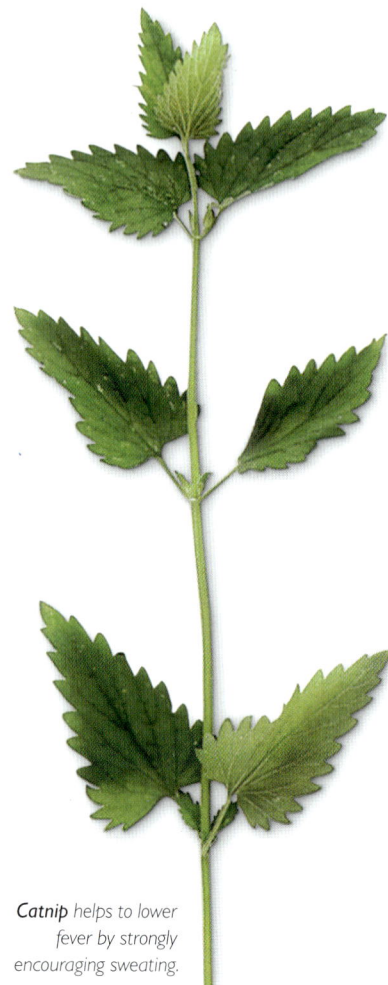

Catnip helps to lower fever by strongly encouraging sweating.

Nicotiana tabacum (Solanaceae)

Tobacco

Description Annual or biennial plant growing to 3 ft (1 m). Has an erect stem, large oval leaves, and pink or white flowers.

Habitat & cultivation Tobacco is native to tropical America. It is now grown worldwide, chiefly for smoking tobacco but also as the source of an insecticide. Leaves for smoking are gathered, dried, and cured.

Parts used Leaves.

Constituents Tobacco contains alkaloids (notably nicotine) and a volatile oil. Nicotine is stimulant and addictive.

History & folklore Even in 17th-century England, opinions on smoking were sharply divided. King James I unsuccessfully tried to ban "a custome loathsome to the eye, hatefully to the nose, harmfull to the braine [and] dangerous to the lungs." In Central America, tobacco was prescribed by the Maya as a treatment for asthma, convulsions, and skin disease. Tobacco has been used as part of rituals in many Indigenous American cultures.

Medicinal actions & uses Tobacco is no longer used medicinally. The dried leaves make a good insecticide, but external application should be avoided as nicotine is readily absorbed through the skin.

Caution Tobacco should not be taken in any form.

Nigella sativa (Ranunculaceae)

Black cumin

Description Annual herb growing to 1 ft (30 cm). Has an upright branching stem, fine deeply cut leaves, gray-blue flowers, and toothed seedpods.

Habitat & cultivation Native to western Asia, black cumin is grown throughout much of Asia and the Mediterranean region for its seeds and as a garden plant. The seeds are gathered once they are ripe.

Parts used Seeds.

Constituents The seeds contain 40% fixed oil, a saponin (melantin), alkaloids, and up to 1.4% volatile oil..

History & folklore Black cumin was found in the tomb of Tutankhamen, but its role in ancient Egypt, medicinal or otherwise, is unknown. Dioscorides, a Greek physician of the 1st century CE, recorded that black cumin seeds were taken to treat headaches, nasal congestion, toothache, and intestinal worms, and, in large quantities, as a diuretic, to promote menstrual periods, and to increase breast milk production.

Medicinal actions & uses Like many culinary herbs, black cumin seeds are beneficial for the digestive system, soothing stomach pain and spasms and easing gas, bloating, and colic. The seeds are also antiseptic and are used to treat intestinal worms, especially in children. Cumin seeds are much used in India to increase the production of breast milk.

Research Recent research indicates that black cumin seed may prove useful in metabolic syndrome, a condition that typically involves raised cholesterol levels, raised blood pressure and late-onset diabetes. The seeds are also antiviral and show promise in the treatment of chronic viral infections, such as hepatitis C.

Caution Love-in-a-mist (*N. damascena*) should not be used as a substitute for black cumin seeds.

Notopterygium incisum (Apiaceae)

Notopterygium root, *Qiang huo* (Chinese)

Description Carrot-family member with an upright ridged stem, deeply cut leaves, and flowers in dense clusters.

Habitat & cultivation Notopterygium root is native to central and western China. The root is unearthed in spring or fall.

Part used Root.

Constituents Notopterygium root contains furanocoumarins, sterols, and a volatile oil.

Medicinal actions & uses Notopterygium root is taken mainly for colds and chills, fevers, headache, general aches and pains, and malaise. The herb is warming and pungent, counters cold and damp conditions, and promotes sweating, especially in fevers. It is also prescribed for neck and back pain.

Caution At high dosage notopterygium root may cause vomiting.

Nymphaea alba (Nymphaeaceae)

White water lily

Description Perennial aquatic plant with deep roots, plate-shaped leaves on long cylindrical stems, and large-petaled white flowers occasionally tinged with pink.

Habitat & cultivation Native to Europe, white water lily is found in ponds and in still water in lakes, rivers, and canals. The rhizome is gathered in the fall.

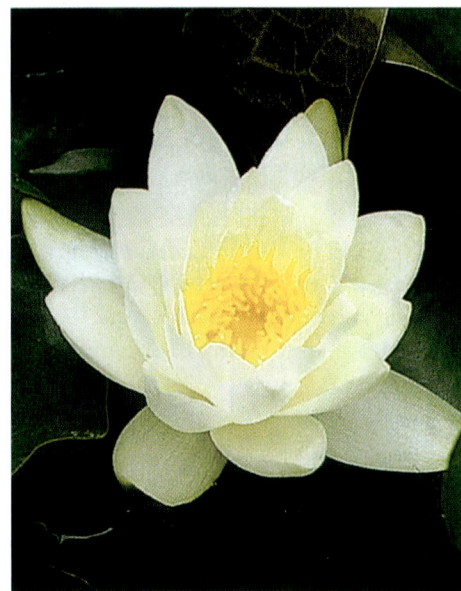

White water lily flowers have a sedative effect, calming nervous tension and anxiety.

Parts used Rhizome, flowers.

Constituents The rhizome contains alkaloids (nymphaeine and nupharine), resin, glycosides, and tannins.

History & folklore According to the 17th-century herbalist Nicholas Culpeper, "The leaves do cool all inflammations … the syrup helpeth much to procure rest, and to settle the brains of frantic persons."

Medicinal actions & uses The rhizome of the white water lily is astringent and antiseptic. A decoction treats dysentery, or diarrhea due to irritable bowel syndrome. White water lily has also been employed to treat chronic bronchitis and kidney pain, and taken as a gargle for sore throats. The rhizome may be used to make a douche for vaginal soreness and discharge, or to make a poultice for boils and abscesses. White water lily flowers have long been reputed to reduce sexual drive. Their generally calming and sedative effect on the nervous system makes them useful in the treatment of insomnia, anxiety, and similar disorders of this nature.

Research Studies suggest that white water lily may, as has been claimed, act as an anaphrodisiac, diminishing sexual drive. The plant has been found to lower blood pressure in animals.

Related species The white pond lily (*N. odorata*) is a close American relative used for much the same purposes. The rhizome of the white lotus (*N. lotus*), native to tropical Africa and Asia, has been used medicinally since the earliest times, and is taken for indigestion, dysentery, and other gastrointestinal problems.

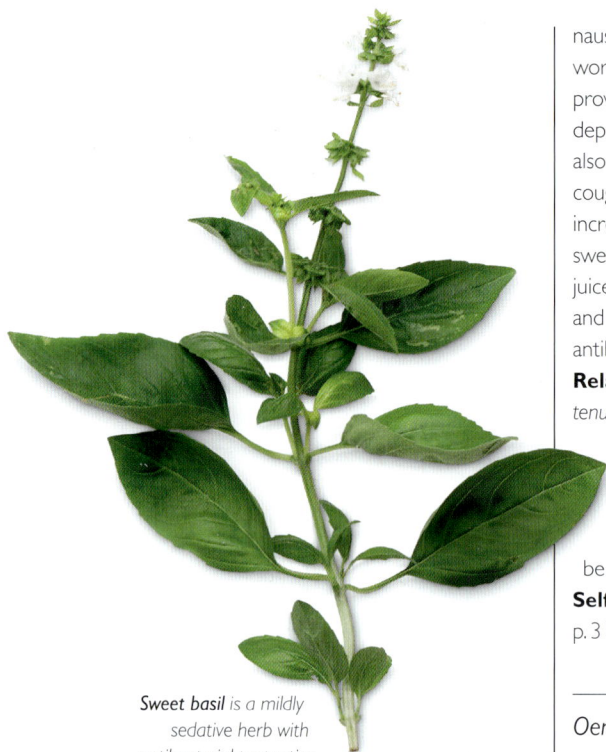

Sweet basil is a mildly sedative herb with antibacterial properties.

Ocimum basilicum (Lamiaceae)

Sweet basil, Basil

Description Strongly aromatic annual growing to 20 in (50 cm). Has shiny oval leaves, a square stem, and small white flowers in whorls.

Habitat & cultivation Sweet basil, also known as basil, is probably native to India. Over 150 varieties are now grown around the world for their distinctive flavor and essential oil. The leaves and flowering tops are gathered as the plant comes into flower.

Parts used Leaves, flowering tops, essential oil.

Constituents Sweet basil contains a volatile oil (about 1%), which consists principally of linalool and methylchavicol, along with small quantities of methyl cinnamate, cineole, and other terpenes.

History & folklore In his 1st-century CE *Materia Medica*, the Greek physician Dioscorides described the African belief that eating sweet basil stopped the pain caused by a scorpion's sting. The herb was used in Roman times to relieve flatulence, to counteract poisoning, as a diuretic, and to stimulate breast milk production. Basil also has a history of use in Ayurvedic medicine.

Medicinal actions & uses Sweet basil acts principally on the digestive and nervous systems, easing flatulence, stomach cramps, colic, and indigestion. It can be used to prevent or relieve nausea and vomiting, and helps to kill intestinal worms. Sweet basil has a mildly sedative action, proving useful in treating nervous irritability, depression, anxiety, and difficulty in sleeping. It may also be taken for epilepsy, migraine, and whooping cough. The herb has been traditionally taken to increase breast milk production. Applied externally, sweet basil leaves act as an insect repellent. The juice from the leaves brings relief to insect bites and stings. Sweet basil has an established antibacterial action.

Related species See also holy basil (*Ocimum tenuiflorum*, p. 116). Bush basil (*O. basilicum* var. *minimum*) has a much milder action than sweet basil, and is used to relieve cramping pain and flatulence.

Caution Sweet basil essential oil should not be taken internally.

Self-help use Minor bites, stings, & swellings, p. 313.

Oenothera biennis (Onagraceae)

Evening primrose

Description Biennial herb growing to 8 in (20 cm). Has red blotches on stem, crinkled lance-shaped leaves, 4-petaled yellow flowers, and elongated seed capsules.

Habitat & cultivation Native to North America, evening primrose is now commonly found in many temperate zones around the world. It thrives on waste ground, especially in dunes and sandy soil. Evening primrose is grown commercially for its seed oil.

Parts used Leaves, stem bark, flowers, seed oil.

Constituents Evening primrose oil is rich in essential fatty acids—linoleic (about 70%) and gammalinolenic acid (about 9%) in particular. Its action mostly depends on the gammalinolenic acid (GLA), which is a precursor of prostaglandin E1. The oil is often combined with vitamin E to prevent oxidation.

Medicinal actions & uses The flowers, leaves, and stem bark of evening primrose have astringent and sedative properties. All three parts have been employed in the treatment of whooping cough. Evening primrose has also been taken for digestive problems and asthma, and used as a poultice to ease the discomfort of rheumatic disorders. The oil, applied externally, is beneficial in the treatment of eczema, certain other itchy skin conditions, and breast tenderness. Taken internally, the oil has an effect in lowering blood pressure, and in preventing the clumping of platelets. The oil is now commonly taken for premenstrual problems, including tension and abdominal bloating, and may prove helpful in conditions as diverse as dry eyes and multiple sclerosis.

Caution Do not take evening primrose oil if suffering from epilepsy.

Ononis spinosa (Fabaceae)

Spiny restharrow

Description Spiny perennial with 3 small leaflets per leaf, bright pink, pealike flowers, and small seed pods.

Habitat & cultivation A relatively common European plant, spiny restharrow thrives in dry grassland and along roadsides.

Part used Root.

Constituents Spiny restharrow root contains phenols, lectins, triterpenoids, and a volatile oil (comprising mainly trans-anethole). It is thought that the volatile oil is diuretic and the remainder of the plant, antidiuretic. A decoction of the root has an antidiuretic effect, as the volatile oil is lost in the steam. If a diuretic is desired, the root is made into an infusion.

Medicinal actions & uses The root is used as a diuretic and to prevent kidney and bladder stones. It is of value in a range of urinary system problems, including stones, gout, and cystitis. For excess fluid retention, spiny restharrow is best taken as a short-term treatment, in the form of an infusion.

Opuntia ficus-indica (Cactaceae)

Prickly pear

Description Perennial cactus growing to 10 ft (3 m). Has large spatula-shaped stems covered in clusters of spines, brilliant yellow flowers, and roundish purple fruit.

Habitat & cultivation Prickly pear is native to Mexico and naturalized in semitropical regions around the world. The fruit is harvested when ripe, the stems when required.

Parts used Flowers, fruit, stems.

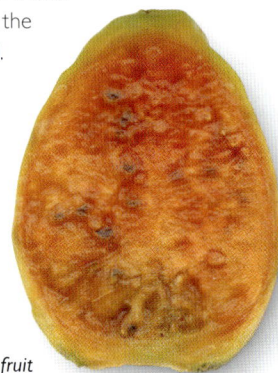

Prickly pear fruit

Constituents The fruit contains mucilage, sugars, vitamin C, and other fruit acids.

History & folklore Prickly pear fruit is used to make conserves and an alcoholic drink in Mexico. The split stems have been bound around injured limbs as a first-aid measure.

Medicinal actions & uses Prickly pear flowers are astringent and reduce bleeding, and are used for problems of the gastrointestinal tract—particularly diarrhea, colitis, and irritable bowel syndrome. The flowers are also taken to treat an enlarged prostate gland. The fruit is nutritious.

Origanum majorana syn. *Majorana hortensis* (Lamiaceae)

Sweet marjoram

Description Woody perennial herb growing to 20 in (50 cm). Has aromatic oval leaves and pinkish-white flowers emerging from the upper leaf axils.

Habitat & cultivation Sweet marjoram is native to countries bordering the Mediterranean. It is much cultivated as a culinary herb, and for its essential oil.

Constituents Sweet marjoram contains about 3% volatile oil (comprising sabinene hydrate, sabinene, linalool, carvacrol, and other terpenes), flavonoids, a wide range of phenolic acids including caffeic and rosmarinic acids, and triterpenoids.

History & folklore In 1597, the herbalist John Gerard made this assessment: "Sweet marjoram is a remedy against cold diseases of the braine and head, being taken anyway to your best liking; put up into the nostrils it provokes sneesing, and draweth forth much baggage flegme; it easeth the toothache being chewed in the mouth."

Medicinal actions & uses Mainly used as a culinary herb, sweet marjoram is also medicinally valuable due to its stimulant and antispasmodic properties. Like oregano (*O. vulgare*, following entry), it treats flatulence, colic, and respiratory problems, but it appears to have a stronger effect on the nervous system than its wild cousin. Sweet marjoram is a good general tonic, helping to relieve anxiety, headaches, and insomnia. The herb is also thought to lower sexual drive.

Research Following longstanding Middle Eastern use of sweet marjoram for gynecological conditions such as vaginitis and polycystic ovary syndrome (PCOS), a small-scale Jordanian clinical trial (2016) found that the herb significantly improved the hormone imbalance associated with PCOS. In a Pakistani (2011) research paper, sweet marjoram essential oil, contrary to expectation, was shown to have greater cytotoxic/anticancer activity than oregano essential oil (see next entry).

Cautions Do not take as a medicine during pregnancy. Do not take sweet marjoram essential oil internally.

Origanum vulgare (Lamiaceae)

Oregano,
Wild marjoram

Description Upright perennial herb growing to about 32 in (80 cm). Has square red stems, elliptical leaves, and clusters of deep pink flowers.

Habitat & cultivation Oregano is native to Europe and naturalized in the Middle East. The plant thrives in chalky soils close to the sea. It is gathered when in flower in summer.

Parts used Aerial parts, essential oil.

Constituents Oregano contains a volatile oil (comprising carvacrol, thymol, beta-bisabolene, caryophyllene, linalool, and borneol), tannins, a wide range of phenolic acids, resin, sterols, and flavonoids.

Oregano's essential oil, well diluted, is a traditional remedy for toothache.

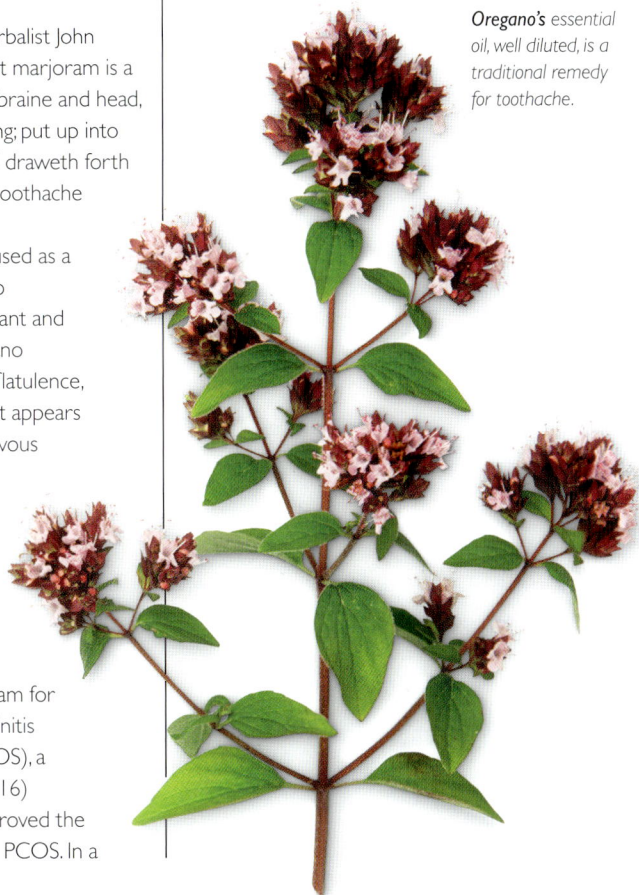

Both carvacrol and thymol are antibacterial and antifungal.

History & folklore Esteemed by the ancient Greeks, oregano was considered a cure-all in medieval times. It was one of the medicinal plants cultivated by early New England colonizers.

Medicinal actions & uses Oregano and its oil are strongly antiseptic with potent activity against many bacteria and fungi, notably *E. coli* and *Candida* strains. It can aid many acute and chronic infections affecting the gastrointestinal and respiratory tracts, especially gastroenteritis, dysentery, bronchitis, coughs, and tonsillitis. Both herb and oil inhibit the gut flora (bacteria naturally occurring within the gut) and have an important role to play in gut dysbiosis, a condition where the presence of harmful gut bacteria leads to symptoms such as gas, bloating, and abdominal discomfort. The diluted oil can be applied to toothache or painful joints.

Cautions Do not take as a medicine during pregnancy. External use may cause irritation of the skin. Do not take essential oil internally.

Orthosiphon aristata (Lamiaceae)

Java tea

Description Shrub growing to about 3 ft (1 m). Has pointed leaves and lilac-colored flowers with very long stamens.

Habitat & cultivation Java tea is native to Southeast Asia and Australia. Now cultivated as a medicinal plant, it is picked as required throughout the year.

Part used Leaves.

Constituents Java tea contains flavones (including sinensetin), a glycoside (orthosiphonin), a volatile oil, and large amounts of potassium.

History & folklore The plant's Dutch Indonesian name, *koemis koetjing* (cat's whiskers), probably derives from its long whiskery stamens.

Medicinal actions & uses Java tea is listed in the French, Indonesian, Dutch, and Swiss pharmacopoeias (official documents containing a list of drugs and their medicinal uses, preparations, and dosages). It is thought to increase the kidneys' ability to eliminate nitrogen-containing compounds. The herb is much used as a diuretic and as a treatment for kidney infections, stones, and poor renal function resulting from chronic nephritis. It is also used to treat cystitis and urethritis.

Research Java tea's diuretic activity has been confirmed in scientific experiments. Extracts significantly increase potassium levels in the urine.

Paeonia officinalis (Paeoniaceae)

Peony

Description Perennial growing to 2 ft (60 cm). Has a tuberous root, upright stems, oval to lance-shaped leaflets, and attractive large red, red-purple or white flowers.

Habitat & cultivation A native of southern Europe, peony grows in mountain woodlands and is widely cultivated. The root is unearthed in the fall.

Part used Root.

Constituents Peony is thought to contain alkaloids, tannins, saponins, flavonoids and triterpenoids, and a volatile oil.

History & folklore Since the time of Hippocrates (470–377 BCE), peony has been used to treat epilepsy. Ibn el Beitar, a medieval Arab physician, recommended a necklace of peony seeds to ward off epilepsy in children. Mrs. Grieve, the author of *A Modern Herbal* (1931), recounted how "in ancient times, peony was thought to be of divine origin, an emanation from the moon, and to shine during the night protecting the shepherds and their flocks."

Medicinal actions & uses Though little used in contemporary European herbal medicine, Peony is greatly valued within Unani herbal medicine from the Middle East. It has anti-inflammatory, antispasmodic, and sedative activity, and is prescribed for conditions as varied as nervous debility, epilepsy, and high blood pressure, and as a heart tonic. The root has also been taken to treat whooping cough, and suppositories are made of the root to relive anal and intestinal spasms.

Related species Chinese peony (*Paeonia lactiflora*, p. 122) is much used in Chinese herbal medicine.

Cautions Take peony only under professional supervision. Do not take during pregnancy.

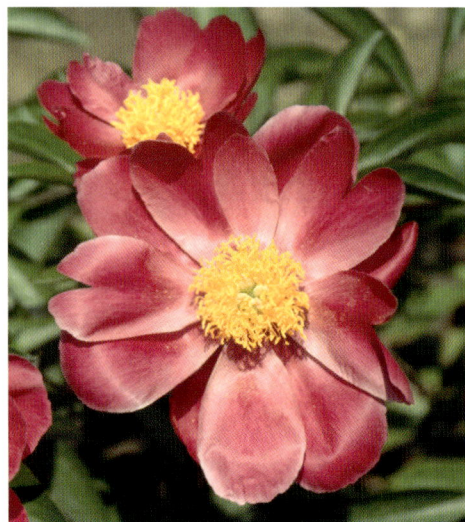

Peony *is named after Paeon, the physician of the Greek gods.*

Panax notoginseng (Araliaceae)

Notoginseng, *San qi* (Chinese)

Description Deciduous perennial with an erect stem growing to 3 ft (1 m), compound leaves, small greenish flowers, and small berrylike fruit.

Habitat & cultivation Native to China, notoginseng is now rare in the wild. It is cultivated commercially in southern and central China. The root is unearthed before flowering or after the fruit has ripened.

Part used Root.

Constituents Notoginseng contains steroidal saponins, polysaccharides, and a flavonoid.

History & folklore Despite its importance as a tonic, notoginseng was only recorded in Chinese herbal medicine in 1578, in the *Compendium of Materia Medica* by Li Shizhen. He described the root as being "more valuable than gold."

Medicinal actions & uses Like ginseng (*P. ginseng*, p. 123), notoginseng is a tonic that supports the function of the adrenal glands, in particular the production of corticosteroids and male sex hormones. Notoginseng also helps to improve blood flow through the coronary arteries, thus finding use as a treatment for arteriosclerosis, high blood pressure, and angina. Notoginseng treats internal bleeding of almost any kind. The herb may also be applied externally as a poultice to help speed the healing of wounds and bruises.

Research Clinical studies have confirmed notoginseng's longstanding reputation as a means to arrest bleeding. A Chinese trial indicated that the herb hastens blood clotting. Another clinical trial and extensive scientific studies, again in China, associated the herb with positive improvements in coronary circulation, in lessening the symptoms of angina, and in the reduction of blood pressure levels. In common with other ginseng-type herbs, notoginseng has been shown to enhance physical performance.

Caution Do not take during pregnancy.

Panax quinquefolium (Araliaceae)

American ginseng

Description Deciduous perennial growing to about 1 ft (30 cm). Has a smooth stem, leaves with oblong to oval leaflets, small greenish flowers, and kidney-shaped scarlet-red berries.

Habitat & cultivation American ginseng is native to North America and the Himalayas. A woodland plant, it is rarely seen in the wild due to over-harvesting. It is cultivated in Wisconsin, China, and France. The root is gathered in the fall.

Part used Root.

Constituents American ginseng contains steroidal saponins, including panaquilon.

History & folklore Indigenous North American peoples may have considered this herb a means to increase female fertility. From the mid-18th century, the collection of the herb for export to China became a virtual gold rush, with so many Indigenous peoples harvesting American ginseng that colonizers reported finding villages almost deserted. The Ojibwa people always planted a seed to replace the herb, but this was not universal practice. American ginseng became rare toward the end of the 19th century.

Medicinal actions & uses The action of American ginseng is presumed to be similar to, but milder than, that of its Chinese cousin, ginseng (*P. ginseng*, p. 123). American ginseng increases the ability to tolerate stress of all kinds. In traditional Chinese medicine, it is employed as a yin tonic, treating weakness, fever, wheezing, and coughs.

Related species See ginseng, notoginseng (*P. notoginseng*, preceding entry), and Siberian ginseng (*Eleutherococcus senticosus*, p. 98).

Caution Do not take during pregnancy.

Papaver rhoeas (Papaveraceae)

Red poppy

Description Delicate hairy-stemmed annual growing to 3 ft (90 cm). Has basal rosette of lance-shaped leaves and deeply incised stem leaves, 4-petaled red flowers with black anthers, and small rounded seed capsules.

Habitat & cultivation Red poppy is native to Europe, North Africa, and temperate regions of Asia, and is naturalized in North and South America. It thrives on cultivated land and on road verges. The flowers are picked in summer.

Parts used Flowers.

Constituents Red poppy contains alkaloids (including papaverine, rhoeadine, isorhoeadine, and many others), meconic acid, mekocyanin, mucilage, and tannin. The alkaloids are similar to those in the opium poppy (*P. somniferum*, see *following entry*), but are much milder.

History & folklore According to Agnus Castus, writing in the 14th century, "If a man hawe ony peyne aboutyn his eyne or if a man hawe a mygreyn tak this herb and stamp it and nedle it with oyle de olywe and anoynt ther-with the forhed and it schal amende the syth and slake the peyne and distroye the mygreyn."

Medicinal actions & uses Red poppy flowers are mildly analgesic and sedative, and have long been used in European herbal medicine, particularly for ailments in children and the elderly. Chiefly employed as a mild pain reliever and as a treatment for irritable coughs, red poppy also helps reduce nervous overactivity. The herb may be used in the treatment of insomnia, general irritability, coughs—especially paroxysmal coughs—and asthma, and is generally given as a syrup.

Related species See also opium poppy (*P. somniferum, following entry*), Mexican poppy (*Argemone mexicana*, p. 175) and Californian poppy (*Eschscholzia californica*, p. 212).

Cautions Use only under professional supervision. All parts of red poppy except the seeds are potentially toxic if eaten.

Papaver somniferum (Papaveraceae)

Opium poppy

Description Thick-stemmed annual growing to about 3 ft (1 m). Has many dull green leaves, solitary pink, purple or white flowers, and globe-shaped seed capsules.

Habitat & cultivation Native to western Asia, opium poppy is now cultivated commercially around the world as the source of morphine and codeine, and as an illegal crop for the production of opium and heroin. During the summer, the seed capsules are cut and the white latex that exudes is gathered the next day and dried.

Part used Latex.

Constituents Opium poppy contains more than 40 opium alkaloids, including morphine (up to 20%), narcotine (about 5%), codeine (about 1%), and papaverine (about 1%). It also contains meconic acid, albumin, mucilage, sugars, resin, and wax. Many of the opium poppy's alkaloids have a well-established therapeutic action. Morphine is one of the most powerful analgesics of all, used extensively in conventional medicine to relieve pain, especially in terminal illness. Codeine is a milder analgesic used for headaches and other pain, and in the symptomatic treatment of diarrhea. Opium's strongly addictive nature is well established.

History & folklore Cultivated for its medicinal properties for at least 4,000 years, the opium poppy was introduced to Greece about 3,000 years ago, and from there spread throughout Europe. It was unknown in China until the 7th century CE, and in Japan until the 15th century. It is mentioned in the Assyrian herbals (c. 1700 BCE), and the Greek physician Dioscorides (40–90 CE) wrote that "a decoction of the leaves and flower heads if drunk

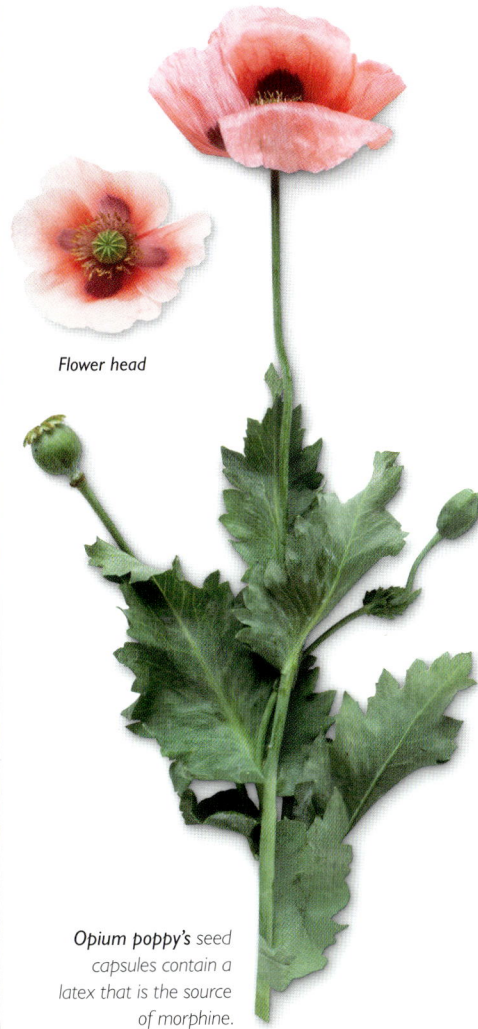

Flower head

Opium poppy's seed capsules contain a latex that is the source of morphine.

and bathed on the head is unrivaled in inducing sleep. The mashed heads, mixed with flour, make a useful plaster in inflammations and St. Anthony's fire [erysipelas, a bacterial infection of the skin]."

Medicinal actions & uses Opium (the dried latex) is a potent narcotic, analgesic and antispasmodic, and has been taken to relieve pain of various kinds. In all the main herbal traditions it is regarded as a powerfully "cold" remedy, reducing physical function and sedating or suppressing nervous activity, pain and coughs. In view of its addictive nature, opium is mainly used after other less powerful analgesics have failed to bring relief. It is also an effective remedy for acute diarrhea and severe coughs. Pharmaceutical drugs produced from opium poppy include morphine and codeine.

Research Much research has been done, confirming most of the uses of opium poppy listed above.

Related species See also red poppy (*P. rhoeas, preceding entry*), Mexican poppy (*Argemone mexicana,*

p. 175) and Californian poppy (*Eschscholzia californica*, p. 212).

Cautions The use of opium poppy cannot be advised even under professional supervision. It is subject to legal restrictions in most countries.

Parietaria officinalis syn. *P. diffusa* (Urticaceae)

Pellitory-of-the-wall

Description Annual growing to 28 in (70 cm). Has deep green leaves, greenish flowers, and small dark seeds.

Habitat & cultivation Native to Europe, this plant is commonplace in southern countries, where it is found on walls and in dry stony sites. It is gathered in summer when in flower.

Parts used Aerial parts.

Constituents Pellitory-of-the-wall contains flavonoids and tannins.

History & folklore For more than 2,000 years, pellitory-of-the-wall has been valued as a diuretic, as a soother of chronic coughs, and as a balm for wounds and burns.

Medicinal actions & uses Pellitory-of-the wall is chiefly employed as a diuretic, demulcent, and stone-preventing herb. In European herbal medicine, it is regarded as having a restorative action on the kidneys, supporting and strengthening their function. It has been prescribed for conditions such as nephritis, pyelitis (inflammation of the kidney), kidney stones, renal colic (pain caused by kidney stones), cystitis, and edema (fluid retention). It is also occasionally taken as a laxative.

Caution Do not take if suffering from hay fever or other allergies.

Paullinia cupana syn. *P. sorbilis* (Sapindaceae)

Guarana

Description Woody vine growing to a height of 33 ft (10 m). Has divided compound leaves, clusters of inconspicuous yellow flowers, and pear-shaped fruit that contains small shiny brown seeds.

Habitat & cultivation Guarana is native to tropical forests of the Brazilian Amazon, and is also cultivated in Brazil. The seeds are gathered when ripe.

Parts used Seeds.

Constituents Guarana contains xanthine derivatives (including up to 7% caffeine, together with theobromine and theophylline), tannins, and saponins. The xanthines are stimulant and diuretic, and reduce fatigue over the short term.

History & folklore In Brazil, guarana is traditionally prepared by roasting, crushing, and drying the seeds. The resulting "cakes" are made into a tea, taken to counter fatigue or to treat diarrhea. Guarana has recently become a popular alternative to coffee.

Medicinal actions & uses Guarana's medicinal uses are similar to those of coffee (*Coffea arabica*, p. 196)—it is taken for headache and migraine, for mild depression, and to boost energy levels. The problems that apply to long-term or excessive consumption of coffee also apply to guarana—both stimulate over the short term but tend to inhibit the body's restorative processes over the longer term. In view of guarana's high tannin content, long-term use is even less advisable, because tannins impair the intestines' ability to absorb nutrients. Nevertheless, guarana is a useful short-term remedy for boosting energy, or for treating a tension headache that cannot be treated with rest. Guarana's astringency also treats chronic diarrhea.

Related species *P. yoco*, native to the Colombian Amazon, is used by Indigenous peoples to reduce fevers, as a stimulant, and as a post-malarial treatment

Cautions Do not take guarana if suffering from cardiovascular disease or from high blood pressure. It should also not be taken during pregnancy or while breastfeeding.

Pausinystalia yohimbe syn. *Corynanthe yohimbe* (Rubiaceae)

Yohimbe

Description Evergreen tree growing to 100 ft (30 m). Has reddish-brown bark, oblong or elliptical leaves, and clusters of small yellow flowers.

Habitat & cultivation Yohimbe is native to the forests of western Africa, especially Cameroon, the Democratic Republic of Congo, and Gabon. The bark is gathered at any time of year.

Part used Bark.

Constituents Yohimbe contains approximately 6% indole alkaloids (including yohimbine), pigments, and tannins. The alkaloids have a cerebral stimulant action at moderate doses, but are highly toxic in large doses.

History & folklore Yohimbe has an ancient reputation in western Africa, especially among the Bantu people, as a male aphrodisiac and mild hallucinogen.

Medicinal actions & uses Yohimbe is little used in herbal medicine owing to its potential toxicity. In western Africa, it is often employed as a stimulant

and as a means to counter erectile dysfunction. Yohimbine has been used in conventional medicine in the treatment of erectile dysfunction.

Cautions Take yohimbe only under professional supervision. The herb is subject to legal restrictions in many countries.

Peganum harmala (Zygophyllaceae)

Harmala,
African rue

Description Multi-branched shrubby perennial growing to 20 in (50 cm). Has deeply cleft linear leaves, white 5-petaled flowers, and rounded 3-celled seed capsules.

Habitat & cultivation Native to the Middle East, North Africa, and southern Europe, harmala is naturalized in other subtropical regions, including Australia. It thrives in saline soil in semidesert areas.

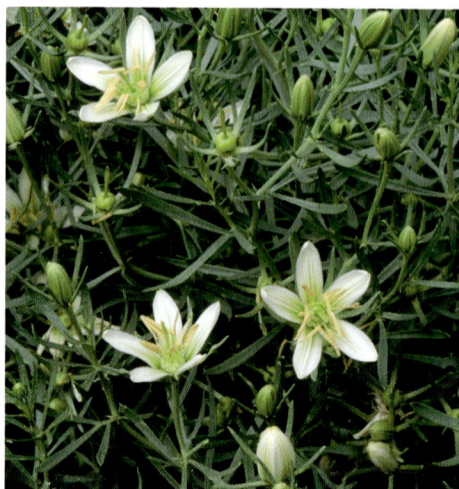

Harmala, which thrives in dry conditions, has been used as an intoxicant in the Middle East.

The seeds are gathered in summer.

Parts used Seeds, root.

Constituents Harmala contains up to 4% indole alkaloids (including harmine, harmaline and harmalol). Harmine has been used to help alleviate the tremors of Parkinsonism.

History & folklore Since the earliest times, harmala has been used in the Middle East as a means to induce intoxication. Known to the Greek physicians Dioscorides (40–9 CE) and Galen (131–200 CE), as well as to their Arabic counterpart Ibn Sina (980–1037 CE), harmala was also used to expel intestinal worms and to promote the onset of menstrual flow.

Medicinal actions & uses Despite its long history as a euphoric and purportedly aphrodisiac herb, harmala is little used in contemporary Western herbal medicine because of its potential toxicity. The seeds have been taken, especially in the Middle East, to treat a very wide range of conditions, including high blood pressure, eye problems, psychiatric disorders, depression, Parkinson's disease, and cancer. In central Asia, the root is a popular medicinal remedy that is used to treat rheumatism and nervous conditions

Research Seed extracts, and key alkaloids within them, have been shown to have wide-ranging effects on the heart and circulation, in part due to increased nitric oxide levels, slowing heart rate, lowering blood pressure, and reducing peripheral vascular resistance (opening up the capillary network).

Caution This plant is potentially very toxic and should not be used under any circumstances.

Pergularia extensa (Asclepiadaceae)

Pergularia

Description Perennial climber with broad oval leaves and small greenish-white flowers

Habitat & cultivation Pergularia is native to India. Its aerial parts are gathered throughout the year.

Parts used Aerial parts.

Constituents Pergularia contains a resin, bitter principles and plant sterols.

Medicinal actions & uses Pergularia is thought to have bitter, expectorant, diuretic, and laxative properties, and is employed in several ways in Indian herbal medicine. It is prescribed as a treatment for bronchitis and asthma. Pergularia is also used as a means to curtail heavy menstrual or non-menstrual uterine bleeding. Juice from the leaves may be applied to relieve the pain and swelling of cysts and rheumatic joints.

Petroselinum crispum (Apiaceae)

Parsley

Description Annual herb growing to 1 ft (30 cm). Has an erect stem, bright green compound smooth or crinkled leaves, small white flowers growing in clusters, and small ribbed seeds.

Habitat & cultivation Parsley is native to Europe and the eastern Mediterranean. Today it is rarely found in the wild, but is cultivated throughout the world as a nutritious salad herb. The leaves may be picked from spring to fall, and the seeds are gathered when just ripe.

Parts used Leaves, root, seeds.

Constituents Parsley contains a volatile oil (including about 20% myristicin, about 18% apiole, and many other terpenes), flavonoids, phthalides, furanocoumarins (including bergapten), vitamins A, C, and E, and high levels of iron. The flavonoids are anti-inflammatory and antioxidant. Myristicin and apiole have diuretic properties. The volatile oil relieves cramping pain and flatulence, and is a strong uterine stimulant.

History & folklore Parsley was known in ancient Greece and Rome—but more as a diuretic, digestive tonic, and menstrual stimulant than as a salad herb. In Rome, parsley was associated with the goddess Persephone, queen of the underworld, and was used in funeral ceremonies. Parsley was introduced to Britain in 1548.

Medicinal actions & uses The fresh leaves are highly nutritious and can be considered a natural vitamin and mineral supplement in their own right. Chewing fresh parsley leaves is a valued remedy for bad breath and halitosis. The seeds have a much stronger diuretic action than the leaves, and may be substituted for celery seeds (*Apium graveolens*, p. 68) in the treatment of gout, rheumatism, and arthritis. Both plants act by encouraging the flushing out of waste products from the inflamed joints, and the waste's subsequent elimination via the kidneys. Parsley root is taken as a treatment for flatulence, cystitis, and rheumatic conditions. Parsley is also valued as a promoter of menstruation, being helpful both in stimulating a delayed period and in relieving menstrual pain.

Cautions Parsley is a safe herb at normal dosage and consumption levels, but excessive quantities of the seeds are toxic. Do not take the seeds during pregnancy or if suffering from kidney disease.

Peucedanum ostruthium syn. *Imperatoria ostruthium* (Apiaceae)

Masterwort

Description Perennial growing to 2 ft (60 cm) with green leaves divided into 3 leaflets with 3 lobes, white flowers on large umbels, and winged seeds.

Habitat & cultivation Native to central and southern Europe and Asia, most often found in the wild. The root is unearthed in the fall or spring.

Part used Root.

Constituents Masterwort contains a volatile oil, mostly sabinene, terpineol, beta-caryophyllene, and humulene, bitter principles, tannins, and coumarins.

History & folklore From the late Middle Ages

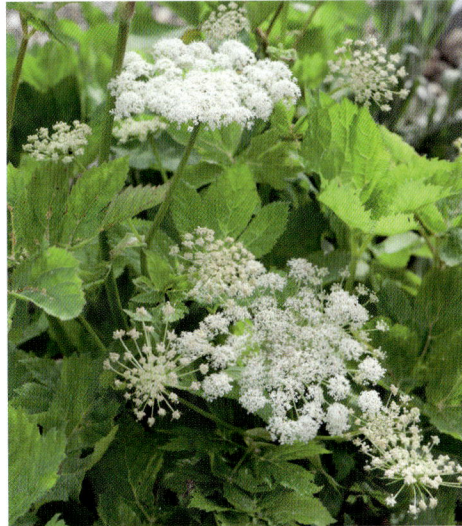

Peucedanum ostruthium has a strong action within the stomach and gut, settling indigestion and relieving wind.

onward, masterwort was held in high regard by herbalists. Pierandrea Mattioli's *Materia Medica* of 1548 explains: "Masterwort powerfully resolves all flatulence in the body, stimulates urine and menstruation, is an admirable remedy for paralysis and cold conditions of the brain, and helps against pestilence and the bites of rabid dogs." A century later, Nicholas Culpeper was no less fulsome in recommending masterwort for rheumatic conditions, shortness of breath, kidney and bladder stones, water retention, "falling sickness," and wounds.

Medicinal actions & uses Masterwort is little used today, but it may well be an herb that bears further investigation. The root is aromatic, warms central areas of the body, and is a bitter tonic. It has a strong action within the stomach and gut, settling indigestion and relieving gas and cramping. Masterwort is also beneficial for chest conditions, and is used for colds, asthma, and bronchitis. It can also be helpful for menstrual problems.

Caution If applied to the skin, masterwort may cause an allergic reaction to sunlight.

Peumus boldus (Apiaceae)

Boldo

Description Strongly aromatic multi-branched evergreen shrub or tree growing to 20 ft (6 m). Has egg-shaped leathery leaves with a lemony scent, clusters of white or yellow bell-shaped flowers, and small yellow berries.

Habitat & cultivation Boldo is native to Chile and Peru, and has become naturalized in the Mediterranean region and the West Coast of North

America. It grows on dry sunny slopes and in mountain pastures in the Andes, where it is widely cultivated. The leaves are gathered throughout the year.

Parts used Leaves.

Constituents Boldo contains 0.7% isoquinoline alkaloids (including boldine), as well as a volatile oil and flavonoids.

History & folklore Boldo is a valued remedy in Latin American herbal medicine and is used by the Araucanian people in Chile as a tonic. Boldo leaves are strongly aromatic and are a common ingredient in southern South American cooking. They have a cinnamon-like aroma.

Medicinal actions & uses Boldo stimulates liver activity and bile flow and is chiefly valued as a remedy for gallstones and liver or gallbladder pain. It is normally taken for a few weeks at a time, either as a tincture or infusion. Boldo is also a mild urinary antiseptic and demulcent and may be taken for infections such as cystitis.

Research A poorly researched herb, laboratory research to date has confirmed that the leaves exert a strong liver-protective activity.

Cautions Do not take during pregnancy. This herb is subject to legal restrictions in some countries.

Pfaffia paniculata (Amaranthaceae)

Suma,
Brazilian ginseng

Description Climbing perennial with a thick rootstock, growing up through rainforest trees into the forest canopy.

Habitat & cultivation Suma is native to rainforests of South America, from Venezuela to southern Brazil.

Parts used Root.

Constituents Suma contains triterpene saponins (pfaffosides), sterols (including beta-ecdysone), and minerals (including significant levels of germanium).

History & folklore Suma has been used by the people of the Amazon rainforest from the earliest times for conditions as varied as wound healing, diabetes, and cancer. Also taken for its aphrodisiac qualities, suma has become a popular herbal medicine in Brazil, where it is known as *para todo* ("for all"), or Brazilian ginseng.

Medicinal actions & uses Suma has many medicinal applications, most centered around three areas of activity: as a hormonal and glandular tonic, as an immune stimulant and detoxifying agent, and in cancer prevention and treatment. Suma is perhaps best known as a male sexual tonic, but it is equally effective for women and has value in treating menstrual and menopausal problems. Suma root enhances nonspecific immunity and has a role to play in treating chronic infection and lowered immune resistance.

Research Research into suma suggests that it can be useful in cancer prevention and treatment; several of the pfaffosides have been shown to prevent tumor growth in laboratory conditions. The pfaffosides are chemically similar to the ginsenosides found in ginseng (Panax ginseng, p. 123), and, like ginseng, suma's acclaimed value as an aphrodisiac appears to have a scientific basis. Male rats with depressed sexual function were observed to become more sexually active on being given a suma extract.

Cautions Avoid in pregnancy and while breast-feeding.

Phaseolus vulgaris (Fabaceae)

French bean, Haricot bean

Description Slender-stemmed, annual climber growing to 13 ft (4 m). Has pointed oval leaflets, curly tendrils, clusters of white or lilac flowers, and a bean pod containing kidney-shaped seeds.

Habitat & cultivation French beans are thought to have originated from South America. Today, varieties are cultivated all over the world. The ripe beans are gathered in summer.

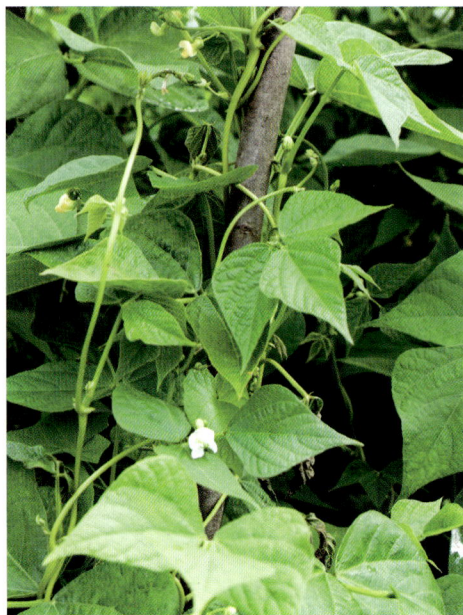

French beans are intensively cultivated all over the world.

Parts used Bean pods, beans.

Constituents French beans contain lectins, saponins, flavonoids, allantoin, amino acids, and sugars.

History & folklore French beans have been used since antiquity to treat diabetes. In *A Modern Herbal* (1931), Mrs. Grieve records that "because of the seed's close resemblance to a male testicle … [ancient Egyptians] made it an object of sacred worship and forbade its use as a food."

Medicinal actions & uses In addition to being an important food in many parts of the world, French beans, and beans in general, offer several health benefits. As part of a balanced nutritious diet, they help to lower high blood pressure and raised cholesterol levels. They are hypoglycemic and promote more stable blood-sugar levels. Like soy (Glycine max, p. 221), they are estrogenic and will help reduce menopausal symptoms. The pods act as a medium-strength diuretic, stimulating urine flow and the clearance of toxins from the body. Powdered beans may be dusted onto eczema to ease itching and dry skin.

Phellodendron amurense (Rutaceae)

Huang bai

Description Deciduous tree growing to 39 ft (12 m). Has compound leaves with 7 lance-shaped leaflets, clusters of green flowers, and round berries.

Habitat & cultivation *Huang bai* is native to China, Japan, and Korea, and is cultivated in northeastern China. The bark of 10-year-old trees is collected in spring.

Part used Bark.

Constituents *Huang bai* contains isoquinoline alkaloids (including berberine), sesquiterpene lactones, and plant sterols. Due to its alkaloid content, *huang bai* is antimicrobial and antibiotic.

History & folklore Listed in the *Divine Husbandman's Classic* (*Shen'nong Bencaojing*), of the 1st century CE, *huang bai* was regarded as an herb to be used with care.

Medicinal actions & uses Strongly bitter, *huang bai* is used within Chinese herbal medicine to "drain damp heat." It is prescribed for conditions such as acute diarrhea, jaundice, vaginal infection (including trichomonas), and certain skin conditions. It is also given for urinary system disorders such as frequent urination, pain, and infection.

Research Clinical trials in China indicate that the bark is useful in the treatment of meningitis and conjunctivitis.

Cautions Take *huang bai* only under professional supervision. Do not take *huang bai* during pregnancy.

Phyllanthus amarus (Euphorbiaceae)

Phyllanthus

Description Slender annual herb, to 2 ft (60 cm) in height, with oval leaves and small yellowish-green flowers.

Habitat & cultivation Phyllanthus is native to the Indian subcontinent and found commonly in central and southern India. The plant is harvested when required.

Parts used Leaves, aerial parts.

Constituents Phyllanthus leaves contain lignans (including phyllanthin and hypophyllanthin), flavonoids, and alkaloids.

Medicinal actions & uses Phyllanthus is a traditional Ayurvedic remedy used to treat liver and cardiovascular problems. It combines well with picrorhiza (Picrorhiza kurroa, p. 255) in treating hepatitis B and other liver disorders.

Research A growing body of research shows that phyllanthus has antiviral activity, specifically against the hepatitis B virus. Research also indicates that the leaves are diuretic, and lower blood pressure and blood-sugar levels. Not all the studies have shown that phyllanthus works effectively in treating hepatitis B, but overall the evidence is positive, with some trials showing significant improvement in measures of infection. In laboratory experiments, phyllanthus inhibits RNA replication of the hepatitis B virus.

Caution Use on professional advice only.

Physalis alkekengi syn. *P. franchetii* (Solanaceae)

Chinese lantern, Winter cherry

Description Perennial herb growing to 32 in (80 cm). Has oval- to diamond-shaped leaves, long-stemmed white flowers, and a translucent papery sheath surrounding an orange-red fruit.

Habitat & cultivation Chinese lantern is native to central and southern Europe and China. It grows wild along damp roadsides. It is widely cultivated in warm temperate and subtropical regions, including North and South America and South Africa. The fruit is gathered once it has ripened in summer.

Parts used Fruit.

Constituents Chinese lantern contains flavonoids, plant sterols, and vitamins A (carotene) and C. The roots contain tropane-type alkaloids, physalin A and B. Water extracts of the plant may have an antiestrogenic effect.

History & folklore The Greek physician Dioscorides (1st century CE) considered Chinese lantern to be medicinally beneficial as a diuretic and a treatment for jaundice. In Spain, a therapeutic wine made with the fruit was taken to treat excess fluid retention and problems of the urinary tract.

Medicinal actions & uses Though commonly eaten as a fruit, Chinese lantern is also a useful diuretic. The fruit is traditionally used within European herbal medicine to treat kidney and bladder stones, fluid retention, and gout. It has also been taken to reduce fever.

Caution The foliage and unripe fruit are harmful if eaten.

Phytolacca americana syn. *P. decandra* (Phytolaccaceae)

Pokeweed

Description Herbaceous perennial growing to 10 ft (3 m). Has alternate lance-shaped leaves, spikes of greenish-white flowers, and clusters of fleshy, purple berries.

Habitat & cultivation Native to North America, pokeweed is now naturalized in the Mediterranean region. It thrives in damp woodland and on waste

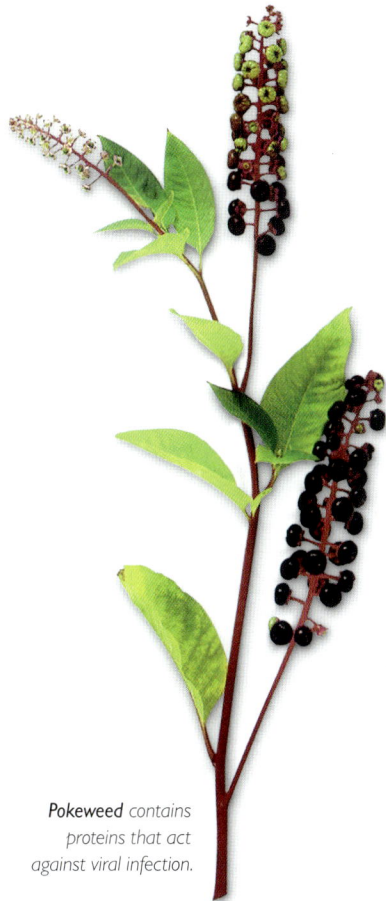

Pokeweed contains proteins that act against viral infection.

ground. The root is unearthed in late fall.

Part used Root.

Constituents Pokeweed contains triterpenoid saponins, lectins, lignans, resin, and mucilage. The triterpenoid saponins are strongly anti-inflammatory, the lignans are antiviral, and the lectins are mitogenic (break up chromosomes).

History & folklore Pokeweed was widely used by Indigenous North American peoples and European colonizers as a poultice for skin diseases, sores, ulcers and tumors. It was also given internally to relieve pain and to induce vomiting. The berries are used in southern Europe to create a deeper red wine color in poor quality wines.

Medicinal actions & uses Pokeweed is strongly anti-inflammatory and is taken internally as a tincture in small amounts to treat rheumatic and arthritic conditions. The root has also been used to treat respiratory tract infections, such as sore throats and tonsillitis, as well as swollen glands and chronic infections. The herb is sometimes prescribed for pain and infection of the ovaries or testes, and as a lymphatic "decongestant," stimulating the clearance of waste products. As a poultice or ointment, it is applied to sore and infected nipples and breasts, acne, folliculitis, fungal infections, and scabies.

Cautions The plant is highly toxic in overdose. Use only under professional supervision. Do not take during pregnancy.

Research Two Chinese species (*P. acinosa* and *P. esculenta*) are used medicinally in a more or less identical way to pokeweed.

Picrasma excelsa syn. *Quassia excelsa* (Simaroubaceae)

Quassia

Description Deciduous tree growing to 100 ft (30 m). Has smooth gray bark, compound leaves, small yellow flowers, and pea-size black fruit.

Habitat & cultivation Native to tropical America and the Caribbean, quassia grows in forests and near water. It is cultivated mainly for medicinal use. The bark is harvested throughout the year.

Part used Bark.

Constituents Quassia contains quassinoid bitter principles (including quassin), alkaloids, a coumarin (scopoletin), and vitamin B_1. Some of the quassinoids have been shown to have cytotoxic (cell-killing) and antileukemic actions.

History & folklore Quassia bark was first introduced into Europe from Suriname, then a Dutch colony, in 1756. The herb is named after Quassi, an Indigenous healer, who told Europeans of its therapeutic value.

Medicinal actions & uses The strongly bitter quassia supports and strengthens weak digestive systems. It increases bile flow and the secretion of salivary juices and stomach acid, and improves the digestive process as a whole. Quassia is commonly used to stimulate the appetite, especially in the treatment of anorexia. Its bitterness has led to it being used for malaria and other fevers, and it is given in the Caribbean for dysentery. The bark has been used in the form of an enema to expel threadworms and other parasites. A decoction of the bark may be used as an insect repellent and to treat head lice.

Cautions Excessive doses may, in some cases, cause digestive irritation, vomiting, and diarrhea. Do not take during pregnancy.

Picrorhiza kurroa (Plantaginaceae)

Picrorhiza

Description Hairy perennial with serrated elliptical leaves and white or lilac flowers growing in spikes.

Habitat & cultivation Picrorhiza is native to the mountains of India and Nepal. The rhizome is gathered in the fall.

Part used Rhizome.

Constituents Picrorhiza contains the bitter glycoside kutkin (composed of picrosides I to III and kutkoside), iridoids, cucurbitacins, and apocynin. Apocynin is powerfully anti-inflammatory and reduces platelet aggregation.

History & folklore Picrorhiza has been used in Ayurvedic medicine as a laxative and bitter tonic since the earliest times.

Medicinal actions & uses In India, picrorhiza is used as a bitter tonic, equivalent in many respects to gentian (*Gentiana lutea*, p. 103), and given for a wide range of digestive and liver troubles, such as indigestion, constipation, jaundice, and hepatitis. In China, it is chiefly employed to treat chronic diarrhea and dysentery. Picrorhiza also helps treat asthma, acute and chronic infections, conditions where the immune system is compromised, and autoimmune diseases, including psoriasis and vitiligo. The herb's traditional use for liver disorders is well founded, and picrorhiza may play an important role in treating liver disease. Demand for picrorhiza is great, exceeding the annual harvest of the rhizome. Due to overharvesting the herb has become endangered in the wild. Alternative herbs such as gentian and Oregon Grape (*Berberis aquifolium*) should be used as appropriate.

Research In 1992 Indian trials, extracts of picrorhiza were shown to boost immunity, and to have a specific action against *Leishmania donovani*, which causes the tropical parasitic disease known as leishmaniasis. Indian research also indicates that picrorhiza is of therapeutic value in the treatment of auto-immune disease.

Caution Picrorhiza should only be taken under professional supervision.

Pimenta officinalis (Myrtaceae)

Allspice

Description Aromatic evergreen tree growing to 39 ft (12 m). Has leathery oblong leaves, clusters of small white flowers, and tiny green berries that turn brown as they become ripe.

Habitat & cultivation Allspice is native to the Caribbean and to Central and South America. The berries are gathered before they are fully ripe because the volatile oil content reduces as they mature.

Parts used Berries, leaves, essential oil.

Constituents Allspice contains volatile oil (about 4%, mostly eugenol—up to 80%), lignins, and terpenoids.

History & folklore Used as a spice in the Caribbean before the arrival of Europeans, allspice is now an ingredient in many well-known sauces, chutneys, and condiments.

Medicinal actions & uses A digestive stimulant, allspice is taken to relieve flatulence and indigestion. It may also be used to treat diarrhea. Allspice is often combined with herbs that have a tonic or laxative effect. The herb has an action that is similar to that of cloves (*Eugenia caryophyllata*, p. 101); both are stimulant, stomach-settling, and antiseptic. Allspice essential oil is markedly antiseptic and analgesic.

Research Taking a lead from allspice's use in Costa Rica as a menopause remedy, scientists found that the berries have a strong estrogenic activity. A 2009 paper suggested that allspice may well help with menopausal symptoms. Studies also indicate that allspice lowers high blood pressure.

Cautions Do not take essential oil internally without professional guidance. Do not take allspice as a medicine during pregnancy.

Pimpinella anisum (Apiaceae)

Anise

Description Erect annual growing to 2 ft (60 cm), with feathery leaves, umbels of yellow flowers, and ridged, gray-green seeds.

Habitat & cultivation Anise is native to the eastern Mediterranean, western Asia and North

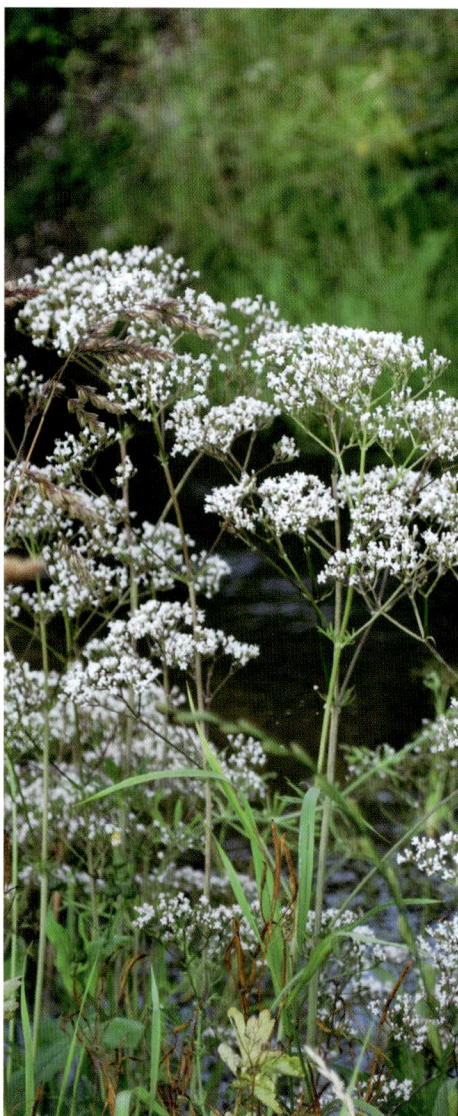

Anise seeds, which benefit the digestion, are harvested when ripe in the fall.

Africa. It is widely cultivated for its seeds, which are used for medicinal purposes and as a flavoring in cooking and alcoholic drinks.

Parts used Seeds, essential oil.

Constituents Anise contains a volatile oil (comprising 70–90% anethole, together with methylchavicol and other terpenes), furanocoumarins, flavonoids, fatty acids, phenylpropanoids, sterols, and proteins. Anethole has an observed estrogenic effect, and the seeds as a whole are mildly estrogenic. This effect may substantiate the herb's use as a stimulant of sexual drive and of breast milk production.

History & folklore After examining the records of Cyprus hospital monastery, historians discovered that anise was used to treat plague and cholera during the Ottoman Period (1571–1878 CE).

Medicinal actions & uses Anise seeds are known for their ability to reduce gas and bloating, and to settle digestion. They are commonly given to infants and children to relieve colic, and to people of all ages to ease nausea and indigestion. Anise seeds' antispasmodic properties make them helpful in countering period pain, asthma, whooping cough, and bronchitis. The seeds' expectorant action justifies their use for these respiratory ailments. Anise seeds are thought to increase breast milk production and may be beneficial in treating impotence and frigidity. Anise essential oil is used for similar complaints, and is also used externally to treat lice and scabies.

Research Anise essential oil has been shown to have significant antifungal activity, including against *Candida albicans*. A 2008 Iranian double-blind clinical trial that postmenopausal women taking an anise extract experienced a significant reduction in hot flash frequency and intensity.

Cautions Do not take anise essential oil internally except under professional supervision. Do not take anise during pregnancy, except in amounts normally used in cooking.

Self-help uses Acidity & indigestion, p. 317; Digestive upsets, gas, & colic, p. 328; Stomach spasm, p. 315; Gas & bloating, p. 316.

Pinguicula vulgaris (Lentibulariaceae)

Butterwort

Description Insectivorous perennial growing to 4 in (10 cm). Has fleshy leaves in a basal rosette and double-lipped, purple-blue flowers.

Habitat & cultivation Native to northern and western Europe, butterwort grows in moorland and on mountains. The leaves are gathered in midsummer.

Parts used Leaves.

Constituents Butterwort contains mucilage, tannins, benzoic acid, cinnamic acid, and valeric acid. Cinnamic acid has antispasmodic properties.

History & folklore Butterwort was much used in Welsh herbal medicine as a purgative. In Norway, the plant has been used to curdle reindeer milk, and medicinally, to treat wounds and ringworm.

Medicinal actions & uses Butterwort is little employed in European herbal medicine today. Its main use is as a cough remedy, with properties similar to those of sundew (*Drosera rotundifolia*, p. 208), another insect-eating plant. Butterwort may be used to treat chronic and convulsive coughs.

Related species The similar *P. grandiflora*, native to the Pyrenees, has been used as a purgative and to treat spasmodic coughs.

Caution Butterwort should only be taken under professional supervision.

Pinus sylvestris (Pinaceae)

Scots pine

Description Coniferous tree growing to 100 ft (30 m). Has reddish-brown bark, pairs of fine, needlelike leaves, yellowish buds in winter, and oval to conical cones.

Habitat & cultivation Native to mountainous regions of Europe and north and west Asia, Scots pine is now found throughout the northern hemisphere. The leaves are gathered in summer. The stems are usually harvested when the tree is felled.

Parts used Leaves, branches, stems, seeds, essential oil.

Constituents The leaves of Scots pine contain a volatile oil (consisting mainly of alpha-pinene), resin, and bitter principles.

History & folklore Pine oil is added to disinfectants and other preparations. The distilled resin produces turpentine.

Medicinal actions & uses Scots pine leaves, taken internally, have a mildly antiseptic effect within the chest, and may also be used for arthritic and rheumatic problems. Essential oil from the leaves may be taken for asthma, bronchitis, and other respiratory infections, and for digestive disorders such as gas. Scots pine branches and stems yield a thick resin, which is also antiseptic within the respiratory tract. The seeds yield an essential oil with diuretic and respiratory-stimulant properties.

Cautions Do not use Scots pine if prone to allergic skin reactions. Do not take the essential oil internally except under professional supervision.

Piper angustifolia (Piperaceae)

Matico

Description Perennial shrub reaching 23 ft (7 m). Has deeply veined aromatic lance-shaped leaves, spikes of tiny yellow flowers, and small black fruit.

Habitat & cultivation Matico is native to mountainous regions of Bolivia, Peru, and Ecuador. It is found in the wild and widely cultivated in these and other countries in tropical South America. The leaves are gathered throughout the year.

Parts used Leaves.

Constituents Matico contains a volatile oil (including camphor, borneol, and azulene), alkaloids, tannins, mucilage, and resins.

History & folklore Matico was and is used by Andean and Amazonian people as a wound-healing remedy and urinary antiseptic. European colonizers learned of it in the 19th century and it became an official drug in some South American pharmacopoeias.

Medicinal actions & uses Matico is an aromatic stimulant, diuretic and astringent used extensively for gastric and intestinal problems, including peptic ulcers, diarrhea, and dysentery. It is commonly used in South American herbal medicine for internal bleeding, particularly within the digestive tract—for example, rectal bleeding and hemorrhoids. It is also taken for bleeding in the urinary tract. Applied externally, a decoction of matico makes a valuable remedy for minor wounds, sore and inflamed skin, and insect bites and stings. The decoction may also be used as either a mouthwash or a douche.

Piper betle (Piperaceae)

Betel

Description Slender climbing vine growing to 16 ft (5 m). Has heart-shaped leaves, tiny yellow-green flowers, and small spherical fruit.

Habitat & cultivation Betel is native to Malaysia and southern India. It is widely cultivated in much of southern Asia, East Africa and Madagascar, and the Caribbean. The leaves are gathered throughout the year and dried for extracts or to use whole.

Parts used Leaves, root, fruit.

Constituents Betel leaves contain up to 1% volatile oil (including cadinene, chavicol, chavibetol and cineole). As with many volatile oils, the percentages are variable. Malaysian samples have been shown to contain up to 69% chavibetol.

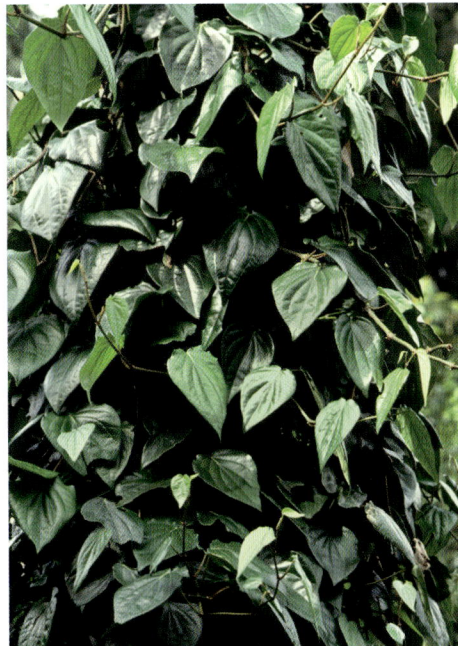

Betel leaves, traditionally chewed with areca nut and lime, give a mild sensation of well-being.

History & folklore Betel leaves, wrapped around areca nut (*Areca catechu*) and lime (*Citrus aurantiifolia*), are known to have been chewed in India and Southeast Asia for several thousand years. Betel leaves are described in the *Mahavasama*, the most ancient Sri Lankan text. Chewing quickly produces a red-stained saliva and does not, despite what is commonly thought, lead to blackened teeth. However, long-term use of betel leaves and areca nut is considered to increase the incidence of cancer of the mouth and tongue.

Medicinal actions & uses Betel leaves are chiefly used as a gentle stimulant, since they apparently induce a mild sensation of well-being. They also affect the digestive system, stimulating salivary secretions, relieving flatulence, and preventing worm infestation. In many Asian traditions, including Ayurvedic medicine, betel leaves are thought to have aphrodisiac and nerve tonic properties. In Chinese herbal medicine, betel root, leaves, and fruit are sometimes used as a mild tonic and stomach-settling herb. The root has been used with black pepper (*P. nigrum*, p. 258) or jequirity (*Abrus precatorius*, p. 162) to produce sterility in women.

Caution The observed increase in the occurrence of oral cancers in regular users makes it unwise to chew betel.

Piper cubeba (Piperaceae)

Cubeb

Description Climbing evergreen perennial growing to 20 ft (6 m). Has oval to oblong leaves, small flowers forming spikes, and round brown fruit.

Habitat & cultivation Native to Indonesia, cubeb is cultivated in much of tropical Asia, especially in the shade of coffee bushes (*Coffea arabica*, p. 196). The fruit is gathered when immature.

Part used Fruit.

Constituents Cubeb contains a volatile oil (up to 20%), a bitter principle (cubebin), an alkaloid (piperidine), resin, and fixed oil.

Medicinal actions & uses Like other members of the pepper family, cubeb has a significant antiflatulent and antiseptic action. The fruit is used medicinally as a means to counter infections of the urinary tract, and has been taken in the past as a treatment for gonorrhea. In addition, the fruit is helpful in relieving digestive problems such as flatulence and bloating. Cubeb is occasionally employed as an expectorant in the treatment of chronic bronchitis.

Cautions Cubeb should not be taken by people suffering from kidney disease or inflammatory conditions of the digestive tract.

Piper nigrum (Piperaceae)

Pepper

Description Perennial woody climber growing to about 16 ft (5 m). Has large oval leaves, spikes of small white flowers, and clusters of small round fruits, which ripen from green to red.

Habitat & cultivation Native to southwestern India, pepper is now cultivated in tropical areas around the world. The fruit is harvested from plants that are at least 3 years old. Green peppercorns are picked unripe and pickled, black peppercorns are picked unripe and dried, red peppercorns are picked ripe and dried, and white peppercorns are picked ripe and soaked in water for 8 days before drying.

Parts used Fruit, essential oil.

Constituents Pepper contains a volatile oil (including beta-bisabolene, camphene, beta-caryophyllene, and many other terpenes and sesquiterpenes), up to 9% alkaloids (especially piperine, which is largely responsible for the herb's acrid taste), about 11% proteins, and small quantities of minerals.

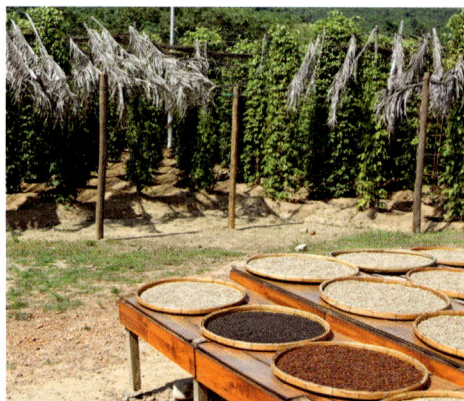

Pepper, here drying after the harvest, is still highly valued both medicinally and in cooking.

History & folklore Cultivated as a spice and a medicine since ancient times, pepper was a vital commodity in world trade for thousands of years. Attila the Hun is reputed to have demanded 3,000 lb (1,360 kg) of pepper as ransom during his siege of the city of Rome (408 CE).

Medicinal actions & uses The familiar sharp taste of pepper reflects the stimulant and antiseptic effect it has on the digestive tract and the circulatory system. Pepper is commonly taken to warm the body, or to improve digestive function in cases of nausea, stomachache, flatulence, bloating, constipation, or lack of appetite. The essential oil eases rheumatic pain and toothache. It is antiseptic and antibacterial, and reduces fever.

Research Piperine, the main active constituent within black pepper, has significant therapeutic benefits, with a 2012 research paper listing "immunomodulatory, antioxidant, anti-asthmatic, anticarcinogenic, anti-inflammatory, anti-ulcer and anti-amoebic properties." Piperine appears to aid the absorption of herbal and chemical medicines, e.g. curcumin (from turmeric, *Curcuma longa*, p. 94), and in some cases, to slow their clearance by the liver.

Caution Do not take the essential oil internally without professional supervision.

Self-help use Back pain, p. 323.

Piscidia erythrina (Fabaceae)

Jamaica dogwood

Description Deciduous tree or shrub growing to 49 ft (15 m). Compound leaves, blue to white flowers with red stripes, and winged seed pods.

Habitat & cultivation Jamaica dogwood is native to the southern US, Central America, northern South America, and the Caribbean. It is grown mainly for its wood, which is used in boat-building. The root bark is stripped when the tree is felled.

Part used Root bark.

Constituents Jamaica dogwood contains isoflavones, phytosterols, tannins, and organic acids. The isoflavones are antispasmodic.

History & folklore The pounded bark and twigs have been used by Indigenous Caribbean and Afro-Caribbean peoples to stupefy fish.

Medicinal actions & uses Jamaica dogwood is a useful and undervalued remedy that acts both as a sedative and as a painkiller. It is chiefly employed in the treatment of insomnia and overexcitability, as it calms mental activity. It is also prescribed for nerve pain, toothache, and period pain. As an antispasmodic, it is useful for treating muscle spasms, especially in the back, and spasmodic respiratory ailments such as asthma and whooping cough.

Cautions Do not take Jamaica dogwood during pregnancy or if you are suffering from cardiovascular problems.

Pistacia lentiscus (Anacardiaceae)

Mastic tree

Description Multi-branched perennial growing to 10 ft (3 m). Has small elliptical leathery leaves, clusters of reddish flowers, and round scarlet fruit that ripens to black.

Habitat & cultivation Mastic tree is native to the Mediterranean region. It grows wild in scrub and on waste ground and is cultivated for its resin, which is collected from incisions made in the bark in summer and fall.

Part used Resin.

Constituents The resin contains alpha- and beta-masticoresins, a volatile oil (comprising mainly alpha-pinene), tannins, masticin, and mastic acid. Pinenes are strongly antiseptic.

History & folklore Mastic resin was used by the ancient Egyptians for embalming the dead.

Medicinal actions & uses In the recent past, mastic resin was little used, but contemporary research indicates that this should be reconsidered. Traditionally mastic extracts have been taken for coughs and bronchitis, and applied to the skin for boils, sores, and ulcers. Recent studies point to the gum resin being useful in treating and preventing atheroma (fatty deposits in the arteries), to have antifungal and liver-protective activity, and to aid in conditions such as arthritis and gout.

Related species The pistachio nut is produced by *P. vera*, also native to the Mediterranean region.

Plantago major (Plantaginaceae)

Common plantain

Description Perennial plant growing to 10 in (25 cm). Has a basal rosette of broad, deeply veined leaves and dense clusters of tiny green flowers on spikes.

Habitat & cultivation Common plantain is native to Europe and temperate regions of Asia. Rarely cultivated, it is normally picked from the wild. The leaves are gathered throughout the summer.

Parts used Leaves.

Constituents Common plantain contains iridoids (such as aucubin), flavonoids (including apigenin), tannins, plant acids, and mucilage. Aucubin increases uric acid excretion by the kidneys; apigenin is anti-inflammatory.

History & folklore In Gaelic, this herb is known as "the healing plant" because it was used in Ireland to treat wounds and bruises. It is a plant that has accompanied European colonization around the world—some Indigenous American peoples called it Englishman's foot," because it seemed to spring up in the footsteps of white colonizers.

Medicinal actions & uses Common plantain quickly staunches blood flow and encourages the repair of damaged tissue. It is possible to use it as a substitute for comfrey (*Symphytum officinale*, p. 142) in treating bruises and broken bones. An ointment or lotion may be used to treat hemorrhoids, fistulas (abnormal passages in the skin), and ulcers. Taken internally, common plantain is diuretic,

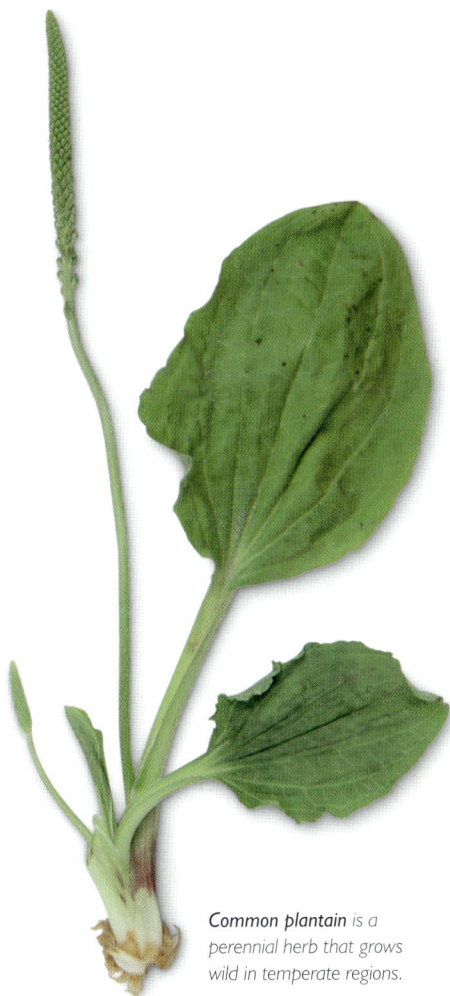

Common plantain is a perennial herb that grows wild in temperate regions.

expectorant, and anti-mucus. It is commonly prescribed for conditions including gastritis, peptic ulcers, diarrhea, dysentery, irritable bowel syndrome, respiratory inflammation, loss of voice, and urinary tract bleeding.

Research A 2021 clinical trial found that 2 g of plantain seed a day over a 12 week period led to a significant improvement in liver enzyme levels, and a reduction in waist circumference, in people with non-alcoholic fatty liver disease.

Related species Ribwort plantain (*P. lanceolata*) is used in the same way as common plantain. *Che qian cao* (*P. asiatica*) is used in Chinese medicine as a diuretic and to counter catarrh.

Self-help uses Allergic rhinitis with catarrh, p. 310; Diarrhea, p. 328.

Plumbago zeylanica (Plumbaginaceae)

Ceylon leadwort

Description Evergreen shrub, often a climber, growing to 16 ft (5 m). Has oval pointed leaves, spikes of 5-petaled white flowers, and angled seed capsules.

Habitat & cultivation Ceylon leadwort is native to southern India and Malaysia, and is now naturalized in much of Southeast Asia and in Africa. The leaves and root are gathered throughout the year.

Parts used Leaves, root.

Constituents Ceylon leadwort contains apthaquinones, including plumbagin, and phytosterols.

History & folklore In Africa, the juice of Ceylon leadwort is used as a tattoo dye.

Medicinal actions & uses Ceylon leadwort root is acrid and stimulates sweating, and is commonly used as a paste for skin infections such as ringworm and scabies. The paste is also applied as a counterirritant to relieve rheumatic aches and pains. In India, extracts of the leaves and root are taken for digestive infections such as dysentery. In Nepal, a decoction of the root is used to treat baldness.

Related species The root of European leadwort (*P. europaea*) has been used to treat toothache and, in the form of a poultice or plaster, back pain and sciatica.

Cautions Use only under professional supervision. Taken internally, the root may be toxic, and may induce abortion. Do not use Ceylon leadwort during pregnancy.

Podophyllum peltatum (Berberidaceae)

American mandrake

Description Perennial plant growing to 16 in (40 cm). Has a forked stem, two deeply lobed umbrella-like leaves, white flowers, and small yellow fruit.

Habitat & cultivation American mandrake is native to northeastern North America. It is commonly found in damp woodland and pastureland. The rhizome is unearthed in the fall.

Part used Rhizome.

Constituents The rhizome of American mandrake contains lignans (especially podophyllotoxin), flavonoids, resin, and gums. The lignans are responsible for the rhizome's purgative action.

History & folklore American mandrake was much used as a purgative, emetic, and worm-expelling herb by Indigenous American peoples. In the US in the 19th century, both herbal and conventional medical practitioners regarded the plant as the safest and most readily available purge.

Medicinal actions & uses Despite 19th-century beliefs in its safety, American mandrake is no longer taken internally on account of its cytotoxic (cell-killing) action. However, applied externally as a poultice, lotion, or ointment, the root can be an effective treatment for all kinds of warts.

Research The lignans in American mandrake—podophyllotoxin in particular—act against tumors and have been extensively researched for their anticancer potential. Semisynthetic derivatives of podophyllotoxin appear to be the most promising, having minimal toxicity.

Related species The Himalayan *P. hexandrum* may have similar actions.

Cautions Do not take internally. The plant is subject to legal restrictions in most countries.

Pogostemon cablin syn. *P. patchouli* (Lamiaceae)

Patchouli

Description Hairy, aromatic perennial growing to 3 ft (1 m). Has square stems, oval leaves, and spikes bearing whorls of white to light-purple flowers.

Habitat & cultivation Native to Malaysia and the Philippines, patchouli is now cultivated in tropical and subtropical regions around the world. The shoots and leaves are picked 2 or 3 times a year.

Parts used Young leaves and shoots, essential oil.

Constituents Patchouli contains a volatile oil comprising mainly the sesquiterpenes patchoulol (35%) and bulnesene.

History & folklore Patchouli has been used extensively in Asian medicine, featuring in the Chinese, Indian, and Arabic traditions. Its most common use has been as an aphrodisiac. The essential oil is widely employed in India as a fragrance and as an insect repellent.

Medicinal actions & uses Patchouli is used in herbal medicine in Asia as an aphrodisiac, antidepressant, and antiseptic. It is also employed for headaches and fever. Patchouli essential oil is used in

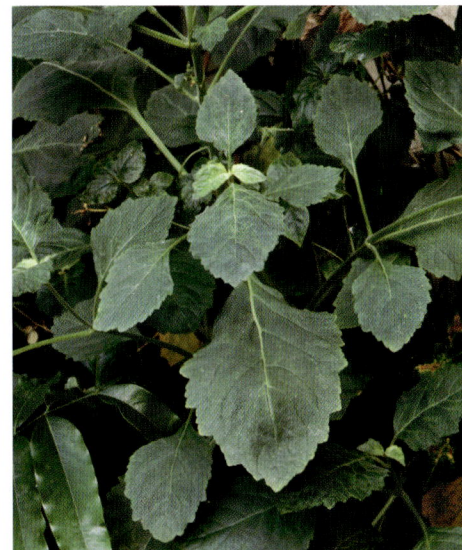

Patchouli is the source of an essential oil.

aromatherapy to treat skin complaints. It is thought to have a regenerative effect on skin tone and to help clear conditions such as eczema and acne. The oil may also be used for varicose veins and hemorrhoids.

Research A 2020 Korean study found that "inhalation of patchouli oil effectively reduced the levels of stress and increased compassion satisfaction in emergency nurses, suggesting that patchouli oil inhalation may improve the professional quality of life of emergency nurses."

Caution Do not take essential oil internally.

Polygala senega (Polygalaceae)

Seneca snakeroot

Description Perennial growing to about 16 in (40 cm). Has narrow lance-shaped leaves with toothed edges, and spikes of whitish-pink flowers.

Habitat & cultivation Seneca snakeroot is native to North America, and found in dry stony open ground and woodland. It is cultivated in western Canada. The root is unearthed in the fall.

Part used Root.

Constituents Seneca snakeroot contains phenolic acids, methyl salicylate, triterpenoid saponins (including sengins), polygalitol, and plant sterols. The triterpenoid saponins promote the clearing of phlegm from the bronchial tubes.

History & folklore This plant's name refers to the Seneca people of North America, who employed the root as a remedy for snake bite. Seneca snakeroot was highly valued as a medicine by both Indigenous peoples and European colonizers. In 1768, Dr. Alexander Garden of Charleston wrote that "The Seneka is the most powerful and efficacious antiphlogistic [fever- and inflammation-reducing substance] attenuant among the Galenical medicines."

Medicinal actions & uses In North American and European herbal medicine, Seneca snakeroot is used as an expectorant to treat bronchial asthma, chronic bronchitis, and whooping cough. The root has a stimulant action on the bronchial mucous membranes, promoting the coughing up of phlegm from the chest. Seneca snakeroot is also thought to encourage sweating and to stimulate the secretion of saliva.

Related species *Yuan zhi* (*P. tenuifolia*), native to China and Japan, has similar constituents. *Yuan zhi* is taken to treat congestion in the chest and to "calm the spirit and quieten the heart." See also milkwort (*P. vulgaris, following entry*).

Cautions Do not take if pregnant. Causes diarrhea and vomiting in excessive doses.

Polygala vulgaris (Polygalaceae)

Milkwort

Description Short perennial with pointed lance-shaped leaves and spikes of small blue, mauve, or white flowers.

Habitat & cultivation Milkwort is common in grassy and moorland areas in much of western and northern Europe. It is gathered from the wild when the plant is in flower in summer.

Parts used Aerial parts, root.

Constituents Milkwort contains triterpenoid saponins, a volatile oil, gaultherin, and mucilage.

History & Folklore Milkwort has been most often used to treat chest problems such as pleurisy and dry coughs. In larger doses, the plant acts as an emetic. In his Irish Herbal (1735), K'Eogh states that "it has a hot dry nature, and it encourages the production of milk in nursing mothers."

Medicinal Actions & Uses While milkwort is infrequently used in European herbal medicine today, it—like Seneca snakeroot (*P. senega*, see preceding entry)—is a valuable herb for the treatment of respiratory troubles such as chronic bronchitis, bronchial asthma, and convulsive coughs, including whooping cough. Milkwort is also thought to have sweat-inducing and diuretic properties.

Polygonatum multiflorum (Liliaceae)

Solomon's seal

Description Perennial growing to about 20 in (50 cm). Has arching stems, alternate elliptical leaves, delicate greenish-white, bell-shaped flowers, and blue-black fruit.

Habitat & cultivation Native to Europe and to temperate regions of Asia and North America, Solomon's seal is quite rare in the wild. However, it is a common ornamental garden plant. The rhizome is unearthed in the fall.

Part Used Rhizome.

Constituents Solomon's seal contains steroidal saponins (similar to diosgenin), flavonoids, and vitamin A.

History & Folklore Solomon's seal has been used in Western herbal medicine since classical times. In China, the herb's first recorded use stretches back to the *Divine Husbandman's Classic (Shen'nong Bencaojing)* of the 1st century CE. In North America, the species *P. biflorum* was known to various Indigenous peoples. The Penobscot people used Solomon's seal as part of a formula for treating gonorrhea.

Medicinal Actions & Uses Like arnica (*Arnica montana*, p. 176), Solomon's seal is believed to prevent excessive bruising and to stimulate tissue repair. The rhizome, which is mainly used in the form of a poultice, has astringent and demulcent actions that undoubtedly contribute to its ability to accelerate healing. Solomon's seal has also been recommended for tuberculosis, as a remedy for menstrual problems, and as a tonic. In Chinese herbal medicine, it is considered a *yin* tonic, and is thought to be particularly applicable to respiratory system problems—sore throats, dry and irritable coughs, bronchial congestion, and chest pain.

Related species Angular or scented Solomon's seal (*P. odoratum*) is used in much the same way as *P. multiflorum*.

Caution Do not take internally except under professional advice. The aerial parts, especially the berries, are harmful if eaten.

Polygonum aviculare (Polygonaceae)

Knotgrass, *Bian xu* (Chinese)

Description Annual creeper growing to 20 in (50 cm). Has lance-shaped leaves and clusters of small pink or white flowers.

Habitat & cultivation Knotgrass is found in temperate regions throughout the world. It thrives on waste ground and along shorelines. The plant is gathered throughout the summer.

Parts used Aerial parts.

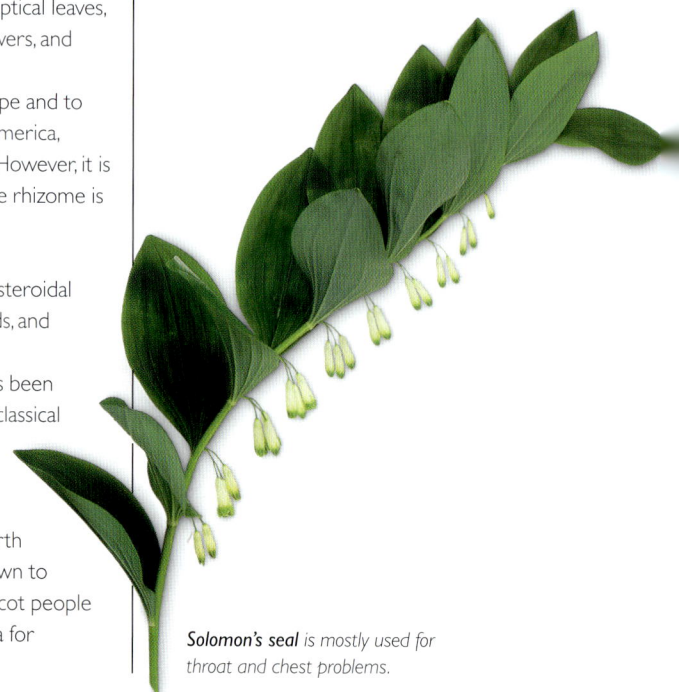

Solomon's seal is mostly used for throat and chest problems.

Constituents Knotgrass contains tannins, flavonoids, polyphenols, silicic acid (about 1%) and mucilage.

History & folklore Knotgrass has been used as a diuretic in Chinese herbal medicine for over 2,000 years. In the Western tradition, the 1st-century CE physician Dioscorides likewise considered knotgrass to be a diuretic, as well as a remedy for heavy menstrual bleeding and snake bite.

Medicinal actions & uses An herb with astringent and diuretic properties, knotgrass is used in European herbal medicine to treat many conditions—diarrhea and hemorrhoids, to expel worms, to staunch bleeding wounds, to reduce heavy menstrual flow, and to stop nosebleeds. Knotgrass is also taken for pulmonary complaints, since its silicic acid content strengthens connective tissue within the lungs. In Chinese medicine, it is given to expel tapeworm and hookworm, to treat diarrhea and dysentery, and as a diuretic, particularly when urination is painful.

Research Chinese research indicates that the plant is a useful medicine for bacillary dysentery. Of 108 people with this disease treated with a paste of knotgrass (taken internally), 104 recovered within 5 days. Results from Iranian laboratory studies indicate that knotgrass stimulates apoptosis (programmed cell death) and might be of use in treating breast cancer.

Related species See also bistort (*P. bistorta*, *following entry*), and *he shou wu* (*P. multiflorum*, p. 129).

Polygonum bistorta (Polygonaceae)

Bistort

Description Perennial growing to 12 in (30 cm). Has long basal leaves, dense spikes of small pink flowers, and dark nutlets.

Habitat & cultivation Native to Europe, Asia, and North America, bistort prefers damp conditions. The leaves are gathered in spring, the rhizome in the fall.

Parts used Leaves, rhizome.

Constituents Bistort contains polyphenols (including ellagic acid), tannins (15–20%), phlobaphenes, flavonoids, and a trace of the anthraquinone emodin.

History & folklore Bistort rhizomes have long been employed for their astringency. As the rhizomes also contain large amounts of starch, they have been steeped in water, roasted, and eaten as a vegetable in Russia and North America. In addition, the young, tender leaves of bistort may be used in salads or, alternatively, cooked in the same way as

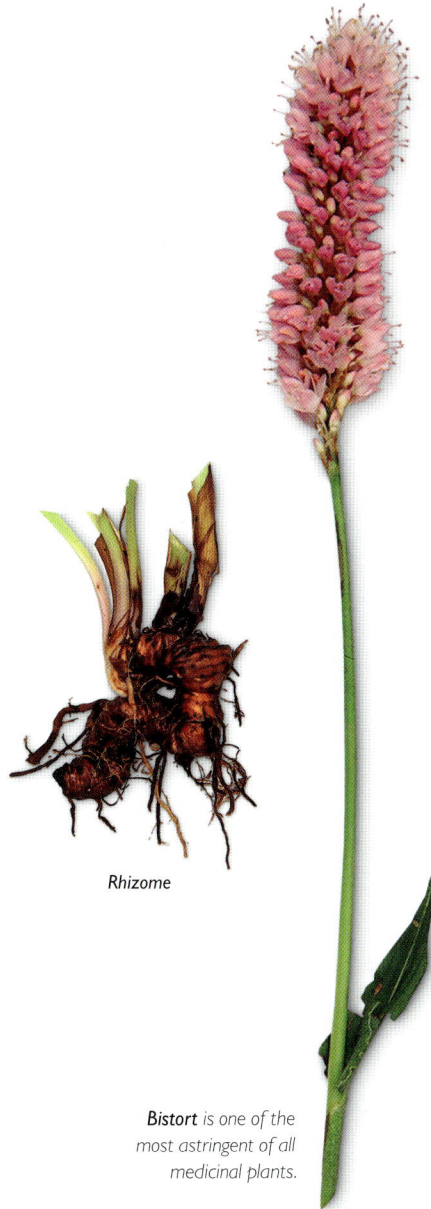

spinach (*Spinacia oleracea*).

Medicinal actions & uses One of the most strongly astringent of all herbs, bistort is used to contract tissues and staunch blood flow. It makes a valuable mouthwash and gargle for treating spongy gums, mouth ulcers, and sore throats, and is also useful as a wash for small burns and wounds, a douche for excessive vaginal discharge, and an ointment for hemorrhoids and anal fissures. Internally, bistort may be taken to treat peptic ulcers, ulcerative colitis, and conditions such as dysentery and irritable bowel that give rise to diarrhea.

Related species *P. hydropiper*, which is native to Europe, has traditionally been used to relieve heavy menstrual bleeding. See also knotgrass (*P. aviculare*, *preceding entry*).

Caution Use bistort internally for no more than 3–4 weeks at a time.

Self-help use Diarrhea, p. 317.

Rhizome

Bistort is one of the most astringent of all medicinal plants.

Polymnia uvedalia (Asteraceae)

Bearsfoot

Description Perennial herb growing to 6½ ft (2 m) with large 3-lobed leaves and yellow flowers.

Habitat & cultivation Bearsfoot is native to the eastern US. It grows from New York southward, preferring rich soil. The root is unearthed in the fall.

Part used Root.

History & folklore Bearsfoot root was used by Indigenous North American peoples as a stimulant and laxative remedy. In the 19th century, it became a widely popular healing herb in North America, having a specific use as a treatment for mastitis (inflammation of the breast tissue).

Medicinal actions & uses Bearsfoot is perhaps best known for its use as a hair tonic, having traditionally been a popular ingredient in hair lotions. It is still used in this way, but today the root is more often taken internally as a treatment for nonmalignant swollen glands and especially for mastitis. The root is thought to have a beneficial effect on the stomach, liver, and spleen, and may be taken to relieve indigestion and counteract liver malfunction.

Polypodium vulgare (Polypodiaceae)

Polypody

Description Delicate perennial fern growing to a height of 1 ft (30 cm). Has slender knotty rhizomes and curving fronds that are dotted with brown spores (sori) on their lower surface.

Habitat & cultivation Native to Europe and northern Asia, polypody is commonly found growing in damp woodland and hedgerows, and on walls. The rhizome is unearthed in the fall.

Part used Rhizome.

Constituents Polypody rhizome contains saponins (based on polypodosapogenin), ecdysteroids, phloroglucins, volatile oil, fixed oil, and tannins.

History & folklore Polypody has been used medicinally in Europe since ancient times. Like mistletoe (*Viscum album*, p. 292), polypody often grows on host trees, for example oak (*Quercus robur*, p. 268). This was thought to impart great medicinal value to the plant. The Greek physician Dioscorides, writing in the 1st century CE, noted that polypody was used to purge phlegm and was an ingredient of a plaster applied to dislocated fingers and to sores that occur between the fingers.

Medicinal actions & uses Polypody stimulates bile secretion and has been used to treat such conditions

261

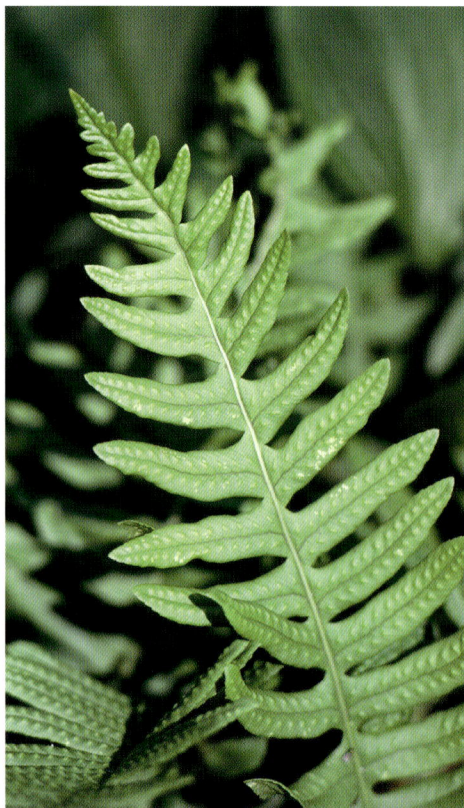

Polypody is often seen growing in damp woodland in Europe and northern Asia.

as hepatitis, jaundice and indigestion. A gentle laxative, polypody makes a safe treatment for constipation in children. The rhizome is also expectorant, having a supportive and mildly stimulating effect on the respiratory system. It may be taken for the relief of catarrh, bronchitis, pleurisy, and dry irritable coughs.

Caution Polypody may cause a skin rash when applied externally.

Pomaderris kumeraho (Rhamnaceae)

Kumarhou

Description Branching tree growing to about 10 ft (3 m). Has shiny leaves and clusters of yellow-white flowers.

Habitat & cultivation Kumarhou is native to New Zealand.

Parts used Aerial parts.

Medicinal actions & uses Kumarhou is a traditional Māori remedy that has been used to treat a wide range of illnesses. Its most common use is as a remedy for problems of the respiratory tract, such as asthma and bronchitis. However, it has also been used in the treatment of indigestion and heartburn,

diabetes, and kidney problems. Kumarhou is considered a detoxifier and "blood cleansing" plant. It is used to treat skin rashes and sores, including lesions produced by skin cancer.

Populus x candicans syn. *P. x gileadensis* (Salicaceae)

Balm of Gilead

Description Deciduous tree growing to 80 ft (25 m). Has heart-shaped leaves, buds producing a sticky resin, and female catkins.

Habitat & cultivation Naturalized in northern temperate regions, balm of Gilead is also cultivated as an ornamental tree. The buds and bark from young branches are collected in spring.

Parts used Buds, stem bark.

Constituents Balm of Gilead buds contain flavonoids, phenolic glycosides (including salicin), and fatty acids. Salicin's analgesic, anti-inflammatory, and fever-reducing actions resemble those of aspirin. Many poplars have a similar chemical profile and are often used interchangeably as medicines.

History & folklore Balm of Gilead has been used for several thousand years to soothe inflamed or irritated skin. The 17th-century herbalist Nicholas Culpeper recorded that "The oyntment called populeon, which is much of this poplar, is singular for all heat and inflammation in any part of the body and tempereth the heat of wounds: It is much used to dry up the milk in women's breasts."

Medicinal actions & uses Balm of Gilead is a common ingredient of cough mixtures. Its expectorant, antiseptic, and analgesic properties make it an excellent remedy for sore throats, dry irritable coughs, bronchitis, and other respiratory ailments. In France and Germany, balm of Gilead is applied as a salve to scrapes, small wounds, chapped and itchy skin, sunburn, chilblains, and hemorrhoids. A preparation of balm of Gilead, applied externally, may also help relieve the pain of rheumatic joints and strained muscles. Culpeper noted the plant is also thought to reduce breast milk production.

Research Studies have demonstrated that balm of Gilead buds have significant expectorant, antibacterial, antifungal, and anti-inflammatory properties. Research into the bud resin of this and other poplar species has been prompted largely by the resin's chemical similarity to propolis, a natural antibiotic resin that is gathered by bees.

Cautions Best avoided while breastfeeding. Do not take if allergic to aspirin.

Self-help use Coughs, p. 320.

Populus tremuloides (Salicaceae)

Quaking aspen

Description Deciduous, spreading tree growing to 65 ft (20 m). Has oval, slightly sticky buds and round, finely toothed leaves that quiver in the wind.

Habitat & cultivation Native to North America, quaking aspen prefers damp and moist areas, and grows alongside rivers and in valleys, hedgerows, and groves. It is also widely cultivated in temperate regions. The bark is collected in early spring.

Part used Bark.

Constituents The bark contains phenolic glycosides (including salicin and populin) and tannins. Salicin and populin are salicylates, substances that have fever-reducing, pain-relieving, and anti-inflammatory properties that are similar to those of aspirin.

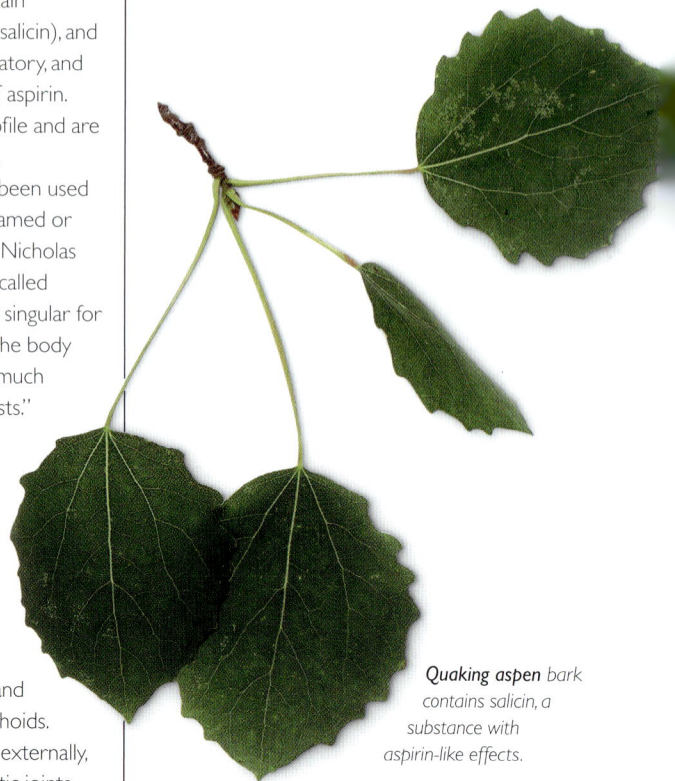

Quaking aspen bark contains salicin, a substance with aspirin-like effects.

History & folklore The Ojibwa people used an oily compound made from quaking aspen and bear fat to treat earache. Other Indigenous American peoples used the bark for a variety of purposes, including as an eyewash for sore eyes.

Medicinal actions & uses Like willow bark (Salix alba, p. 133), quaking aspen bark has widely recognized anti-inflammatory and pain-relieving properties. It is often taken to treat arthritic and rheumatic aches and pains. It is also used to lower fever, especially when this condition is associated with rheumatoid arthritis. Being stimulant, quaking aspen bark acts as a tonic remedy in the treatment of anorexia and other debilitated states. The bark's significant astringent and antiseptic qualities make it useful for treating diarrhea and the symptoms of irritable bowel syndrome. It is also used to treat urinary tract infections.

Caution Do not take quaking aspen if sensitive or allergic to aspirin.

Portulaca oleracea (Portulacaceae)

Purslane

Description Succulent annual plant growing to 6 in (15 cm). Has small, thick rounded leaves and small yellow flowers growing in clusters.

Habitat & cultivation Native to Europe and Asia, purslane is now one of the most widely distributed plants, growing from Australia and China to the Americas. Often found growing near water, it is gathered throughout the summer. Wild purslane is the variety chiefly used as a medicine; the golden variety, *P. oleracea* var. *sativa*, is cultivated mostly as a kitchen potherb.

Parts used Aerial parts.

Constituents Purslane contains flavonoids, alkaloids, fatty acids (including omega-3 oils). terpenoids, polysaccharides, vitamins A, B₁, and C, proteins, and minerals (especially calcium). It is one of the richest vegetable sources of omega-3 essential fatty acids, with significant levels of alpha-linolenic, gamma-linolenic and linoleic acids.

History & folklore Purslane's use as a medicinal herb in Europe, Iran, and India dates back at least 2,000 years, and it was probably eaten as a vegetable well before then. In ancient Rome, purslane was used to treat headaches, stomach ache and dysentery, intestinal worms, and lizard bite.

Medicinal actions & uses Purslane has long been considered valuable in the treatment of urinary and digestive problems. The diuretic effect of the juice makes it useful in the alleviation of bladder ailments, for example difficulty in passing urine. The plant's mucilaginous properties also make it a soothing remedy for gastrointestinal problems such as dysentery and diarrhea. In Chinese herbal medicine, purslane is employed for similar problems and, additionally, for appendicitis. The Chinese also use the plant as an antidote for wasp stings and snake bite. Used as an external wash, the juice or a decoction relieves skin ailments such as boils and carbuncles, and also helps to reduce fever.

Research Purslane is being intensively researched. Extracts of the herb show antioxidant, anti-inflammatory, analgesic, and antidiabetic activity,

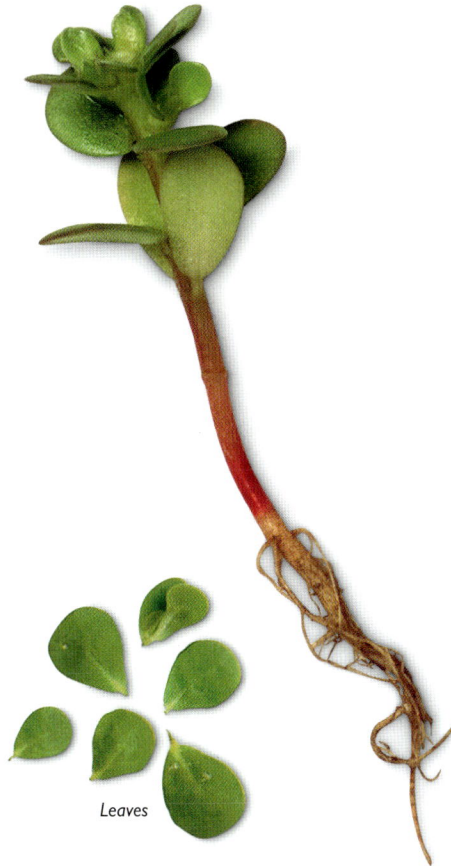

Leaves

Purslane *is a good source of vitamins and calcium. It also has antibiotic properties.*

underlining that fact that purslane is valuable as food and as medicine. The alkaloids have neuroprotective activity and inhibit acetylcholinesterase, making the herb theoretically useful in neurodegenerative conditions such as Parkinson's and Alzheimer's disease.

Caution Purslane should not be taken as a medicine during pregnancy.

Potentilla anserina (Rosaceae)

Silverweed

Description Perennial plant growing to 16 in (40 cm). Has toothed compound leaves that are silvery on the underside, and 5-petaled yellow flowers.

Habitat & cultivation Silverweed is found in Europe, Asia, and North America, where it flourishes in dry grassy places. The aerial parts are collected in late summer, the root at the same time or in the fall.

Parts used Aerial parts, root.

Constituents Silverweed contains 2–10% ellagitannins, flavonoids, choline and bitters.

History & folklore William Withering, the 18th-century doctor who discovered the cardiotonic effects of foxglove (*Digitalis purpurea*,

p. 207), recommended a teaspoon of dried leaves to be taken at 3-hour intervals to assuage bouts of malarial fever.

Medicinal actions & uses Silverweed's main medicinal value lies in its astringent and anti-inflammatory activity. It makes an effective gargle for sore throats, and is a helpful remedy for diarrhea. Less astringent than its close relative tormentil (*P. erecta*, see *following entry*), it also has a gentler action within the gastrointestinal tract. It is used externally as a lotion or ointment for bleeding hemorrhoids.

Caution Use internally for more no more than 3–4 weeks at a time.

Potentilla erecta syn. *P. tormentilla* (Rosaceae)

Tormentil

Description Downy creeping perennial growing to 4 in (10 cm). Has leaves bearing 5 leaflets, and many 4-petaled yellow flowers.

Habitat & cultivation Native to temperate regions of Asia and Europe, tormentil thrives in grassy sites and on heaths and moorland. The aerial parts of tormentil are harvested in summer and the root is gathered in the fall.

Parts used Aerial parts, root.

Constituents Tormentil contains 15–20% tannins, catechins, ellagitannins, and a phlobaphene.

History & folklore According to the 17th-century herbalist Nicholas Culpeper, the herb "is most excellent to stay all kinds of fluxes of blood or humours in man or woman, whether it be at nose, mouth, belly, or any wound in the veins or elsewhere."

Medicinal actions & uses Containing even more tannins than oak bark (*Quercus robur*, p. 268), all parts of tormentil are strongly astringent, finding use wherever this action is required. The plant makes a beneficial gargle for throat infections, and an effective mouthwash for treating mouth ulcers and infected gums. Tormentil may be taken for conditions that give rise to diarrhea, such as irritable bowel syndrome, colitis, ulcerative colitis, and dysentery, and for rectal bleeding. Applied externally as a lotion or ointment, tormentil helps relieve hemorrhoids (especially those that are bleeding). In the form of a lotion, tormentil is used to help staunch wounds and protect areas of damaged or burned skin.

Caution Use internally for more no more than 3–4 weeks at a time.

Research Recent studies suggest that while Tormentil root acts to staunch bleeding and promote tissue repair—in line with traditional use, it also has an antithrombotic effect (prevents blood clot formation) similar in strength to aspirin.

Primula veris (Primulaceae)

Cowslip, Primula

Description Hairy perennial growing to 4 in (10 cm). Has a basal rosette of slightly rough oblong leaves. Stems bear clusters of bright yellow, bell-shaped flowers.

Habitat & cultivation Cowslip grows in Europe and western Asia, preferring fields and pastures with chalky soils. The flowers and leaves are gathered in spring and summer, the root in the fall. This increasingly rare plant should not be picked from the wild.

Parts used Flowers, leaves, root.

Constituents Cowslip contains triterpenoid saponins, flavonoids, phenols, tannins, and a trace of volatile oil. The flavonoids, mainly in the flowers, are antioxidant, anti-inflammatory and antispasmodic. The triterpenoid saponins, which are concentrated in the root (5–10%), are strongly expectorant.

History & folklore This plant is so closely associated with springtime that it is known as primavera (spring) in Spanish and Italian. Cowslip has long been reputed to preserve beauty. The 16th-century herbalist William Turner wrote:"Some weomen … sprinkle ye floures of cowslip with whyte wine and after … wash their faces with that water to … make them fayre in the eyes of the worlde rather than in the eyes of God, whom they are not afryd to offend."

Medicinal actions & uses Cowslip is an underused but valuable plant. The root is strongly expectorant, stimulating a more liquid mucus and so easing the clearance of phlegm. It is given for chronic coughs, especially those associated with chronic bronchitis and mucus congestion. The root is also thought to be mildly diuretic and antirheumatic and to slow blood clotting. The leaves have similar properties to the root, but are weaker in action. The flowers are believed to be sedative and are recommended for overactivity and sleeplessness, particularly in children. Cowslip flowers' antispasmodic and anti-inflammatory properties make them potentially useful in the treatment of asthma and other allergic conditions.

Cautions Do not take cowslip during pregnancy, if allergic to aspirin or if taking anticoagulant medication. Excessive doses can cause vomiting and diarrhea.

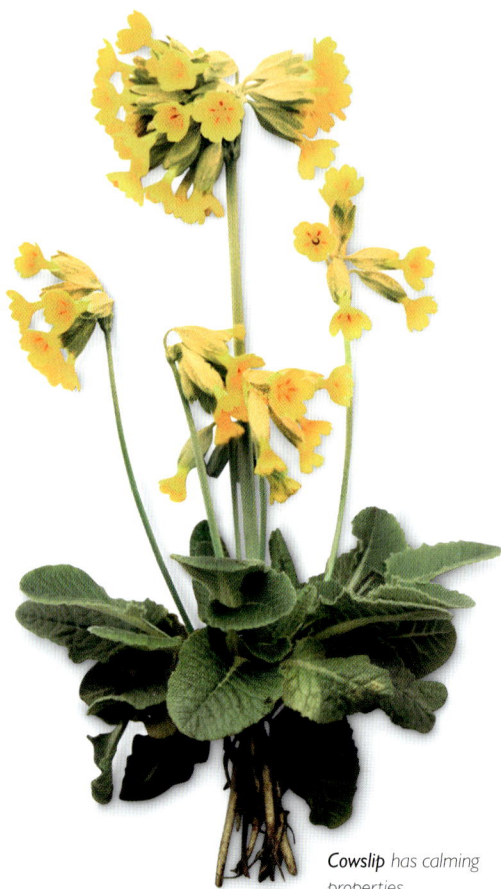

Cowslip has calming properties.

Prunella vulgaris (Lamiaceae)

Self-heal

Description Creeping perennial, growing to 20 in (50 cm) tall, with pointed oval leaves and violet-blue or pink flowers.

Habitat & cultivation Native to Europe and Asia, self-heal can be found in temperate regions worldwide. It is a wayside plant, growing in meadows and by roadsides, and thrives in sunny areas. Rarely cultivated, self-heal can easily be grown from seed or by root division. The aerial parts are picked in summer when in flower.

Parts used Aerial parts.

Constituents Self-heal contains entacyclic triterpenes, tannins, caffeic and rosmarinic acids, and vitamins B_1, C, and K.

History & folklore As its name indicates, self-heal has been used for centuries to staunch bleeding and heal wounds. The 17th-century herbalist John Gerard wrote:"there is not a better wounde herbe in the world than that of selfe-heale."

Medicinal actions & uses Self-heal is an undervalued astringent and wound-healer with tonic activity. In common with other members of the mint family, such as rosemary (*Rosmarinus officinalis*, p. 132) and sage (*Salvia* spp., p. 135), it has powerful antioxidant and tissue-protective activity—making it potentially of value in many chronic illnesses. Its antioxidant and astringent activity makes it beneficial in conditions such as sore throat, inflammatory bowel disease, and diarrhea, and to heal internal bleeding. Externally, a lotion can be applied to treat leukorrhea (vaginal discharge). In Chinese medicine, self-heal is taken with *ju hua* (*Chrysanthemum* × *morifolium*, p. 83) for fevers, headaches, dizziness, and vertigo, and is thought to cool "liver fire."

Research Several clinical trials have studied the effect of a combination of self-heal and thyroxine (a thyroid hormone) in the treatment of thyroid disease. Lower levels of thyroxine were required for effective treatment, with a reduced frequency of side effects. Thyroid nodules, where present, were reduced in size.

Prunus armeniaca (Rosaceae)

Apricot

Description Sturdy deciduous tree growing to 33 ft (10 m). Has finely serrated oval leaves, clusters of white (or, rarely, pink) 5-petaled flowers, and lightly freckled pale yellow to deep purple fruits.

Habitat & cultivation Native to China and Japan, apricot is now cultivated in Asia, North Africa, and California. The fruit is collected when ripe in late summer.

Parts used Fruit, seeds, bark.

Constituents Apricot fruit contains fruit sugars, vitamins, and iron. The seeds contain up to 8% amygdalin, the cyanogenic glycoside that yields laetrile and hydrocyanic (prussic) acid. The bark contains tannins.

History & folklore In India and China, the apricot has been appreciated for well over 2,000 years. Dong Feng, a physician who practiced at the end of the 2nd century CE, is said to have asked for his payment in apricot trees.

Medicinal actions & uses Apricot fruit is nutritious, cleansing, and mildly laxative. A decoction of the astringent bark soothes inflamed and irritated skin conditions. Though the seeds contain highly toxic prussic acid, they are prescribed in small amounts in the Chinese tradition as a treatment for coughs, asthma, and wheezing, and for excessive mucus production and constipation. An extract from the seeds, laetrile, has been used in Western medicine as a controversial (and illegal in the US) treatment for cancer. The seeds also yield a fixed oil, similar to almond oil (from P. amygdalus), that is often used in the formulation of cosmetics.

Research Chinese trials show that apricot seed paste helps combat vaginal infection.

Caution Apricot seeds are highly toxic in all but the smallest amounts and should not be consumed.

Prunus avium & P. cerasus (Rosaceae)

Sweet cherry, & Sour cherry

Description Deciduous shrub or tree growing to 26 ft (8 m). It has reddish-brown bark, oval to elliptical leaves, clusters of 2–6 white flowers, and almost spherical red fruit.

Habitat & cultivation Native to southwestern Asia, cherry is naturalized in Europe and cultivated in temperate regions around the world. The stems and ripe fruit are collected in summer.

Parts used Stems, fruit.

Constituents Cherry stems contain phenols, including salicylic acid, and tannins. Cherry fruit contains anthocyanins and flavonoids, including quercetin, carotenoids, sugars, fruit acids, vitamin C, and melatonin.

History & folklore The 16th-century herbalist John Gerard recorded the French custom of hanging cherries in houses to ward off fever.

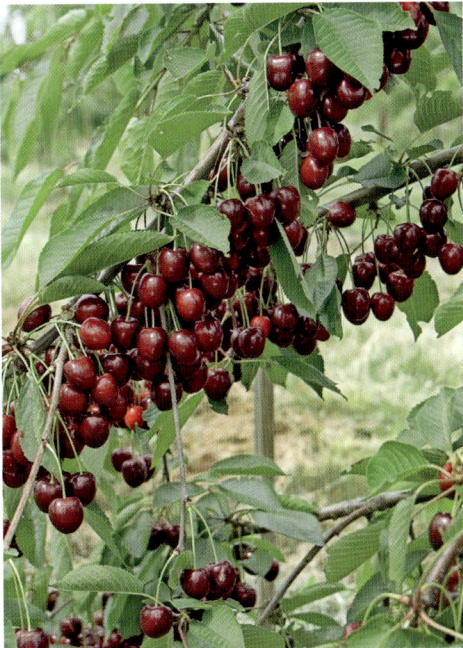

Sweet cherry fruit and stems have been harvested for medicinal use since classical times.

Medicinal actions & uses In European herbal medicine, cherries and cherry stems have long been used for their diuretic and astringent properties. They have been prescribed for cystitis, nephritis, and urinary retention, and for arthritic problems, notably gout. Cherries and cherry juice can be useful in treating gout and arthritic problems. Their fruit sugar content makes them mildly laxative.

Research In a 2012 American-Australian clinical study involving 633 people with gout, the risk of an acute gout attack was reduced by 35% for those taking cherry extract. One laboratory study concluded that the anti-inflammatory activities of anthocyanins within cherry fruit are comparable to those of ibuprofen.

Caution The seeds are toxic and should not be consumed.

Prunus mume (Rosaceae)

Asian plum, *Wu mei* (Chinese)

Description Deciduous tree growing to 33 ft (10 m). Has pointed oval to elliptical leaves, white flowers, and yellow fruit.

Habitat & cultivation Native to China, Asian plum grows wild and is planted in the southern and eastern provinces. The fruit is picked in late spring.

Part used Fruit.

Constituents Asian plum contains fruit acids and sugars, vitamin C and plant sterols.

Medicinal actions & uses The sour-tasting astringent Asian plum is used in Chinese medicine to counter diarrhea and dysentery, to stop bleeding, and to ease coughs. It may also be effective in expelling hookworms. Externally, a plaster of the fruit is applied to the sites of removed corns and warts to hasten healing.

Research Laboratory research undertaken in China indicates that the fruit of Asian plum has antibiotic properties.

Prunus serotina (Rosaceae)

Wild cherry

Description Deciduous tree growing to 100 ft (30 m). Has elliptical to oblong leaves, white flowers, and purple-black fruit.

Habitat & cultivation Native to North America, wild cherry grows throughout much of the US. It is cultivated in central Europe for its timber. The bark is collected in late summer and early fall.

Part used Inner bark.

Constituents Wild cherry contains prunasin (a cyanogenic glycoside that yields hydrocyanic acid), benzaldehyde, eudesmic acid, coumarins and tannins. Prunasin reduces the cough reflex.

History & folklore Cherokee women traditionally took wild cherry bark to ease labor pain. Other

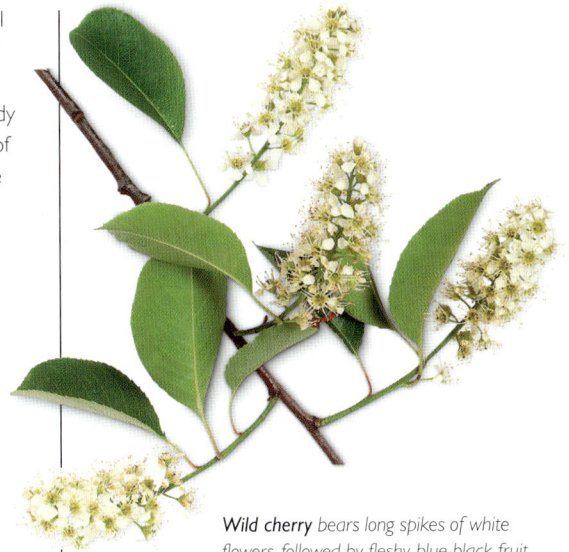

Wild cherry bears long spikes of white flowers, followed by fleshy, blue-black fruit.

indigenous American peoples used it in the treatment of coughs and colds, hemorrhoids, and diarrhea. European colonizers learned of the bark's medicinal properties, and in the 19th century it became a widely used remedy.

Medicinal actions & uses Figuring in official pharmacopoeias and much used in the Anglo-American tradition, wild cherry bark is an effective remedy for chronic dry and irritable coughs. It combines well with mullein (Verbascum thapsus, p. 291) as a treatment for asthma and whooping cough. The astringent bark also helps treat indigestion and the symptoms of irritable bowel syndrome, especially when these conditions are of nervous origin.

Caution Wild cherry bark is highly toxic in excessive doses.

Psoralea corylifolia (Fabaceae)

Bu gu zhi

Description Perennial growing to 3 ft (90 cm). Has oval leaves, yellow cloverlike flowers, and black seed pods containing yellow-black seeds.

Habitat & cultivation *Bu gu zhi* is native to southern and southeastern Asia and cultivated in China. The fruit is gathered when ripe in the fall.

Parts used Seeds.

Constituents The seeds contain a volatile oil, flavonoids, a flavone and furanocoumarins.

History & folklore In the Chinese tradition, *bu gu zhi* has long been considered a tonic remedy. It was first documented in *Grandfather Lei's Discussion of Herb Preparations*, which was written in about 490 CE.

Medicinal actions & uses Valued as a *yang* tonic, *bu gu zhi* is taken in China to treat impotence and premature ejaculation and to improve vitality. The seeds are also used to counter debility and other problems reflecting "kidney *yang* deficiency," such as lower back pain, frequent urination, incontinence, and bed-wetting. *Bu gu zhi* is used externally to treat skin conditions such as psoriasis, alopecia (loss of hair), and vitiligo (loss of skin pigmentation). In Vietnam, a tincture of the seeds is used in the treatment of rheumatism.

Research Studies in China indicate that this herb is of value in the treatment of skin disorders, including vitiligo.

Caution Applied externally, this herb may sensitize the skin, resulting in an allergic reaction to sunlight.

Pterocarpus marsupium (Fabaceae)

Kino

Description Handsome deciduous tree growing to 52 ft (16 m). Has leaves with 5–7 oval leathery leaflets, and numerous small yellow or white flowers.

Habitat & cultivation Native to Sri Lanka, India, Malaysia and the Philippines, kino grows in tropical rainforests. The tree is cultivated for its timber and for the sap ("kino") that exudes from cuts made in the trunk. The sap is collected year round.

Part used Sap.

Constituents Kino contains tannins, flavonoids and marsupsin.

Medicinal actions & uses Kino is a strongly astringent herb that tightens the mucous membranes of the gastrointestinal tract. Kino relieves chronic diarrhea and the irritation caused by intestinal infection and colitis. Though its taste is unpleasant, this herb makes a good mouthwash and gargle. It is widely used in Asia as a douche for excessive vaginal discharge.

Research Clinical trials have found that the herb is therapeutically useful in treating the early stages of non-insulin-dependent diabetes.

Ptychopetalum olacoides syn. *P. uncinatum* (Oleaceae)

Muira puama

Description Tree growing to 49 ft (15 m) with a gray trunk, dark brown leaves, white flowers, and orange-yellow fruits.

Habitat & cultivation Muira puama is native to Brazilian rainforests, especially the Rio Negro and Amazonas regions.

Part used Root, bark, wood.

Constituents Muira puama contains esters and plant sterols.

Medicinal actions & uses Muira puama has long been used in Amazonian medicine as a tonic and aphrodisiac. Considered useful as an aid for impotence, it is thought to help with both physical and psychological aspects of the problem. It is also used to treat or prevent baldness. The bark is strongly astringent and is employed as a gargle for sore throats and taken in the form of an infusion in order to treat diarrhea and dysentery.

Related species *Liriosma ovata*, another Brazilian tree, is also known as muira puama, but has quite distinct chemical constituents.

Pueraria montana var. *lobata* (Fabaceae)

Kudzu,
Ge gen (Chinese)

Description Deciduous climber growing to 100 ft (30 m). Has leaves with 3 broadly oval leaflets, curling tendrils, and spikes of pea-type purple flowers.

Habitat & cultivation Native to China, Japan, and eastern Asia, kudzu is naturalized in the US. It is cultivated in the central and eastern provinces of China. The root is unearthed in spring or fall.

Parts used Root, flower.

Constituents Kudzu contains triterpenoid saponins, isoflavones, and phytosterols. The isoflavones are estrogenic.

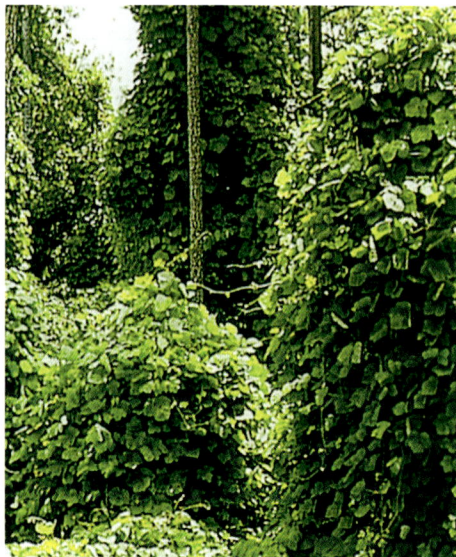

Kudzu is used in China to treat alcoholism and is an ingredient in a remedy for hangovers.

History & folklore From the 6th century BCE onward, Chinese herbalists have considered kudzu to be a remedy for muscular pain and a treatment for measles. Zhang Zhongjing (150–c.219 CE) recommended kudzu if the patient "has a stiff back and muscles, does not breathe easily, and is susceptible to wind." Kudzu leaves, buds, and sprouts have been consumed as a vegetable in Korea.

Medicinal actions & uses In China, kudzu is frequently used as a remedy for measles, often in combination with *sheng ma* (*Cimicifuga foetida*). Kudzu is also given for muscle aches and pains, especially when they are linked with fever or are affecting the neck and upper back. The root may be taken to treat symptoms of headache, dizziness, or numbness caused by high blood pressure. Kudzu also treats diarrhea and dysentery. Kudzu flowers are traditionally taken to treat alcohol intoxication and hangovers, and are thought to increase the rate of clearance of alcohol from the body, aiding recovery from intoxication. Kudzu root, however, is thought to act in a more or less opposite way—it slows the liver's ability to break down (and clear) alcohol from the system. Kudzu root may therefore increase the risks associated with alcohol consumption, and should not be taken as a "hangover cure."

Research Chinese studies indicate that kudzu increases cerebral blood flow in patients with arteriosclerosis, and eases neck pain and stiffness. US research indicates that kudzu may suppress the desire for alcohol.

Related species The closely related *P. mirifica* and *P. tuberosa* have been investigated for their contraceptive effect. Kudzu appears to protect the skin from sun induced ultraviolet radiation.

Pulmonaria officinalis (Boraginaceae)

Lungwort

Description Perennial growing to 1 ft (30 cm). Has broad oval basal leaves, smaller upper leaves mottled with white spots, and clusters of pink-purple flowers.

Habitat & cultivation Lungwort is native to Europe and the Caucasus. It flourishes in mountain pastures and in damp sites. The leaves are gathered in late spring.

Parts used Leaves.

Constituents Lungwort contains allantoin, flavonoids, tannins, mucilage, and saponins. Pyrrolizidine alkaloids occur in the roots, but in negligible quantities in the leaves.

History & folklore According to the medieval Doctrine of Signatures, which held that a plant's appearance pointed to the ailment it treated, lungwort was effective for chest ailments because its

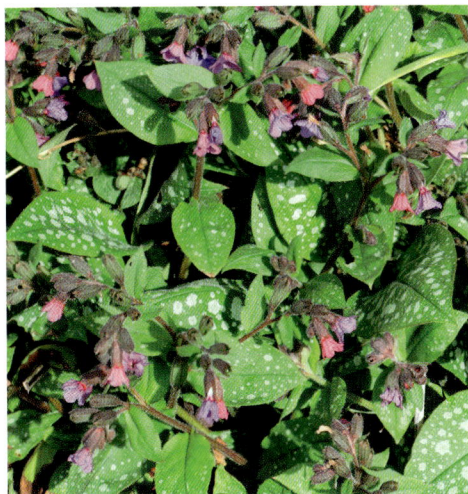

Lungwort's speckled leaves were once considered a sign of its ability to cure lung problems.

leaves were said to resemble lung tissue.

Medicinal actions & uses Given its high mucilage content, lungwort is considered a useful remedy for chest conditions, and it is particularly beneficial in cases of chronic bronchitis. It combines well with herbs such as mullein (Verbascum thapsus, p. 291) as a treatment for chronic coughs (including whooping cough), and it can be taken for asthma. Lungwort can also be used as a treatment for sore throats and congestion. In the past, lungwort was given for the coughing up of blood arising from tubercular infection. Lungwort leaves are astringent, and have been applied externally to stop bleeding.

Caution Lungwort is subject to legal restrictions in some countries.

Pulsatilla chinensis (Ranunculaceae)

Chinese anemone, *Bai tou weng* (Chinese)

Description Perennial herb growing to 10 in (25 cm). Has erect downy stems, compound leaves, bell-shaped flowers, and feathery seed heads.

Habitat & cultivation Chinese anemone is native to eastern Asia, and is found in Mongolia, China, and Japan. The root is unearthed either before the plant comes into flower in spring, or in the fall.

Part used Root.

Constituents Chinese anemone contains lactones (including protoanemonin and anemonin), pulsatoside, and anemonol.

History & folklore Chinese anemone root was first documented in Chinese medicine in the Divine Husbandman's Classic (*Shen'nong Bencaojing*), an

herbal written in the 1st century CE.

Medicinal actions & uses Chinese anemone is thought to clear toxicity and to lower fever. It is most commonly taken as a decoction to counter infection within the gastrointestinal tract. The root is also used to treat malarial fever and vaginal infections.

Research Chinese studies have shown the root to be potentially valuable as a treatment for amoebic dysentery.

Related species See pasqueflower (*Anemone pulsatilla*, p. 172).

Caution Take Chinese anemone only under professional supervision.

Punica granatum (Lythraceae)

Pomegranate

Description Deciduous shrub or tree growing to 20 ft (6 m). Has branches tipped with spines, whorls of lance-shaped leaves, scarlet flowers, and leathery-rinded round fruit containing many pulp-covered seeds.

Habitat & cultivation Native to southwestern Asia, pomegranate has become naturalized in Europe. The tree is widely cultivated for its fruit, which is gathered in the fall when it is ripe. The bark is also gathered in the fall.

Parts used Juice, fruit pulp, rind, bark.

Constituents The fruit and juice contain pelletierene alkaloids, elligatannins (up to 25%), and triterpenoids. The alkaloids are highly toxic.

History & folklore In 1500 BCE, the pharaoh Thutmose reputedly brought back pomegranate to Egypt from Asia. Prized as a fruit, it was also sought after as a remedy for worms. The Greek physician Dioscorides, in the 1st century CE, knew of the herb's ability to expel worms, but this attribute was subsequently forgotten in Europe for nearly 1,800 years. In the early 19th century, after an Indian herbalist used pomegranate to cure an Englishman of tapeworms, English doctors in India became interested in pomegranate and its medicinal properties were investigated.

Medicinal actions & uses Until recently, the chief medicinal value of pomegranate was as a deworming agent, with the rind and bark being considered specific remedies for tapeworm infestation. Now, pomegranate juice is widely available and known for its positive effects on the heart and circulation. Like other medicinal plants with a high anthocyanidin content, pomegranate fruit and juice have potent protective activity on all aspects of the circulation, supporting

healthy circulation and countering local inflammatory activity, which damages the inner lining of the blood vessels. The juice is commonly taken to help with cardiovascular problems, including high blood pressure, capillary fragility, angina, and congestive heart failure. It also appears to help prevent dental plaque.

Research In recent years, there has been significant interest in the medicinal properties of pomegranate fruit and juice. As above, pomegranate has a strongly beneficial activity on the cardiovascular system, but it also appears to have an unusually wide range of potential therapeutic properties, including antibacterial, antiseptic, anti-inflammatory, and estrogenic activity. James A. Duke, a former USDA botanist, has described it as an "antimenopausal fruit." Pomegranate shows signs of having anticancer activity and has been recommended as a preventative and treatment for prostate cancer. In laboratory studies, pomegranate seed oil has been shown to inhibit the development of skin cancer. New potential uses are likely to emerge over time.

Cautions Do not use the rind or bark unless under professional supervision. This plant, and especially its bark extracts, is subject to legal restrictions in some countries.

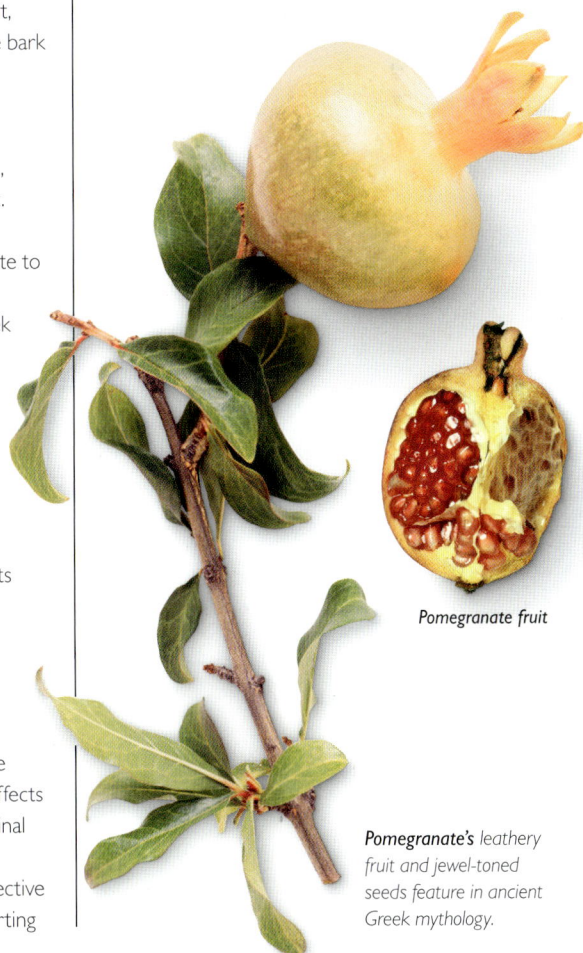

Pomegranate fruit

Pomegranate's leathery fruit and jewel-toned seeds feature in ancient Greek mythology.

Pygeum africanum (Boraginaceae)

Pygeum

Description Evergreen tree growing to 115 ft (35 m). Has oblong leaves, white flowers, and red berries.

Habitat & cultivation Pygeum is native to Africa. It is still harvested from the wild, but severe shortages have led to the establishment of plantations.

Part used Bark.

Constituents Pygeum contains phytosterols (beta-sitosterol), triterpenes (ursolic and oleanolic acids), long-chain alcohols (n-tetracosanol), as well as tannins.

Medicinal actions & uses In conventional medicine in France, the fat-soluble extract of pygeum bark has become the primary treatment for an enlarged prostate gland. A decoction of the bark may reduce the severity of chronic prostate inflammation, and it may also help reverse male sterility when this is due to insufficient prostate secretions. In combination with other plants, pygeum may be valuable in the treatment of prostate cancer.

Research Trials carried out since the 1960s, many of them in France, have established that pygeum extract has positive effects on the prostate gland. Specifically, the extract increases glandular secretions and reduces levels of cholesterol within the organ. In some Western countries, surgery is the main option for enlarged prostates, but in France pygeum is prescribed in 81% of cases.

Related species The fruit kernels of the Asian *P. gardneri* are used to poison fish.

Caution Only take pygeum bark under professional supervision.

Quercus robur (Fagaceae)

English oak

Description Slow-growing, long-lived deciduous tree reaching 150 ft (45 m). Has deeply lobed leaves, long catkins, and green to brown fruit (acorns).

Habitat & cultivation English oak grows throughout the northern hemisphere, in woods and forests, and along roadsides. The bark is collected in spring and the fruit is harvested in the fall.

Parts used Bark, galls (growths produced by insects or fungi).

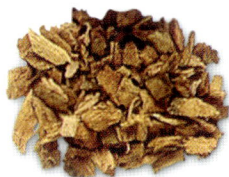

Oak bark

Constituents English oak bark contains 15–20% tannins (including phlobatannin, ellagitannins, and gallic acid). Oak galls contain about 50% tannins.

History & folklore Sacred to the Druids, the oak tree has been esteemed in European herbal medicine for its astringent bark, leaves, and acorns.

Medicinal actions & uses English oak bark, prepared as a decoction, is often used as a gargle to treat sore throats and tonsillitis. It may also be applied as a wash, lotion, or ointment to treat conditions such as hemorrhoids, anal fissures, small burns, or other skin problems. Less commonly, a decoction of the bark is taken in small doses to treat diarrhea, dysentery, and rectal bleeding. Powdered oak bark may be sniffed to treat nasal polyps, or sprinkled on eczema to dry the affected area.

Caution Do not take oak bark internally for more than 4 weeks at a time.

Self-help use Hemorrhoids, p. 312.

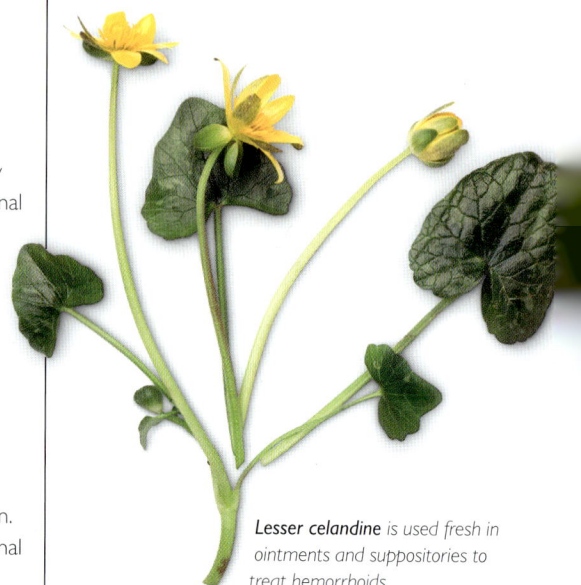

Quillaja saponaria (Rosaceae)

Soap bark

Description Evergreen tree growing to 65 ft (20 m). Has glossy oval leaves, white flowers, and star-shaped fruit.

Habitat & cultivation Soap bark is native to Chile and Peru, and is cultivated in California and India. The bark is gathered throughout the year.

Part used Inner bark.

Constituents Soap bark contains up to 10% triterpenoid saponins, calcium oxalate, and tannins. The saponins are strongly expectorant and can cause inflammation of the digestive tract.

History & folklore In Peru and Chile, soap bark has traditionally been used by Andean peoples as an alternative to soap. The bark has been used medicinally as an expectorant remedy.

Medicinal actions & uses Soap bark has a long tradition of use as a treatment for chest problems. Its strong expectorant effect is beneficial in the treatment of bronchitis, especially in the early stages of the illness. Like other medicinal plants that contain saponins, soap bark stimulates the production of a more fluid mucus in the airways, facilitating the clearing of phlegm through coughing. Soap bark is useful for treating any condition featuring congested mucus within the chest, but it should not be used for dry irritable coughs. Soap bark is also used externally, appearing in the formulations of dandruff shampoos.

Cautions Use only under professional supervision. As soap bark is irritant to the digestive tract, internal use must be carefully monitored.

Ranunculus ficaria (Ranunculaceae)

Lesser celandine, Pilewort

Description Mat-forming perennial growing to 6 in (15 cm). Has small tubers, fleshy heart-shaped leaves, and shiny-petaled, brilliant yellow flowers.

Habitat & cultivation Lesser celandine is native to western Asia, North Africa, and Europe. Commonly found in woods, roadsides, and bare open spaces, it is collected when in flower in spring.

Parts used Aerial parts.

Constituents Lesser celandine contains saponins, protoanemonin and anemonin, tannins, and vitamin C.

History & folklore Lesser celandine has been used from the earliest times as a medicine for the relief of hemorrhoids and ulcers. In medieval times it was believed that simply carrying lesser celandine on one's person was sufficient to cure hemorrhoids.

Medicinal actions & uses Lesser celandine's principal use is an ointment or suppository for treating hemorrhoids.

Related species Various other *Ranunculus* species have been used in herbal medicine, even though all are toxic and irritant to a greater or lesser degree. In North America, the Meskwaki people used the flowers and stigma of the yellow water crowfoot (*R. delphinifolius*) as a snuff to provoke sneezing, and mixed it with other herbs to treat respiratory conditions such as mucus and nasal congestion.

Caution Do not take lesser celandine orally.

Self-help use Hemorrhoids, p. 312.

Lesser celandine is used fresh in ointments and suppositories to treat hemorrhoids.

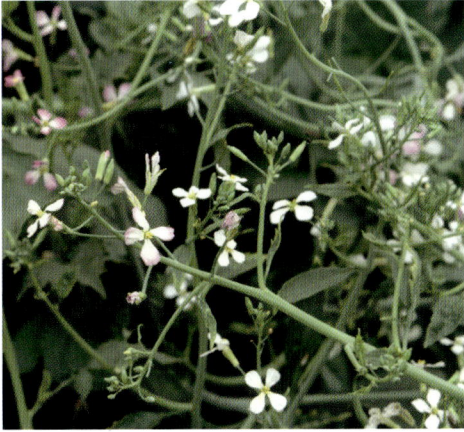

Radish has been used since the 7th century to aid the digestion.

Raphanus sativus (Brassicaceae)

Radish

Description Bristly annual growing to about 3 ft (1 m). Has a swollen taproot, deeply cut compound leaves, pale violet to lilac flowers, and cylindrical seed pods.

Habitat & cultivation Radish is believed to be native to southern Asia. Cultivated varieties are grown around the world both as vegetables and for medicinal use. The root is unearthed in the fall.

Part used Root.

Constituents Radish contains glucosilinates, which yield a volatile oil, raphanin, phenolic compounds, and vitamin C. Raphanin is antibiotic; the phenolic compounds are antioxidant. The leaves are a highly nutritious and underused food.

History & folklore Herodotus (c.485–c.425 BCE) wrote that the builders of the pyramids in ancient Egypt were paid in radishes, onions, and garlic. In Egypt, the plant was used as a vegetable and a medicine. In ancient Rome, radish oil was applied to treat skin diseases. In China, radish was listed in the *Tang Materia Medica* (659 CE) as a digestive stimulant.

Medicinal actions & uses Radish stimulates the appetite and digestion. The common red radish is eaten as a salad vegetable and an appetizer. The juice of the black radish is drunk to counter gassy indigestion and constipation. Black radish juice has a tonic and laxative action on the intestines, and indirectly stimulates the flow of bile. Consuming radish generally results in improved digestion, but some people are sensitive to its acridity and robust action. In China, radish is eaten to relieve abdominal distension. The root is also prepared "dry-fried" to treat chest problems.

Caution Avoid if you have gall stones.

Rauvolfia serpentina (Apocynaceae)

Indian snakeroot, *Sarpagandha* (Hindi)

Description Evergreen shrub growing to 3 ft (1 m). Has whorls of elliptical leaves, tiny pink and white tubular flowers, and glossy red berries.

Habitat & cultivation Indian snakeroot is native to much of southern and southeastern Asia, including India, Malaysia, and Indonesia. It is widely cultivated for medicinal use, notably in India and the Philippines. The root of plants at least 18 months old is unearthed in late winter.

Part used Root.

Constituents Indian snakeroot contains a complex mixture of indole alkaloids, including reserpine, rescinnamine, ajmaline, and yohimbine. Ajmaline has been used to regulate heartbeat.

History & folklore Indian snakeroot is listed in the *Charaka Samhita*, the earliest Ayurvedic medical text (c.400 BCE). The plant has been used since at least that time to treat mental illness and insomnia. Indian snakeroot's status as a healing plant was first recorded in Europe in 1785, but it was not until 1946 that conventional Western medicine recognized the herb's efficacy. After that date, the whole plant, and its reserpine extract in particular, were widely used in conventional medicine to lower high blood pressure and lessen the symptoms of mental illness.

Medicinal actions & uses Indian snakeroot is useful in the treatment of high blood pressure and anxiety. The root has a pronounced sedative and depressant effect on the sympathetic nervous system. By reducing the system's activity, the herb brings about the lowering of blood pressure. It may also be used to treat anxiety and insomnia, as well as more serious mental health problems such as psychosis and schizophrenia. Indian snakeroot is a slow-acting remedy and it takes some time for its effect to become fully established.

Research As indicated above, Indian snakeroot and its alkaloids have been extensively researched since the 1930s. Despite concerns raised in the medical journal *The Lancet* in 1974, there is little evidence to show that the root has serious side-effects at normal dosage.

Related species The West African species *R. vomitoria* is used as a sedative, aphrodisiac, and anticonvulsant in traditional African medicine.

Cautions Take only under professional supervision. Indian snakeroot is subject to legal restrictions in some countries.

Rhamnus frangula syn. *Frangula alnus* (Rhamnaceae)

Alder buckthorn

Description Deciduous shrub or small tree growing to 16 ft (5 m). Has smooth brown bark, oval to elliptical leaves, white flowers in late spring, and small round berries ripening from yellow to black.

Habitat & cultivation Alder buckthorn grows in Europe (except for the Mediterranean region and the extreme north), and in northeastern parts of the US. It prefers marshy woodland. The bark of trees at least 3–4 years old is collected in late spring and early summer, and is dried and stored for at least 1 year before use.

Part used Bark.

Constituents Alder buckthorn contains 3–7% anthraquinones (including frangulin and emodin), anthrones, anthranols, an alkaloid (armepavine), tannins, and flavonoids. The anthrones and anthranols induce vomiting, but the severity of their effect lessens after long-term storage. The anthraquinones found in alder buckthorn and closely related species act on the wall of the colon, stimulating a bowel movement approximately 8–12 hours after ingestion.

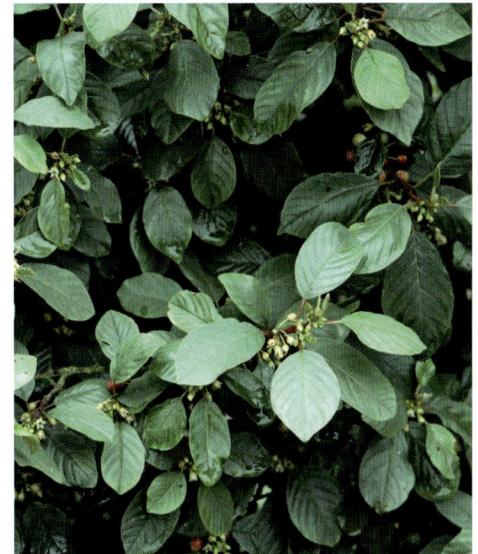

Alder buckthorn bark is toxic when fresh but is safe to use once dried and stored for a year.

Medicinal actions & uses Alder buckthorn is a laxative and a cathartic, and is most commonly taken as a treatment for chronic constipation. Once dried and stored, it is significantly milder than senna (*Cassia senna*, p. 80) or common buckthorn (*R. catharticus*) and may be safely used over the long term to treat constipation and to encourage the return of regular bowel movements. Alder buckthorn is a particularly beneficial remedy if the muscles of the colon are weak, and if there is poor bile flow. The plant should not be used for constipation caused by excessive tension in the colon wall.

Related species Cascara sagrada (*R. purshiana*), native to woodlands along the Pacific coast of North America, is used medicinally in much the same way as alder buckthorn. Common buckthorn (*R. catharticus*), a European native, is today used mainly in veterinary medicine.

Cautions Use only dried bark that has been stored for at least a year, as the fresh bark is violently purgative. The berries may also be harmful if eaten.

Rhaponticum carthamoides syn. *Leuzia carthamoides* (Asteraceae)

Maral root

Description Maral root is an herbaceous perennial growing up to 32 in (80 cm). Recognizable as a typical thistle, it has an upright main stem, long divided leaves and large purple compound flowers atop the main stem.

Habitat & cultivation Maral root is native to central Asia, as far east as Siberia and Xinjiang, in China. It is a rare plant and critically endangered in the wild. Only cultivated plants should be used.

Parts used Root and rhizome; leaf extracts are also now being used.

Constituents Maral root contains steroids, flavonoids, phenolic acids, polyacetylenes, sesquiterpene lactones, triterpenoids, and volatile oil.

History & folklore Maral root is named after the maral deer that graze on the plant. The plant has a long history of medicinal use in Siberia and was first researched in the former Soviet Union in the 1940s for its tonic and adaptogenic properties. It is included in the *Russian Pharmacopoeia,* 14th edition (2018).

Medicinal actions & uses Little known in western Europe and North America, maral root—like Korean ginseng (*Panax ginseng* p. 123)—is an adaptogen, a medicine with a nonspecific activity on the body that improves its resistance to all kinds of stress. This includes exposure to cold, overwork, and lowered immune resistance, as well as emotional stress. Maral root is classically taken to support recovery from physical and mental exhaustion, whether due to post-viral fatigue syndrome, over-training, or nervous exhaustion. It has immune modulating activity, strengthening immune function and by encouraging protein formation promotes muscle bulk.

Research Over 117 research papers have been published on maral root, mostly in Russia.

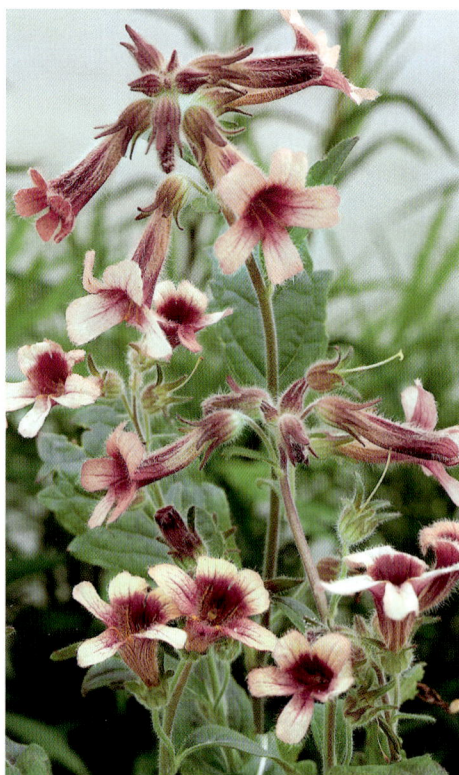

Rehmannia's appearance gave rise to its Western folk name "Chinese foxglove."

Rehmannia glutinosa (Scrophulariaceae)

Rehmannia, *Di huang* (Chinese)

Description An important Chinese tonic herb, rehmannia has figured extensively in many traditional herbal formulas and has an ancient history: it was referred to by Ge Hong, the 4th-century CE Chinese physician and alchemist. Rehmannia is a "longevity" herb and has a marked tonic action on the liver and kidneys. Research has confirmed its traditional use, showing that it protects the liver and is useful for hepatitis.

Habitat & cultivation Rehmannia grows wild on sunny mountain slopes in northern and northeastern parts of China, especially in Henan province. Rehmannia can be cultivated, in which case it is propagated from seed sown in the fall or spring. The root is harvested in the fall, after the plant has flowered.

Part used Root.

Constituents Iridoids, polysaccharides, phytosterols, phenethyl glycosides.

History & folklore Raw & prepared root is used in Chinese herbal medicine, the root (*di huang*) is known as sheng di huang when it is eaten raw and

shu di huang when it has been cooked in wine. The former is the most commonly taken remedy. Both are *yin* tonics (see p. 44), but have different therapeutic indications. The raw root "cools the blood," and is given to help lower fever in acute and chronic illnesses. Its cooling nature is reflected in its use for problems such as thirst and a red tongue that arise from "heat patterns." *Sheng di huang* is useful for treating people with impaired liver function and is used specifically to treat hepatitis and other liver conditions. This preparation is used specifically for blood loss and "blood deficiency" states such as irregular and heavy menstrual bleeding. It is warming rather than cooling, and is considered to be a prime kidney tonic. Rehmannia is used to treat high blood pressure. Interestingly, while sheng di huang appears to raise blood pressure, shu di huang has the opposite effect. Rehmannia is a traditional and valuable tonic for old age. It is considered to help prevent senility. The herb is an ingredient of many famous herbal formulas, most notably "the pill of eight ingredients," which contemporary Chinese herbalists consider to "warm and invigorate the *yang* of the loins."

Related species *R. lutea* is used in Chinese herbal medicine as a diuretic.

Research Listed in the *Chinese Pharmacopoeia,* rehmannia has many potential uses, mostly due to its anti-inflammatory and tonic or restorative effects. Chronic conditions for which some level of research evidence exists include rheumatoid arthritis, chronic kidney disease, asthma, and other allergic conditions such as urticaria. Rehmannia also has liver protective activity and supports adrenal gland function. More than 100 clinical trials in China have established that rehmannia has bone stabilizing properties and can prove an effective remedy in osteoporosis.

Self-help uses Heavy menstrual bleeding, p. 325. Weakened liver & metabolism, p. 329.

Rhus glabra (Anacardiaceae)

Smooth sumac

Description Deciduous shrub growing to a height of about 6 1/2 ft (2 m). Has straggling branches, compound leaves in pairs, large clusters of greenish-red flowers, and downy deep red berries.

Habitat & cultivation Native to North America, smooth sumac is found on the borders of woods, along fences and roadsides, and in neglected sites. The root bark is collected in the fall, the berries when ripe in late summer.

Parts used Root bark, berries.

Constituents Smooth sumac contains tannins. Its other constituents are unknown.

History & folklore Indigenous peoples across North America used smooth sumac and closely related species to treat hemorrhoids, rectal bleeding, dysentery, venereal disease, and bleeding after childbirth. John Josselyn, a 17th-century New England naturalist, observed: "the English use to boyl [the plant] in beer, and drink it for colds; and so do the Indians [sic], from whom the English had the medicine."

Medicinal actions & uses The astringent root bark of smooth sumac is often used as a decoction. It is taken to alleviate diarrhea and dysentery, applied externally to treat excessive vaginal discharge and skin eruptions, and used as a gargle for sore throats. The berries are diuretic, help reduce fever, and may be of use in type 2 diabetes. The berries are also astringent and can be used as a gargle for both mouth and throat complaints.

Related species Sweet sumac (*R. aromatica*) has a similar range of uses. Poison ivy (*R. toxicodendron*) was formerly used in herbal medicine as a treatment for rheumatism, paralysis, and certain skin disorders. It is itself highly irritant to the skin, and causes severe dermatitis.

Ricinus communis (Euphorbiaceae)

Castor oil plant

Description Evergreen shrub growing to about 33 ft (10 m) in its natural state, but a much smaller annual when cultivated. Has large, palm-shaped leaves, green female flowers, and prickly red seed capsules.

Habitat & cultivation Castor oil plant is probably native to eastern Africa. It is cultivated in hot climates around the world. The seed capsules are gathered throughout the year when nearly ripe and are then put out in the sun to mature.

Parts used Seed oil, seeds.

Constituents The seeds contain 45–55% fixed oil, which consists mainly of glycerides of ricinoleic acid, ricin (a highly toxic protein), ricinine (an alkaloid), and lectins. The seeds are highly poisonous—2 are sufficient to kill an adult—but the toxins do not pass into the expressed oil.

History & folklore Castor oil has been used medicinally for about 4,000 years. Until recently, it was a common remedy given regularly to children "to help keep the system clear." Owing to its unpleasant taste, castor oil is remembered as the bane of many childhoods.

Medicinal actions & uses Castor oil is well known for its strongly laxative (and, in higher doses, purgative) action, prompting a bowel movement about 3–5 hours after ingestion. The oil is so effective that it is regularly used to clear the digestive tract in cases of poisoning. Castor oil is well tolerated by the skin, and it is sometimes used as a vehicle for medicinal and cosmetic preparations. In India, the oil is massaged into the breasts after childbirth to stimulate milk flow. Indian herbalism uses a poultice of castor oil seeds to relieve swollen and tender joints. In China, the crushed seeds are used to treat facial palsy.

Cautions Do not ingest the seeds, which are extremely poisonous. Do not take castor oil during pregnancy, and do not take more often than once every few weeks as a treatment for constipation.

Rosa canina (Rosaceae)

Dog rose

Description Climbing perennial growing to a height of 10 ft (3 m). Has curved thorns, leaves with 2–3 pairs of toothed leaflets, pink or white flowers, and scarlet fruit (called "hips").

Habitat & cultivation Native to Europe, temperate areas of Asia, and North Africa, dog rose grows in hedgerows and thickets and in open areas. The fruit is picked in the fall.

Part used Hips.

Constituents Dog rose hips contain vitamins C (up to 1.25%), A, B1, B2, B3, and K, flavonoids, tannins (2–3%), invert sugar, pectin, plant acids, polyphenols, carotenoids, volatile oil, and vanillin.

History & folklore The hips of the dog rose were a popular sweetmeat in the Middle Ages. The plants were not esteemed to the same degree as were cultivated roses (*R. gallica*, following entry), but dog

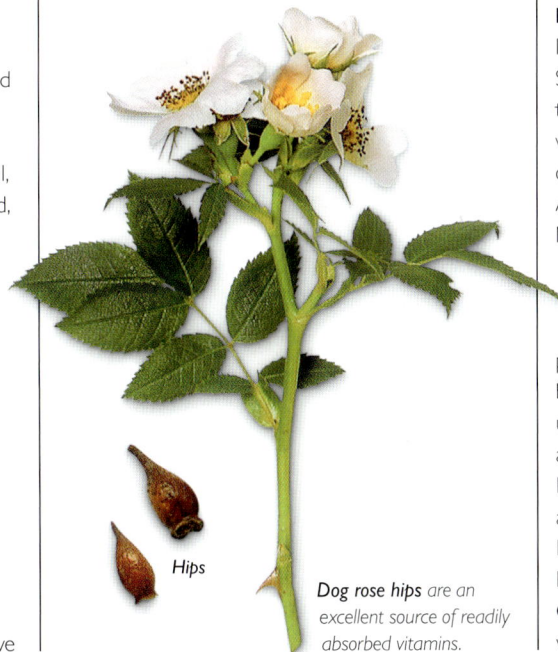

Hips

Dog rose hips are an excellent source of readily absorbed vitamins.

rose was valued as the source of a widely used folk remedy for chest problems.

Medicinal actions & uses Dog rose hips have extremely high levels of vitamins. When consumed fresh, they provide vitamins and other nutrients in a form that is readily absorbed by the body. This makes rose-hip syrup a nourishing drink for young children. The tannin content of rose hips makes them a gentle remedy for diarrhea. The hips are mildly diuretic.

Research Clinical studies investigating the use of rose-hip extracts for osteoarthritis, rheumatoid arthritis, and lower back pain have produced mixed results. Some have shown positive benefits, others none. It is likely that some people will benefit more than others, and given that rose-hip extracts are very safe, rose hips and rose-hip extract are well worth trying for arthritic conditions.

Rosa gallica (Rosaceae)

Rose

Description Deciduous shrub growing to about 5 ft (1.5 m). Has a smooth stem, sharp thorns, serrated leaves with 2–3 pairs of leaflets, semi-double deep pink or red flowers, and scarlet hips.

Habitat & cultivation Native to the Middle East, the rose is not now found in the wild except as a garden escape. It has been cultivated for at least 3,000 years. The flowers are gathered in summer.

Parts used Flowers, essential oil.

Constituents Rose contains a volatile oil consisting of geraniol, nerol, citronellol, geranic acid and other terpenes, and many other substances.

History & folklore The rose comes originally from Iran and has been cultivated there since antiquity. Sappho, the 6th-century bce Greek poet, described the red rose as the "Queen of flowers." In Rome, it was much used in festivities and the petals were consumed as food. Rosewater was prepared by the Arab physician Ibn Sina (980–1037 CE). During the Middle Ages and the Renaissance, the rose was esteemed as a remedy for depression.

Medicinal actions & uses The rose is currently little used in herbal medicine, but it is probably time for a reevaluation of its medicinal benefits. The essential oil, called "attar of rose," is used in aromatherapy as a mildly sedative, antidepressant, and anti-inflammatory remedy. Rose petals and their preparations have a similar action. They also reduce high cholesterol levels. Rosewater is mildly astringent and makes a valuable lotion for inflamed and sore eyes.

Caution Do not take the essential oil internally without professional supervision.

Rubia tinctorum (Rubiaceae)
Madder

Description Evergreen perennial growing to 3 ft (1 m). Has whorls of finely toothed lance-shaped leaves, greenish-white flowers, and black berries containing 2 seeds.

Habitat & cultivation Madder is native to southern Europe, western Asia, and North Africa. It flourishes on waste ground and on roadsides, and amid rubble. The root is unearthed in the fall.

Part used Root.

Constituents Madder contains anthraquinone derivatives (including ruberythric acid, alizarin, and purpurin), an iridoid (asperuloside), resin, and calcium.

History & folklore Throughout history, madder has been used principally as a red dye for a variety of fabrics. In the ancient world, madder root was taken medicinally to treat jaundice, sciatica, and paralysis, and it was also used as a diuretic. When ingested, madder imparts its distinctive color to bones, milk, and urine, and it probably owed much of its reputation as a diuretic to this property.

Medicinal actions & uses Madder fell largely out of use in the 19th century, and is now only rarely employed to treat kidney and bladder stones.

Rubus fruticosus (Rosaceae)
Blackberry

Description Sprawling prickly shrub growing to 13 ft (4 m). Has palm-shaped leaves with 3–5 lobes, white to pale pink flowers and clusters of black berries.

Habitat & cultivation Native to temperate areas of Europe, blackberry is naturalized in the Americas and in Australia. It is commonly found along roads, on waste ground, and in woodlands. The leaves are gathered in summer, the berries in summer and fall.

Parts used Leaves, berries.

Constituents Blackberry leaves contain tannins, flavonoids, and gallic acid. The fruit contains anthocyanins, pectin, fruit acids, and vitamin C.

History & folklore As early as the 1st century CE, the physician Dioscorides recommended ripe blackberries in a gargle for sore throats. In European folk medicine, blackberry leaves have long been used for washing and staunching wounds. Arching blackberry runners that had rooted at both ends were credited with magical properties. In England, for example, children with hernias were pushed under arched runners for a magical cure.

Medicinal actions & uses Blackberry leaves are strongly astringent and may be used as a mouthwash to strengthen spongy gums and ease mouth ulcers, as a gargle for sore throats, and as a decoction to relieve diarrhea and hemorrhoids. Like many red or purple fruits, such as bilberry (*Vaccinium myrtillus*, p. 151), blackberry fruit and juice has significant antioxidant and anti-inflammatory activity, helping to maintain a healthy circulation.

Related species See raspberry (*R. idaeus*, following entry).

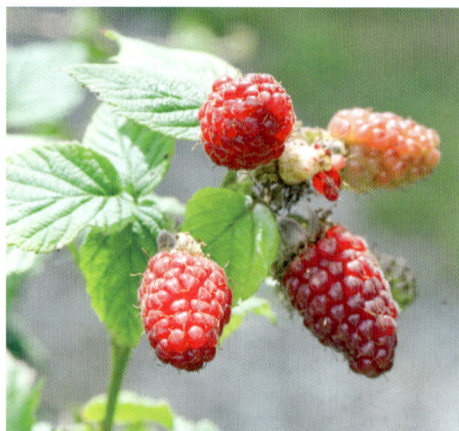
Raspberry leaves and fruit have been used since classical times as an astringent remedy.

Rubus idaeus (Rosaceae)
Raspberry

Description Deciduous shrub growing to 6½ ft (2 m). Has woody stems with prickles, pale green leaves with 3–7 leaflets, white flowers, and red berries.

Habitat & cultivation Native to Europe and Asia, raspberry now grows wild and is cultivated in many temperate regions. The leaves are collected in early summer, the fruit when ripe in summer.

Parts used Leaves, fruit.

Constituents The fruit contains polyphenols, especially anthocyanins, which have antioxidant and anti-inflammatory activity, pectin, fruit sugars, and acids. Raspberry seed oil is rich in vitamin E, carotenes, and essential fatty acids, and is increasingly used in cosmetic skin products.

History & folklore In 1735, the Irish herbalist K'Eogh described uses for raspberry: "an application of the flowers bruised with honey is beneficial for inflammations of the eyes, burning fever and boils … The fruit is good for the heart and diseases of the mouth."

Medicinal actions & uses Raspberry leaves are mainly used to encourage easy labor. While the specific mode of action is unknown, the leaves are thought to strengthen the longitudinal muscles of the uterus, increasing the force of contractions and thereby hastening childbirth. A decoction of raspberry leaves may be used to relieve diarrhea. The leaves also find use as an astringent external remedy—as an eyewash for conjunctivitis, a mouthwash for mouth problems, or a lotion for ulcers, wounds, or excessive vaginal discharge.

Research A laboratory study in 2012 found that a raspberry fruit extract reduced joint inflammation, cartilage damage, and bone resorption.

Caution Do not take medicinally during the early stages of pregnancy.

Self-help use Preparing for childbirth, p. 327.

Rumex acetosella (Polygonaceae)
Sheep's sorrel

Description Slender low-growing perennial. Has arrow-shaped leaves and terminal spikes bearing small green flowers that turn red as their seeds ripen.

Habitat & cultivation Sheep's sorrel is found in most temperate regions of the world. It grows on waste ground and in meadows, and is gathered in early summer.

Parts used Aerial parts.

Constituents Sheep's sorrel contains oxalates and anthraquinones (including chrysophanol, emodin, and physcion).

History & folklore Sheep's sorrel is an ingredient in what has become a somewhat notorious anticancer remedy, derived from an indigenous North American herbal formula, and known as "Essiac". Essiac also includes includes burdock (*Arctium lappa*, p. 69) and slippery elm (*Ulmus rubra*, p. 149). Western herbalists learned of it early in the 20th century, after a Canadian nurse observed the recovery from breast cancer of a patient who had taken the formula. Essiac has since had a checkered history. Despite attempts to initiate proper clinical trials, none has yet been undertaken.

Medicinal actions & uses Sheep's sorrel is a detoxifying herb, the fresh juice having a pronounced diuretic effect. Like other members of the dock family, sheep's sorrel is mildly laxative, and holds potential as a long-term treatment for chronic disease, in particular that of the gastrointestinal tract.

Related species Sorrel (*R. acetosa*) is a European relative that is also taken for its detoxifying effect. *See also* yellow dock (*R. crispus, following entry*) and Chinese rhubarb (*Rheum palmatum*, p. 130).

Caution Sheep's sorrel should not be taken by anyone with a tendency to develop kidney stones.

Rumex crispus (Polygonaceae)

Yellow dock, Curled dock

Description Perennial, growing to 3 ft (1 m), with lance-shaped leaves and many small green flowers arranged in whorls on the upper part of the stem.

Habitat & cultivation A common wayside plant in many regions of the world, yellow dock thrives in ditches, on verges and in open areas, and barely needs cultivation. The roots are dug up in the fall, chopped, and dried.

Parts used Root.

Constituents Yellow dock contains anthraquinones (about 2.5%), tannins (3–6%), flavonoids and oxalates.

Medicinal actions & uses Though a valuable herb, yellow dock is not often used on its own, being combined with other alterative herbs such as burdock root (*Arctium lappa*, p. 69) and dandelion root (*Taraxacum officinale*, p. 145) for long-term toxic conditions. Its gentle laxative action makes it a valuable remedy for constipation, particularly when combined with changes to the diet such as increased bulk and fiber. By stimulating large intestine function, the feces are eliminated more efficiently, with reduced reabsorption of waste products, a form of toxicity that tends to occur in a poorly functioning colon. Yellow dock is also thought to improve the flow of bile, which further contributes to its detoxifying activity. It is also typically taken for skin conditions such as acne, eczema, and fungal infections, and for arthritic problems.

Research The anthraquinones are purgative and laxative (see *Cassia senna*, p. 80), but this activity is tempered by the tannins, which counter the irritant effect of the anthraquinones within the gut. The presence of oxalates suggests that yellow dock is best avoided in gout and kidney stones. The leaf has high levels of oxalates, and poisoning and death have resulted from eating the leaves as a salad vegetable.

Caution Best avoided during pregnancy and while breast-feeding.

Ruscus aculeatus (Asparagaceae)

Butcher's broom

Description Bushy evergreen perennial growing to 3 ft (1 m). Has leaflike leathery branches with a terminal spine, greenish-white flowers, and shiny red berries.

Habitat & cultivation Butcher's broom is found throughout much of Europe, western Asia, and North Africa. It is a protected species, growing wild in woodland and on uncultivated ground. Cultivated plants are gathered in autumn when in fruit.

Parts used Aerial parts, rhizome.

Constituents Butcher's broom contains saponin glycosides, including ruscogenin and neoruscogenin. These constituents have a structure similar to that of diosgenin, found in wild yam (*Dioscorea villosa*, p. 95). They are anti-inflammatory and cause the contraction of blood vessels, especially veins.

History & folklore Much used in antiquity, butcher's broom was described by the 1st century CE Greek physician Dioscorides as having the ability to promote urine flow and menstrual bleeding. The plant's name comes from its use as a broom in butchers' shops in Europe up until the 20th century.

Medicinal actions & uses Though little used in Anglo-American herbal medicine, butcher's broom is now a common remedy in Germany for venous problems. It has been shown to have a directly positive effect on varicose veins and hemorrhoids, preventing increased tensing of the veins and helping the return of excess fluid into the veins. Extracts can be taken orally or applied to affected legs.

Research A growing body of research is demonstrating that butcher's broom is a valuable medicine for venous disorders. In a clinical trial, patients with varicose veins who applied a butcher's broom extract to their legs showed a contraction of 1.25 mm in their femoral artery within 2¹/₂ hours. A paper published in the *Journal of Complementary and Alternative Medicine* in 2000 identifies butcher's broom as having great potential as a medicine for orthostatic hypotension (a specific form of low blood pressure).

Caution Do not take butcher's broom if suffering from high blood pressure.

Ruta graveolens (Rutaceae)

Rue

Description Strongly aromatic evergreen perennial growing to 3 ft (1 m). Has fleshy 3-lobed leaves, yellow-green 5-petaled flowers, and round seed capsules.

Habitat & cultivation Rue grows in the Mediterranean region, preferring open sunny sites. It is also cultivated in many parts of the world as both a garden ornamental and a medicinal plant. The aerial parts are gathered in summer.

Parts used Aerial parts.

Constituents Rue contains about 0.5% volatile oil (including 50–90% 2-undecanone), flavonoids (including rutin), furanocoumarins (including bergapten), and about 1.4% furoquinoline alkaloids (including fagarine, arborinine, skimmianine, and others). Rutin has the effect of supporting and strengthening the inner lining of blood vessels and reducing blood pressure.

History & folklore In ancient Greece and Egypt, rue was employed to stimulate menstrual bleeding, to induce abortion, and to strengthen the eyesight.

Medicinal actions & uses Rue is chiefly used to encourage the onset of menstruation. It stimulates the muscles of the uterus and promotes menstrual blood flow. In European herbal medicine, rue has also been taken to treat conditions as varied as hysteria, epilepsy, vertigo, colic, intestinal worms, poisoning, and eye problems. The latter use is well founded, as an infusion used as an eyewash brings quick relief to strained and tired eyes, and reputedly improves the eyesight. Rue has been used to treat many other conditions, including multiple sclerosis and Bell's palsy.

Research Rue is currently being investigated for its potential use as an anticancer treatment.

Related species The related species, *R. chalepensis*, which is also native to the Mediterranean region, is

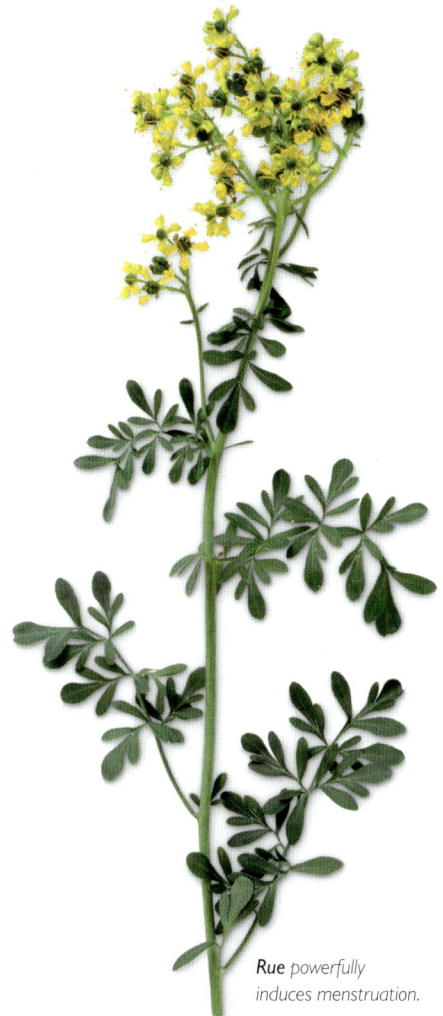

Rue *powerfully induces menstruation.*

used to expel worms, to promote menstrual flow, and to soothe sore eyes.

Cautions Rue is toxic in excess. Never take during pregnancy. The fresh plant frequently causes dermatitis, so wear gloves while handling it. Taken internally, rue may cause an allergic skin reaction to sunlight.

Salvia hispanica (Lamiaceae)

Chia seed

Description Chia is an annual herbaceous plant growing to 3 ft (1 m), with toothed vivid green leaves and clusters of small purple to white flowers. The gray/brown oval seeds are about $^1/_{25}$ in (1 mm) in diameter.

Habitat & cultivation Native to Mexico and central America, chia is a subtropical plant that prefers a sandy well-drained soil. It is now widely cultivated throughout Latin America and in Australia, and can be grown from seed in a greenhouse.

Parts used Seeds.

Constituents Chia seeds have an unusually high omega-3 fatty content—60% alpha-linolenic acid. They also contain dietary fiber (35%), protein, minerals, phenolic acids, flavonoids, isoflavones, and sterols.

History & folklore Chia seed has formed a key part of the traditional diet in Mexico and Central America for over 5,000 years. The seed and its oil were used as food, medicine, and cosmetics by the Maya, Aztecs, and other Indigenous peoples. Chia production was suppressed after the Spanish conquest, due to the use of chia oil and seed in the religious ceremonies of Indigenous American peoples. The word *chia* comes from *chian*, the Nahuatl word for the plant, meaning "oily."

Medicinal actions & uses Chia is another ancient food and medicine that has been "rediscovered." Its high essential fatty acid and fiber content—it has twice the level of fiber found in oat bran (*Avena sativa* p. 179)—make it a valuable, nutritious food. At the same time, it acts as a prebiotic within the digestive tract, promoting a healthy gut microbiome and slowing the absorption of fats and sugars. Chia can therefore prove a useful addition to the diet for people with type 2 diabetes and raised cholesterol levels. Some of the phenolic constituents in the seeds relax the muscle walls of arteries, so the seeds are probably helpful in treating high blood pressure as well.

Related species Many sage (*Salvia*) species have medicinal use. See also Sage (*S. officinalis* p.135), Chinese sage (*S. miltiorrhiza* p. 134), and Clary sage (next entry).

Salvia sclarea (Lamiaceae)

Clary sage

Description Square-stemmed biennial growing to 3 ft (1 m). Has hairy wrinkled leaves and whorls of pale blue flowers.

Habitat & cultivation Native to southern Europe and the Middle East, clary sage is now cultivated in France and Russia for its essential oil. It prefers sunny conditions and dry soil. It is gathered in summer, usually in its second year.

Parts used Aerial parts, seeds, and the essential oil.

Constituents Clary sage contains 0.1% volatile oil (consisting mainly of linalyl acetate and linalool), diterpenes, and tannins.

History & folklore Clary sage has been perceived both as a weaker version of its close relative, sage (*S. officinalis*, p. 135), and as a significant herb in its own right. Since the seeds were once commonly used to treat eye problems, clary sage was also known as "clear eye."

Medicinal actions & uses An antispasmodic and aromatic plant, clary sage is used today mainly to treat digestive problems such as gas and indigestion. It is also regarded as a tonic, calming herb that helps relieve period pain and premenstrual problems. Owing to its estrogen-stimulating action, it is most effective when levels of this hormone are low. The plant can therefore be a valuable remedy for complaints that are associated with menopause, particularly hot flashes.

Cautions Do not take clary sage essential oil internally. Do not use clary sage during pregnancy.

Sanguinaria canadensis (Papaveraceae)

Blood root

Description Perennial plant growing to 6 in (15 cm). Has palm-shaped leaves and solitary flower stems bearing attractive white flowers with 8–12 petals.

Habitat & cultivation Native to northeastern North America, bloodroot grows in shady woods. It is cultivated as a garden plant. The rhizome is unearthed in summer or fall.

Part used Rhizome.

Constituents Bloodroot contains isoquinoline alkaloids, notably sanguinarine (1%), and many others, including berberine. Sanguinarine is a strongly expectorant substance that also has antiseptic and local anesthetic properties.

History & folklore Bloodroot was a traditional remedy of Indigenous American peoples, who used it to treat fevers and rheumatism, to induce vomiting,

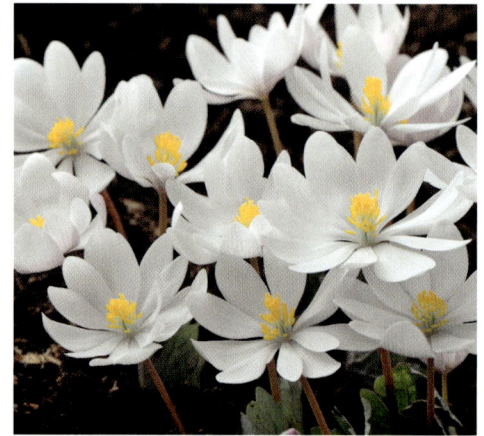

Bloodroot was used by Indigenous American peoples to treat fevers and rheumatism.

and as an element in divination. The rhizome's bright red juice has been used as a rouge. From 1820 to 1926, bloodroot was listed as an expectorant in the *Pharmacopoeia of the United States*.

Medicinal actions & uses In contemporary herbal medicine, bloodroot is chiefly employed as an expectorant, promoting coughing and the clearing of mucus from the respiratory tract. The plant is prescribed for chronic bronchitis and—as it also has an antispasmodic effect—for asthma and whooping cough. Bloodroot may also be used as a gargle for sore throats, and as a wash or ointment for fungal and viral skin conditions such as athlete's foot and warts.

Cautions Take only under professional supervision and do not exceed the dose. Bloodroot induces vomiting in all but very small doses, and at excessive doses it is toxic. Do not take during pregnancy, while breastfeeding, or if suffering from glaucoma.

Sanguisorba officinalis syn. *Poterium officinalis* (Rosaceae)

Greater burnet

Description Perennial herb growing to 2 ft (60 cm). Has long-stalked compound leaves with 13 leaflets, and purple flowers.

Habitat & cultivation Native to Europe, North Africa, and temperate regions of Asia, greater burnet flourishes in damp pastures, especially in mountainous regions. It is cultivated as a fodder crop and as a salad vegetable, and is gathered in summer.

Parts used Aerial parts, root.

Constituents Greater burnet contains tannins, including sanguisorbic acid dilactone (a phenolic acid), and gum.

History & folklore In Europe, greater burnet has long been used as a fodder for animals and as an ingredient in beer-making. As its Latin name implies, it has also been employed as a wound healer: *sanguis* means "blood" and *sorbeo* means "I staunch."

Medicinal actions & uses Greater burnet is still used to slow or arrest blood flow. In both the Chinese and European traditions, it is taken internally to treat heavy periods and uterine hemorrhage. Externally, a lotion or ointment may be used for hemorrhoids, burns, wounds, and eczema. Greater burnet is also a valuable astringent and is employed for a variety of gastrointestinal problems, including diarrhea, dysentery, and ulcerative colitis, particularly if accompanied by bleeding.

Research Chinese research indicates that the whole herb heals burns more effectively than the extracted tannins. Patients suffering from eczema showed marked improvement when treated with an ointment made from greater burnet root and petroleum jelly.

Sanicula europaea (Apiaceae)

Sanicle

Description Perennial growing to 16 in (40 cm). Has long-stalked, palm-shaped, shiny leaves, with clusters of pale pink to greenish-white flowers.

Habitat & cultivation Found throughout most of Europe and western and central Asia, sanicle is common in woodland areas, particularly in damp shady sites. It is collected in summer.

Parts used Aerial parts.

Constituents Sanicle contains up to 13% saponins, allantoin, a volatile oil, tannins, chlorogenic and rosmarinic acid, mucilage, and vitamin C. Allantoin increases the healing rate of damaged tissue. Rosmarinic acid is anti-inflammatory.

History & folklore Sanicle derives from *sanus*, meaning "whole" or "sound" in Latin. St. Hildegard of Bingen (1098–1179), who wrote the earliest extant description of sanicle's use in healing wounds, states of the herb that it "is hot, and there is much purity in it, and its juice is sweet and healthful, that is wholesome." During the 15th and 16th centuries sanicle became a popular herbal medicine. The 17th-century English herbalist Nicholas Culpeper praised sanicle's ability "to heal all green wounds speedily, or any ulcer, imposthumes, or bleedings inwardly," and compared its benefits to those of comfrey (*Symphytum officinale*, p. 142) and self-heal (*Prunella vulgaris*, p. 264).

Medicinal actions & uses With its longstanding reputation for healing wounds and treating internal bleeding, sanicle is a potentially valuable plant, but it is little used in contemporary herbal medicine. Sanicle may be used to treat bleeding within the stomach or intestines, the coughing up of blood, and nosebleeds. It may also be of use in treating diarrhea and dysentery, bronchial and congestive problems, and sore throats. This herb is traditionally thought to be detoxifying and has also been taken internally for skin problems. Externally, sanicle may be applied in the form of a poultice or ointment for the treatment of wounds, burns, chilblains, hemorrhoids, and inflamed skin.

Santalum spp. (Santalaceae)

Sandalwood, Chandan

Description Semiparasitic evergreen tree growing to 33 ft (10 m). Has lance-shaped leaves, clusters of pale yellow to purple flowers, and small, nearly black fruit.

Habitat & cultivation Native to eastern India, sandalwood is cultivated in Southeast Asia for its wood and essential oil. The trees are felled throughout the year.

Parts used Wood, essential oil.

Constituents Sandalwood contains 3–6% volatile oil (which consists predominantly of the sesquiterpenols alpha- and beta-santalol), resin, and tannins.

History & folklore Sandalwood's aroma has been highly esteemed in China and India for thousands of years. The wood is often burned as incense and plays a part in Hindu ritual. The heartwood is most often used in perfumery, but it has also been taken as a remedy in China since around 500 CE.

Medicinal actions & uses Sandalwood and its essential oil are used for their antiseptic properties in treating genitourinary conditions such as cystitis and gonorrhea. In Ayurvedic medicine, a paste of the wood is used to soothe rashes and itchy skin. In China, sandalwood is held to be useful for chest and abdominal pain.

Caution Do not take sandalwood essential oil internally.

Saponaria officinalis (Caryophyllaceae)

Soapwort

Description Perennial growing to a height of 3 ft (1 m). Soapwort has lance-shaped leaves and clusters of delicate pink 5-petaled tubular flowers.

Habitat & cultivation Native to temperate regions of Europe, Asia, and North America, soapwort thrives in open woodland areas and on railroad embankments and waste ground. It has been widely cultivated as a garden plant. The herb is gathered while in flower in summer; the root is unearthed in the fall.

Parts used Root, aerial parts.

Constituents All parts of soapwort contain saponins (around 5%), resin, and a small quantity of volatile oil.

History & folklore Soapwort has mostly been used as a substitute for soap, especially in washing clothes. Boerhaave (1668–1738), a Dutch physician, recommended soapwort as a treatment for jaundice.

Medicinal actions & uses Soapwort's main internal use is as an expectorant. Its strongly irritant action within the gut is thought to stimulate the cough reflex and increase the production of a more fluid mucus within the respiratory passages. Consequently, the plant is prescribed for bronchitis, coughs, and some cases of asthma. Soapwort may be taken for other problems, including rheumatic and arthritic pain. A decoction of the root, and, to a lesser extent, an infusion of the aerial parts of the herb, make soothing washes for eczema and other itchy skin conditions.

Cautions Soapwort is a potentially toxic herb. Take internally only under professional supervision.

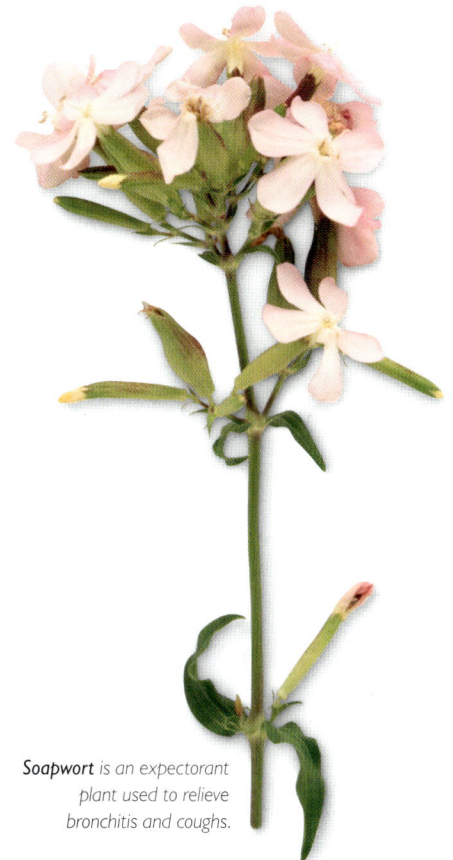

Soapwort is an expectorant plant used to relieve bronchitis and coughs.

Sargassum fusiforme (Sargassaceae)

Hai zao
Hijiki (Japanese)

Description Brown seaweed (alga) with long thin fronds.

Habitat & cultivation *Hai zao* is found along the coastlines of China and Japan, where it is often seen floating in large masses. It is gathered throughout the year.

Part used Whole plant.

Constituents *Hai zao* contains polysaccharides, alginic acid, and significant levels of potassium and iodine.

History & folklore Wang Tao, an 8th-century Chinese physician, recommended *hai zao* for goiter (an enlargement of the thyroid gland due to iodine deficiency). *Hai zao* is eaten as a vegetable in Chinese and Japanese cuisine.

Medicinal actions & uses *Hai zao* is used in a similar way to its European counterpart, the seaweed bladder wrack, or kelp (*Fucus vesiculosus*, p. 218). In Chinese medicine, it is given principally to treat thyroid problems caused by low iodine levels within the body. The herb also helps to combat other thyroid conditions that produce enlargement of the gland, for example Hashimoto's thyroiditis. *Hai zao* is prescribed to treat cases of scrofula (enlargement of the lymph glands in the neck due to tubercular infection) and edema (fluid retention).

Research Chinese research indicates that *hai zao* has antifungal and immunomodulating activity.

Related species In Chinese medicine, *S. fusiforme* is used interchangeably with *S. pallidum*.

Caution Do not take *hai zao* for thyroid problems without professional supervision.

Satureja montana (Lamiaceae)

Winter savory

Description Semi-evergreen aromatic herb growing to 16 in (40 cm). Has lance-shaped leaves and white-pink flowers appearing in clusters.

Habitat & cultivation Native to southern Europe, winter savory thrives in sunny, well-drained sites. It is commonly cultivated as a garden herb. The flowering tops are collected in summer.

Parts used Flowering tops, essential oil.

Constituents Winter savory contains about 1.6% volatile oil, composed mainly of carvacrol, p-cymene, linalool, and thymol.

History & folklore Winter savory was classified as

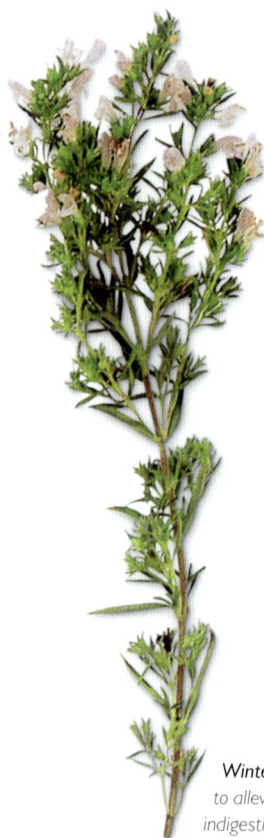

Winter savory helps to alleviate flatulence, indigestion, and colic.

"heating and drying" by the classical physicians Dioscorides and Galen, and was thought to have therapeutic benefits similar to those of thyme (*Thymus vulgaris*, p. 147).

Medicinal actions & uses Winter savory is most often used in cooking, but it also has marked medicinal benefits. It settles gas and stimulates the digestion, helping to alleviate flatulence and colic. It is warming and has been taken for chest infections and bronchitis. The essential oil is strongly antibacterial and may be used to treat candidiasis and other fungal conditions.

Related species Summer savory (*S. hortensis*) is a similar herb that has a milder essential oil. Calamint (*Calamintha ascendens*, p. 181) is another close relative.

Cautions Do not take the essential oil internally without professional supervision. Do not take winter savory during pregnancy.

Saussurea lappa syn. *S. costus* (Asteraceae)

Kuth

Description Upright perennial herb growing to 10 ft (3 m). Has heart-shaped leaves and blue-black flower heads.

Habitat & cultivation Native to the Indian subcontinent, kuth is most commonly found in mountainous areas of Kashmir. The root is gathered in the fall.

Parts used Root, essential oil.

Constituents Kuth contains a volatile oil (consisting of terpenes, sesquiterpenes, and aplotaxene), an alkaloid (saussarine), and a resin. Saussarine depresses the parasympathetic nervous system.

History & folklore Kuth root has been used in Indian medicine for at least 2,500 years. It has also been exported to China and the Middle East. The fragrant root is often used in perfumery. In India, it is valued as an aphrodisiac and for its reputed ability to prevent gray hair.

Medicinal actions & uses Kuth is used in the Ayurvedic and Unani Tibb traditions in India for its tonic, stimulant, and antiseptic properties. The root is commonly taken, in combination with other herbs, for respiratory system problems such as bronchitis, asthma, and coughs. It is also used to treat cholera.

Related species *S. amara* is used in Mongolian herbal medicine to treat bacterial infections and gallbladder disease.

Caution Do not take kuth essential oil internally.

Schizonepeta tenuifolia (Lamiaceae)

Jing jie

Description Perennial plant growing to 26 ft (8 m) with upright square stems, lance-shaped leaves, and whorls of small flowers.

Habitat & cultivation Native to the Far East, *jing jie* is widely cultivated in eastern China. The aerial parts of the plant are gathered in the fall.

Parts used Aerial parts.

Constituents *Jing jie* contains a volatile oil, the main constituents of which are menthone and limonene.

Medicinal actions & uses In the Chinese tradition, *jing jie* is valued as an aromatic and warming herb. It is taken to alleviate skin conditions such as boils and itchiness. *Jing jie* also induces sweating and is used to treat fever and chills, and as a remedy for measles. It is often combined with *bo he* (*Mentha haplocalyx*, p. 240).

Research Chinese studies have confirmed *jing jie's* ability to increase blood flow in the vessels just beneath the skin.

Scolopendrium vulgare (Polypodiaceae)

Hartstongue

Description Evergreen fern growing to 2 ft (60 cm). Has long, tongue-shaped fronds with twin rows of spores on the underside.

Habitat & cultivation Hartstongue is found throughout much of Europe, North Africa, East

Asia, and North America. It prefers shaded sites in woodlands and on banks and walls. The fronds are gathered throughout the summer.

Parts used Fronds.

Constituents Hartstongue contains tannins, mucilage, and flavonoids (including leucodelphidin).

History & folklore Hartstongue has been prescribed as a treatment for diarrhea and dysentery for at least 2,000 years. In Wales and the Scottish Highlands, it was traditionally used as a poultice for wounds, scalds, and burns, and as an ointment for hemorrhoids. In Japan, the fronds were smoked by the Ainu people.

Medicinal actions & uses Hartstongue was valued in the past for its ability to heal wounds, but today it is employed chiefly as a mild astringent. It is sometimes used in the treatment of diarrhea and IBS, and it may be of benefit to the liver and spleen. Hartstongue appears to have expectorant properties, and it is also mildly diuretic.

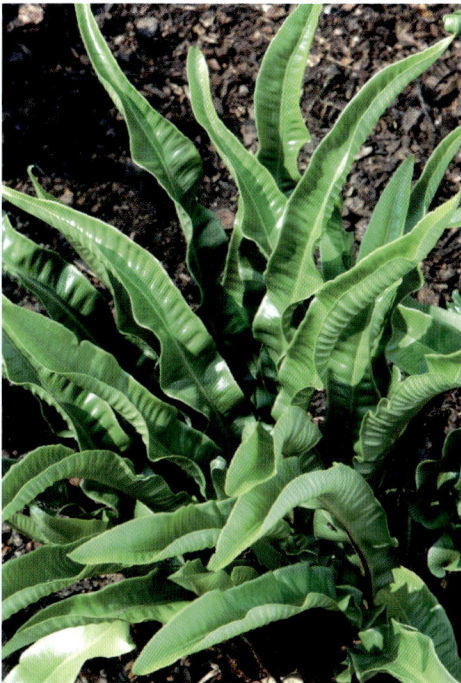

Hartstongue is found growing in shady woodland sites across the northern hemisphere.

Scrophularia nodosa (Scrophulariaceae)

Figwort

Description Upright perennial herb growing to 3 ft (1 m). Has a square stem, oval leaves, small round brown flowers in clusters, and green seed capsules.

Habitat & cultivation Native to Europe, Central Asia, and North America, figwort thrives in wet or damp places, in open woodland, on riverbanks, and alongside ditches. The herb is gathered in the summer while in flower.

Parts used Aerial parts.

Constituents Figwort contains iridoids (including aucubin, harpagoside, and acetyl harpagide), flavonoids, cardioactive glycosides, and phenolic acids. Harpagoside and harpagide are thought to account for its anti-arthritic activity.

History & folklore Figwort's genus name, *Scrophularia*, alludes to the plant's age-old use as a treatment for scrofula. In this condition, the lymph nodes of the neck, infected with tuberculosis, swell to form hard protruding lumps beneath the skin. Figwort root resembles these swollen glands and therefore, according to the Doctrine of Signatures (which holds that a plant's appearance indicates the ailments it treats), the herb was considered to be an appropriate remedy for treating scrofula. Indeed, in the 16th and 17th centuries, figwort was esteemed as the best medicinal plant to help relieve all manner of swellings and tumors.

Medicinal actions & uses Figwort is an herb that supports detoxification of the body and may be used as a treatment for various types of skin conditions. Taken internally as an infusion or applied externally, figwort is of value in treating chronic skin diseases such as eczema and psoriasis. Applied externally, it will also help speed the healing of burns, wounds, hemorrhoids, and ulcers. The traditional use of figwort as a treatment for swellings and tumors continues in Europe to this day. The herb is also mildly diuretic, and it is reputed to be effective when used to expel worms.

Related species Water figwort (*S. aquatica*), another plant that is native to Europe, has similar properties, as does the American *S. marylandica*. In China, *S. ningopoensis* is used to treat infections and to clear toxicity.

Caution Do not take figwort if suffering from a heart condition.

Selenicereus grandiflorus (Cactaceae)

Night-blooming cereus

Description Climbing multi-branched perennial cactus with upright cylindrical stems and aerial roots. Produces large flower buds opening into night-blooming white flowers that grow to 8 in (20 cm) across, and red oval fruit.

Habitat & cultivation Native to Mexico and Central America, night-blooming cereus is now rarely found in the wild. It is cultivated both as an

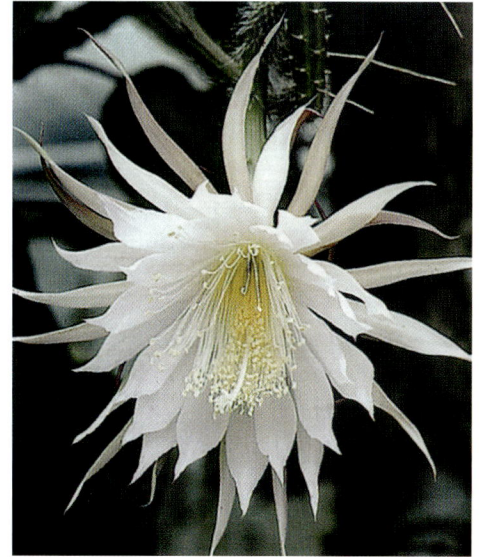

Night-blooming cereus has spectacular flowers that open at dusk and close at dawn.

ornamental and a medicinal plant. The flowers and young stems are gathered in summer.

Parts used Flowers, young stems.

Constituents Night-blooming cereus contains alkaloids (including cactine), flavonoids (isorhamnetin), and a pigment. Cactine's cardiotonic effect is considered similar to that of cardiac glycosides (see foxglove, *Digitalis* species, p. 207).

Medicinal actions & uses As it is in short supply, night-blooming cereus is little used at present, but it is a valuable remedy for the heart. It stimulates the action of the heart, increasing the strength of contractions while slowing heart rate. It is prescribed as a treatment for various conditions, including angina and low blood pressure, and is often given as a tonic during recovery from a heart attack. In the Caribbean, the juice of the whole plant is used to expel worms, and the stems and flowers are used in the treatment of rheumatism.

Cautions Take only under professional supervision. Excessive doses may cause stomach upset and hallucinations.

Sempervivum tectorum (Crassulaceae)

Houseleek

Description Succulent perennial growing to 4 in (10 cm). Has round rosettes of leaves, and flowering stems bearing clusters of bell-shaped red flowers.

Habitat & cultivation The herb is native to central and southern Europe and now grows wild in northern Europe, North Africa, and western Asia, preferring sandy dry soil. Houseleek is widely

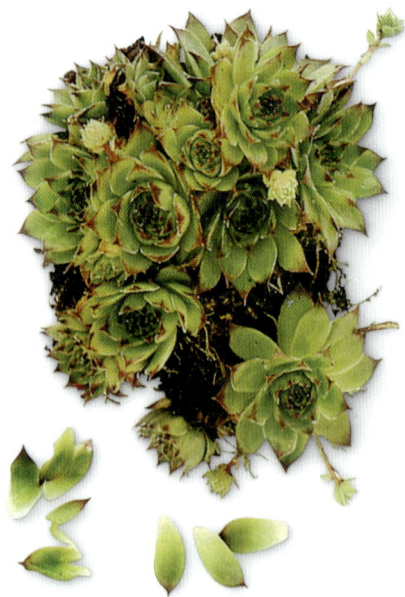

Houseleek's succulent leaves contain tannins and mucilage, both soothing to the skin.

cultivated as a garden plant. The leaves are picked in summer

Parts used Leaves, leaf juice.

Constituents Houseleek contains polyphenols, including procyanidins and mucilage.

History & folklore The Frankish King Charlemagne (742–814 CE) told his subjects to plant houseleek on their roofs, as the plant reputedly warded off lightning and fire.

Medicinal actions & uses Houseleek leaves and their juice are used for their cooling and astringent effect, being applied externally to soothe many skin conditions, including burns, wounds, boils, and corns. As with many other remedies that are both astringent and soothing, houseleek simultaneously tightens and softens the skin. Traditionally, the leaves have been chewed to relieve toothache, and the juice has been sniffed to stop nosebleeds. Houseleek is still used externally, but internal use of this herb is not advised because in large doses it will induce vomiting.

Caution Do not take houseleek internally.

Senecio aureus syn. *Packera aurea*

Life root

Description Upright perennial growing to 3 ft (1 m). Has lance-shaped leaves and clusters of yellow daisy-type flowers.

Habitat & cultivation Native to eastern North America, life root is found in marshes, and on damp ground and riverbanks. The aerial parts are gathered in summer.

Parts used Aerial parts.

Constituents Life root contains a volatile oil, pyrrolizidine alkaloids (including senecine, senecionine, and otosenine), tannins, and resin. In isolation, the pyrrolizidine alkaloids are highly toxic to the liver.

History & folklore The Catawba people of North America used life root as a remedy for gynecological problems in general, and to relieve labor pains in particular.

Medicinal actions & uses Until recently, life root was employed in Anglo-American herbalism much as it was in earlier times—as a means to induce menstrual periods and to bring relief to menopausal complaints. Today, the plant is recommended only for external use, as a douche for excessive vaginal discharge.

Related species Ragwort (*S. jacobaea*) has traditionally been used as a poultice or lotion to relieve rheumatic aches and pains.

Cautions Do not take life root internally. The plant is subject to legal restrictions in some countries.

Senegalia catechu syn. *Acacia catechu*

Black catechu, Cutch

Description Tree growing to 49 ft (15 m) with thorny branches and divided, feathery leaves.

Habitat & cultivation Native to India, Myanmar (Burma), Sri Lanka, and East Africa, this tree is cultivated for its timber. It grows to altitudes of 4,900 ft (1,500 m).

Parts used Bark, heartwood, leaves, shoots.

Constituents The shiny, black-brown extract of leaves and young shoots, which is called "cutch," becomes a brittle solid when dried, and is the form in which black catechu is generally sold. Cutch contains 25–60% tannins, 20–30% mucilage, flavonoids, and resins.

Medicinal actions & uses Black catechu is a strong astringent and clotting agent. It helps reduce excess mucus in the nose, the large intestine, or vagina. It is also used to treat eczema, hemorrhages, diarrhea, and dysentery. It may be used as an infusion, tincture, powder, or ointment. A small piece of cutch dissolved in the mouth is an excellent remedy for bleeding gums and canker sores. The powder and tincture are also applied to infected gums and have been used to clean the teeth. In Ayurvedic medicine, decoctions of the bark and heartwood are used for sore throats.

Research Cutch has been shown to lower blood pressure.

Related species See also gum arabic (*V. nilotica* p.290).

Cautions Do not take for more than 2–3 weeks at a time, or if suffering from kidney inflammation. There are some countries where cutch is subject to legal restrictions.

Self-help use Diarrhea, p. 317.

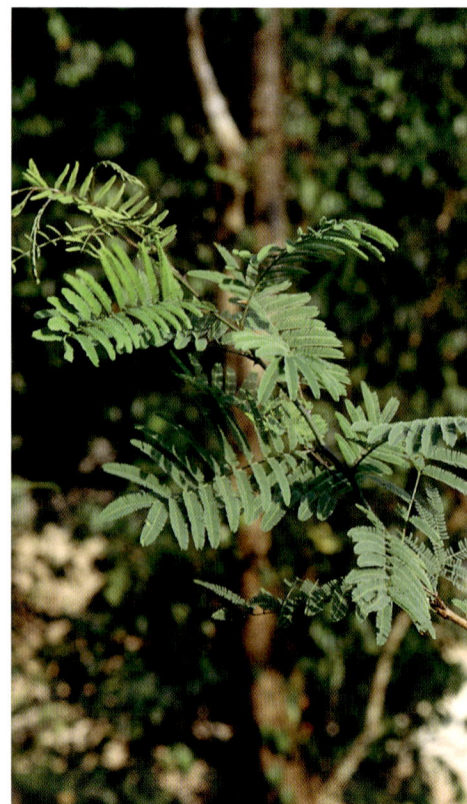

Black catechu is an astringent and antiseptic.

Sesamum indicum (Pedaliaceae)

Sesame, *Hei zhi ma*

Description Erect annual growing to 6½ ft (2 m). Has lance-shaped to oval leaves, white, pink, or mauve flowers, and oblong seed capsules bearing many small gray seeds.

Habitat & cultivation Native to Africa, sesame is cultivated in tropical and subtropical areas around the world. The root is unearthed in summer; the seeds are collected after the seed capsules have turned brown-black.

Parts used Seeds, seed oil, root.

Constituents The seeds are highly nutritious and contain about 55% oil (mainly polyunsaturated fats),

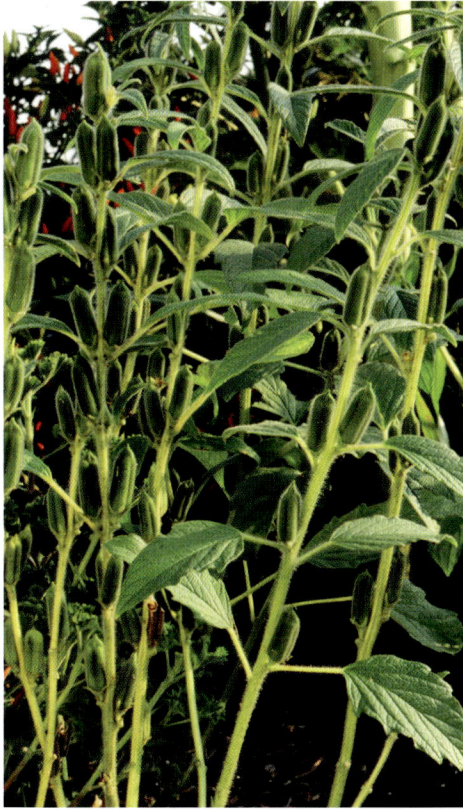

Sesame seeds are a rich source of unsaturated fatty acids and calcium.

about 20% protein, lignans (notably sesamin and sesamolin), vitamins B₃ and E, and minerals. The lignans are thought to lower blood cholesterol levels and blood pressure.

History & folklore Sesame was one of the plants found in the tomb of Tutankhamen (1370–1352 BCE). In ancient Egypt, the nutritionally valuable seeds were eaten and also pressed to yield oil, which was burned in lamps and used to make ointments. Sesame has long been considered to have magical powers, and the phrase "Open sesame!" from the *Arabian Nights* remains a well-known magical command. The Middle Eastern confection halvah is made from crushed and sweetened sesame seeds.

Medicinal actions & uses Sesame is principally used as a food and flavoring agent in China, but it is also taken to redress "states of deficiency," especially those affecting the liver and kidneys. The seeds are prescribed for problems such as dizziness, tinnitus (ringing in the ears), and blurred vision (when due to anemia). Owing to their lubricating effect within the digestive tract, the seeds are also considered a remedy for "dry" constipation. The seeds have a marked ability to stimulate the production of breast milk. Sesame seed oil benefits the skin and is used as a base for cosmetics. It can be used to treat fungal skin problems such as athlete's foot.

Research Research suggests that sesame seeds have antibacterial and antifungal activity. They also lower cholesterol and support levels of "good cholesterol" (HDL)."

Smilax spp. (Liliaceae)

Sarsaparilla

Description Perennial woody climber growing to 16 ft (5 m). Has broadly ovate leaves, tendrils, and small greenish flowers.

Habitat & cultivation Sarsaparilla species are found in tropical rainforests and in temperate regions in Asia and Australia. The root is gathered throughout the year.

Part used Root.

Constituents Sarsaparilla contains 1–3% steroidal saponins, phytosterols (including beta- and e-sitosterol), about 50% starch, resin, sarsapic acid, and minerals. Despite the herb's reputation for being testosterogenic, the steroidal saponins and sterols are estrogenic and anti-inflammatory. The saponins also have antibiotic activity.

History & folklore Brought from the New World to Spain in 1563, sarsaparilla was heralded as a cure for syphilis, reportedly having been used in the Caribbean with some success. The claims, however, were grossly inflated and the herb's popularity soon waned. In Mexico, sarsaparilla has traditionally been used to treat a variety of skin problems. Before it was replaced by artificial agents, sarsaparilla root was the original flavoring for root beer.

Medicinal actions & uses Sarsaparilla is anti-inflammatory and cleansing, and the herb can bring relief to skin problems such as eczema, psoriasis, and general itchiness, and help treat rheumatism, rheumatoid arthritis, and gout. Its estrogenic action makes it beneficial in premenstrual problems, and menopausal conditions such as debility and depression. Indigenous Amazonian peoples take sarsaparilla to improve virility and to treat menopausal problems. In Mexico, the root is still frequently consumed for its reputed tonic and aphrodisiac properties.

Research Some of the steroidal saponins have been shown to bind to toxins within the gut, reducing their absorption into the bloodstream. This may account for sarsaparilla's usefulness in autoimmune conditions such as psoriasis, rheumatoid arthritis, and ulcerative colitis, which can be associated with this sort of toxicity. Clinical research in China suggests that sarsaparilla might hold potential in the treatment of leptospirosis, a rare disease transmitted to humans by rats, and the acute stage of syphilis.

Solanum dulcamara (Solanaceae)

Bittersweet

Description Slender-stemmed, woody climber growing to 13 ft (4 m). Has deeply lobed oval leaves, dark purple flowers with yellow anthers, and scarlet oval berries.

Habitat & cultivation Native to Europe, North Africa, and northern Asia, this herb has been naturalized in North America. A common wayside plant, it flourishes on waste ground. The twigs are collected in spring or fall, and the root bark in the fall.

Parts used Twigs, root bark.

Constituents Bittersweet contains steroidal alkaloids (including solasodine and soldulcamaridine), steroidal saponins, and about 10% tannins.

History & folklore The Swedish botanist Carolus Linnaeus (1707–1778) considered the herb to be a valuable remedy for fever and inflammatory disorders. The name bittersweet possibly refers to the initial bitter taste of the berries, followed by a sweet aftertaste.

Medicinal actions & uses This plant has stimulant, expectorant, diuretic, detoxifying, and antirheumatic properties. It appears to be most effective taken internally to treat skin problems such as eczema, itchiness, psoriasis, and warts. A decoction of the twigs, applied as a wash, may also help lessen the severity of these conditions. The herb may also be taken to relieve asthma, chronic bronchitis, and rheumatic conditions, including gout.

Caution Bittersweet is toxic in excess. Take only under professional supervision.

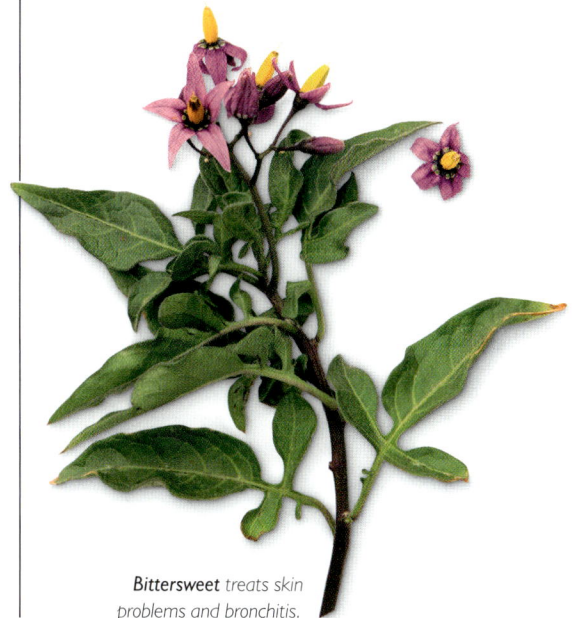

Bittersweet treats skin problems and bronchitis.

Solanum melongena (Solanaceae)

Eggplant,
Aubergine

Description An erect, herbaceous perennial growing to 28 in (70 cm). Has slightly woolly leaves, violet flowers, and large purple fruit.

Habitat & cultivation Native to India and Southeast Asia, the eggplant is now cultivated in many tropical areas and also grown under glass in cooler climates. The fruit is gathered when ripe in summer or fall.

Parts used Fruit, fruit juice, leaves.

Constituents Eggplant contains proteins, carbohydrates, and vitamins A, B_1, B_2, and C.

History & folklore Eggplant has been cultivated as a food in southern and eastern Asia since ancient times.

Medicinal actions & uses Eggplant fruit helps to lower blood cholesterol levels and is suitable as part of a diet to help regulate high blood pressure. The fruit can be applied fresh as a poultice for hemorrhoids, but it is more commonly used in the form of an oil or ointment. The fruit and its juice are effective diuretics. A soothing, emollient poultice for the treatment of burns, abscesses, cold sores, and similar conditions can be made from eggplant leaves. The mashed fruit can also be applied to sunburn.

Research Ongoing research suggests that eggplant may be a useful food/medicine in treating high cholesterol levels or disordered blood fats. It might also help as part of a regime to treat metabolic syndrome, a disease that typically involves high blood pressure, raised cholesterol levels, late onset diabetes, and obesity. Two small clinical trials found that eggplant lowered total cholesterol levels.

Caution Eggplant leaves are toxic and should only be used externally.

Solanum tuberosum (Solanaceae)

Potato

Description Perennial growing to 3 ft (1 m). Has branching stems with compound leaves, white or purple flowers, green berries, and swollen tubers (potatoes).

Habitat & cultivation Native to Chile, Bolivia, and Peru, the potato plant with its many varieties is cultivated around the world. The tuber is normally unearthed from fall to early spring.

Part used Tuber.

Constituents Potato contains starch, large amounts of vitamins A, B_1, B_2, C, and K, minerals (especially

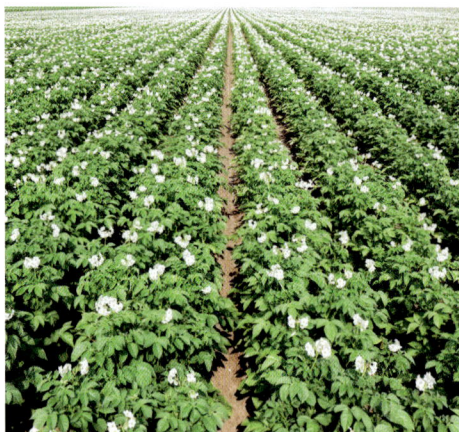

Potato can be helpful in relieving the painful symptoms of a gastric ulcer.

potassium), and very small quantities of atropine alkaloids. One property of these alkaloids is the reduction of digestive secretions, including acids produced in the stomach.

History & folklore Many different potato species and varieties were cultivated by the Quechua and Aymara peoples of the central Andes. In the early 16th century, the potato was introduced into Europe by Spanish voyagers returning from the New World. It was not until \the 18th century that the potato became a staple ingredient in the European diet.

Medicinal actions & uses Taken in moderation, potato juice can be helpful in the treatment of peptic ulcers, bringing relief from pain and acidity. The juice or the mashed pulp may be used externally to soothe painful joints, headache, backache, skin rashes, and hemorrhoids. Potato skins are used in India to treat swollen gums and to heal burns.

Related species The root of the Brazilian *S. insidiosum* is used as a diuretic and stomach-supporting remedy.

Cautions All parts of the plant except the tuber are poisonous. Excessive doses of potato juice are toxic. Do not drink the juice of more than one large potato per day.

Solidago virgaurea (Asteraceae)

Goldenrod

Description Perennial plant growing to 28 in (70 cm). Has toothed leaves and branched spikes of golden-yellow flowers.

Habitat & cultivation Native to Europe and Asia and naturalized in North America, goldenrod prefers open areas, waste ground, and hillsides. It is gathered in summer while in flower.

Parts used Aerial parts.

Constituents Goldenrod contains saponins, diterpenes, phenolic glucosides, acetylenes, cinnamates, flavonoids, tannins, hydroxybenzoates, and inulin. The saponins are antifungal.

History & folklore The herbalist John Gerard commented wryly in 1597 that "goldenrod has in times past been had in greater estimation and regard than in these days: for within my remembrance, I have known the dry herb which came from beyond the seas, sold … for half a crown an ounce. But since it was found in Hampstead wood [London] … no man will give half a crown for an hundredweight of it: which plainly setteth forth our inconstancy and sudden mutability, esteeming no longer of any thing (how precious soever it may be) than whilst it is strange and rare." Four hundred years on, one can only agree.

Medicinal actions & uses Antioxidant, diuretic, and astringent, goldenrod is a valuable remedy for

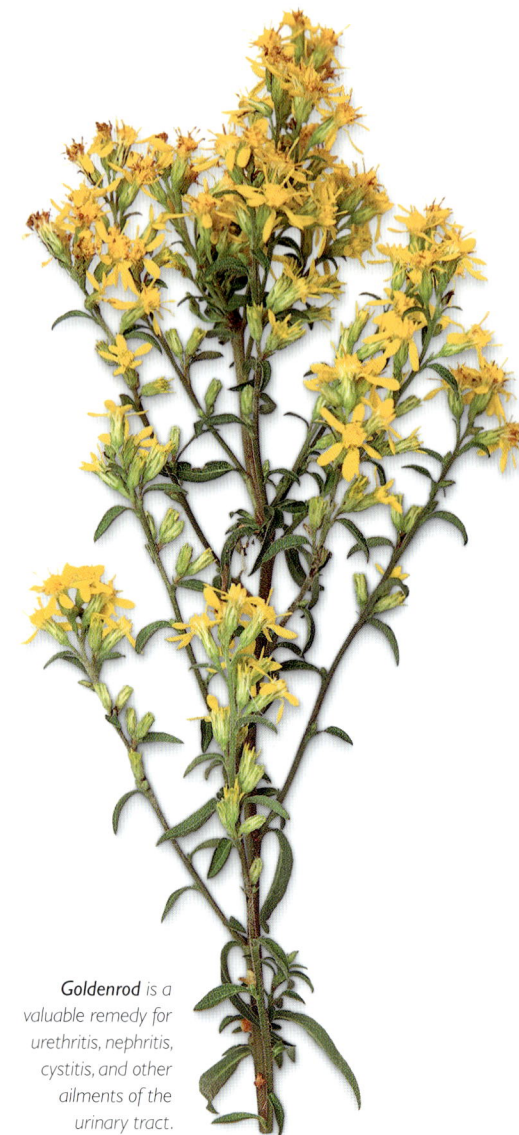

Goldenrod is a valuable remedy for urethritis, nephritis, cystitis, and other ailments of the urinary tract.

urinary tract disorders. It is used both for serious ailments such as nephritis, and for more common problems like cystitis. The herb also has a reputation for helping to flush out kidney and bladder stones. Goldenrod's saponins act specifically against the *Candida* fungus, the cause of vaginal yeast infection and oral thrush. The herb can also be taken for conditions such as sore throats, chronic nasal congestion, and diarrhea. Due to its mild action, goldenrod is used to treat gastroenteritis in children. Externally, it may be used as a mouthwash or douche for thrush.

Related species Various *Solidago* species are used medicinally in North America. Several species, including Canadian goldenrod (*S. canadensis*), have been taken to relieve colds, fevers, and chest pain. Sweet-scented goldenrod (*S. odora*) was listed as a stimulant, carminative, and diaphoretic (sweat-inducer) in the US *Pharmacopoeia* from 1820 to 1882.

Self-help uses Allergic rhinitis with congestion, p. 310; Urinary infections, p. 324.

Sorbus aucuparia (Rosaceae)

Rowan,
Mountain ash

Description Deciduous tree growing to 39 ft (12 m). Has reddish bark, compound leaves, clusters of small white flowers, and clusters of round red-orange fruit (berries).

Habitat & cultivation Rowan grows in woodlands throughout the Northern Hemisphere. It is also cultivated as an ornamental tree.

Part used Fruit.

Constituents The fruit contains tannins, sorbitol, malic and sorbic acids, sugars, and vitamin C. The seeds contain cyanogenic glycosides, which, in a reaction upon contact with water, produce the extremely poisonous prussic acid.

History & folklore In the Scottish Highlands, this tree was believed to be a reliable antidote to witchcraft. Highlanders planted it near their houses, and cowherds believed that by using a rowan switch to drive their cattle they could protect them from evil influences. The fruit has long been used to make preserves and alcoholic drinks.

Medicinal actions & uses The astringent rowan is most often taken as a jam or an infusion to treat diarrhea and hemorrhoids. In addition, infusions may be used as a gargle for sore throats and as a wash to treat hemorrhoids and excessive vaginal discharge.

Caution Remove the toxic seeds prior to using the fruit as a medicine or a food.

Spigelia marilandica (Loganiaceae)

Indian pink

Description Perennial plant with oval to lance-shaped leaves, spikes of brilliant red-pink flowers, and a double seed capsule.

Habitat & cultivation Native to the southern regions of the US, Indian pink flourishes in dry rich soil in clearings and along woodland borders. The root is unearthed in the fall.

Part used Root.

Constituents Indian pink contains alkaloids (mainly spigeleine), a volatile oil, tannin, and resin. Spigeleine is emetic and irritant to the stomach.

History & folklore Indian pink was used extensively by Indigenous American peoples as a worm-expelling herb. It was gathered for trade with white colonizers by the Creek and Cherokee peoples. From the late 18th century onward, Indian pink became one of the chief deworming herbs used in North America and Europe.

Medicinal actions & uses Indian pink is used today solely to expel intestinal worms—particularly tapeworms and roundworms. It is prescribed with other herbs such as senna (*Cassia senna*, p. 79) and fennel (*Foeniculum vulgare*, p. 217) to ensure the elimination of both the worms and the root itself, which is potentially toxic if it is absorbed through the gut.

Related species Several *Spigelia* species act as worm-expelling herbs, for example *S. flemmingania*, native to Brazil, and *S. anthelmia*, native to the Caribbean, Venezuela, and Colombia. *S. anthelmia* also contains isoquinoline alkaloids and is used in the treatment of heart disease.

Caution Only use Indian pink with the supervision of a professional practitioner.

Stachys officinalis syn. *S. betonica* (Lamiaceae)

Betony

Description Mat-forming perennial growing to a height of 2 ft (60 cm). Has toothed elliptical leaves and spikes of pink or white flowers.

Habitat & cultivation Betony grows throughout most of Europe, and occurs in Asia as far east as the Caucasus, where it is found in meadows, heathland, and hilly areas. The aerial parts are collected when the plant is in flower during early summer.

Parts used Aerial parts.

Constituents Betony contains alkaloids (including stachydrine and betonicine), as well as phenolic compounds, betaine, choline, and tannins.

History & folklore Betony has been regarded as a panacea since classical times, even attributed with the ability to ward off evil spirits. Antonius Musa, physician to Emperor Augustus (63 BCE–14 CE), claimed that betony would cure 47 different illnesses. The herb has always been particularly valued as a remedy for headaches.

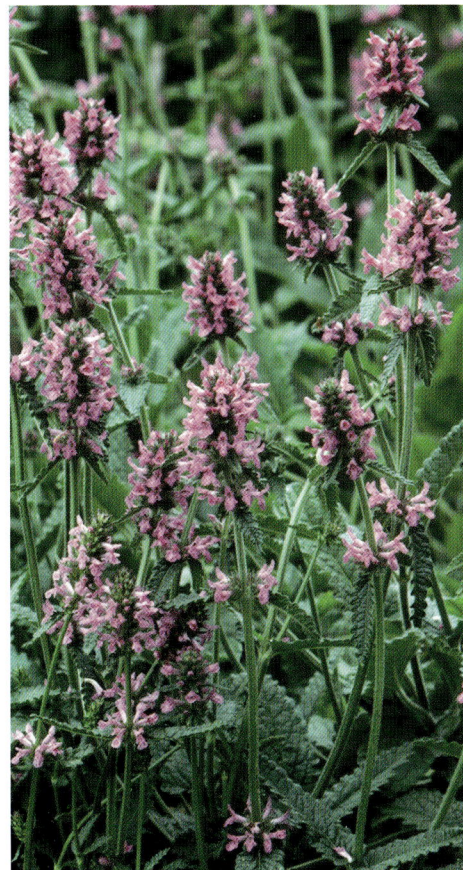

Betony is an age-old headache remedy. Its name may derive from the Celtic for "good head."

Medicinal actions & uses No longer regarded as a panacea, betony nevertheless has real value as a remedy for headaches and facial pain. The plant is also mildly sedative, relieving nervous stress and tension. In British herbal medicine, betony is thought to improve nervous function and to counter overactivity. It is taken to treat "frayed nerves," premenstrual complaints, poor memory, and tension. The plant has astringent properties, and in combination with other herbs, such as comfrey (*Symphytum officinale*, p. 142) and linden flowers (*Tilia* species, p. 286), it is effective against sinus headaches and congestion. Betony may be taken alone or with yarrow (*Achillea millefolium*, p. 60) to help staunch nosebleeds. Betony is also mildly bitter. It stimulates the digestive system and the liver, and has an overall tonic effect on the body.

Caution Do not take betony if you are pregnant.

Stellaria media (Caryophyllaceae)
Chickweed

Description Sprawling perennial growing to about 6 in (15 cm). Has hairy stems, oval leaves, and starlike white flowers

Habitat & cultivation Native to Europe and Asia, chickweed is now found in most regions of the world. It grows easily in waste ground, and is generally regarded as a troublesome weed. The plant is harvested in summer.

Parts used Aerial parts.

Constituents Chickweed contains triterpenoid saponins, coumarins, flavonoids, carboxylic acids, and vitamin C. The saponins may account for the herb's ability to help reduce itchiness.

History & folklore Dioscorides, a Greek physician writing in the 1st century CE, described chickweed's applications as follows: "it [chickweed] may usefully be applied with corn meal for inflammation of the eyes. The juice may also be introduced into the ear in earache." Apart from its medicinal uses, chickweed is a tasty and nutritious vegetable.

Medicinal actions & uses Chickweed is chiefly used to treat irritated skin, being applied as juice, poultice, ointment, or cream. In certain cases, chickweed may soothe severe itchiness where all other remedies have failed. It is often used to relieve eczema, varicose ulcers, and nettle rash (hives). An infusion of the fresh or dried plant may be added to a bath, where the herb's emollient properties will help to reduce inflammation—in rheumatic joints,

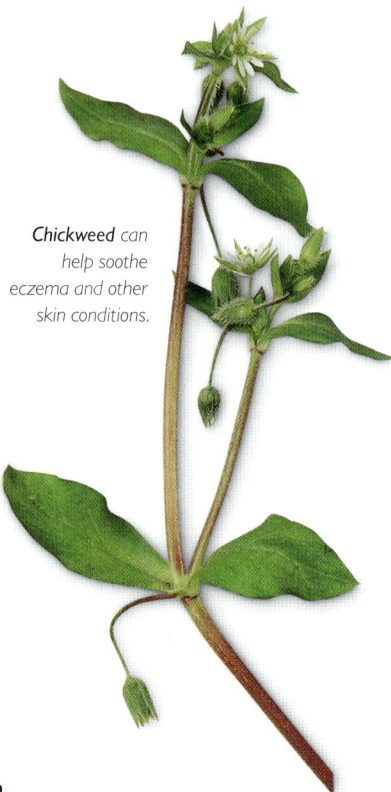

Chickweed can help soothe eczema and other skin conditions.

for example—and encourage tissue repair. Chickweed may also be taken internally to treat chest ailments. There is some suggestion that chickweed has an anti-obesity action.

Cautions If taken in excessive doses, chickweed may cause diarrhea and vomiting. Do not take during pregnancy.

Self-help uses Eczema, p. 310; Diaper rash & inflamed skin rashes, p. 328; Nettle rash, p. 313.

Stillingia sylvatica (Euphorbiaceae)
Queen's delight

Description Perennial growing to 4 ft (1.2 m). Has leathery leaves, yellow flowers without petals, and 3-lobed fruit.

Habitat & cultivation Queen's delight is native to the southeastern US. where it prefers sandy soils. The root is unearthed in the fall.

Part used Root.

Constituents Queen's delight contains diterpenes, fixed oil, volatile oil, resin, and tannins. The fresh root is considered to be most active.

History & folklore Queen's delight was used by Indigenous American peoples as a purgative, a treatment for skin eruptions, and a remedy for venereal disease. Creek women who had just given birth took a decoction of the root or were bathed with an infusion. Queen's delight was included in the *Pharmacopoeia of the United States* from 1831 to 1926.

Medicinal actions & uses Queen's delight appears to promote general detoxification. It is taken internally to help clear constipation, boils, weeping eczema, and scrofula (tubercular infection of the lymph glands of the neck). The root is also taken to treat bronchitis and throat infection. Externally, it is applied as a lotion to hemorrhoids, eczema, and psoriasis.

Cautions Use only under professional supervision. Queen's delight is emetic and purgative in large doses.

Strychnos nux-vomica (Loganiaceae)
Nux vomica

Description Evergreen tree growing to 49 ft (15 m). Has glossy oval leaves, tubular white flowers, and yellow fruit containing 5–8 disk-shaped seeds.

Habitat & cultivation Nux vomica is native to Southeast Asia. It grows wild and is cultivated commercially. The seeds are gathered when mature.

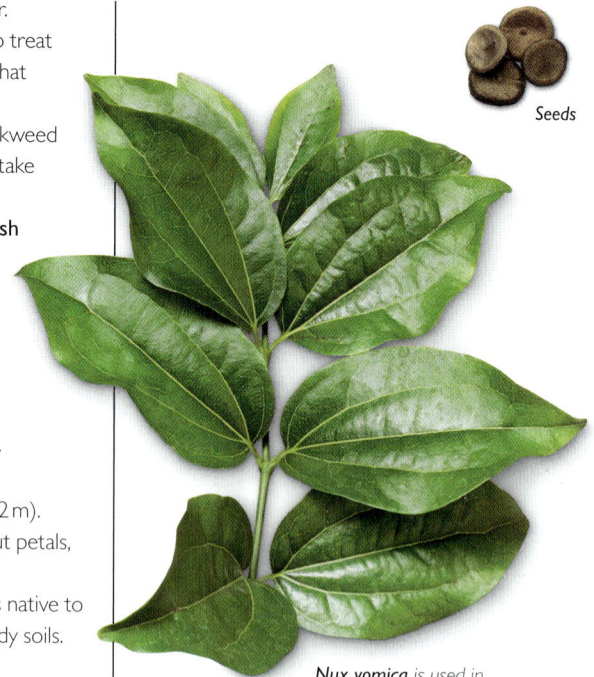

Seeds

Nux vomica is used in homeopathic preparations.

Parts used Seeds.

Constituents Nux vomica contains 3% indole alkaloids (predominantly strychnine, with many others), loganin, chlorogenic acid, and fixed oil. Strychnine is a lethal poison, producing intense muscle spasms.

History & folklore Nux vomica seeds were first brought to Europe in the 15th century, probably as a poison for game and rodents. In 1640, the seeds were first used in European medicine, as a stimulant.

Medicinal actions & uses Though rarely used internally due to its toxicity, nux vomica can be an effective nervous system stimulant, particularly in the elderly. In Chinese herbal medicine the seeds are used externally to relieve pain, to treat various types of tumors, and to relieve paralysis, including Bell's palsy (facial paralysis). Nux vomica is a common homeopathic remedy prescribed mainly for digestive problems, sensitivity to cold, irritability, and melancholia.

Research In a Chinese clinical trial, a paste made from nux vomica seeds was applied to 15,000 patients with Bell's palsy. The treatment was reported to have been effective in more than 80% of the cases.

Related species Many *Strychnos* species are equally potent and have been used as arrow poisons.

Cautions Take nux vomica only in homeopathic preparations. This herb and strychnine are subject to legal restrictions in most countries.

Styrax benzoin (Styracaceae)

Benzoin gum

Description Shrubby deciduous tree growing to 30 ft (9 m). Has pointed oval leaves and clusters of white, fragrant, bell-shaped flowers.

Habitat & cultivation Native to Southeast Asia, benzoin grows in tropical rainforests. It is also cultivated for its gum, which exudes from incisions made in the bark of trees that are at least 7 years old.

Part used Gum.

Constituents Benzoin gum contains variable quantities of cinnamic, benzoic, and sumaresinolic acid esters, free acids (such as benzoic acid), benzaldehyde, and vanillin.

Medicinal actions & uses Benzoin gum is strongly antiseptic and astringent. It may be used externally on wounds and ulcers to tighten and disinfect the affected tissue. When taken internally, benzoin gum acts to settle cramping, to stimulate coughing, and to disinfect the urinary tract. Benzoin gum is an ingredient of Friar's Balsam, an antiseptic and expectorant steam inhalation for sore throats, head and chest colds, asthma, and bronchitis.

Sutherlandia frutescens (Fabaceae)

Sutherlandia,
Balloon pea

Description A medium-size shrub growing up to 4 ft (1.2 m) in height, with fine grayish-green pinnate leaves, orange red flowers, and black seeds contained within distinctive balloon-shaped pods.

Habitat & cultivation Native to southern Africa, sutherlandia grows primarily in the Cape but can be found as far north as Botswana and Namibia. It is readily cultivated from seed, and though a subtropical plant is hardy down to −50°C. Plants collected in the wild vary widely in their chemical profiles.

Parts used Leaves and young stems

Constituents A relatively poorly understood herb, sutherlandia's main active constituents are triterpenoid saponins, flavonoids, L-canavinine, gamma-aminobutyric acid (GABA) and pinitol. L-canavinine has anticancer activity, pinitol is antidiabetic, and GABA has a direct anti-anxiety effect within the body.

History & folklore The Khoisan and other Indigenous peoples of southern Africa are thought to have used sutherlandia over many generations for its wide-ranging therapeutic benefits. The first recorded use of the herb to treat cancer is in 1895.

Medicinal actions & uses A key traditional medicine in southern Africa, sutherlandia is used to treat many varied conditions, including fever, indigestion, peptic ulcer, dysentery, cancer (prevention and treatment), diabetes, kidney and liver disorders, heart failure, and urinary tract infection. As an adaptogen, it supports the body in enduring stress of all kinds and can help with anxiety and depression—due in part to its GABA content. In South Africa, it is commonly taken alongside retroviral treatment by people with HIV for its antiviral, tonic, and restorative effects.

Related species Several closely related species, including *Sutherlandia microphylla*, are used interchangeably with sutherlandia.

Cautions Do not take in pregnancy or if breastfeeding. In view of its ability to interact negatively with prescribed drugs, it is best taken on professional advice.

Swertia chirata (Gentianaceae)

Chiretta,
Chirayata (Hindi)

Description Annual, growing to about 3 ft (1 m), with a much-branched stem, smooth, pointed, lance-shaped leaves, and numerous purple-tinged, pale green flowers.

Habitat & cultivation Chiretta grows at high altitudes in northern India and Nepal. The whole herb is harvested while in flower.

Parts used Whole herb.

Constituents Chiretta contains xanthones, bitter iridoids (including amarogentin), alkaloids, and flavones.

History & folklore Chiretta was a common treatment for malaria, until Peruvian bark (*Cinchona* spp., p. 84) became readily available in Europe and Asia.

Medicinal actions & uses A strongly bitter herb, chiretta is powerful medicine for a weak stomach, especially when linked to nausea, indigestion, and bloating. It is taken in small, frequent doses to improve appetite and digestive function. For hiccups, small, frequent doses are taken with honey. Like most bitters it reduces fever, cooling the body and increasing blood flow to the liver. In Ayurvedic medicine the herb is used for *pitta* (fire) conditions, and is best known as the major herb in *mahasudarshan churna*—a standard mixture of more than 50 herbs prescribed for fevers such as malaria, liver problems, gallstones, and indigestion. Recently it has been used with other herbs to treat allergies.

Research The xanthones are thought to be antituberculous and antimalarial. Amarogentin has a protective action on the liver.

Caution Avoid in digestive hyperacidity.

Symplocarpus foetidus (Araceae)

Skunk cabbage

Description Unpleasant-smelling perennial plant growing to 30 in (75 cm). Has a thick tuberous rootstock, cabbage-like leaves, and small purple flowers on a hooded spike.

Habitat & cultivation Native to northern North America, skunk cabbage thrives in meadows, swamps, and marshes. The root and rhizome are collected in fall or early spring.

Parts used Root, rhizome.

Constituents Skunk cabbage contains a volatile oil, serotonin (5HT), and resins.

History & folklore The Winnebago and Dakota peoples used the expectorant and antispasmodic skunk cabbage root to treat asthma and bronchitis. The root was also employed as a poultice to draw splinters and thorns, to heal wounds, and to relieve headaches. It was much used in America in the 19th century.

Medicinal actions & uses Skunk cabbage continues to be used primarily as an expectorant, treating cases of asthma, bronchitis, and whooping cough. It is also taken for upper respiratory problems such as nasal congestion and hay fever. Less commonly, skunk cabbage is used as a treatment for epilepsy, headaches, vertigo, and rheumatic problems, and to stop bleeding.

Cautions Handling fresh skunk cabbage may cause the skin to blister. Excessive doses can bring on nausea and vomiting, headaches, and dizziness.

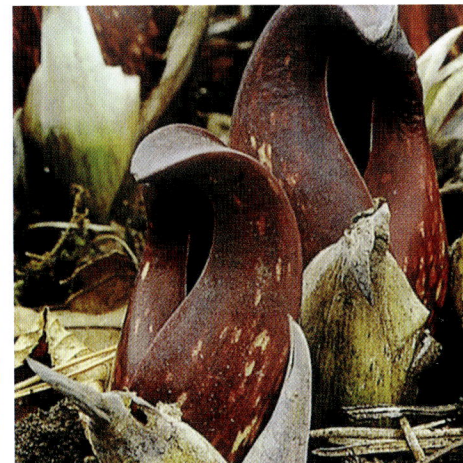

Skunk cabbage is a foul-smelling plant with a powerful expectorant action.

Syzygium cumini (Myrtaceae)

Jambul

Description Evergreen tree growing to 33 ft (10 m). Has lance-shaped leaves and green-yellow flowers.

Habitat & cultivation A native of southern Asia and Australia, jambul is now also found in tropical regions of Africa. The tree is cultivated commercially for its fruit and is propagated from seed or semi-ripe cuttings in summer. It requires well-drained soil and plenty of sun. The fruit is harvested when ripe.

Parts used Fresh and dried fruit, seeds.

Constituents Jambul contains triterpenes, anthocyanins, flavonoids, and volatile oil.

History & folklore Jambul is a typical example of a medicinal plant that is both food and medicine. The fruit when ripe has the scent and taste of a ripe apricot and is eaten as a preserve. While both fruit and seed have a tonic and astringent effect on the digestion, the seeds have long traditional use in Ayurveda as a preventative and treatment for diabetes.

Medicinal actions & uses Following traditional use, jambul continues to be employed for a wide variety of health problems. The powdered seed is commonly taken to treat diabetes and the frequent urination that accompanies it, as well as a remedy for mouth ulcers, stomachache, diarrhea, dysentery, and worms. Case reports over the last 100 years and more recent pharmacological research supports the use of jambul for diabetes and poor blood glucose control. It is thought to lower blood-sugar levels by about 30%.

Related species Many other closely related species have notable therapeutic activity. Cloves (*Eugenia caryophyllata*, p. 101) are taken for digestive problems and to treat infection. *Syzygium gerrardii* from South Africa and *Luma chequen* from Chile are used to treat coughs and congestion.

Tamarindus indica (Fabaceae)

Tamarind

Description Evergreen tree growing to 80 ft (25 m). Has fine compound leaves, clusters of orange-yellow flowers, and brittle gray-brown seed pods (fruit) containing up to 12 round seeds.

Habitat & cultivation While native to Madagascar, the tamarind is now cultivated in many of the world's tropical regions, including the Caribbean, India, Southeast Asia, and China.

Parts used Fruit, leaves, seeds.

Constituents Tamarind contains 16–18% plant acids (including nicotinic acid—vitamin B$_3$), a volatile oil (with geranial, geraniol, and limonene), sugars, pectin, 0.8% potassium, and fats. Vitamin C was formerly believed to be among the constituents of tamarind, but this is now being disputed.

History & folklore Sailors ate tamarind fruit as a nourishing complement to their otherwise starchy diet, in the belief that eating the fruit would prevent scurvy. However, it appears that tamarind does not in fact contain vitamin C. Tamarind is a major ingredient in many chutneys and condiments, notably Worcestershire sauce.

Medicinal actions & uses Tamarind is a wholesome and cleansing fruit that improves digestion, relieves gas, soothes sore throats, and acts as a mild laxative. However, mixed with cumin and sugar, tamarind is also prescribed as a treatment for dysentery. It is given for loss of appetite and nausea, and as a stomach tonic and mild laxative. It may help with nausea and vomiting in pregnancy. In southern India, tamarind soup is taken to treat colds and other ailments that produce excessive phlegm. In Chinese medicine, it is considered a cooling herb, appropriate for treating "summer heat." The fruit is also given for loss of appetite, for nausea and vomiting in pregnancy, and for constipation. The seeds' traditional use as an antivenin in snake bite has been partly confirmed in laboratory research.

Self-help use Sore throats, p. 321

Tanacetum vulgare (Asteraceae)

Tansy

Description Strongly aromatic perennial growing to 3 ft (1 m). Has an erect stem, feathery compound leaves, and clusters of yellow disk-shaped flower heads.

Habitat & cultivation Found throughout temperate zones in the northern hemisphere, tansy grows on waste ground, alongside roads, and close to water. The flowering tops are collected as the flowers open in summer.

Parts used Flowering tops.

Constituents Tansy contains a volatile oil, which includes significant levels of thujone and camphor, sesquiterpene lactones, flavonoids, and resin. The volatile oil strongly induces menstruation.

History & folklore While it is not mentioned in surviving classical texts, tansy was described by medieval herbalists, notably St. Hildegard of Bingen (12th century). Ever since that time, tansy has been used most commonly as a worm-expelling plant. In England, tansy puddings were consumed during Lent.

Medicinal actions & uses Tansy is little used today because of its potential toxicity. When the plant is

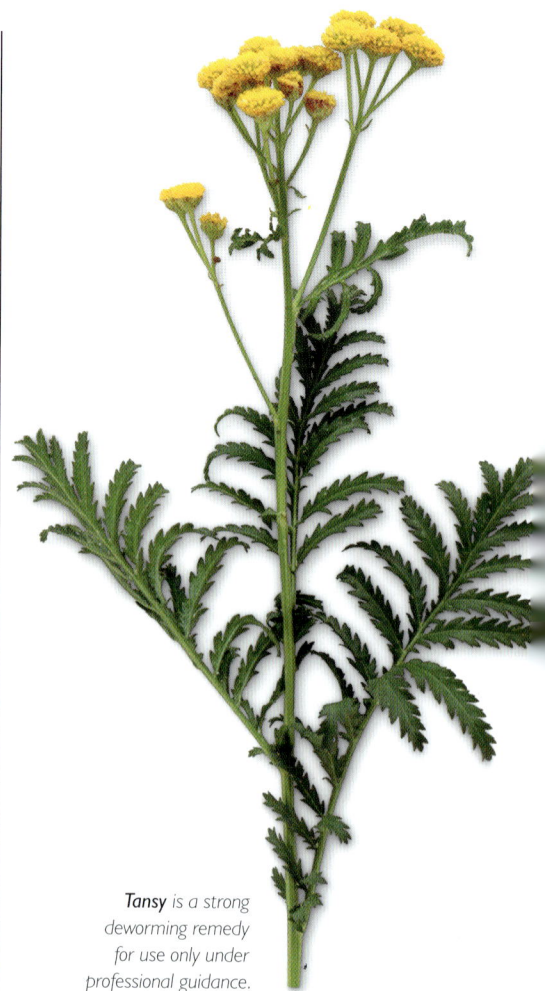

Tansy is a strong deworming remedy for use only under professional guidance.

taken, it is chiefly in order to expel intestinal worms, and, to a lesser degree, to help stimulate menstrual bleeding. Tansy may be used externally to kill scabies, fleas, and lice, but even external application of tansy preparations carries the risk of toxicity.

Cautions Use only under professional supervision. Tansy is possibly unsafe for internal and external use, and should never be taken during pregnancy. The plant, and especially its essential oil, are subject to legal restrictions in some countries.

Taxus baccata (Taxaceae)

Yew

Description Slow-growing evergreen tree reaching 80 ft (25 m) in height. Has rust-red bark and flattened, dark green needlelike leaves. The female trees produce fleshy red cuplike fruit.

Habitat & cultivation Yew grows throughout northern temperate zones. More often found in cultivation than in the wild, it prefers lime-rich soil. The leaves are gathered in spring.

Part used Leaves.

Constituents Yew contains a mixture of alkaloids known as taxine, and also diterpenes (including taxol in some varieties), lignans, tannin, and resin.

History & folklore The yew tree was sacred to the Druids, who are believed to have considered it an emblem of immortality. The Druids planted yews in holy sites, a practice that continued with the coming of Christianity. Many medieval churchyards contain ancient yews, some thought to be over 2,000 years old. In the Middle Ages, the best longbows were made from yew wood, as were magic wands.

Medicinal actions & uses Though yew has been used in small doses to treat rheumatic and urinary problems, its extreme toxicity makes it an unsafe medicinal plant.

Research Taxol inhibits cell division, and has thus been extensively researched for its use as an anticancer drug. Taxol is most commonly found in the Pacific yew (*T. brevifolia*), though some varieties of *T. baccata* also contain the substance. Studies have been conducted since the 1980s in search of potential cancer treatments.

Caution Yew is extremely toxic. Do not take under any circumstances.

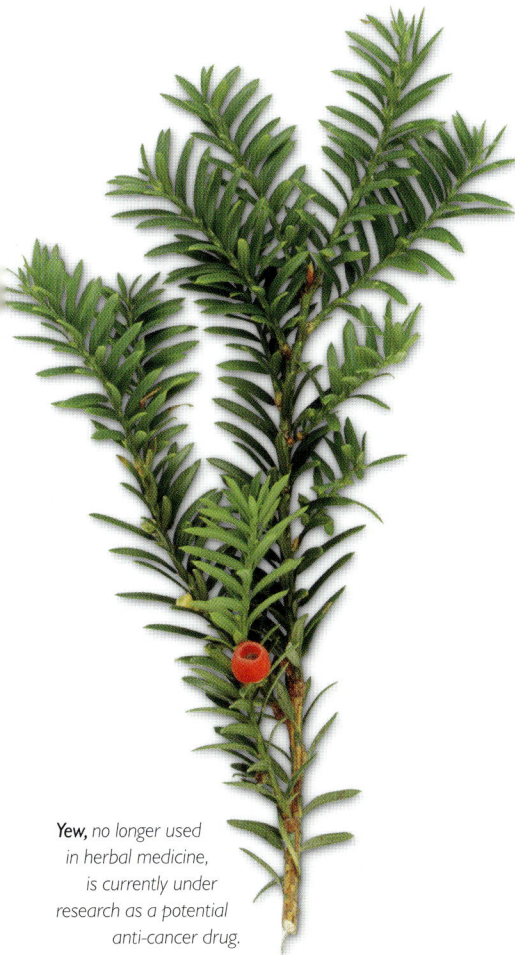

Yew, no longer used in herbal medicine, is currently under research as a potential anti-cancer drug.

Terminalia bellirica (Combretaceae)

Beleric myrobalan

Description Evergreen tree with clusters of oval leaves, spikes of small greenish unpleasant-smelling flowers, and hairy brown fruit.

Habitat & cultivation Beleric myrobalan is native to India, Malaysia, and the Philippines. It is found in forests and is cultivated for its astringent fruit, which is gathered both immature and ripe.

Part used Fruit.

Constituents The fruit contains tannins and anthraquinones.

Medicinal actions & uses Beleric myrobalan fruit is astringent, tonic, and laxative. It is principally employed as a treatment for digestive and respiratory problems. In Indian herbal medicine, the ripe fruit is taken for diarrhea and indigestion, and the unripe fruit is used as a laxative for chronic constipation. It forms part of the classic Ayurvedic *Triphala* formula, chiefly used as a bowel tonic. Beleric myrobalan is also often used to treat upper respiratory tract infections that cause symptoms of sore throats, hoarseness, and coughs.

Related species Many *Terminalia* species are used to make astringent remedies, and also for their timber. See chebulic myrobalan (*T. chebula*, following entry).

Caution Do not take during pregnancy.

Terminalia chebula (Combretaceae)

Chebulic myrobalan

Description Evergreen tree growing to 65 ft 20 m). Has egg-shaped leaves, white flowers in terminal spikes, and small, 5-ribbed fruit.

Habitat & cultivation Native to Central Asia and India, chebulic myrobalan is found throughout Iran, Pakistan, and India. The fruit is collected when ripe.

Part used Fruit.

Constituents Chebulic myrobalan contains triterpenes, polyphenols, a coumarin (chebulic acid), resin, and fixed oil.

History & folklore Chebulic myrobalan has been used in Indian medicine for several thousand years, and the fruit has long been considered a prime remedy for all manner of digestive problems.

Medicinal actions & uses Laxative and astringent, the fruit gently improves bowel regularity without excessively irritating the colon. It forms part of the classic Ayurvedic *Triphala* formula, used chiefly as a bowel tonic. Like Chinese rhubarb (*Rheum palmatum*, p. 130), chebulic myrobalan may be used as a treatment for diarrhea and dysentery. The fruit's tannins protect the gut wall from irritation and infection, and tend to reduce intestinal secretions. Likewise, the fruit helps to counter acidic indigestion and heartburn. A decoction of chebulic myrobalan may be used as a gargle and mouthwash, as a lotion for sore and inflamed eyes, and as a douche for vaginitis and excessive vaginal discharge. The fruit has been also shown to have liver-protective and antidiabetic properties.

Caution Do not take chebulic myrobalan during pregnancy.

Theobroma cacao (Sterculiaceae)

Cacao, Cocoa

Description Evergreen tree growing to 26 ft (8 m). Has pale brown bark, glossy oval leaves, clusters of small yellow flowers, and large, pear-shaped, red-yellow seed pods.

Habitat & cultivation Native to Mexico and Central America, cacao is now a major crop throughout the tropics. The seed pods are harvested several times a year and are cut directly from the trunk of the tree (where they grow). One pod contains up to 50 beans, with roughly 900 weighing 2¼ lb (1 kg). According to the World Cocoa Foundation, world production of cacao in 2012 was more than 3.8 million tons.

Part used Seeds.

Constituents The unprocessed seed pulp contains high levels of polyphenols (mostly proanthocyanidins and catechins), xanthines (including caffeine), a fixed oil, and many constituents responsible for chocolate's flavor. Due to fermentation and the processing involved, chocolate has significantly reduced levels of polyphenols. Minute quantities of endorphins (powerful painkillers that occur naturally within the body) are also present in cacao.

History & folklore The word *chocolate* derives from *chócolatl*, the name given to this tree by the Aztecs. In 1720, Cotton Mather, an American preacher and natural historian, praised cacao, writing that the plant "supplies the Indian [sic] with bread, water, wine, vinegar, brandy, milk, oil, honey, sugar, needles, thread, linen, clothes, caps, spoons, besoms, baskets, paper, and nails; timber, coverings for their houses; masts, sails, cordage for their vessels; and medicine for their diseases; and what can be desired more?"

Medicinal actions & uses Though cacao is most often used as a food, it also has therapeutic value as a nervous system stimulant. In Central America and the Caribbean, the seeds are taken as a heart and kidney tonic. The plant may be used to treat angina, and as a diuretic. Cacao butter (the fixed oil) makes a good lip salve and is often used as a base for suppositories and pessaries.

Research The potent mix of polyphenols in the unprocessed seed pulp has been the main focus of research into cacao. These have a protective activity on the heart and blood vessels, particularly supporting the capillaries or microcirculation. Cacao consumption is linked with lower blood pressure and cholesterol levels, as well as a reduced risk of coronary heart disease and stroke. It also appears to have an antidiabetic activity, stimulating the pancreas to regulate blood sugar levels more effectively. Other potential uses of cacao that have been investigated include the prevention of tooth decay, as an aid to weight loss, as a cancer-preventative food within the diet, and as a treatment for chronic fatigue.

Thuja occidentalis (Cupressaceae)
Arborvitae

Description Evergreen tree growing to 33 ft (10 m). Has scalelike leaves, male and female flowers, and small, egg-shaped cones.

Habitat & cultivation Native to the northeastern US and also known as white cedar, arborvitae flourishes in wet, marshy ground and along riverbanks. It has become a popular ornamental tree in Europe. The leaves are gathered in summer.

Parts used Leaves.

Constituents Arborvitae contains a volatile oil (up to 60% thujone), coumarins, flavonoids (including procyanidin), tannins, and polysaccharides.

History & folklore Many Indigenous American peoples prized arborvitae as a medicine for fever, headaches, coughs, swollen hands, and rheumatic problems. The herb was burned as a smudge (smoky fire) for its scent and to ward off evil spirits. The 19th-century Eclectic herbalists used arborvitae as a remedy for bronchitis, rheumatism, and uterine cancer. Arborvitae has also been used to treat the side-effects of the smallpox vaccination.

Medicinal actions & uses Arborvitae has an established antiviral activity. It is most often used to treat warts and polyps, being prescribed both internally and externally for these conditions. It is also used as part of a regime for treating cancer—especially cancer of the uterus. Arborvitae makes an effective expectorant and anticatarrhal remedy, and may be used to treat acute bronchitis and other respiratory infections. It induces menstruation and can be taken to bring on delayed periods, though this use is inadvisable if menstrual pain is severe. Arborvitae is diuretic and is used to treat acute

cystitis and bed-wetting in children. Extracts of the herb may be painted on painful joints or muscles as a counterirritant, improving local blood supply and easing pain and stiffness.

Cautions Take only under professional supervision. Do not take arborvitae during pregnancy or while breastfeeding.

Self-help use Warts, p. 314.

Thymus serpyllum (Lamiaceae)
Wild thyme

Description Tuft-forming evergreen herb growing to a height of 3 in (7 cm). Has square stems, small aromatic oval leaves, and spikes of bright mauve flowers.

Habitat & cultivation Native to Europe, thyme prefers heaths, moorland, and barren places. The herb is collected when in flower in summer.

Parts used Flowering tops.

Constituents Wild thyme contains a volatile oil (with thymol, carvacrol and linalool), flavonoids, caffeic acid, tannins, and resin. The volatile oil's properties are similar to, but less potent than, those of thyme oil (from *Thymus vulgaris,* p. 147).

History & folklore The 17th-century herbalist Nicholas Culpeper advised taking wild thyme to treat internal bleeding, coughing, and vomiting. He noted that "it comforts and strengthens the head, stomach, reins [ureters] and womb, expels wind and breaks the stone." Carolus Linnaeus, the 18th-century Swedish naturalist, used the plant to treat headaches and hangovers.

Medicinal actions & uses Like its close relative thyme (*Thymus vulgaris*, p. 147), wild thyme is antiseptic and antifungal. It may be taken as an infusion or syrup to treat flu and colds, sore throats, coughs, whooping cough, chest infections, and bronchitis. Wild thyme has anticatarrhal properties and helps clear a stuffy nose, sinusitis, ear congestion, and related complaints. It has been used to expel threadworms and roundworms in children, and is used to settle gas and colic. Wild thyme's antispasmodic action makes it useful in relieving period pain. Externally, it may be applied as a poultice to treat mastitis (inflammation of the breast), and an infusion may be used as a wash to help heal wounds and ulcers. Wild thyme is also used in herbal baths and pillows.

Related species See thyme (*T. vulgaris*, p. 147).

Caution For worms in children, use only under professional supervision.

Tilia spp. (Tiliaceae)
Linden, Lime

Description Deciduous trees growing to a height of 100 ft (30 m), with smooth gray bark, heart-shaped leaves, and clusters of pale yellow flowers with winglike bracts.

Habitat & cultivation Native to Europe, linden is found in the wild, but is also much planted in gardens and along roads. The flowers are collected in summer.

Parts used Flowers and bracts.

Constituents Linden contains flavonoids (especially quercetin and kaempferol), caffeic and other acids, mucilage (about 3%), tannins, volatile oil (0.02%-0.1%), and traces of benzodiazepine-like compounds. The flavonoids improve circulation.

History & folklore Greek myth recounts how Philyra, a nymph, was raped by the god Cronus in the guise of a horse, and eventually gave birth to the famed centaur, Chiron. Philyra was so devastated that she begged the gods not to leave her among mortals. The gods granted her wish by transforming her into a linden tree.

Medicinal actions & uses Linden is an antispasmodic, sweat-inducing, and sedative remedy. It relieves tension and sinus headaches, helping to calm the mind and allow easy sleep. Linden is an excellent remedy for stress and panic, and is used specifically to treat nervous palpitations. The flowers bring relief to colds and flu by reducing nasal congestion and soothing fever. Linden flowers are commonly taken to lower high blood pressure, particularly when there are emotional factors involved. The flowers are used over the long term to treat high systolic blood pressure associated with arteriosclerosis. Because of their emollient quality, linden flowers are used in France to make a lotion for itchy skin.

Related species The Mexican and North American linden (*Tilia americana*) has similar properties to its European cousins.

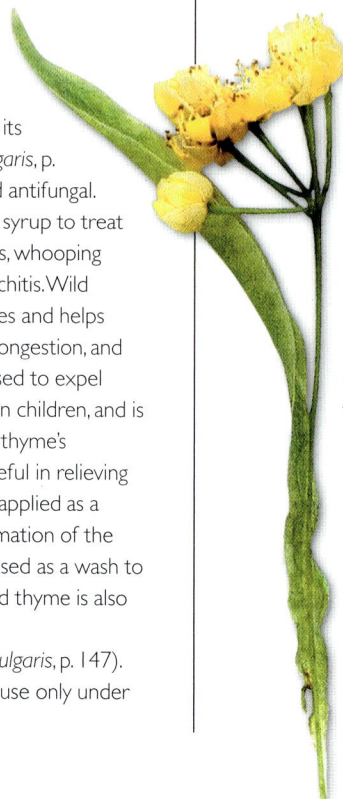

Linden flowers from several species, including Tilia europaea, are used in herbal medicine.

Trifolium pratense (Fabaceae)
Red clover

Description Perennial herb growing to 16 in (40 cm). Has a hairy upright stem, leaves with 3 (or, rarely, 4) oval leaflets with a white crescent marking, and pink to purple egg-shaped flower heads.

Habitat & cultivation Native to Europe and Asia, and naturalized in North America and Australia, red clover is widely cultivated for hay and as a nitrogen-fixing crop. The flower heads are collected when newly opened in summer.

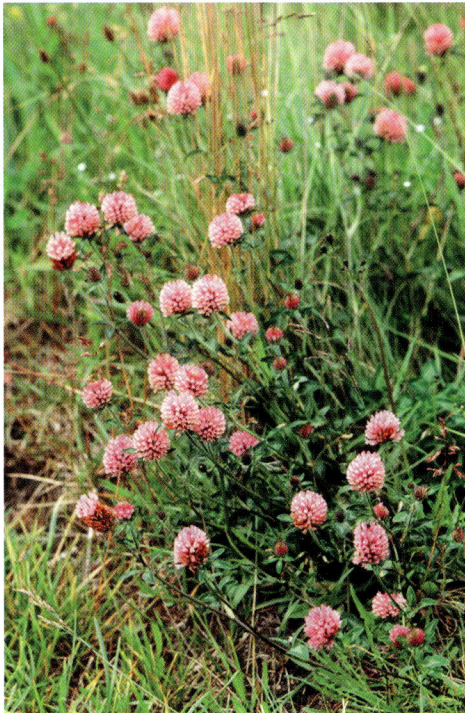

Red clover is a common wayside plant, but it is also cultivated as a fodder crop.

Parts used Flower heads.

Constituents Red clover contains volatile oil, including benzyl alcohol and methyl salicylate, isoflavones, coumarins, and cyanogenic glycosides. The isoflavones occur at relatively high levels and are phytoestrogenic. The isolated isoflavones are marketed as a treatment for menopausal problems.

History & folklore This herb has traditionally been used to treat breast cancer. A concentrated decoction was applied to the site of the tumor in order to encourage it to grow outward and clear the body.

Medicinal actions & uses Red clover is used to treat skin conditions, normally in combination with other purifying herbs such as burdock (*Arctium lappa*, p. 69) and yellow dock (*Rumex crispus*, p. 273). It is also expectorant and may be used for spasmodic coughs. Red clover's significant phytoestrogenic activity has led to increasing use of the herb to relieve menopausal symptoms. In most cases it will be preferable to use extracts of red clover flowers rather than the isoflavones on their own.

Research The isoflavones have an established phytoestrogenic activity. Red clover isoflavones have been shown to have not only therapeutic use during menopause, helping to reduce the impact of falling estrogen levels, but also to exert a protective effect on the heart and circulation in menopausal women with low estrogen levels. Early-stage research points to the isoflavones countering bone loss, making them potentially of use in osteoporosis. Due to the isoflavones' ability to "compete" with the body's own estrogen, it is now thought that red clover may be helpful in both preventing and treating breast cancer.

Trigonella foenum-graecum (Fabaceae)
Fenugreek

Description Strongly aromatic annual growing to about 32 in (80 cm). Has trifoliate leaves, yellowish-white pealike flowers, and sickle-shaped pods.

Habitat & cultivation Native to North Africa and countries bordering the eastern Mediterranean, fenugreek grows on waste ground and is widely cultivated, notably in India. The seeds are collected during the fall months.

Part used Seeds.

Constituents Fenugreek contains a volatile oil, alkaloids (including trigonelline), saponins (based on diosgenin), flavonoids, mucilage (about 27%), protein (about 25%), fixed oil (approximately 8%), vitamins A, B$_1$, and C, and minerals.

History & folklore The Egyptian Ebers papyrus, which dates from c. 1500 BCE, records a prescription for burns that includes fenugreek. The seeds were also used in ancient Egypt to induce childbirth. In the 5th century BCE the Greek physician Hippocrates considered fenugreek to be a valuable soothing herb. Dioscorides, writing in the 1st century CE, recommended fenugreek as a remedy for all manner of gynecological problems, including infection of the uterus and inflammation of the vagina and vulva.

Medicinal actions & uses Fenugreek is much used in herbal medicine in North Africa, the Middle East, and India, being esteemed as a remedy for a wide variety of conditions. The nourishing seeds are given during convalescence and to encourage weight gain, especially in anorexia. They are also helpful in lowering fever, with some authorities comparing their ability to that of quinine. The seeds' soothing effect makes them of value in treating gastritis and gastric ulcers. They are used to induce childbirth and to increase breast milk production. Fenugreek is also thought to be antidiabetic and to lower blood cholesterol levels. Externally, the seeds may be applied as a paste to treat abscesses, boils, ulcers, and burns, or used as a douche for excessive vaginal discharge.

Research Research indicates that fenugreek seed (preferably powdered) can prove effective in controlling insulin resistance and late-onset diabetes. The seeds help to stabilize blood-sugar levels, though the recommended dosage of seed required is unclear. The seeds also lower blood cholesterol levels. Other potential uses for the seeds include cramping period pains, polycystic ovary syndrome (PCOS), and Parkinson's disease. An Iranian clinical trial in 2014 found that 1⁄10 oz (2–3 g) of powdered seed helped to reduce menstrual cramps.

Caution Do not take during pregnancy.

Trillium erectum (Liliaceae)
Bethroot

Description Attractive perennial with an erect stem growing to 16 in (40 cm). Has 3 wavy leaves and an unpleasant-smelling, 3-petaled, red to yellow flower.

Habitat & cultivation Native to North America, bethroot grows in shady areas in woodlands. The rhizome is usually unearthed after the leaves have dropped in the fall.

Part used Rhizome.

Constituents Bethroot contains steroidal saponins (such as trillin), tannin, resin, fixed oil, and a trace of volatile oil.

History & folklore Various *Trillium* species were used by Indigenous American peoples to aid childbirth, to treat irregular menstrual periods, period pain and excessive vaginal discharge, and, as a poultice, to soothe sore nipples.

Medicinal actions & uses Bethroot is a valuable remedy for heavy menstrual or intermenstrual bleeding, helping to reduce blood flow. It is also used to treat bleeding associated with uterine fibroids. Bethroot may also be taken for bleeding within the urinary tubules and, less commonly, for the coughing up of blood. It remains a valuable herb in facilitating childbirth. A douche of bethroot is useful for excessive vaginal discharge and yeast infections.

Caution Do not take during pregnancy except under professional supervision.

Tropaeolum majus (Tropaeolaceae)

Nasturtium

Description Climbing annual growing to 10 ft (3 m). Has straggling stems, rounded leaves, and orange to yellow trumpet-shaped flowers with a long spur.

Habitat & cultivation Native to Peru, nasturtiums flourish in sunny sites. They are grown as an ornamental and as a salad herb. All parts of the plant are harvested in summer.

Parts used Flowers, leaves, seeds.

Constituents Nasturtiums contain glucosinolates, sulfur glycosides, glucotropaeolin, flavonoids, spilantolic acid, and iodide. Glucotropaeolin is converted into mustard oils by gut bacteria and acts as an antibiotic within the urinary and respiratory systems.

History & folklore The nasturtium has long been used in Andean herbal medicine as a disinfectant and wound-healing herb, and as an expectorant to relieve chest conditions.

Medicinal actions & uses All parts of the nasturtium appear to have antibiotic activity. An infusion of the leaves may be used to increase resistance to bacterial infections and to clear nasal and bronchial congestion—apparently the remedy both reduces congestion formation and stimulates the clearing and coughing up of

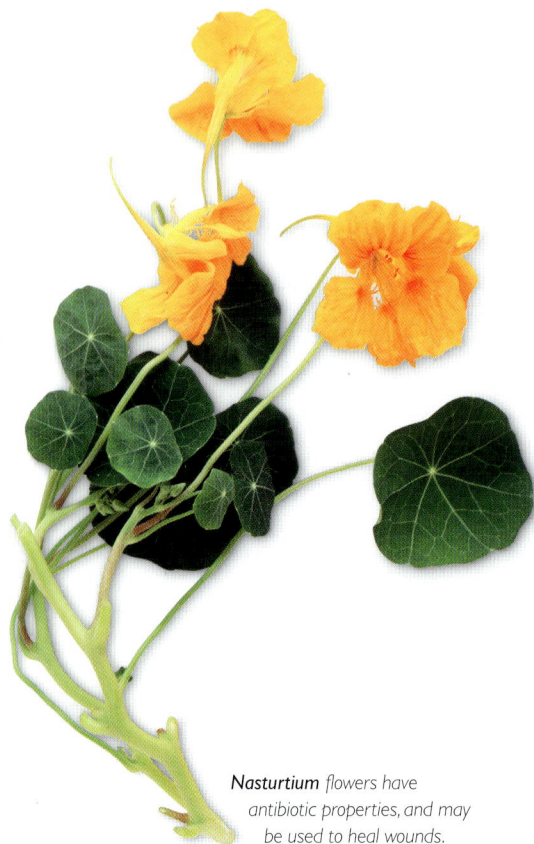

Nasturtium flowers have antibiotic properties, and may be used to heal wounds.

phlegm. It can also prove useful in bacterial cystitis and it makes an effective antiseptic wash for external application. The juice of the plant has been taken internally for the treatment of scrofula (tubercular infection of the lymph nodes). The piquant-tasting leaves and flowers (and juice) of nasturtium are high in vitamin C, and make a good salad vegetable, while the ground seeds have purgative properties.

Tsuga canadensis (Pinaceae)

Eastern hemlock

Description Evergreen tree growing to 100 ft (30 m). Has reddish-brown bark, short narrow needle leaves, and small male and female cones.

Habitat & cultivation Canada hemlock is native to eastern parts of North America, growing in woodland and marshy sites. The bark is collected from mature trees throughout the year.

Part used Bark.

Constituents Canada hemlock contains volatile oil (with alpha-pinene, bornyl acetate, and cadinene), 10–14% tannins, and resin.

History & folklore Indigenous American peoples may have given Canada hemlock to the explorer Jacques Cartier in 1535. He and his crew, exploring the St. Lawrence River, had fallen sick with scurvy, but all made a quick recovery upon taking a decoction of leaves and bark. Many Indigenous American peoples used the bark to treat wounds.

Medicinal actions & uses The bark of Canada hemlock is astringent and antiseptic. A decoction may be taken to treat diarrhea, colitis, diverticulitis, and cystitis. Externally, Canada hemlock can be employed as a douche to treat excessive vaginal discharge, yeast infection, and a prolapsed uterus; as a mouthwash and gargle for gingivitis and sore throats; or as a wash to cleanse and tighten wounds.

Tussilago farfara (Asteraceae)

Coltsfoot

Description Perennial herb growing to 12 in (30 m). Has flowering stems with purple scales, yellow-gold flowers, and heart-shaped leaves.

Habitat & cultivation Indigenous to Europe and northern Asia, and naturalized in North America, coltsfoot is a common plant often found along roadsides and on verges and waste ground. The flowers are gathered in late winter, the leaves in summer.

Parts used Leaves, flowers.

Constituents Coltsfoot contains flavonoids, about 8% mucilage (polysaccharides), 10% tannins, pyrrolizidine alkaloids, vitamin C, and zinc. The pyrrolizidine alkaloids may have a toxic effect on the liver, but are largely destroyed when the parts are boiled to make a decoction. The polysaccharides are anti-inflammatory and immunostimulant. The flavonoids are anti-inflammatory and antispasmodic.

History & folklore For at least 2,500 years, coltsfoot has been taken as a cough remedy and smoked as a means to ease breathing. Dioscorides, a Greek physician of the 1st century CE, recommended it for dry coughs, and "for those who are unable to breathe except standing upright."

Medicinal actions & uses Coltsfoot has been one of the most popular European remedies for treating chest problems, leaves and flowers traditionally being taken for chest conditions such as bronchitis and asthma. It has been a common ingredient in herbal cough remedies, and as a syrup was given to soothe children's coughs. However, in view of the potential toxicity of the alkaloids present in coltsfoot (particularly in the flowers), it is no longer considered a safe herb to use.

Cautions Coltsfoot is thought to be potentially toxic, do not use internally. It is subject to restrictions in some countries.

Tylophora asthmatica (Asclepiadaceae)

Asmatica, Indian lobelia

Description Perennial twining climber with lance-shaped leaves and greenish flowers producing many flat seeds.

Habitat & cultivation Native to the Indian subcontinent, asmatica grows wild on the plains of India. The leaves are gathered when the plant is in flower.

Part used Leaves.

Constituents Asmatica contains alkaloids (including tylophorine), flavonoids, sterols, and tannins. Tylophorine has anti-inflammatory and antitumor properties.

History & folklore Asmatica is used in Ayurvedic medicine to induce vomiting and expectoration, and to treat dysentery and rheumatic conditions.

Medicinal actions & uses Considered a specific remedy for asthma, asmatica may relieve symptoms for up to 3 months. It is also beneficial in cases of hay fever, and is prescribed for acute allergic problems such as eczema and hives. It holds potential as a treatment for chronic fatigue syndrome and other immune system disorders. Asmatica may relieve rheumatoid arthritis, and may also be of value in the treatment of cancer.

Research Extensive laboratory and clinical research in India has established that asmatica is an effective remedy for asthma. In the 1970s, a number of clinical trials showed that a majority of asthmatic patients taking the herb for just 6 days gained relief from asthma for up to a further 12 weeks. However, subsequent studies have failed to reproduce these results. The leaves produce side-effects including nausea and vomiting.

Caution Take asmatica only under professional supervision.

Typha angustifolia (Typhaceae)
Cattail,
Pu huang (Chinese)

Description Stout upright plant growing to a height of 6½ ft (2 m). Has long, flat, narrow leaves rising parallel to the stem, a distinctive brown cylindrical head of female flowers, and straw-colored male flowers immediately above.

Habitat & cultivation Cattail flourishes in marshes, swamps, and other freshwater sites in both temperate and tropical zones, and is cultivated. The pollen is shaken off the plant while it is in bloom.

Part used Pollen.

Constituents Cattail contains isorhamnetin, pentacosane, and sterols.

History & folklore The pollen is highly inflammable and has been used in the manufacture of fireworks. The root is edible and has been eaten in times of famine. The young shoots can be eaten raw or cooked in spring, and are said to taste like asparagus (Asparagus officinalis, p. 178). Although "bulrushes" (the British and Irish name for cattails) are mentioned in the Bible, it is likely the plant being referred to is actually *Cyperus papyrus*.

Medicinal actions & uses In Chinese herbal medicine, the astringent pollen has been employed chiefly to stop internal or external bleeding. The pollen may be mixed with honey and applied to wounds and sores, or taken orally to reduce internal bleeding of almost any kind—for example, nosebleeds, uterine bleeding, or blood in the urine. The pollen is now also used in the treatment of angina (pain in the chest or arm due to lack of oxygen to the heart muscle). In India, the dried pollen has been used for kidney stones, to treat nosebleeds and internal bleeding, as well as for painful menstruation. Cattail does not appear to have been used as a medicine in the European herbal tradition.

Research Chinese research suggests that cattail

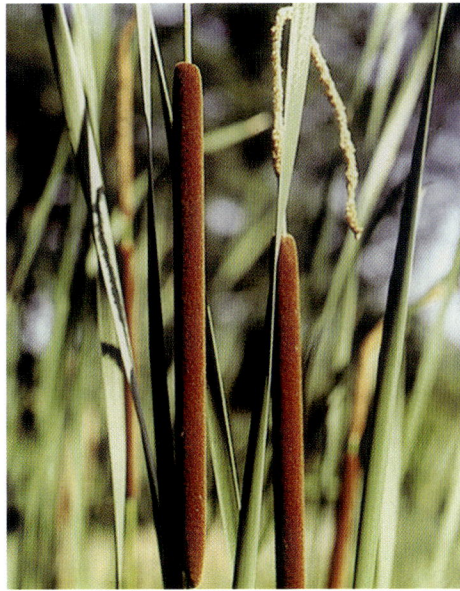

Cattail or pu huang *is used to staunch wounds and stop internal bleeding.*

pollen protects blood vessels from inflammation and acts as an immunosuppressant.

Caution Do not take during pregnancy.

Uncaria rhynchophylla (Rubiaceae)
Gou teng

Description Climbing perennial growing to 33 ft (10 m). Has opposite lance-shaped leaves, thorns, and composite flower heads.

Habitat & cultivation Native to China and Southeast Asia, *gou teng* is cultivated in the southern and eastern provinces of China. The stems and thorns are collected in fall and winter.

Parts used Stems, thorns.

Constituents *Gou teng* contains indole alkaloids, flavonoids, triterpenoid, and polysaccharides.

History & folklore The first recorded use of *gou teng* in Chinese medicine is in the *Miscellaneous Records* (c.500 CE).

Medicinal actions & uses *Gou teng* is a sedative and antispasmodic, and is mainly used to ease symptoms such as tremors, seizure, spasms, headache, and dizziness. It is also prescribed for infantile convulsions. In Chinese herbal medicine it "extinguishes [internal] wind [gas] and stops tremors." It is also used by the Chinese to reduce high blood pressure and excess liver "fire."

Research Chinese tests on laboratory animals indicate that *gou teng* lowers blood pressure, reduces anxiety, and has notable sedative activity.

Related species Like *gou teng*, pale catechu

(*U. gambier*) contains a constituent that lowers blood pressure. See also cat's claw (*U. tomentosa, following entry*).

Caution Take *gou teng* only under professional supervision.

Uncaria tomentosa (Rubiaceae)
Cat's Claw,
Una de gato

Description Climbing vine growing to 100 ft (30 m) or more, with stems up to 8 in (20 cm) in diameter, large, glossy leaves, and sharp hooks (the "cat's claws").

Habitat & cultivation A native of tropical rainforests in the central and eastern Andes, especially Peru, Ecuador, and Colombia, cat's claw has also been found in Guatemala, Costa Rica, and Panama. Until recently, the root bark was the part most commonly used as medicine. However, by the early 1990s collection from the wild threatened the species' survival. Only the stem bark, from ecologically sustainable sources, should be used.

Parts used Stem bark.

Constituents Cat's claw contains pentacyclic oxindole alkaloids (POA), tetracyclic oxindole alkaloids (TOA) in one chemotype only, triterpenoid glycosides, sterols, flavonoids, and tannins, including epicatechin and proanthocyanidins.

History & folklore Known by the Ashaninka and other Indigenous peoples of central Peru for its power in regulating illness, cat's claw has long been used since the earliest times to treat serious illness, from asthma and diabetes to arthritis and cancer. Indigenous healers are able to distinguish between what are botanically identical plants, selecting those that have a low TOA content and are therefore most likely to prove effective in strengthening immunity.

Medicinal actions & uses Like echinacea (*Echinacea* spp., p. 96), with which it combines effectively, cat's claw supports a weakened immune system, and can reinvigorate the body's efforts to counter infection and inflammation. The herb's antioxidant activity also helps to contain the widespread cellular damage that occurs in chronic degenerative disease. Conditions that may benefit include infections such as chronic fatigue syndrome and HIV/AIDS; chronic inflammatory diseases such as rheumatoid arthritis and ulcerative colitis; and asthma. Cat's claw may also be taken to help prevent cancer, particularly breast cancer, and is useful in countering the damaging effects of chemotherapy.

Research Investigations into the root and stem

bark have established that cat's claw has potent anti-inflammatory, antioxidant and immune-stimulant activity. The POAs and water extracts of the bark stimulate production of white blood cells and nonspecific immune resistance, and appear to inhibit tumor development and growth; extracts of the bark are strongly anti-inflammatory and may inhibit inflammatory gene expression. Nevertheless, the bark's medicinal activity probably results from the synergistic effect of several compounds, including the tannins. Clinical research in Peru indicates that cat's claw may have use in the treatment for HIV and AIDS. Of the two types of cat's claw, only the one containing POAs should be used as medicine, since the TOAs may suppress immune function. Cat's claw has a contraceptive activity. A small-scale clinical trial in Brazil found that patients with advanced cancer had more energy and some improvement in quality of life when taking a cat's claw extract.

Caution Avoid taking Cat's Claw during pregnancy and while breastfeeding.

Urginea maritima syn. *Drimia maritima*
(Asparagaceae)

Squill

Description Perennial growing to 5 ft (1.5 m) from a large white or red bulb. Has a single flowering stem, a rosette of large basal leaves, and a dense spike of white flowers.

Habitat & cultivation Native to southern Spain, the Canary Islands, and South Africa, squill is cultivated in the Mediterranean region. The bulb of the white (but not the red) variety is unearthed in late summer.

Part used Bulb.

Constituents Squill contains cardiac glycosides (0.15–2.4% bufadienolides, including scillaren A), flavonoids, stigmasterol anthocyanidins, and mucilage. The cardiac glycosides are strongly diuretic and relatively quick-acting. They do not have the same cumulative effect as those present in foxglove (*Digitalis purpurea*, p. 207).

History & folklore Squill appears in the Egyptian Ebers papyrus (c. 1500 BCE). In Greece it was used by Pythagoras and Hippocrates in the 6th and 5th centuries BCE.

Medicinal actions & uses Squill is a diuretic, emetic, cardiotonic, and expectorant plant that finds use in a wide range of conditions. It makes a good diuretic in cases of water retention. Since its active constituents do not accumulate to a great degree within the body, it is a potential substitute for foxglove in aiding a failing heart. At low dosage, squill is an effective expectorant. At higher doses, the herb

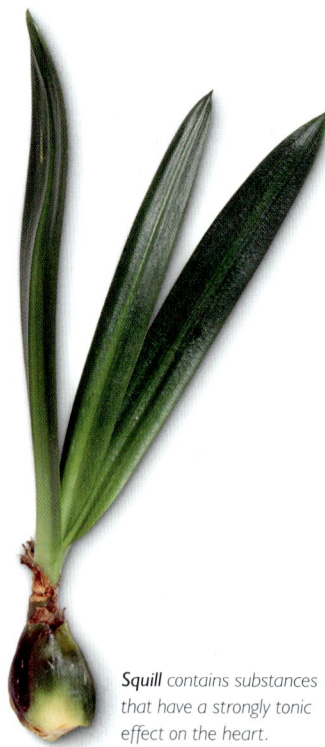

Squill contains substances that have a strongly tonic effect on the heart.

acts as an emetic. Squill is also used in homeopathic preparations.

Caution Use only under professional supervision. Squill is toxic in excessive doses.

Vaccinium macrocarpon (Ericaceae)

Cranberry

Description Small, slender, evergreen shrub, growing to 1 ft (30 cm), with oval, dark green leaves, pink flowers, and round or slightly pear-shaped red berries.

Habitat & Cultivation Native to eastern North America and northern Asia, cranberry thrives in acidic soils and in wet, boggy ground. It is widely cultivated in the northeastern US.

Parts used Berry (fruit).

Constituents Cranberry contains tannins (catechins, proanthocyanidins, and polyphenols), flavonoids, and vitamin C.

History & folklore Best known as the key ingredient in cranberry sauce, cranberries were first used by Indigenous American peoples as a food and for a range of conditions such as fever, liver disorders, and stomach problems. The plant was first cultivated in Britain in 1808 by the English botanist Joseph Banks, and in the US—now the principal grower of cranberries—in the 1840s.

Medicinal actions & uses A classic remedy for urinary tract infections, cranberry can be used both to prevent and to treat problems such as cystitis and urethritis. Taken as berries, juice, or extract, it will

help to disinfect the urinary tubules and may be taken for problems associated with poor urinary flow such as enlarged prostate, as well as bladder infections. In cases of acute infection, cranberry is likely to work better in combination with herbs such as buchu (*Agathosma betulina*, p. 75) and uva-ursi (*Arctostaphylos uva-ursi*, p. 174). though cranberry is probably most useful when taken as a juice or extract long-term as a preventative in those prone to urinary tract infection.

Research Over 10 clinical trials have investigated the effectiveness of cranberry in treating urinary infections, with mixed results. One trial found that cranberry juice reduced the need for antibiotics in women suffering from chronic urinary tract infection. It seems likely that cranberry works by making it more difficult for bacteria to cling to the urinary tract wall, and infection is therefore more easily flushed out. The proanthocyanidins and catechins are probably responsible for this action.

Caution In kidney disease, use only on professional advice.

Vachellia nilotica syn. *Acacia nilotica* (Fabaceae)

Gum arabic, Babul

Description Tree growing to 65 ft (20 m) with hard, rust-brown bark and feathery leaves. Small, bright yellow flower heads produce pods up to 6 in (15 cm) long.

Habitat & cultivation Gum arabic is native to North Africa. Today it is commonly found in Egypt and is cultivated in India.

Part used Bark.

Constituents Gum arabic contains tannins (12–20%), mucilage, and flavonoids.

History & folklore In ancient Egypt, the wood of the gum arabic tree was used to make dwellings, wheels, and tool handles. The leaves, flowers, and pods were used to expel worms, heal wounds, alleviate diarrhea, and suppress the coughing up of blood.

Medicinal actions & uses Strongly astringent, gum arabic is used to contract and toughen mucus membranes throughout the body, for instance as a mouthwash/gargle for bleeding gums and sore throat. It may be taken internally to help relieve diarrhea. In India and many parts of Africa, gum arabic is used to treat more severe illness, especially diabetes, liver disease and some types of cancer.

Research Clinical studies indicate that gum arabic is clinically effective in treating periodontal infections, and has significant antidiabetic activity. A 2021 research paper concluded that gum arabic is strongly antiviral and shows signs of being effective in treating hepatitis C (HCV) infection.

Related species Australian wattle (*A. decurrens*), native to Australia, is used in much the same way as gum arabic. See also black catechu (*A. catechu*, p. 278)

Cautions Do not take gum arabic internally for more than 2–3 weeks. *Vachellia* and *Acacia* species are subject to legal restrictions in some countries.

Verbascum thapsus (Scrophulariaceae)

Mullein

Description Upright biennial growing to 6½ ft (2 m). Has slightly hairy, gray-green, oval to lance-shaped leaves, and spikes of bright yellow flowers.

Habitat & cultivation Mullein is native to central and southern Europe and western Asia. It is now also naturalized in many other temperate regions. Mullein grows on open uncultivated land and along roadsides. The leaves and flowers are collected during the summer.

Parts used Leaves, flowers.

Constituents Mullein contains mucilage, flavonoids, triterpenoid saponins, volatile oil, and tannins.

History & folklore Mullein was once credited with magical as well as medicinal virtues. John Gerard, a 16th-century herbalist, expressed doubts about the former: "there be some who think that this herbe being carryed aboute one, doth help the falling sickness … which thing is vaine and superstitious." However, he did affirm mullein's value as a cough medicine.

Medicinal actions & uses Mullein is a valuable herb for coughs and congestion, and is a specific treatment for tracheitis and bronchitis. The leaves and the flowers may be used as an infusion to reduce mucus formation and stimulate the coughing up of phlegm. Mullein combines well with other expectorants such as elecampane (*Inula helenium*, p. 111) and thyme (*Thymus vulgaris*, p. 147).

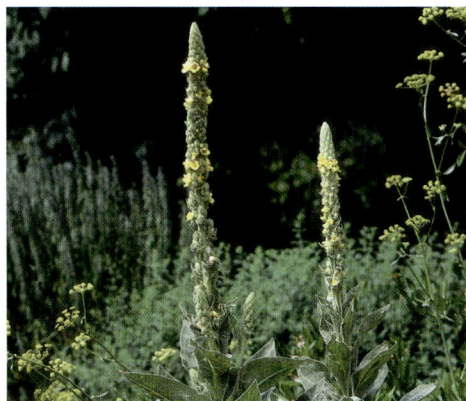

Mullein is a good expectorant remedy for coughs and other chest problems.

Applied externally, mullein is emollient and makes a good wound healer. In Germany, the flowers are steeped in olive oil, and the resulting fixed oil is used as a remedy for ear infections and hemorrhoids.

Veronica officinalis (Plantaginaceae)

Speedwell

Description Creeping hairy perennial growing to 20 in (50 cm). Has oval leaves and darkly veined lilac flowers.

Habitat & cultivation A common wild plant in Europe and North America, speedwell is most often found on heaths and in dry grassy places. It is picked in summer.

Parts used Aerial parts.

Constituents Speedwell contains iridoid glycosides (including aucubin), acetopenone glucosides, and flavonoids (including apigenin and scutellarin).

History & folklore Speedwell was formerly considered a useful diuretic and expectorant. It was much used to treat congestion, coughs, and chronic skin conditions. It was also given to counter nervous exhaustion due to excessive mental activity or concentration. However, in 1935, the French medicinal plant specialist Leclerc stated that "the infusion has no more virtue than the hot water used to prepare it."

Medicinal actions & uses Speedwell is now considered to have only a slight therapeutic effect. It is little used today.

Viburnum prunifolium (Adoxaceae)

Black haw

Description Deciduous shrub growing to 16 ft (5 m). Has serrated oval leaves, clusters of white flowers, and blue-black berries.

Habitat & cultivation Native to central and southern North America, black haw grows in woodland. The branch bark is stripped in the spring or fall, the root bark in the fall only.

Parts used Bark, root bark.

Constituents Black haw contains coumarins (including scopoletin and aesculetin), salicin, 1-methyl-2,3-dibutyl hemimellitate, viburnin, plant acids, a trace of volatile oil, and tannin.

History & folklore The Catawba people used black haw bark to treat dysentery. In the 19th century, the bark was considered to be a uterine tonic, and a decoction was commonly used to help arrest hemorrhage of the uterus.

Medicinal actions & uses Black haw is

---

antispasmodic and astringent, and is regarded as a specific treatment for menstrual pain. Echoing its 19th-century applications, the bark is also used to treat other gynecological conditions, such as prolapse of the uterus, heavy menopausal bleeding, morning sickness, and threatened miscarriage. Black haw's antispasmodic property makes it of value in cases where colic or other cramping pain affects the bile ducts, the digestive tract, or the urinary tract.

Related species The closely related *V. rufidulum* was used by the Menominee people to treat cramps and colic. See also cramp bark (*Viburnum opulus*, p. 154).

Caution People who are allergic to aspirin should not take black haw.

Self-help use Period pain, p. 325.

Vinca minor (Apocynaceae)

Lesser periwinkle

Description A mainly ground-hugging evergreen shrub arching to 18 in (45 cm). Has rooting stems, shiny elliptical leaves, and 5-petaled, violet-blue flowers.

Habitat & cultivation Native to Europe, lesser periwinkle grows in along roadsides and woodland borders. It is also cultivated as a garden plant. The leaves are gathered in spring.

Parts used Leaves.

Constituents Lesser periwinkle contains about 7% indole alkaloids (including vincamine, vincine, and vincaminine), a bisindol alkaloid (vincarubine), and tannins. Vincamine increases blood flow and oxygen supply to the brain.

History & folklore In his *Herbarium*, the 2nd-century CE Roman writer Apuleius describes lesser periwinkle's virtues "against the devil sickness and demoniacal possessions and against snakes and wild beasts." He also specifies the rituals used in harvesting the herb: "This wort thou shalt pluck thus, saying, 'I pray thee, *vinca pervinca*, thee that art to be had for thy many useful qualities … outfit me so that I be shielded and ever prosperous and undamaged by poisons and by water.' When thou shalt pluck this wort, thou shalt be clean of every uncleanness, and thou shalt pick it when the moon is nine nights old."

Medicinal actions & uses Lesser periwinkle is employed as an astringent and blood-staunching herb. Its astringency makes it a useful mouthwash for sore throats, gingivitis, and mouth ulcers. Its staunching ability is effective against internal bleeding, heavy menstrual bleeding, and nosebleeds. Since vincamine was discovered in the leaves, lesser periwinkle has been used to treat arteriosclerosis and for dementia due to insufficient blood flow to the brain.

Related species Greater periwinkle (*V. major*) also has similar astringent activity. See also Madagascar periwinkle (*V. rosea, following entry*).

Caution Do not take during pregnancy.

Vinca rosea (Apocynaceae)

Madagascar periwinkle

Description Fleshy perennial growing to 32 in (80 cm). Has glossy oval leaves and bright, white to red 5-petaled flowers.

Habitat & cultivation Thought to be a native of Madagascar, this herb is now common in many tropical and subtropical regions worldwide. It is cultivated commercially as a garden ornamental. The herb and root are gathered in summer.

Parts used Aerial parts, root.

Constituents Madagascar periwinkle contains over 70 different indole alkaloids, including vinblastine, vincristine, alstonine, ajmalicine, leurocristine, and reserpine.

Medicinal actions & uses This plant is used in folk medicine in the Philippines as a remedy for diabetes. In the Caribbean, the flowers are used as a soothing eyewash.

Research Madagascar periwinkle's traditional use as a treatment for diabetes has led to extensive investigation into its properties. Vincristine and vinblastine are powerful anticancer agents, and are two of the most important medicinal compounds found in plants in the last 40 years. Vincristine is a standard treatment for Hodgkin's disease, and vinblastine for childhood leukemia. While extracts from Madagascar periwinkle have been shown to lower blood-sugar levels, simple preparations of the whole plant may not be effective.

Caution Take Madagascar periwinkle only under professional supervision.

Viola odorata (Violaceae)

Sweet violet

Description Creeping perennial growing to 6 in (15 cm). Has toothed oval leaves, and attractive, violet-blue or white flowers with a 5-petaled corolla.

Habitat & cultivation Native to much of Europe and Asia, sweet violet is a common wayside plant also found along roadsides and in woodlands. The flowers and leaves are collected in spring, the root in the fall.

Parts used Flowers, leaves, root.

Constituents Sweet violet contains phenolic glycosides (including gaultherin), saponins (myrosin and violin), flavonoids, an alkaloid (odoratine), and mucilage.

History & folklore In classical myth, sweet violet was associated with death, but classical physicians also knew it as an effective emetic and cough remedy. The 17th-century herbalist Nicholas Culpeper stated that: "All the violets are cold and moist while they are fresh and green, and are used to cool any heat or distemperature of the body either inwardly or outwardly."

Medicinal actions & uses Sweet violet flowers and leaves have a gentle expectorant and demulcent action and they induce light sweating. They are often used as an infusion or syrup for treating coughs, chest colds and congestion. They are used in British herbalism to treat breast and stomach cancer. The root is a much stronger expectorant and, at higher doses, is emetic.

Research Iranian researchers investigated the use of two drops of sweet violet essential oil applied to the nostrils as a remedy for insomnia. The study, which lasted a month, found positive improvements in sleep measurements in those using the oil. A 2015 study of children with asthma concluded that sweet violet syrup helped to reduce symptoms of dry irritable cough.

Related species The related dog violet (*V. canina*) has approximately the same uses as sweet violet. The Chinese *V. yedoensis* is prescribed for hot swellings and tumors, mumps, and abscesses. See also heartsease (*V. tricolor, following entry*).

Viola tricolor (Violaceae)

Heartsease

Description Annual, biennial, or perennial plant growing to 15 in (38 cm). Has lobed, oval leaves and handsome violet, yellow, and white pansy-type flowers.

Habitat & cultivation Heartsease is native to Europe, North Africa, and temperate regions of Asia, and has become naturalized in the Americas. It thrives in many habitats, from grassy mountainous areas to coastal sites, and is also cultivated as a garden plant. The aerial parts are gathered in summer.

Parts used Aerial parts.

Constituents Heartsease contains saponins, flavonoids, salicylates, mucilage, gums, and a resin

History & folklore K'Eogh wrote in his 1735 *Irish Herbal* that heartsease flowers "cure convulsions in children, cleanse the lungs and breast and are very good for fevers, internal inflammations and wounds".

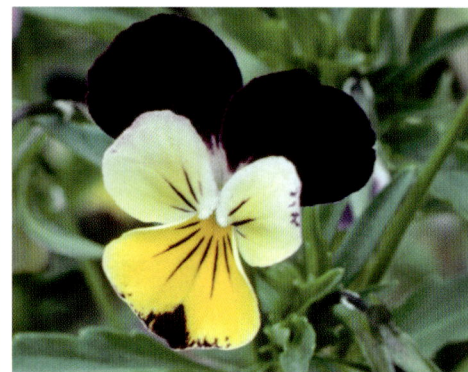

Heartsease grows wild in temperate areas, and is widely cultivated as a garden plant.

Medicinal actions & uses In Western herbal medicine, heartsease is used as an anti-inflammatory and purifying herb and is taken for skin conditions such as eczema. An infusion also makes a useful wash for itchiness. Being expectorant, heartsease is used to treat bronchitis and whooping cough. The plant's established diuretic action makes it useful for treating rheumatism, cystitis, and difficulty in passing urine.

Research Recent research has found that heartsease has potential anticancer properties. It promoted programmed cell death (apoptosis) and inhibited blood vessel growth (angiogenesis), both important anticancer effects. A clinical trial in children with asthma found that heartsease syrup helped to control dry irritable cough alongside prescribed medication for asthma.

Self-help use Hives, p. 313.

Viscum album (Loranthaceae)

European mistletoe

Description Parasitic evergreen shrub that forms bunches up to 10 ft (3 m) across on host trees. Has narrow leathery leaves, yellowish flowers in clusters of 3, and sticky, round, white berries.

Habitat & cultivation Native to Europe and northern Asia, European mistletoe grows on host trees, especially apple trees (*Malus* species). It is harvested in the fall.

Parts used Leaves, branches, berries.

Constituents Mistletoe contains glycoproteins, polypeptides (viscotoxins), lectins, flavonoids, caffeic and other acids, lignans, acetylcholine, and, in the berries, polysaccharides. Viscotoxins inhibit tumors and stimulate immune resistance.

History & folklore In Norse mythology, a mistletoe bough was used to slay Balder, the god of peace. The plant was subsequently entrusted to the goddess of love, and kissing under it became obligatory.

Medicinal actions & uses European mistletoe is chiefly used to lower blood pressure and heart rate, ease anxiety, and promote sleep. In low doses it also relieves panic attacks and headaches, and improves the ability to concentrate. The plant is also prescribed for tinnitus and epilepsy. It may be used to treat hyperactivity in children. In anthroposophical medicine, extracts of the berries are injected to treat cancer.

Research European mistletoe's efficacy as an anticancer treatment has been subject to significant research. There is no doubt that certain constituents, especially the viscotoxins, exhibit an anticancer activity, but the value of the whole plant in cancer treatment is not yet fully accepted.

Caution European mistletoe, and especially the berries, is highly toxic. Take only under professional supervision.

Vitis vinifera (Vitaceae)

Grape

Description Deciduous climber with erect stems, tendrils, palm-shaped leaves, clusters of small pale green flowers, and bunches of fruit (grapes) that vary in color from green to black.

Habitat & cultivation Native to southern Europe and western Asia, grapes are cultivated in warm temperate regions throughout the world for their fruit and to produce wine. The leaves are collected in summer, the fruit in the fall.

Parts used Leaves, fruit, seeds, sap.

Constituents Grapes contain flavonoids, tannins, tartrates, inositol, carotenes, choline, and sugars. The fruit contains tartaric and malic acids, sugars, pectin, tannin, flavone glycosides, anthocyanins (in red leaves and red grapes), vitamins A, B_1, B_2, and C, and minerals. The anthocyanins reduce capillary permeability.

History & folklore Nicholas Culpeper in 1652

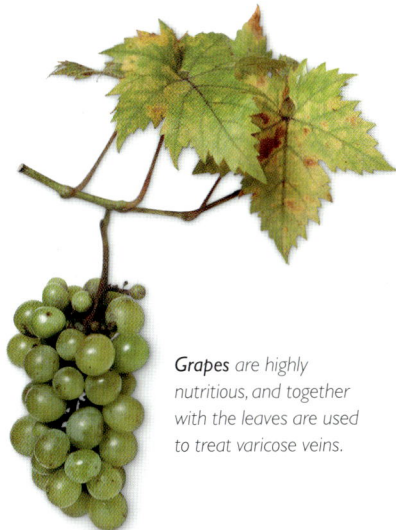

Grapes are highly nutritious, and together with the leaves are used to treat varicose veins.

extolled the virtues of the grape vine, describing it as "a most gallant tree of the sun very sympathetical to the body of man, and that's the reason spirit of wine is the greatest cordial amongst all vegetables."

Medicinal actions & uses Grape leaves, especially the red leaves, are astringent and anti-inflammatory. They are taken as an infusion to treat diarrhea, heavy menstrual bleeding, and uterine hemorrhage, as a wash for mouth ulcers, and as a douche for vaginal discharge. Red leaves and grapes are helpful in the treatment of varicose veins, hemorrhoids, and capillary fragility. The sap from the branches is used as an eyewash. Grapes are nourishing and mildly laxative and they support the body through illness, especially of the gastrointestinal tract and liver. Because the nutrient content of grapes is close to that of blood plasma, grape fasts are recommended for detoxification. The dried fruit (raisins or currants) is mildly expectorant and emollient, with a slight effect in easing coughs. Wine vinegar is astringent, cooling, and soothing to the skin.

Research Grape-seed extract has potent antioxidant and circulatory-protective activity. It appears to normalize blood pressure and heart rate, working best as a preventative, antiaging remedy that supports healthy circulation. One study found grape-seed extract reduced leg swelling in healthy women required to sit for long periods of time at work. Recent studies also indicate that grape-seed extract can be useful in nonalcoholic fatty liver disease and type 2 diabetes.

Wolffia globosa, (Araceae)

Mankai
Asian watermeal

Description Mankai is a duckweed, a cultivated variety of a tiny Asian aquatic plant, its green stemless frond being less than $1/25$ in (1 mm) in diameter. It is thought to be the world's smallest vegetable.

Habitat & cultivation Native to fresh waters in eastern Asia, mankai's very high protein and nutrient content has led to selected varieties being cultivated hydroponically in aquatic greenhouses. When dry, mankai is about 45% protein, and has a similar protein content to egg.

Parts used Whole plant.

Constituents Mankai contain proteins, vitamin A, B12 and folate, E; iron, magnesium and zinc; omega-3 fatty acids, phenolic acids and flavonoids. The B12 has been shown to be well absorbed in clinical trials to date.

History & folklore Mankai is used as a nutritious

protein-rich ingredient in Korean and Thai cooking.

Medicinal actions & uses Mankai is essentially a food and rich source of protein, vitamins, minerals and omega-3 fatty acids. However, its combination of nutrients and directly medicinal compounds means that it can be useful both in aiding weight loss and regulating blood glucose levels. Additionally, research suggests that mankai has a beneficial action on the gut microbiome, supporting healthy gut bacteria and digestive function.

Ziziphus jujuba (Rhamnaceae)

Jujube,
Da zao (Chinese)

Description Spiny deciduous tree growing to approximately 26 ft (8 m). Has oblong, bluntly toothed leaves, clusters of small greenish-yellow flowers, and reddish-brown or black oval fruit up to 1 in (3 cm) long.

Habitat & cultivation Native to China, Japan, and Southeast Asia, the jujube is widely cultivated in tropical and subtropical regions of Asia and the Mediterranean. The fruit is collected in early fall.

Part used Fruit.

Constituents Jujube contains saponins, bioflavonoids, polyphenols, polysaccharides, volatile oil, mucilage, vitamins A, B_2, and C, in addition to calcium, phosphorus, and iron. It contains 20 times more vitamin C than citrus fruit.

History & folklore Used in Chinese herbal medicine for at least 2,500 years, jujube has a pleasant, sweet taste and high nutritional value. It is mentioned in the *Classic of Odes*, a 6th-century BCE anthology of Chinese poetry.

Medicinal actions & uses Jujube is both a delicious fruit and an effective herbal remedy. It aids weight gain, improves muscular strength, and increases stamina. In Chinese medicine, jujube is prescribed as a *qi* tonic to strengthen liver function. Mildly sedative and anti-allergenic, it is given to reduce irritability and restlessness. It is also used to improve the taste of unpalatable prescriptions.

Research In Japan, jujube has been shown to increase immune-system resistance. In China, laboratory animals fed a jujube decoction gained weight and showed improved endurance. In one clinical study, 12 patients with liver ailments were given jujube, peanuts, and brown sugar nightly. In 4 weeks, their liver function had improved.

Related species The sedative *Z. spinosa* is used in Chinese medicine to "nourish the heart and quieten the spirit."

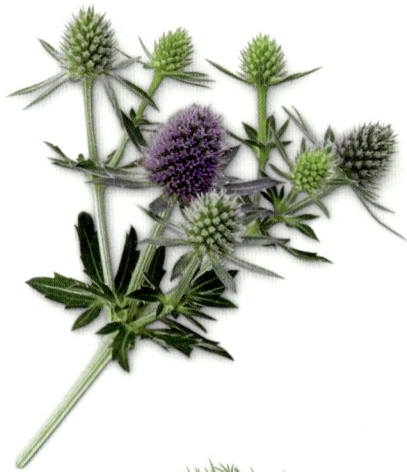

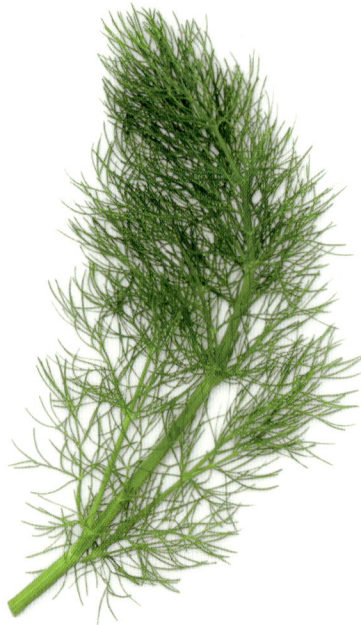

Herbal remedies <u>for</u> home use

Herbal medicines have been used since the earliest times. They are a vital part of our natural and medical heritage, and there is immense satisfaction to be had in growing, harvesting, and processing herbs for home use. Taken sensibly, and with the respect due to medicines of all kinds, medicinal plants can greatly improve health. This section provides practical cultivation advice and step-by-step instructions on how to make and use safe and effective herbal remedies for a range of common ailments, from allergies and digestive complaints to skin conditions and stress-related disorders.

Growing medicinal plants

Growing medicinal plants may be more time-consuming than buying them, but it brings with it the unique pleasure of producing your own herbal remedies. Many medicinal herbs are easy to grow and will flourish indoors on a windowsill or in the garden, providing a year-round supply of fresh, sweet-smelling natural medicines.

The medicinal herb garden

Planning an herb garden depends on a range of factors including the space available, exposure, soil, conditions, and climate. As a starting point, details of ten of the most common and useful medicinal plants for growing in temperate climates are given in the chart below. Some of them, such as thyme (*Thymus vulgaris*, p. 147) and sage (*Salvia officinalis*, p. 135), may be grown indoors. A number of other medicinal herbs, including German chamomile (*Chamomilla recutita*, p. 82), lady's mantle (*Alchemilla vulgaris*, p. 167), and lavender (*Lavandula officinalis*, p. 112) also grow well in a temperate climate and are well worth cultivating. If in doubt about how to care for plants or what will grow well in your garden, consult a nursery.

Outdoor gardens Choose a range of hardy herbs to grow in your garden that will establish themselves easily and produce plenty of foliage that can be harvested. Plant exotic or less hardy herbs in sheltered sunny sites or in containers.

Container gardens Many medicinal plants such as peppermint (*Mentha* x *piperita*, p. 118) or bay laurel (*Laurus nobilis*, p. 232) can be grown in pots, hanging baskets, or window boxes. Care must be taken to prevent them from drying out or becoming pot-bound (when the plant becomes too large for the container). Less hardy plants should be moved to sheltered sites or indoors during winter.

Growing plants under cover Sheltered gardening offers the opportunity to grow more unusual plants. Use the greenhouse to cultivate exotic plants, such as lemon grass (*Cymbopogon citratus*, p. 203), for medicinal and culinary use, as well as for growing seedlings to be planted outdoors. Tender plants, such as holy basil (*Ocimum tenuiflorum*, p. 120), thrive indoors, and some indoor plants, such as aloe vera (*Aloe vera*, p. 64), have the added advantage of absorbing polluting chemicals from the air.

Buying medicinal herbs

Reputable herb nurseries are the best place to buy herbs when particular varieties or species are required. Be clear about what plants you want before visiting the nursery. When buying for medicinal use, purchase the standard medicinal, rather than an improved or ornamental variety.

Cultivation

Bear in mind the following points when planning the garden and choosing herbs.

Site The majority of medicinal plants prefer a sunny exposure and moderately well-drained soil. It is possible to improve a site, for example by planting hedges as windbreaks. Choose sheltered, sunny corners for delicate and half-hardy herbs, and avoid planting on land formerly used for industrial purposes, which may be contaminated.

Temperature Some plants tolerate only very specific temperature ranges, and many herbs, such as rosemary (*Rosmarinus officinalis*, p. 132), are only half-hardy and will not survive exposure to deep or long periods of frost. Protect tender and half-hardy plants from the wind to avoid the windchill factor. Spring is the best time to plant most herbs. Wintering plants in a greenhouse or cool indoor site is often the only way to keep subtropical plants in cool temperate climates, while other herbs will thrive indoors all year round in a warm, sunny position.

Soil Soils vary greatly depending on the proportions of sand, silt, and clay content. Sandy soils drain easily and need feeding, while clay soils can become waterlogged and require drainage.

Pruning Pruning is used to remove dead wood and improve the shape, size, and quality of growth. It is an important garden activity and needs to be done correctly for different woody plants to benefit—check the best time of year for each plant. Deadheading plants, especially shrubs, encourages fresh growth. Pruning and tidying the garden regularly also reduces pests and diseases.

Watering Water well after planting and then, if needed, once a week (rather than a little each day) in the morning or early evening. Do not overwater as many herbs produce medicinally active constituents in dry conditions. Water dry potted plants thoroughly before planting.

Weeding & fertilizing Weeding is necessary since weeds compete with other plants for nutrients and water. Keep beds and containers as free from weeds as possible. Most medicinal herbs should not be fed or mulched as this tends to reduce their therapeutic strength. However, sandy soils should be fed with a good-quality fertilizer to maintain the nutrients in the soil.

Pests & diseases Use only organic methods to treat pests, diseases, and insect infestation. Aphids can be eradicated using soapy water or water in which garlic skins have been soaked for 2 days. Separate any infected plants to prevent further contamination.

Propagation methods

There is a wide variety of propagation methods. Choose the one most suited to the plant. When planting, prepare the ground in advance, taking into account the requirements of the individual plant, and the soil, site, and time of year, as well as the anticipated size of the mature plant.

Seed Seeds can be sown either in containers or in prepared soil in open ground. It is important to time the sowing of seeds to enable seedlings to be planted outdoors when weather and soil become sufficiently warm. Annuals and biennials can be grown with ease from seed and will grow vigorously throughout the summer. Check the germination requirements of perennials before buying seeds, as some varieties germinate easily, while others, such as Siberian ginseng (*Eleutherococcus senticosus*, p. 98), can be far more difficult.

Cuttings This is one of the most popular methods of propagation. It is suitable for woody perennial herbs. Cuttings are usually taken from the stem, although some plants may also be propagated from roots. Choose young, healthy plants and take the cutting just below a leaf and stem joint using a clean,

sharp knife. Strip off the lowest leaves and dip the stem in hormone rooting preparation before inserting it in suitable soil mix. Some plants are very difficult to propagate this way, so check before attempting this method.

Root division This is an easy way to propagate plants that form clumps. Divide spring-flowering herbaceous plants in the fall, and fall-flowering herbaceous plants in spring. Carefully lift a mature plant, divide it into smaller sections, and replant both the new and the mature plant.

Plants from produce Purchase pots of culinary herbs from a grocery or supermarket, split the seedlings into 3 to 4 small clumps, and pot them separately. Fresh roots, such as ginger (*Zingiber officinale*, p. 159), or bulblets, such as garlic (*Allium*

sativum, p. 63), can be planted in pots or in prepared ground outside, if temperature allows.

Layering Layering involves encouraging a shoot or stem to form roots by making a small slit in its underside and burying it, with the growing tip above ground. When the layer roots emerge, remove and pot. "Mound layering" is suitable for woody herbs such as sage (*Salvia officinalis*, p. 135). Pile free-draining soil over the base of the plant, and when the layered stems form new roots, remove and pot.

Offsets Offsets are produced from most herbs that grow from a bulb or corm, such as garlic (*Allium sativum*, p. 63). These can be detached during dormancy and replanted.

Useful herbs to grow

PLANT	WHEN TO PLANT	CULTIVATION METHOD	CONDITIONS & CARE	MEDICINAL USES
Aloe vera (*Aloe vera*, p. 64)	spring/fall	offsets	sunny site indoors; pot as needed; do not overwater	fresh plant gel for minor burns and wounds
Comfrey (*Symphytum officinale*, p. 142)	spring/fall	seed/division	warm sunny site; moist soil	ointment or poultice for sprains and bruises (use the leaf only)
Calendula (*Calendula officinalis*, p. 77)	spring/fall	seed	well-drained soil; full sun; remove dead flower heads	cream for cuts, scrapes, inflamed skin; infusion for fungal infections
Feverfew (*Tanacetum parthenium*, p. 144)	fall/spring	seed/cutting/ division	well-drained or dry, stony soil in sun	fresh leaf or tincture for headaches and migraines
Lemon balm (*Melissa officinalis*, p. 117)	spring/fall	seed/cutting/ division	moist soil in sun; cut back after flowering	infusion for anxiety, poor sleep, and nervous indigestion; lotion for cold sores
Peppermint (*Mentha x piperita*, p. 118)	spring/fall	cutting/division	sunny but moist site; do not allow to dry out	infusion for indigestion and headaches; lotion for itchy skin
Rosemary (*Rosmarinus officinalis*, p. 132)	spring/fall	seed/cutting	sunny sheltered site; protect with burlap in winter	infusion as a stimulating nerve tonic and to aid weak digestion
Sage (*Salvia officinalis*, p. 135)	fall/spring	seed/cutting/ layering	well-drained or dry, sunny, sheltered site	infusion for sore throats, mouth ulcers, and diarrhea
St. John's wort (*Hypericum perforatum*, p. 110)	spring/fall	seed/division	well-drained to dry soil with sun or partial shade	tincture for depression and menopause; infused oil is antiseptic and heals wounds
Thyme (*Thymus vulgaris*, p. 147)	spring/summer	seed/cutting/ division	well-drained soil, may need a layer of gravel; sunny site	infusion for coughs, colds, and chest infections; lotion for fungal infections

Harvesting & Processing

Although there are some herbs that may be collected year round, most have a particular growing season and must be harvested and either used immediately or preserved for use in the following year. See the individual entries on pp. 60–293 for harvesting times. Herbs need to be processed quickly to prevent deterioration and retain their healing action.

Harvesting from the wild

Wild plants offer a free and natural source of herbal remedies. Furthermore, active constituents are often more highly concentrated in wild plants since the herb is likely to be growing in its preferred habitat.

Identification Proper identification of wild plants is essential. Use a field or wildflower guide to help you. If in doubt, do not pick the plant, as poisoning can result from misidentification.

Ecological & legal factors While common species, such as nettle (*Urtica dioica*, p. 150), may be readily harvested from the wild, many rarer species are under great pressure due to the lack of a suitable habitat. In many countriesit is illegal to uproot any wild plant, and certain species may be protected. Although gathering medicinal plants such as gentian (*Gentiana lutea*, p. 103) may be legal in some countries, it will only reduce their future chances of survival in the wild. Never pick rare or uncommon plants from the wild, even if they are locally plentiful,

and do not collect more than you will use. Do not harvest bark from the wild. Before harvesting, consider where the plant is growing and whether it could be contaminated by pollution. Do not collect from roadsides, close to factories or in areas where crop spraying has occurred.

Harvesting from your garden

Cultivated herbs provide a ready supply of fresh material in a controlled environment. Cut perennials carefully so that plants can quickly regrow. Some plants, such as lemon balm (*Melissa officinalis*, p. 117), provide two or more crops per year.

General advice Harvesting medicinal herbs requires careful planning to ensure the parts are processed in peak condition and fast enough to retain their active ingredients.

Equipment Ideally, use a wooden tray or open basket for collecting herbs. This prevents the plant being crushed. In the wild, a non-nylon rucksack or sack may be more

appropriate. Always cut with a sharp knife or scissors to minimize damage to the plant and try to handle plants as little as possible. Wear gloves if gathering prickly or allergenic plants, such as rue (*Ruta graveolens*, p. 273).

What to look for Collect material from healthy plants, free from insect damage and pollution. It is important to discard damaged plants as they can lead to disease or decay in dried plant material. Do not mix cut plant material to avoid mistakes in identification.

When to harvest Gather herbs in dry weather, preferably on a sunny morning after the dew has evaporated. Picking when the plant is at its peak of maturity ensures that it will have a high concentration of active constituents. Unless otherwise stated in the individual plant entries on pp. 60–293, leaves are best collected as they open during the spring or summer months, flowers as they start to bloom, fruit and berries just as they become ripe, and roots in the fall once the plant has drawn its vitality back beneath ground. Bark must be gathered with great care if the shrub or tree is to survive—in most cases, harvest it in spring or fall.

The correct medicinal part In many cases, different parts of the same plant, for example the leaves and seeds, can have quite different actions and uses. Make sure that you harvest the correct medicinal part of the plant for your purposes.

Processing quickly Only collect plant material that you will be able to use or process immediately after harvesting because fresh plant material deteriorates very quickly and the medicinally active constituents are often the first to be affected. In particular, aromatic herbs can lose their volatile oils within hours. Salad leaves and culinary herbs are best eaten right away to make the most of their nutrients, although they can be stored for a few days in a plastic bag filled with air in a refrigerator.

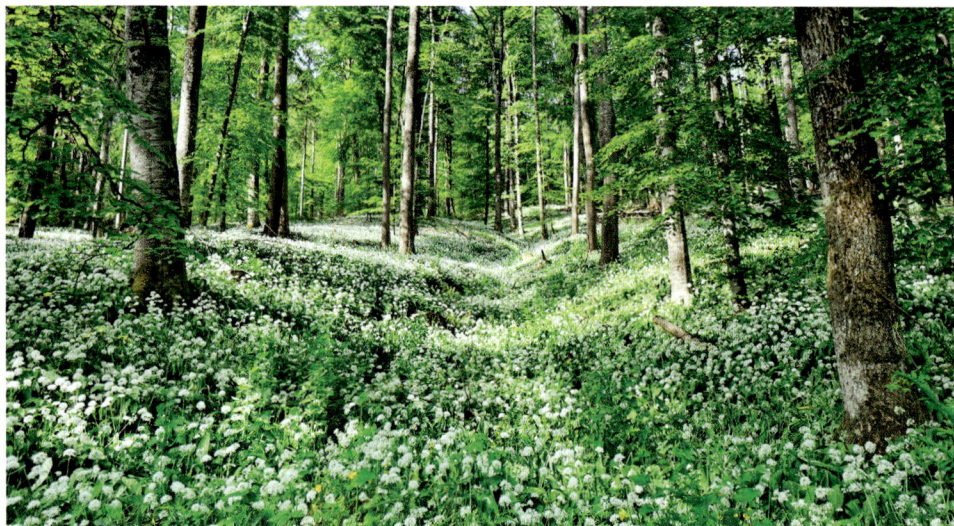

Ramsons can be found carpeting shady sites in damp woods in Europe. The bulb and aerial parts are harvested in early summer for their antibiotic, healing properties.

Storing herbs

It is vital to store dried herbs properly or they will not last. Leaves, flowers, roots, and other parts should be stored in sterilized, dark glass containers with airtight lids. They may also be stored in new brown paper bags, which must be kept dry and away from light. Metal and plastic containers are inadvisable because they may contaminate the herb. If stored in a cool, dark place, herbs can be kept for about 12 months after harvesting. Herbs frozen in plastic bags can be used for up to 6 months. Label the container with the herb, source, date of harvesting, and strength of preparation if appropriate. Watch out for insect infestation. If this occurs, discard all affected material and sterilize the container.

Processing

Herbs can be preserved in a number of ways, the simplest being air or oven drying. A warm, dry place such as an airing cupboard is ideal. Use plain paper for drying herbs, never printed newspaper. Dried herbs can be stored for many months in a dark glass jar or a brown paper bag (see p. 299).

Aerial parts These include all the parts of the plant growing above ground—stems, leaves, flowers, berries, and seeds. The stems are normally cut 2–4 in (5–10 cm) above ground shortly after the plant has begun to flower, when it is putting most effort into growth. Perennials may be cut higher above ground to encourage further crops. Remove and dry large flowers and leaves separately; smaller ones can be dried on the stem.

• Hang bunches of about 8–10 stems in a warm (but not hot), well-ventilated, dark place. Ensure that the stems and leaves are not too tightly packed together to enable air to circulate freely around them.

• Once brittle but not bone dry, separate small stems, leaves, flowers, and seeds from the stems by rubbing the bunches over a large sheet of plain paper.

• Carefully pour the dried material into a dark glass jar or a brown paper bag.

Large flowers In most cases, flowers are picked just after they have opened. Sometimes only specific parts of the flower are used, such as the petals of calendula (*Calendula officinalis*, p. 77), while other flowers are used whole.

• Separate large flower heads from stems and remove any insects or dirt. Place the flowers on absorbent paper on a tray in a dry place, allowing sufficient room between them for air to circulate.

• Once dry, store flower heads in a brown paper bag or dark glass jar. Remove calendula petals from the central part of the flower before storing.

Small flowers Small blooms can be picked with the stalk attached and separated later. Hang small flowers, such as lavender (*Lavandula officinalis*, p. 112), upside down in a paper bag, or suspended over a tray (see drying seeds below). If the stems are fleshy, dry as for large flowers, above.

Fruit & berries Harvest fruit and berries in early fall when ripe but still firm. If left to become over-ripe, they may not dry properly. They can be picked individually or in bunches.

• Place berries or fruit on absorbent paper on trays. Put in a warmed oven (turned off) with the door ajar for 3–4 hours. Move to a dry, warm, dark site and turn occasionally. Discard any moldy berries or fruit.

Roots, rhizomes, tubers, & bulbs

The underground parts of the plant are usually gathered in the fall after the aerial parts have withered or become inactive and before the soil is waterlogged or frozen. Many roots may also be collected in early spring before the aerial parts begin to grow. Dig deeply around the root, prying it out of the ground. Some tap roots are difficult to uproot completely. Remove the required amount and replant the remaining root.

• Shake off any soil and wash thoroughly in warm water, removing any small, unwanted side roots or damaged soft spots. Chop into small slices or pieces with a sharp knife.

• Spread out the root pieces on absorbent paper on a tray and place in a warmed oven (turned off) with the door ajar for 2–3 hours. Move to a warm place until dry.

Seeds Collect ripe seed pods, capsules, or flowering stems in late summer before the seeds have been scattered. For tiny seeds, hang small bunches of seed heads upside down over a paper-lined tray, or place in a paper bag. Allow to dry and gently shake. Remove larger seeds by hand when dry.

Sap & gel Only harvest sap from your own garden. Collect sap in the spring as it rises, or as it falls in the fall. Trees such as silver birch (*Betula pendula*, p. 182) produce huge quantities of sap if tapped, although this reduces the tree's vitality. Bore a deep hole into the trunk—no more than a quarter of its diameter—and place a collecting cup under the hole. In spring, quarts of sap may be produced, and it is essential to stop the hole with resin or wood filler after about a quart (liter) of fluid has been removed. Collect milky juices or latex from plants such as dandelion (*Taraxacum officinale*, p. 145) by squeezing the stems over a bowl. Wear gloves, because latex or sap can be corrosive. The gel from aloe vera (*Aloe vera*, p. 64) is scraped out after slicing the leaf lengthwise and peeling back the edges.

Bark Only harvest bark from your own shrubs or trees as it carries the risk of losing the whole plant through over-stripping or "ringing" (removing a whole band of bark). It is best to collect bark from outlying branches, which can then be pruned back. If stripping bark from a plant, gather it in the fall when the sap is falling. Remove insects, lichen, and moss from the bark, cut it into small pieces, and place it on a tray to dry.

Other ways to preserve herbs

Apart from simply air-drying herbs, there are a number of other ways to preserve their medicinal benefits.

Dehumidifying An effective but expensive way to dry herbs is to use a dehumidifier, which literally sucks water out of the plant. The dehumidifier should be placed in a more or less sealed small room in which the herbs are hung in loose bunches or placed on mesh trays.

Freeze-drying Freeze-drying retains color and flavor but is more suited to culinary than to medicinal herbs. Whole sprigs of herbs can be frozen in plastic bags. There is no need to defrost before use as the leaves crumble easily when still frozen. Chickweed (*Stellaria media*, p. 282) can also be frozen and used topically for itchy and weeping skin conditions. Many plants may be juiced (see p. 307), frozen as ice cubes, and thawed as required.

Microwaving It is possible to dry herbs in a microwave oven, though this is not recommended. The cut parts should be spread out on parchment paper and dried in the microwave according to the manufacturer's guidelines.

Making herbal remedies

Medicinal herbs can be made into a variety of formulations—from infusions, decoctions and tinctures, to oxymels and elixirs. The following pages give simple step-by-step instructions on making common herbal preparations. Making herbal medicine is not difficult, but it can be time-consuming—if you lack time or equipment, buy ready-made remedies from a herbal supplier (see *Buying herbal medicines*, p. 296).

Identification

Before using medicinal plants that have been collected from the wild, it is essential that they be correctly identified. If in doubt, do not use the herb. The wrong identification of herbs has led to many cases of poisoning. Foxglove leaves (*Digitalis purpurea*, p. 207), for example, are often mistaken for comfrey (*Symphytum officinale*, p. 142).

Utensils

Use glass, enamel, or stainless steel pots and pans, wooden or steel knives and spatulas, and plastic or nylon sieves. A wine press is useful for making tinctures. Do not use aluminum utensils, as this potentially toxic element is easily absorbed by herbs.

Sterilization

All utensils used to make herbal remedies should be sterilized for at least 30 minutes in a well-diluted sterilizing solution, such as the type used for a baby's bottle. After soaking, rinse thoroughly with boiled water and dry in a hot oven or wash in a dishwasher. Proper sterilization maintains hygiene and prevents remedies, especially creams and syrups, from becoming moldy.

Weights & measures

For most purposes, ordinary kitchen scales are suitable, although electronic scales are more accurate. Metric measurements of grams and liters are generally much easier to use than imperial measures when making remedies. If it is difficult to weigh a small quantity, such as 10 g, on your scales, measure double the weight; i.e., 20 g, then halve the quantity. Liquids can be measured in a kitchen measuring jug, although conical or straight-sided glass measures are more accurate. Very small volumes of liquid can be measured in drops (see *Measuring Remedies*, right).

Storage

Different preparations may be kept for varying periods of time before they begin to lose their medicinal properties. Infusions should be made fresh each day and decoctions must be consumed within

Measuring remedies

1 ml	= 20 drops
5 ml	= 1 teaspoon
15 ml	= 1 tablespoon
150 ml	= 1 herbal cup
250 ml	= 1 cup

Never exceed the quantity of herbs used or the recommended dosage. Although these measurements are approximate, they are accurate enough for most purposes and are used as standard throughout this book. The number of drops to 1 ml depends on the caliber of the pipette (or size of the dropper tip) being used. This can be checked by counting the number of drops required to fill a 5 ml measuring spoon (this book assumes that 100 drops is equal to 5 ml) and then adjusting the drop dosage as necessary.

48 hours. Store both in a refrigerator or cool place. Tinctures and other liquid preparations, such as syrups and essential oils, need to be stored in dark glass bottles in a cool environment away from sunlight, but can be kept for a number of months or years. Ointments, creams, and capsules are best kept in dark glass jars, although plastic containers are also acceptable. See also *Storing Herbs*, p. 299.

The basic first aid kit

Adding herbal remedies to the conventional first aid kit in your home increases the options available to you and your family when accidents happen or illness strikes. The 13 remedies in this first aid kit can generally be found in pharmacies, herbal stores, and health food stores. Alternatively, some can be made at home, as detailed on the following pages. *Check any cautions for each herb before use.*

Lavender (*Lavandula officinalis*, p. 112) essential oil for insect bites and stings, burns, and headaches

Comfrey (*Symphytum officinale*, p. 142) ointment for bruises and sprains, and for healing fractures

Calendula (*Calendula officinalis*, p. 77) cream for inflamed or minor wounds, skin rashes, and sunburn

Myrrh (*Commiphora myrrha*, p. 89) tincture for sore throats and acne

Thyme (*Thymus vulgaris*, p. 147) syrup for coughs, colds, and chest infections

Witch hazel (*Hamamelis virginiana*, p. 106) distilled water for healing cuts and scrapes

Arnica (*Arnica montana*, p. 176) cream for painful bruises and muscle pain

Garlic (*Allium sativum*, p. 63) capsules for infections; the oil from the capsules for earache

Valerian (*Valeriana officinalis*, p. 152) tablets for stress and insomnia

Tea tree (*Melaleuca alternifolia*, p. 116) essential oil is antiseptic and antifungal

Feverfew (*Tanacetum parthenium*, p. 144) capsules for headaches and migraines

Slippery elm (*Ulmus rubra*, p. 149) powder for coughs and digestive upsets

Echinacea (*Echinacea* spp., p. 96) capsules for colds, flu, and infections

Thermometer

Bandages

Infusions

An infusion is the simplest way to prepare the more delicate aerial parts of plants, especially leaves and flowers, for use as a medicine or as a revitalizing or relaxing drink. It is made in a similar way to tea, using either a single herb or a combination of herbs, and may be drunk hot or cold.

The medicinal value of many herbs lies chiefly in their volatile oils, which will disperse into the air if a lid is not used. This is especially important in the case of German chamomile (*Chamomilla recutita*, p. 82). Use a teapot, or place a lid or saucer over a cup if making a small quantity. Use water that has just boiled. Popular herbal teas, such as German chamomile, are often taken as much for their refreshing taste as for their medicinal value and can be safely consumed in quantities of up to 5 or 6 cups a day. Some herbs, however, such as yarrow (*Achillea millefolium*, p. 60), are significantly stronger and must be taken in less frequent doses. Other herbs, such as feverfew (*Tanacetum parthenium*, p. 144), are so strong that they are not suitable for use in infusions. Always check the recommended dosage and quantity of herb to use, as infusions have medicinal actions and can produce unwanted effects at the wrong dosage.

Standard quantity

Cup 1 tsp (2–3 g) dried or 2 tsp (4–6 g) fresh herb (or mixture of herbs) to a cup of water (this makes 1 dose)

Pot 20 g dried herb or 30 g fresh herb (or a mixture of different herbs) to 2 cups (500 ml) of water

Pot infusion

Warm the pot, then add the herb. Pour in water that has just boiled, replace the lid, and infuse for 10 minutes. Strain some of the infusion into a cup. A teaspoon of honey may be added if desired.

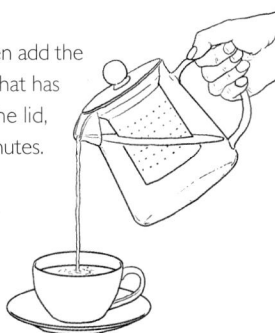

Cup infusion

1 Place the herb in the strainer of the teacup and place the strainer in the cup. Fill the cup with freshly boiled water.

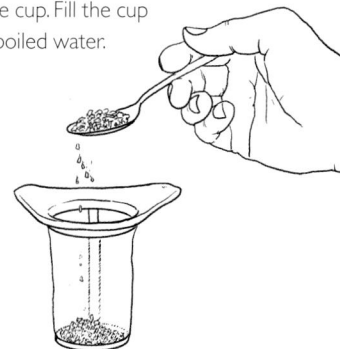

2 Cover the cup with the lid and infuse for 5–10 minutes before removing the tea strainer. Add a teaspoon of honey to sweeten, if desired.

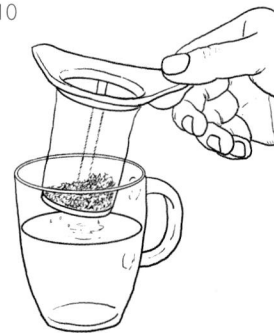

Decoctions

Roots, bark, twigs, and berries usually require a more forceful treatment than leaves or flowers to extract their medicinal constituents. A decoction involves simmering these tougher parts in boiling water. Fresh or dried plant material may be used and should be cut or broken into small pieces before decocting. Like infusions, decoctions can be taken hot or cold.

Decoctions are generally made using roots, bark, and berries, but sometimes leaves and flowers may be included. Add these more delicate parts of a plant once the heat is turned off and the decoction has finished simmering and is beginning to cool. Then strain and use as required.

Chinese decoctions

In traditional Chinese medicine, decoctions are the main way in which herbal medicines are prepared. Large quantities of herb are often used to produce a highly concentrated liquid, or the decoction is further reduced so that there is only ¾ cup (200 ml) of liquid remaining. This increases the preparation's concentration. This process is useful for astringent barks such as babul (*Vachellia nilotica*, p. 290) and common oak (*Quercus robur*, p. 268), which may be used externally to tighten gums or wash weeping skin rashes. (Do not take internally.)

Standard quantity

20 g dried or 40 g fresh herb (or mixture of herbs) to 3 cups (750 ml) cold water, reduced to about 2 cups (500 ml) after simmering (this makes 3–4 doses)

Standard dosage Take 3–4 doses (2 cups/500 ml) each day.

Storage Store in a covered jug in a refrigerator or cool place for up to 48 hours.

Making decoctions

1 Place the herbs in a saucepan. Cover with cold water and bring to a boil. Simmer for about 20–30 minutes, until the liquid is reduced by about one-third.

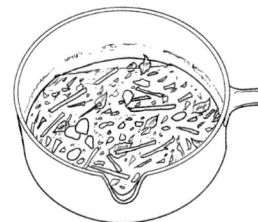

2 Strain the liquid through a sieve into a jug. Pour the required amount into a cup, then cover the jug and store in a cool place.

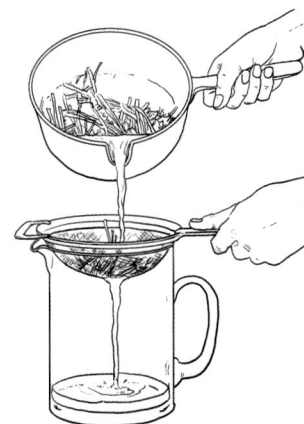

301

Tinctures

Tinctures are made by soaking an herb in alcohol. This encourages the active plant constituents to dissolve, giving tinctures a relatively stronger action than infusions or decoctions. They are convenient to use and last up to two years. Tinctures can be made using a jug and a jelly bag, instead of a wine press. Although mainly used in European, American, and Australian herbal medicine, tinctures play a part in most herbal traditions.

Tinctures are strong preparations, and it is essential to check the recommended dosage. Never use industrial alcohol, methylated spirits (methyl alcohol) or rubbing alcohol (isopropyl alcohol) in tinctures.

Alcohol-reduced tinctures

Alcoholic tinctures should sometimes be avoided, for example during pregnancy or a gastric inflammation. Adding 1 tsp (5 ml) of tincture to a small glass of almost boiling water and leaving it for 5 minutes allows the alcohol to evaporate. To make nonalcoholic tinctures, replace the alcohol with vinegar or glycerol.

Tincture ratios

Tinctures are made in different strengths, expressed as ratios. In this book, a 1:5 ratio (1 part herb to 5 parts alcohol) is used, unless otherwise stated.

Standard quantity

200 g dried or 300 g fresh herb chopped into small pieces to 1 quart (1 liter) alcohol—vodka of 35–40% alcohol is ideal, although rum hides the taste of bitter or unpalatable herbs
Standard dosage Take 1 tsp (5 ml) 2–3 times a day diluted in 1 tbsp plus 1 tsp (25 ml) of water or fruit juice.
Storage Store in sterilized, dark glass bottles in a cool dark place for up to 2 years.

Making tinctures

1 Place the herb in a large, clean glass jar and pour on the alcohol, ensuring that the herb is covered. Close and label the jar. Shake well for 1–2 minutes and store in a cool dark place for 10–14 days, shaking the jar every 1–2 days.

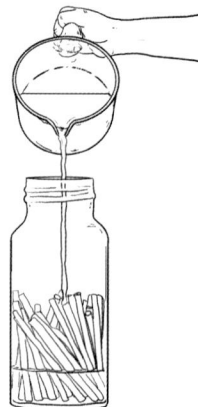

2 Set up the wine press, placing a muslin or nylon mesh bag securely inside. Pour in the mixture and collect the liquid in the jug.

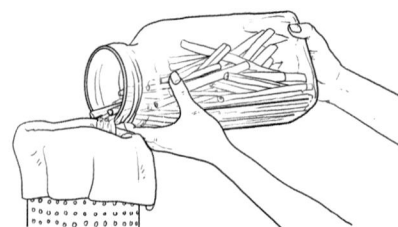

3 Slowly close the wine press, extracting the remaining liquid from the herbs until no more drips appear. Discard the leftover herbs.

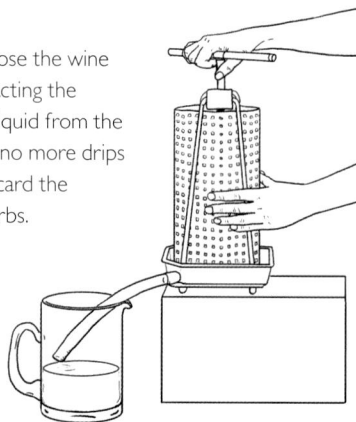

4 Pour the tincture into clean, dark glass bottles using a funnel. When full, stopper with a cork or screw top and label the bottles.

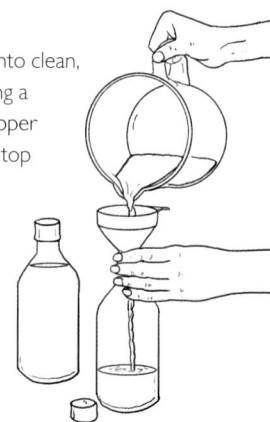

Capsules & powders

Powdered herbs are most easily taken as capsules but can be sprinkled on food or taken with water. Externally, they can be applied as a dusting powder to the skin or mixed with tinctures as a poultice (see p. 305).

Reputable herbal suppliers are the best place to buy powdered herbs and, in general, the finer the powder the better the grade and quality. Gelatin or vegetarian capsule cases are also available from specialist outlets. Powdered slippery elm (*Ulmus rubra*, p. 149) makes a useful base for poultices (see p. 305), and astringents such as witch hazel (*Hamamelis virginiana*, p. 106) may be applied to weeping skin or mixed into ointments (see p. 305) for hemorrhoids and varicose veins.

Standard quantity

Fill size 00 capsules, which contain approximately 250 mg of powdered herb
Standard dosage Take 2–3 capsules twice a day.
Storage Store in airtight, dark glass containers in a cool place for up to 3–4 months.

Making capsules

1 Pour the powder into a saucer and slide the capsule halves toward one another, scooping up the powder (or use a capsule-making tray).

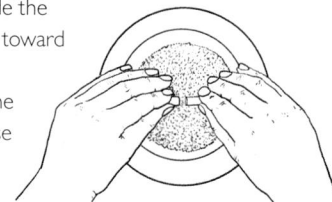

2 When the halves of the capsule are full of powder, slide them together without spilling the powder, and store.

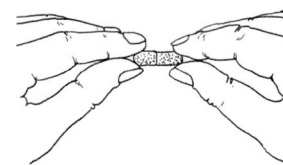

Tonic wines

Tonic wines are an agreeable way to take strengthening and tonic herbs to increase vitality and improve digestion. Neither strictly medicinal, nor simply appealing to the palate, they are easy to prepare at home. Tonic wines are made by steeping tonic herbs, such as *dong quai* (*Angelica sinensis*, p. 67), or bitter herbs, such as southernwood (*Artemisia abrotanum*, p. 176), in red or white wine for several weeks.

A simple and effective way to make a tonic wine is in a jar or a ceramic vat with a tap at the base to enable the wine to be drawn off without disturbing the herbs. Wine can be added periodically to keep the herbs covered, although, in time, this will reduce the wine's tonic effectiveness. If exposed to the air, the herbs may get moldy, making the remedy not only ineffective but unsafe to take.

Herbal wines

Herbal wines are made by fermenting the herb in the same way that wine is produced from grapes. With the correct equipment this is a simple process, but fermentation alters the activity of the herbs and tends to reduce their medicinal value.

Standard quantity
100 g dried or 200 g fresh tonic herbs or 25 g dried bitter herbs and 1 quart (1 liter) of red or white wine
Standard dosage Drink ⅓ cup (70 ml) each day before a meal.
Storage Use a ceramic vat with a tap at its base, or a sterilized glass jar. Store for 3–4 months, ensuring wine covers the herbs. If the herbs become moldy, discard the remedy.

Making tonic wines

1 Place the herb in a large, clean jar or vat. Pour in enough wine to cover the herb completely. Close the jar securely, shake carefully, and leave to stand.

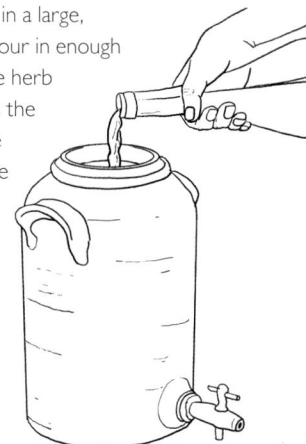

2 Allow the wine to mature over 2–6 weeks, then take a dose from the tap or jar. Regularly top off the mixture with wine.

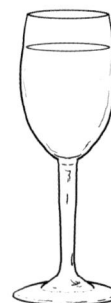

Syrups

Honey and unrefined sugar are effective preservatives and can be combined with infusions or decoctions to make syrups and cordials. They have the additional benefit of having a soothing action, and therefore make a perfect vehicle for cough mixtures as well as relieving sore throats. With their sweet taste, syrups can disguise the taste of unpalatable herbs and are therefore greatly appreciated by children.

A syrup is made with equal proportions of an herbal infusion or decoction and honey or unrefined sugar. When making an infusion or decoction for a syrup, it needs to be infused or simmered for the maximum time to optimize its medicinal action. Infusions should be infused for 15 minutes and decoctions should be simmered for 30 minutes. Press the soaked herb through the strainer or sieve to remove as much liquid as possible. Small amounts of neat tincture can be added to the cooled syrup to increase its effectiveness.

Syrups made with tinctures

Syrups may also be made with tinctures instead of infusions or decoctions. Combine 500 g of honey or unrefined sugar with 1 cup (250 ml) of water. Gently heat until all the sugar or honey has dissolved and the mixture has thickened. Remove from the heat. Once cool, stir 1 part of the tincture, or mixture of tinctures, into 3 parts of the syrup and bottle as directed opposite.

Standard quantity
2 cups (500 ml) infusion or decoction (see p. 301), infused or heated for the maximum time (see left); 500 g honey or unrefined sugar
Standard dosage Take 1–2 tsp (5–10 ml) 3 times a day.
Storage Store in dark glass bottles with cork tops in a cool place for up to 6 months.

Making syrups

1 Pour the infusion or decoction into a pan. Add the honey or sugar. Gently heat, stirring constantly until all the honey or sugar has dissolved and the mixture has a syrupy consistency. Remove from the heat and cool.

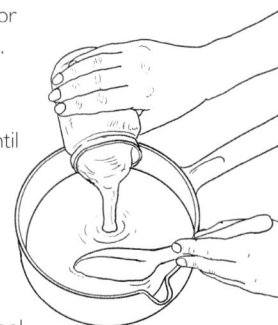

2 Pour the cooled syrup into sterilized glass jars using a funnel and store in a cool, dark place. Seal the jars with cork stoppers, because syrups are prone to ferment and may explode if kept in screw-topped bottles.

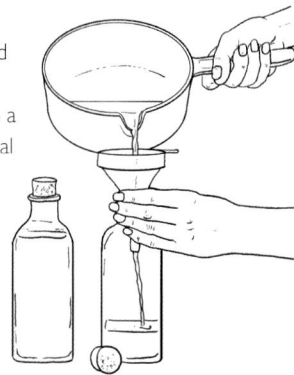

Infused oils

Infusing an herb in oil allows its active, fat-soluble ingredients to be extracted; hot infused oils are simmered, while cold infused oils are heated naturally by the sun. Both types of oil can be used externally as massage oils or added to creams and ointments. Infused oil should not be confused with essential oil, which is an active constituent naturally present in a plant and has specific medicinal properties and a distinct aroma. Essential oil may be added to an infused oil to increase its medicinal efficacy.

Hot infused oils

Although hot infused oils can last up to a year, they are most potent when used fresh. If only using infused oils occasionally, make a smaller quantity than the standard amount with the same proportion of herb to oil. The wine press may be replaced with a jug—when cool enough to touch, squeeze the oil through the jelly bag as illustrated in *Cold Infused Oils* below.

Many herbs make effective hot infused oils, especially spicy herbs such as ginger (*Zingiber officinale*, p. 159), cayenne (*Capsicum frutescens*, p. 79), and pepper (*Piper nigrum*, p. 250). These oils can be rubbed into the skin to relieve rheumatic and arthritic pain, improve local blood flow, and relax muscles. Other hot infused oils from leafy herbs, such as comfrey (*Symphytum officinale*, p. 142), speed wound healing. Oil infused with mullein (*Verbascum thapsus*, p. 291) is used for earache and ear infections, and chickweed (*Stellaria media*, p. 282) ointment may be produced from a hot infused oil (see p. 305).

Standard quantity (infused oils)

250g dried or 500g fresh herb to 3 cups (750ml) olive, sunflower, or other good-quality vegetable oil
Storage Store in sterilized, airtight, dark glass bottles for up to 1 year; for the best results, use within 6 months.

Making hot infused oils

1 Stir the chopped herb and oil together in a glass bowl over a saucepan of boiling water. Cover and simmer gently for 2–3 hours.

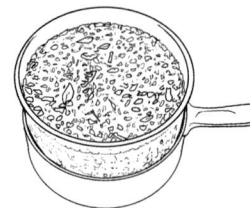

2 Remove from the heat and allow the mixture to cool, then pour into the wine press (or jug if not available) with a jelly bag in place. Collect the strained oil in a jug, pressing all the liquid out of the herb.

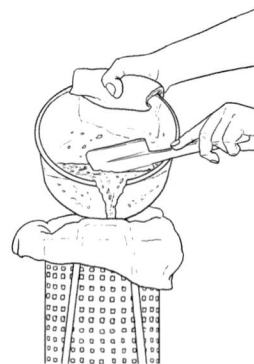

3 Pour the infused oil into clean, dark glass bottles, using a funnel. Seal and label each bottle.

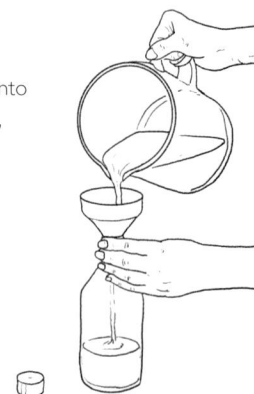

Cold infused oils

Making a cold infused oil is a slow process and involves leaving a jar packed with herbs and oil to stand for several weeks. Sunlight encourages the plant to release its active constituents into the oil. It is the most suitable method of oil infusion for fresh plant material, especially the more delicate parts, such as flowers. St. John's wort (*Hypericum perforatum*, p. 110), calendula (*Calendula officinalis*, p. 77), and melilot (*Melilotus officinalis*, p. 240) are three of the most commonly produced cold infused oils. St. John's wort oil is anti-inflammatory and analgesic, and may be applied topically or taken internally (after consulting an herbalist) for peptic ulceration.

Olive oil is particularly suitable for cold infusion as it rarely turns rancid. The intensity of sunlight and length of time an herb is infused affects the concentration of its medicinal constituents. For greater strength, add the extracted oil to a fresh supply of herbs and infuse again.

Making cold infused oils

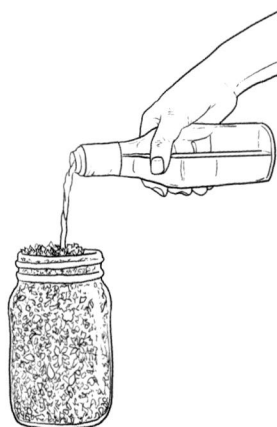

1 Place the herb in a clear glass jar. Pour in oil until it completely covers the herb, close the jar, and shake well. Place the jar in a sunny spot, such as on a windowsill, and leave for 2–6 weeks.

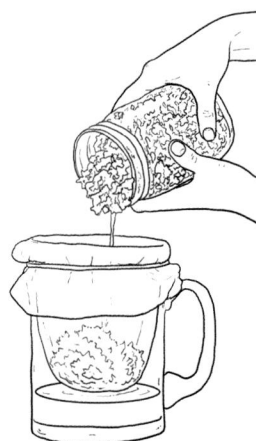

2 Pour the oil and herb mixture into a jelly bag, secured to the rim of a jug or bowl with string (or use a wine press as pictured above in hot infused oils). Allow the oil to filter through the bag.

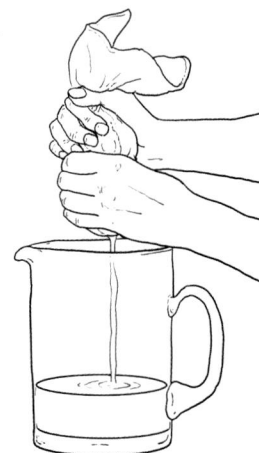

3 Squeeze out the remaining oil from the bag. Pour the infused oil into dark glass bottles, label, and store. Alternatively, repeat the whole process with the infused oil and fresh herbs.

Ointments

Ointments contain oils or fats heated with herbs and, unlike creams, contain no water. As a result, ointments form a separate layer on the surface of the skin. They protect against injury or inflammation of damaged skin and carry active medicinal constituents, such as essential oils, to the affected area. Ointments are useful in conditions such as hemorrhoids or where protection is needed from moisture, as in chapped lips and diaper rash.

Ointments can be made with dozens of bases and they vary in consistency, depending on the constituents and proportions used. The simplest way to make a soft, all-purpose ointment is to use petroleum jelly or soft paraffin wax (other methods are explained below). Petroleum jelly is impermeable to water and provides a protective barrier for the skin. Single herbs or mixtures of herbs may be used as required, provided they are finely cut, and essential oil can be stirred into the ointment just before straining.

Different consistencies

A solid and relatively grease-free ointment will spread easily and is useful for preparations such as lip balms. This may be made by using alternatives to mineral oils. Melt 140g of coconut oil with 120g of beeswax and 100g of powdered herb. Simmer gently for 90 minutes in a glass bowl set in a pan of boiling water or a double boiler, then strain and pour into jars.
A less solid ointment, for conditions such as skin rashes, may be made by combining olive oil and beeswax. Melt 60g of beeswax with 2 cups (500ml) of olive oil and 120g of dried or 300g of fresh herb in a glass bowl. Cover and place in a warm oven for 3 hours, then remove, strain, and pour into jars. This ointment can also be made by combining 2 cups (500ml) of hot infused oil (see p. 304) with 60g of melted beeswax.

Standard quantity

60g dried or 150g fresh herb (or mixture of herbs) to 500g of petroleum jelly or soft paraffin wax
Standard application Apply a little 3 times a day.
Storage Store in sterilized, dark glass jars with lids for up to 3 months.

Making ointments

1 Melt the petroleum jelly or wax in a glass bowl set in a pan of boiling water, or use a double boiler. Add the finely cut herb and simmer for 15 minutes, stirring continuously.

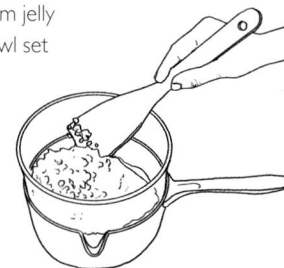

2 Pour the herb mixture into a jelly bag secured to the rim of a jug with string, and allow the liquid to filter through.

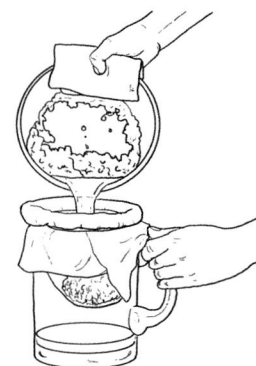

3 Wearing rubber gloves, squeeze as much of the hot herb mixture as possible through the bag into the jug. Quickly pour the molten ointment into jars before it sets in the jug. Place the lid on each jar without securing it firmly. When cool, tighten the lids and label.

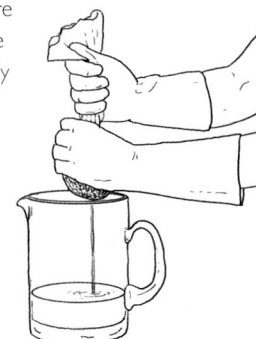

Poultices

A poultice is a mixture of fresh, dried, or powdered herbs that is applied to an affected area. Poultices are used to ease nerve or muscle pains, sprains, or broken bones, and to draw pus from infected wounds, ulcers, or boils.

A poultice of self-heal (*Prunella vulgaris*, p. 264) relieves sprains and fractures, while St. John's wort (*Hypericum perforatum*, p. 110) can help ease muscle or nerve pains.

Drawing boils & infected wounds

Slippery elm powder (*Ulmus rubra*, p. 149) mixed with calendula (*Calendula officinalis*, p. 77) tincture or myrrh (*Commiphora myrrha*, p. 89) tincture makes a useful poultice for drawing boils and wounds.

Standard quantity

Sufficient herb to cover the affected area
Standard application Apply a new poultice every 2–3 hours. Repeat as often as required.

Making poultices

1 Simmer the herb for 2 minutes. Squeeze out any excess liquid, rub some oil on the affected area to prevent sticking, and apply the herb while hot.

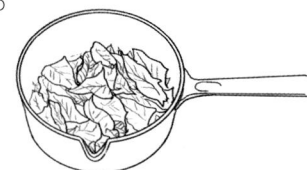

2 Bandage the herb securely in place using gauze or cotton strips. Leave on for up to 3 hours, as required.

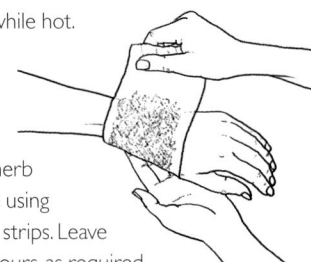

Creams

Making a cream involves combining oil or fat and water in an emulsion. If the process is rushed, the oil and water may separate. Unlike ointments, creams blend with the skin and have the advantage of being cooling and soothing while at the same time allowing the skin to breathe and sweat naturally. They can, however, deteriorate quite quickly and are best stored in dark, airtight jars in a refrigerator.

Small quantities of additional ingredients such as tinctures, powders, and essential oils can be added to a cream before or after it is put in jars. Adding an essential oil, such as 1 ml of tea tree (*Melaleuca alternifolia*, p. 116), to ½ cup (100 ml) of cream, counters mold growth and lengthens shelf life, as does 1 tsp (5 ml) of borax. Other recipes for making cream use infusions, tinctures, or infused oils.

Standard quantity
30 g dried or 75 g fresh herb, 150 g emulsifying wax, 70 g glycerin, and ⅓ cup (80 ml) water
Standard dosage Rub a little into the affected area 2–3 times a day.
Storage Store in sterilized, airtight, dark glass jars in a refrigerator for up to 3 months.

Making creams

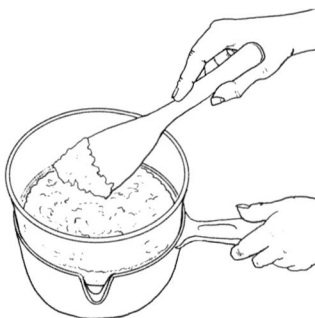

1 Melt the emulsifying wax in a glass bowl set in a pan of boiling water, or a double boiler. Add the glycerin, water, and herb while stirring, and simmer for 3 hours.

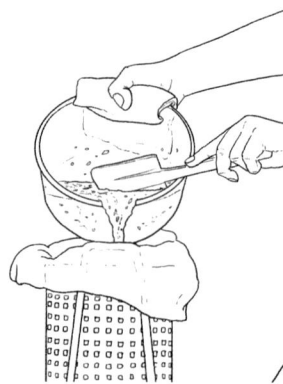

2 Strain the mixture through a wine press or a jelly bag. Stir slowly but continuously until it cools and sets.

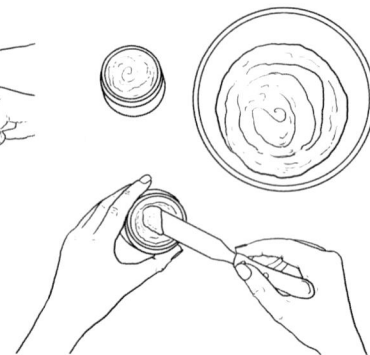

3 With a small knife or spatula, place the set cream into dark glass jars. Tighten the lids and label. Store in a refrigerator as soon as possible.

Compresses & lotions

Lotions are water-based herbal preparations such as infusions, decoctions, or diluted tinctures that are used to bathe inflamed or irritated skin. Compresses are cloths soaked in a lotion and held against the skin. Lotions and compresses are both simple ways to use herbs externally and can be very effective in relieving swelling, bruising, and pain, soothing inflammation and headaches, and cooling fevers.

After an accident or sports injury, bruising and swelling can often be reduced or prevented if a hot compress is swiftly applied, provided the skin is unbroken. Cold compresses are particularly useful in soothing inflammation, cooling fevers, and easing headaches. Both hot and cold compresses should be frequently soaked and reapplied for maximum benefit.

Applying a lotion
As specified, make an infusion or decoction (see p. 301), and strain it well. Alternatively, dilute a tincture with water. Soak a clean cloth in the lotion and wring it out thoroughly. Then gently bathe the affected area with the cloth (rather than laying it on the skin as you would a compress).

Standard quantity of lotion
2 cups (500 ml) infusion or decoction, or 5 tsp (25 ml) tincture in 2 cups (500 ml) water
Standard application of compress or lotion
Use as required. Prepare a fresh compress or lotion when it cools (if hot) or when it dries (if cool).
Storage Store lotions in sterilized bottles, with lids, in a refrigerator for up to 2 days.

Applying a compress

1 Wash your hands thoroughly and soak a soft cloth or clean washcloth in the lotion. Wring out the excess liquid. Before applying, rub some oil on the affected area to prevent sticking.

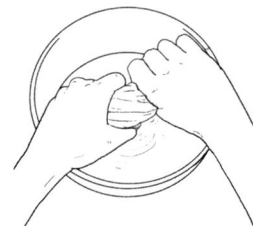

2 Place the compress against the affected area. For pain and swellings, secure the compress with plastic film and safety pins and leave for up to 1–2 hours. Reapply as required.

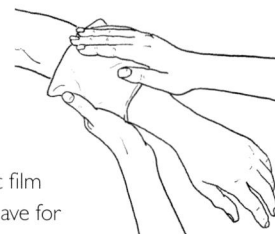

Other preparations

Different herbal preparations suit different ailments. Most of the following preparations provide localized relief. Steam inhalations, for example, help clear various respiratory complaints; gargles and mouthwashes soothe sore throats and mouth ulcers; massage oils can ease aching muscles; and skin washes relieve inflamed skin conditions.

Steam inhalations

Steam inhalations are an effective way to clear congestion and relieve sinusitis, hay fever, and bronchial asthma. The combination of steam and antiseptic ingredients clears the airways throughout the respiratory system.

To make Pour 1 quart of freshly boiled water into a large bowl, add 5–10 drops of essential oil, and stir well. Alternatively, make an infusion of 25 g of herb to 1 quart of water, brew for 15 minutes, and pour into a bowl. Cover the head and bowl with a towel, close the eyes, and inhale the steam for about 10 minutes or until the preparation cools. After a steam inhalation, it is advisable to stay in a warm room for 15 minutes to allow the airways to adjust and any congestion to clear.

Powders

Most dried herb material can be powdered using a pestle and mortar, or a coffee grinder, though it is often better to buy industrially ground powders that have a fine consistency. Powders are versatile but will decay more quickly than cut material. Store in the fridge in a closed container. Powdered herbs can be added to foods, smoothies and drinks.

To make Beet (*Beta vulgaris*, p. 182) and hawthorn leaf (*Crataegus* spp., p. 91) powders, for example, can be routinely added to food or a smoothie to maintain a healthy circulation and lower high blood pressure. Add ½–1 tsp of each and stir in well.

Gargles & mouthwashes

Gargles and mouthwashes usually contain astringent herbs, which tighten the mucous membranes of the mouth and throat. Astringent herbs such as rhatany (*Krameria triandra*, p. 230) and myrrh (*Commiphora myrrha*, p. 89), can be made more palatable and more effective for sore throats by adding a little licorice (*Glycyrrhiza glabra*, p. 105) or a pinch of cayenne pepper (*Capsicum frutescens*, p. 79) to the preparation. As gargles and mouthwashes are made from infusions, decoctions, or diluted tinctures, they can generally be swallowed for internal treatment. Ensure you do not exceed the daily internal dose of an herb.

To make Make an infusion (*see* p. 301) but allow it to stand for 15–20 minutes in order to increase its astringency. Strain, then gargle, or rinse the mouth with a cupful. Alternatively, use a decoction (p. 301) or dilute about 1 tsp (5 ml) of tincture in ⅓ cup (100 ml) of hot water and use in the same way. Repeat as often as required unless specified.

Pessaries & suppositories

Pessaries and suppositories are waxy pellets containing essential oil or fine powder. They are used when oral medicine is likely to be broken down during digestion before reaching its intended site. Pessaries are inserted into the vagina and suppositories into the anus, where they melt at body temperature. The herb is quickly absorbed into the bloodstream, providing fast relief. It is best to buy ready-made suppositories.

To make pessaries Use a pessary mold or make 24 molds from cooking foil shaped around a thimble. Mix 10 g of soft soap, 2 tbsp plus 2 tsp (50 ml) of glycerin and 2 tbsp (40 ml) of methylated spirits and pour into the molds. Leave for a few minutes to coat the molds, then pour out the excess and leave to harden. Melt 20 g of cocoa butter, remove from the heat, and add 30 drops of essential oil or 5 g of powder. Pour into the shells and leave to set for 3 hours, before removing the pessaries. Store in a cool place in a pot lined with greaseproof paper for up to 3 months.

Essential oils

Essential oils can be used in massage to soothe minor aches and pains. Before use, they should be diluted with a carrier oil as they can irritate the skin. Essential oils deteriorate rapidly after dilution, so it is best to mix small quantities as you need them.

For massage Mix 5–10 drops of essential oil with 1 tbsp of carrier oil, such as wheatgerm or almond oil, and massage gently into the skin.

Oil burner Use 5–10 drops of neat essential oil mixed with water. Burn for 30 minutes.

Baths & skin washes

Herbal baths and skin washes can relieve many conditions, including aching limbs and stuffy sinuses. They are made from diluted essential oils or infusions. Eyebaths soothe sore, inflamed, or irritated eyes.

To make an herbal bath Add 2 cups (500 ml) of strained infusion (see p. 301) or 5–10 drops of essential oil to a running bath.

To make a skin wash Make an infusion, strain it, and bathe the affected area.

To make an eyebath Make a small quantity of an infusion or use an herbal teabag. Strain the liquid carefully into a sterilized eyebath. Alternatively, add 2–3 drops of a tincture to an eyebath filled with water that has just boiled. Allow to cool and place the eyebath firmly over the eye. Tip the head back and bathe the eye by continuously blinking. Repeat up to 3 times a day.

General cautions Eyebaths should be very weak, so as not to sting the eyes. Always use boiled, cooled water in a sterilized container. Do not bathe eyes over a period of more than 2–3 weeks at a time. If bathing eyes frequently, add a tiny pinch of salt to each eyebath to counter leaching of salts and minerals from the eye.

Cold macerations

Heat destroys the active constituents of some herbs, and a cold maceration is more appropriate than a decoction.

To make Pour 2 cups (500 ml) of cold water over 25 g of herb and leave to stand overnight. Strain and use as you would a decoction

Juices

The juices extracted from many herbs can be taken internally or applied externally.

To make Pulp the plant, preferably using a mechanical juicer. Otherwise use a food processor. Squeeze the pulp through a jelly bag to collect the juice. Some herbs need to be cooked in order to extract their juice.

Smoothies

Smoothies are a very convenient way to take gentle-acting herbs such as maca (*Lepidium meyenii*, p. 233) and peppermint (*Mentha* x *piperita*, p. 118). A whole range of vegetables, fruits, herbs, spices, seeds, and powders can be blended together to make a nutritious and pleasant tasting drink. Use fresh herbs where possible.

To make Select the herbs and work out how much to use of each—usually ½ tsp dried, 1 tsp fresh. Blend in with vegetables and fruits that complement the herbs and make the drink palatable.

Using herbal remedies safely

One reason that herbal remedies are so popular is that plant medicines are safer and cause fewer side effects than conventional ones. However, herbal remedies are not always safe, and—like medicines of every kind—they need to be used with care.

What can go wrong?

Following a few simple rules will normally ensure that the worst that happens when taking an herbal medicine is that there is no improvement in your condition. Nevertheless, there are situations in which herbal remedies can cause damage, and several medicinal herbs have been shown to interact with conventional medicines. In very rare circumstances people have become seriously ill or have died from taking herbal medicines, though in almost every case the problem has resulted from one of the following safety factors being ignored. If at any time you think that you are reacting badly to an herbal medicine, stop taking it immediately, and contact a qualified herbalist or naturopath, or your doctor.

How problems can occur

The wrong herb is used due to mistaken identification. Usually, when herbs are bought over the counter you have no need to worry, as the necessary checks have been made to ensure it has been correctly identified. If you are harvesting herbs from the wild, you must be certain what herb it is that you are collecting. For example, ragwort (*Senecio jacobaea*), which is very toxic to the liver, can easily be mistaken for St. John's wort (*Hypericum perforatum*, p. 110): both grow in open areas and produce clusters of bright yellow flowers in the summer. In rare cases, the physical act of picking certain highly toxic herbs could be dangerous, because absorption takes place across the skin. Hemlock (*Conium maculatum*, p. 198), for example, is so toxic that serious side effects can result from simply handling the plant.

The wrong part of an herb is used. It is important to use the correct part of the herb. Sometimes one part of a plant is safe, while all other parts are poisonous. For example, while the potato tuber (*Solanum tuberosum*, p. 280) makes good, nutritious food, all other parts of the plant are highly toxic.

Poor-quality material is used or the herb has been poorly prepared. If you are making up your own remedy, follow the recommended methods for storage and preparation (see *Harvesting & Processing*, pp. 298–299). If buying over the counter, check the section on *Quality Control* (see p. 17) for advice on purchasing good-quality products.

The wrong herbal remedy is being used. You can avoid this problem if you stick to using well-known herbs and take them to treat the conditions for which they are usually recommended. Ginger (*Zingiber officinale*, p. 159) and sweet flag (*Acorus calamus*, p. 163) both help to relieve nausea and indigestion, but ginger is an altogether safer medicine—it is better known, is a common treatment for motion and morning sickness, and, unlike sweet flag, has no known side effects.

The herbal remedy interacts with other medicines. Herbal remedies are medicines, so it should come as no surprise that conventional medicines can interact with them. Several herbs are known to interact with conventional medicines. St. John's wort, for example, speeds up the rate at which the liver breaks down a range of drugs, including certain antibiotics, anti-epileptics, and immune-suppressants. This reduces their effectiveness within the body, and in extreme situations could threaten life. It is also inadvisable to take St. John's wort at the same time as other antidepressants. A number of herbs, notably dong quai (*Angelica sinensis*, p. 67), interact with anticoagulant drugs, such as warfarin and clopidogrel. These drugs are prescribed to prevent blood clotting. Herbal products containing these herbs will interact with anticoagulants and increase the risk of internal or external bleeding. Always tell health-care professionals what medicines you are using—both herbal and conventional. If you are taking medicines prescribed by your doctor, it is always sensible to seek advice before starting to take herbal remedies.

The herbal remedy causes an allergic reaction. By and large, allergic reactions to herbs result from touching the herb (contact dermatitis) and from breathing in pollen or powdered herb (airborne allergies). Some plants are well known for causing contact dermatitis—rue (*Ruta graveolens*, p. 273) for example—and should not be handled by those prone to allergies. Some powdered herbs can stimulate sneezing attacks in the sensitive—for example linden (*Tilia* spp., p. 286). In some cases, herbal medicines may trigger allergic reactions within the body. If you are prone to allergies it is advisable to see a qualified herbalist before taking all but the most common herbs. In the case of a severe allergic reaction, call 911.

Other treatment is needed. Sometimes herbal medicine is not the appropriate form of treatment. If you have an acute illness or injury, are seriously ill, or do not recover as expected after taking an herbal remedy, *do not delay*—seek professional advice or emergency treatment.

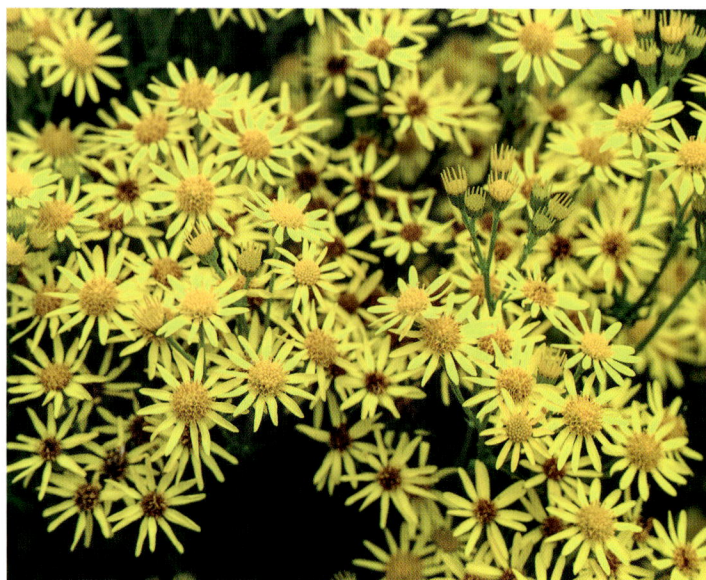

Ragwort is a toxic plant and, with its yellow flowers, easily mistaken for St. John's wort.

Remedies for common ailments

Herbal knowledge is continuing to grow as more people choose herbs as an alternative to pharmaceutical drugs. The following remedies are safe and effective treatments for a range of common ailments; but, like all medicines, they must be treated with respect. The suggestions given here are mostly quite straightforward. However, if you are unsure about what to do, always seek professional advice (see p. 330). For instructions on how to make herbal preparations, see pp. 300–307.

Essential information

Before using remedies read the following.

Dosage

• Except in *Infants & Children* (see p. 328), all dosages given are for adults.

• Do not exceed the stated dose; doubling it will *not* make the medicine twice as effective.

• Before taking a remedy, check the cautions in the relevant herb entry (see pp. 60–293).

• Where different forms of a remedy are given (e.g. take tincture or infusion), the first is preferable.

How long to take remedies

Take remedies until symptoms disappear. If there is no improvement within 2–3 weeks, if the condition worsens, or if in doubt, consult a professional practitioner (see p. 330).

Professional advice

• Advice is given on when to seek professional guidance. Consult a professional if taking a remedy for over 3 weeks.

Infants & children

• Do not give infants under 6 months any internal herbal (or other) medicine without professional advice.

• *Infants & Children*, p. 328, gives children's dosages. Remedies elsewhere can be used for children under 12. Reduce doses as follows:

• 6–12 months old—$\frac{1}{10}$ adult dose

• 1–6 years old—$\frac{1}{3}$ adult dose

• 7–12 years old—$\frac{1}{2}$ adult dose.

Older people

Older adults, due to slower metabolism, may require less than the standard dose. Those over 70 should usually take $\frac{3}{4}$ of the adult dose.

Pregnancy

• During the first 3 months of pregnancy, avoid all medicines, herbal or otherwise, unless absolutely essential.

• Avoid alcoholic tinctures in pregnancy.

• The herbs mentioned in *Pregnancy* (see p. 327) are safe to use. Many of the remedies elsewhere in this section are also safe, but some are not. *Always check the cautions for the remedy and in the relevant herb entry (see pp. 60–293) before taking an herb during pregnancy.*

Prescription medicine

As explained opposite, some herbs are known to interact with pharmaceutical drugs; others may interact in as-yet unknown ways. If you are taking a prescribed medicine, consult a professional practitioner before taking an herb, and do not discontinue any medicine without their advice.

Herbal preparations

• All quantities are for dried herbs unless specified.

• Where more than one part of an herb is used, the instructions specify which part to use. Only use that part. Do not use seeds sold for horticultural purposes.

• Unless specified otherwise, preparations are made with standard quantities of dried herb, as follows:

Infusions (to make, see p. 301). Use a teaspoon of herb to a cup of water, or make enough for 3–4 doses using 20 g of herb to 2 cups (500 ml) of water. Use a covered container to retain the herb's valuable volatile oils.

Decoctions (to make, see p. 301). Use 20 g herb to 3 cups (750 ml) of water.

Inhalations (to make, see p. 307). Add 5–10 drops essential oil to 1 quart (1 liter) of steaming hot water or use an infusion.

Lotions (to make, see p. 306). Use 2 cups (500 ml) infusion or decoction, or 5 tsp (25 ml) tincture diluted in 2 cups (500 ml) of water.

Tablets or capsules (to make, see p. 302). Many herbs are available over the counter in both forms. Take according to the instructions on the packet.

Tinctures (to make, see p. 302). Some tinctures are available ready-made. Take tinctures with cold water unless specified. Sometimes the number of drops recommended is given as a range, e.g. 20–40 drops. In these cases, start with the lowest amount and increase by 5–10 drops per dose as required.

Essential oils

Do not take essential oils internally unless advised to do so by a professional practitioner. For external use, dilute essential oils with a carrier oil, such as sunflower or almond, in a ratio of 1 part essential oil to 20 parts carrier oil; e.g., 5 drops essential oil

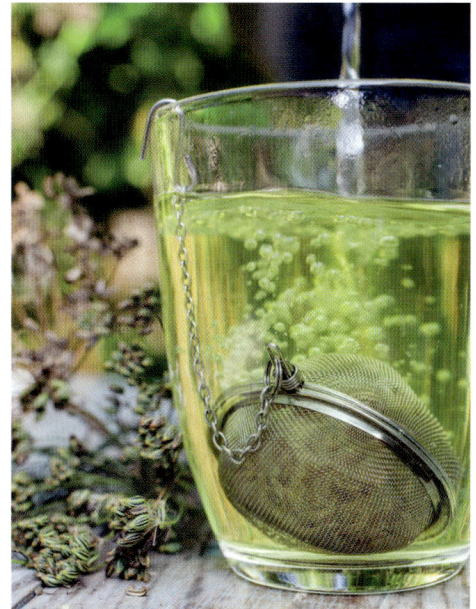

Infusions make effective remedies; some are also relaxing or refreshing drinks.

to 1 tsp (5 ml) carrier oil. For a bath, add 5–10 drops of neat essential oil to the running water. To use essential oils in massage, see p. 307.

Other information

For other preparations, weighing & measuring, and equipment, see pp. 301–307.

Self-help

Lifestyle, diet and exercise advice is given in this section. In general, these suggestions do not provide a "quick-fix" solution and need to be followed long term if they are to be effective. They should be used in addition to the recommended herbal remedy. By ensuring that your body has the right nutrition and level of fitness, you protect yourself against many ailments such as infections and circulatory problems, as well as increase your chances of a speedy and effective recovery.

Allergies

Allergies often develop when the body's immune system overreacts to an external irritant such as pollen, insect stings, and certain plants, or internal substances such as chemicals and foods. The allergens trigger a reaction in those who have a built-in or natural sensitivity. In the long term, allergies are treated by both reducing contact with allergens (if known) and working to reduce the body's oversensitivity. Herbal remedies can bring relief to some allergic states and are helpful in gradually reducing allergic reactions. See also *Skin Rashes*, p. 313.

Seek immediate professional advice for:

- Life-threatening allergies, such as asthma. Consult a professional practitioner prior to taking any herbal remedies for such conditions
- Any allergy that shows signs of deterioration after taking an herbal remedy
- Severe pain in the respiratory tract

Allergic rhinitis, including hay fever

Allergic rhinitis is an umbrella term for allergic reactions to irritants such as pollution, dust, or pollen. Allergic rhinitis may occur year round, while hay fever is usually caused by seasonal grass or pollens. Symptoms include sneezing; copious nasal mucus; sinus congestion; watery, irritated eyes; and even asthma-like wheezing. Self-treatment will help relieve mild conditions, but for severe attacks, consult a professional practitioner who can prescribe herbs such as *ma huang* (*Ephedra sinica*, p. 99). See also *Congestion, Sinus Problems, & Earache*, p. 322.

Diet
Reduce your intake of or cut out mucus-forming foods such as dairy, eggs, sugar, white flour, fatty foods, and alcohol.

General remedies
Herbs Nettle (*Urtica dioica*, p. 150), elderflower (*Sambucus nigra*, p. 136)
Remedy Make a nettle infusion. Take 1⅔–2⅓ cups (450–600ml) a day for 3 months at a time. Alternatively, make an infusion with 1 tsp of each herb to 1¼ cups (300ml) of water and take daily for 3 months at a time.

Herb Baikal skullcap (*Scutellaria baicalensis*, p. 138)
Remedy Make a decoction from the herb and take 1¼ cups (300ml) a day.

Hay fever
Herb Elderflower (*Sambucus nigra*, p. 136)
Remedy Make an infusion and take 1¼–1⅔ cups (300–450ml) a day. Take for a few months before, as well as during, the hay fever season.

Allergic rhinitis with congestion
Herbs Eyebright (*Euphrasia* spp., p. 214), common plantain (*Plantago major*, p. 258), goldenrod (*Solidago virgaurea*, p. 280), boneset (*Eupatorium perfoliatum*, p. 213)
Remedy Make an infusion with one or a mixture of all of the herbs and drink up to 1⅔ cups a day.
Note Use this remedy especially for copious, watery mucus.

Herbs Echinacea (*Echinacea* spp., p. 96), marsh mallow (*Althaea officinalis*, p. 169), elderflower (*Sambucus nigra*, p. 136), thyme (*Thymus vulgaris*, p. 147)
Remedy Take 1 tsp of equal parts of each tincture 3 times daily with warm water.
Note Use this remedy especially for thick yellow/green mucus and sinus congestion.

Eczema

Characterized by red, inflamed skin, eczema causes irritation, flaking, scaling, and tiny blisters. Although it is often the result of an allergic reaction to certain substances, eczema can also be inherited, result from prolonged contact with an irritant, or it may simply appear for an unknown reason. It is best to consult a professional practitioner as eczema is difficult to self-treat. However, the following remedies, taken for at least a week, can bring relief. Two remedies may be used at once. Chickweed reduces soreness or itchiness, and oats can be used to impart a soothing, emollient effect to bathwater. See also *Skin Rashes*, p. 313.

Self-help
To avoid scratching, cover the affected area with an absorbent, nonirritating material such as cotton.
General caution If there is no improvement, or if the condition deteriorates, consult a professional practitioner.

General remedies
Herbs Peppermint (*Mentha × piperita*, p. 118), chickweed (*Stellaria media*, p. 282)
Remedy 1 Make peppermint lotion by infusing 1 tsp of herb to ¾ cup (150ml) of water. Leave for 10 minutes, then strain and cool. Use to wash gently over the affected skin 2–3 times a day.
Remedy 2 Apply chickweed ointment, cream, or freshly squeezed juice up to 5 times a day.
Option Add 2 drops of peppermint oil to 1 tsp of any of the chickweed preparations.

Herb Gotu kola (*Centella asiatica*, p. 81)
Remedy Dust the affected area with powder 2–3 times a day. Alternatively, mix the powder with enough water to make a thick paste and spread over the affected area 1–2 times a day.

Eczema with weeping skin
Herb Witch hazel (*Hamamelis virginiana*, p. 106)
Remedy Apply lotion or cream up to 5 times a day (the lotion is preferable). Alternatively, make a decoction with 2 tsp of leaves to ¾ cup (150ml) of water. Leave for 15 minutes, strain, and cool. Use as a wash up to 5 times a day.
Herb German chamomile (*Chamomilla recutita*, p. 82)
Remedy Make an infusion using 50g of herb to 3 cups (750ml) of water. Apply directly to the itchy area when cool, or add the hot infusion to a warm bath and soak in it for at least 20 minutes.

Herb Oats (*Avena sativa*, p. 179)
Remedy Fill a muslin (or similar) bag with milled oats and place under a hot tap while running a bath. Relax in the bath for 5–10 minutes.

Mild asthma, wheezing, & shortness of breath

Asthma is usually triggered by an allergic reaction to substances such as pollen, dust, animal hair, or certain foods, but may also be related to an infection. The listed remedies will relieve immediate symptoms, but in order to find the cause of your ailment, or for long-term treatment, it is best to consult an herbalist. All the herbal remedies that are suggested here can be taken alongside conventional treatment. Herbs such as nettle, thyme, cramp bark, and echinacea help to ease breathing, while essential oil of German chamomile reduces inflammation.
General caution Seek professional help for asthma. Do not stop using steroidal or other inhalants. Their use should be phased out gradually and only with professional guidance.

Wheezing & shortness of breath
Herbs Nettle (*Urtica dioica*, p. 150), thyme (*Thymus vulgaris*, p. 147)
Remedy Make an infusion using 15 g of each herb to 3 cups of water and drink throughout the day.

Herb German chamomile (*Chamomilla recutita*, p. 82)
Remedy Make an infusion with 2 heaping tsp of the herb to ¾ cup (150 ml) of water and leave to stand for 10 minutes in a covered saucepan. Remove the lid, inhale the steam, and strain and drink the tea.
Option Use the essential oil in a steam inhalation, or inhale 2 drops of undiluted oil placed on a handkerchief.

Herb Baikal skullcap (*Scutellaria baicalensis*, p. 138)
Remedy Make a decoction and take up to 1¼ cups (300 ml) a day.

Breathing difficulty & tight chest
Herb Cramp bark (*Viburnum opulus*, p. 154)
Remedy Take 1 tsp of tincture with water up to 8 times a day for 3 days, then reduce the dose to a maximum of 1 tsp 3 times a day for 7 days.

Mild bronchial asthma from colds & chest infections
Herb Echinacea (*Echinacea* spp., p. 96)
Remedy Take tablets or capsules, or ½ tsp of tincture with water 2–3 times a day.

Circulatory problems

To maintain good health, the body's ten trillion cells need to be bathed in fluid that brings them vital nutrients and removes waste products. When this process is undermined by poor circulation, the body may react with conditions such as raised blood pressure, which places a long-term strain on the heart. A high-vegetable, low-sugar diet and regular aerobic exercise help to keep the heart active and the arteries clear of fatty deposits that can clog up their linings. A number of herbs act preventively to sustain good circulation—few more so than garlic (*Allium sativum*, p. 63).

Seek immediate professional advice for:

- Severe chest pain
- Palpitations lasting several minutes
- Hot, swollen, or ulcerated tender veins, or dark red discoloration of the skin or veins
- Fainting or dizziness with weakness, numbness, or tingling in any part of the body

Anemia

There are several types of anemia. Iron deficiency anemia, caused by blood loss from a wound or menstrual bleeding, can be countered with herbs. Bitter herbs, such as gentian, improve the absorption of nutrients, and nettle contains plenty of iron. Increase your intake of other green herbs that contain iron.
General caution Seek professional advice to determine the type of anemia you have before home treatment.

General remedies
Herbs Gentian (*Gentiana lutea*, p. 103), wormwood (*Artemisia absinthium*, p. 70)

Remedy Take 2–5 drops of either tincture with water, half an hour before meals.
Caution Do not take wormwood during pregnancy.

Herb Chiretta (*Swertia chirata*, p. 283)
Remedy Take 5–10 drops of tincture with water 3 times a day before meals.

Anemia due to heavy menstrual bleeding
Herb Nettle (*Urtica dioica*, p. 150)
Remedy Make an infusion using 25 g of herb to 3 cups (750 ml) of water. Sip the whole dose at intervals throughout the day.
See also *Heavy Menstrual Bleeding*— Four Things Soup remedy, p. 325.

High blood pressure & arteriosclerosis

Mild cases of high blood pressure and arteriosclerosis (hardening of the arteries) can benefit from herbs. Garlic thins the blood, reduces fatty deposits, and lowers blood pressure; beets and ginkgo aid circulation, reduce blood pressure, and prevent arteriosclerosis; and ginger improves circulation, especially to the capillaries.
General caution Seek professional advice, especially if already taking medication for a circulatory condition.

Before taking any herbal remedies, see pages 300 & 308–309

General remedies

Herbs Garlic (*Allium sativum*, p. 63), beet (*Beta vulgaris*, p. 182), pomegranate (*Punica granatum*, p. 267)
Remedy Take a garlic tablet or eat 1–2 fresh garlic cloves each day. Drink ½ cup (125 ml) of beet or pomegranate juice once a day.
Note These are most effective when used to support a healthy circulation and prevent illness.

Herb Ginkgo (*Ginkgo biloba*, p. 104)
Remedy Take tablets or ½ tsp of fluid extract with water twice a day for approximately 2–3 months at a time.

Herb Ginger (*Zingiber officinale*, p. 159)
Remedy Grate 1 tsp of fresh ginger into your food each day.

Palpitations & panic attacks

Palpitations occur when the heart suddenly beats faster or irregularly. They can result from stress, anxiety, and nervous tension; however, they may also be caused simply by drinking too much caffeine (in tea, coffee, and cola drinks). In rare cases, palpitations indicate a heart problem. They are a key symptom of panic attacks, which are characterized by sudden, acute feelings of fear and anxiety. Linden flowers and valerian root are especially relaxing and calming for the nervous system, specifically helping to reduce underlying anxiety.
General caution Seek immediate professional advice if palpitations last for several minutes.

Palpitations

Herb Linden (*Tilia* spp., p. 286)
Remedy Make an infusion with up to 20 g of linden to 3 cups (750 ml) of water. Divide into 3–4 doses and drink throughout the day.

Herb *Dan shen* (*Salvia miltiorrhiza*, p. 134)
Remedy Make a decoction and take 3–4 doses during the day for up to 1 week. Alternatively, take half the daily dose for up to 2–3 weeks.
Cautions Do not take *dan shen* with anticoagulant or antiplatelet drugs, or during pregnancy.

Panic attacks

Herbs Linden (*Tilia* spp., p. 286), valerian (*Valeriana officinalis*, p. 152)
Remedy Make an infusion using 1 tsp of linden and ½ tsp of powdered valerian to ¾ cup (150 ml) of water. Drink 2⅓ cups (600 ml) a day.

Herbs Motherwort (*Leonurus cardiaca*, p. 232), linden (*Tilia* spp., p. 286)
Remedy Make an infusion of motherwort or make an infusion using ½ tsp of each herb to 1 cup (150 ml) of water. Drink up to 4 cups (600 ml) of either remedy a day.
Caution Do not take motherwort during pregnancy.

Cold extremities & chilblains

Poor circulation can cause discomfort and painful chilblains (sores caused by poor local blood flow) on the fingers and toes. By stimulating the circulation and getting more "warmth" into the system with herbs and exercise, the blood flow to the hands and feet is improved. Hot, acrid herbs, such as cayenne or ginger, stimulate the flow of blood through the arteries, helping to prevent the development of chilblains.

Exercise

Aerobic exercise is often the key to improving this condition.
General caution Seek professional advice if fingers and toes frequently become cold and numb.

Poor circulation to the hands & feet

Herb Cayenne (*Capsicum frutescens*, p. 79)
Remedy Take cayenne tablets in winter.
Option Add a pinch of cayenne powder or cayenne sauce to every main meal.
Cautions Do not take tablets during pregnancy.

Herbs Cramp bark (*Viburnum opulus*, p. 154), northern prickly ash (*Zanthoxylum americanum*, p. 157)
Remedy 1 Make a decoction using 15 g of cramp bark to 3 cups (750 ml) of water and take 3 doses each day.
Remedy 2 Mix 5 g of prickly ash and 10 g of cramp bark and make a decoction using 3 cups (750 ml) of water. Take 3 doses each day.
Caution Do not take prickly ash during pregnancy.

Chilblains

Herbs Ginger (*Zingiber officinale*, p. 159), lemon (*Citrus limon*, p. 86), echinacea (Echinacea spp., p. 96)
Remedy (Internal) Grate 1 tsp of fresh ginger into your food each day. Alternatively, drink ¼ cup (70 ml) of ginger wine each day.
Remedy (External) Apply either fresh ginger, lemon juice, or neat echinacea tincture to unopened chilblains twice a day.
Note The external remedy helps to prevent blistering and weeping. Once the blister opens you can continue to apply, but it will sting upon contact.

Varicose veins & hemorrhoids

Varicose veins result from a weakness, or increased pressure, in the veins. This causes the thin supporting walls of the veins to bulge out, resulting in distended veins and the pooling of blood. Hemorrhoids are usually caused by constipation. Many herbs can be of use in relieving these conditions. Distilled witch hazel is an excellent astringent, and yarrow has healing, astringent, and anti-inflammatory properties.

Self-help

Home treatment should aim to relieve pressure on the veins. Varicose vein sufferers should avoid tight clothing around the waist or legs. To ease hemorrhoids, try to maintain regular bowel movements (see *Constipation & Diarrhea*, p. 317).
General caution Do not massage varicose veins.

Varicose veins

Herbs Witch hazel (*Hamamelis virginiana*, p. 106), calendula (*Calendula officinalis*, p. 77)
Remedy Gently apply distilled witch hazel or witch hazel cream or ointment to the affected area 1–2 times a day, or combine equal parts of the creams of both herbs and apply 1–2 times a day.
Note This remedy is particularly effective on painful varicose veins.

Herb Yarrow (*Achillea millefolium*, p. 60)
Remedy (External) Wash varicose veins in a cool infusion, or apply the ointment 1–2 times a day.
Remedy (Internal) Make an infusion and leave for 10 minutes. Take ¾–1¼ cups (150–300 ml) a day for up to 10 weeks.
Caution Do not take yarrow during pregnancy.

Hemorrhoids

Herbs Witch hazel (*Hamamelis virginiana*, p. 106), lesser celandine (*Ranunculus ficaria*, p. 268), common oak (*Quercus robur*, p. 268), calendula (*Calendula officinalis*, p. 77)
Remedy 1 Apply either distilled witch hazel or witch hazel ointment, or lesser celandine ointment, 1–2 times a day.
Remedy 2 Mix 1 tsp of common oak bark powder with 2½ tbsp of calendula ointment and apply 1–2 times a day.

Difficult passage of the stool & painful hemorrhoids

Herb Slippery elm (*Ulmus rubra*, p. 149)
Remedy Take either slippery elm "food" (see *Acidity & Indigestion*, p. 307) or tablets.
Herb Psyllium (*Plantago* spp., p. 128)
Remedy Take 1–2 tsp of seeds soaked in ¾ cup (150 ml) of water overnight, twice a day.

Skin problems

The largest organ of the body, the skin protects against heat, cold, infection, and trauma from the outside world. Although continuously shedding its surface, the skin needs regular cleansing and nourishing to remain healthy. Its ability to resist injury and recover from damage largely depends on the health of the body as a whole. While many minor skin problems respond promptly to simple external remedies, severe or chronic skin conditions need internal treatment and usually require professional advice. See also *Eczema*, p. 310.

Seek immediate professional advice for:

- Changes to freckles, moles, or warts
- Sudden swelling or allergic reaction
- Non-minor burns, including sunburn
- Shingles or suspected shingles
- Boils that do not disperse or burst
- Serious wounds, scrapes, bruising, bites, and stings

Minor bites, stings, & swellings

Inflamed, swollen areas of skin are a common reaction to bites and stings. Although they can be very uncomfortable, most only cause local itching and inflammation, which usually subside within a few hours. All the remedies listed will help to ease irritation and soreness. For the most effective relief, use both an external and internal remedy. Lavender relieves irritation as well as being an insect repellent, aloe vera is soothing and healing, and both calendula and St. John's wort reduce inflammation. Echinacea stimulates the immune system and nettle is anti-allergenic.

General cautions Seek immediate professional attention if prone to, or if there are signs of, extreme allergic reactions, or if there is a sting in the mouth and the throat starts to swell. Some stings and animal bites are poisonous and may need inoculations and immediate medical attention.

External remedies

Herb Lavender (*Lavandula officinalis*, p. 112)
Remedy Rub fresh leaves, neat tincture, or essential oil on and around the bite or sting.
Other uses This will also repel insects.

Herbs Sweet basil (*Ocimum basilicum*, p. 248), holy basil (*Ocimum tenuiflorum*, p. 120), sage (*Salvia officinalis*, p. 135), thyme (*Thymus vulgaris*, p. 147)
Remedy Apply freshly squeezed juice from the leaves of one of the herbs.

Herbs Aloe vera (*Aloe vera*, p. 64), calendula (*Calendula officinalis*, p. 77), St. John's wort (*Hypericum perforatum*, p. 110)
Remedy Apply either aloe vera gel; calendula ointment, cream, lotion, or tincture; or St. John's wort oil. To make the calendula lotion, infuse 2 heaping tbsp of calendula in ¾ cup (150 ml) of water. Strain, cool, then apply.
Option Add 5 drops each of lavender (*Lavandula officinalis*, p. 112) and German chamomile (*Chamomilla recutita*, p. 82) essential oils to 1 tsp of one of the above preparations.
Caution Do not apply chamomile oil in pregnancy.
Tip Apply neat lemon juice (*Citrus limon*, p. 86) if there is nothing else available.

Internal remedies

Herb Nettle (*Urtica dioica*, p. 150)
Remedy Make an infusion and drink 1⅔ cups (450 ml) a day, or take 1 tsp of tincture with water 3 times a day for up to 3 days.

Herb Echinacea (*Echinacea* spp., p. 96)
Remedy Take tablets or tincture.

Skin rashes, minor burns, & sunburn

More annoying than debilitating, skin rashes and minor burns, including sunburn, usually clear up without assistance, although herbal treatment can speed recovery.

Hives (urticaria) are usually caused by an allergic reaction, but can also be triggered by heat, cold, or sunlight. They only last for a few hours but will often recur. For the most effective relief, apply chickweed cream and take one of the internal remedies.

Skin rashes have many causes, such as allergy, infection, irritation, bites, stings, and temperature changes. Use these remedies to alleviate itchiness and swelling.

Small-scale burns usually respond well to herbal medicine, but even small burns may be deep and can quickly become infected. Before using a remedy, bathe the burned area in clean, cold water and keep the area cool for up to 3 hours with a clean cotton cloth that has been soaked in cold water.

General cautions If there is any sign of infection seek professional advice.

Hives (Urticaria)

Herbs Nettle (*Urtica dioica*, p. 150), heartsease (*Viola tricolor*, p. 292), calendula (*Calendula officinalis*, p. 77)
Remedy (Internal) Drink an infusion of 5 g of each herb and 3 cups (750 ml) of water regularly during the day. Repeat for 1 week. If symptoms persist, take for another week.

Herbs Dandelion (*Taraxacum officinale*, p. 145), yellow dock (*Rumex crispus*, p. 273), burdock (*Arctium lappa*, p. 69)
Remedy (Internal) Make a decoction with 5 g of each root to 3 cups (750 ml) of water. Drink 1¼ cups (300 ml) a day and repeat for at least 1 week.
Caution Do not take yellow dock in pregnancy.

Herb Chickweed (*Stellaria media*, p. 282)
Remedy (External) Apply cream as required.

Inflamed skin rashes

Herbs Calendula (*Calendula officinalis*, p. 77), comfrey (*Symphytum officinale*, p. 142)
Remedy Apply calendula or comfrey ointment, cream, or lotion to troubled areas 2–4 times a day. For the lotion, make an infusion, strain, cool, and then apply.
Caution Do not apply comfrey to broken skin.

Weeping skin

Herbs Aloe vera (*Aloe vera*, p. 64), witch hazel (*Hamamelis virginiana*, p. 106)
Remedy Apply aloe vera gel or distilled witch hazel or witch hazel ointment to the affected area 2–4 times a day

Before taking any herbal remedies, see pages 300 & 308–309

Minor wounds & bruises

Minor wounds, bruises, and grazes are part of everyday life, and the remedies listed make effective home treatments. Witch hazel is a very good astringent for minor scrapes, bruises, and swellings, protecting and soothing the damaged area. Arnica can be used to relieve bruising, pain, and swelling, and it combines well with witch hazel. Wounds can be cleansed with aloe vera gel which, like comfrey, is an excellent wound healer. Comfrey ointment is helpful in clearing old scars. See also *Sprains & fractures*, p. 322.

General caution Seek immediate medical attention for serious or deep wounds, bruising, or scrapes, especially if the pain has not considerably lessened after 24 hours.

Cleansing wounds

Herb Yarrow (*Achillea millefolium*, p. 60)
Remedy Make a yarrow lotion, allow to cool, and use as a wash.

Herb Calendula (*Calendula officinalis*, p. 77)
Remedy Make a calendula lotion with 2 heaping tsp of herb to ¾ cup (150 ml) of water, or use the tincture neat or diluted in water. Apply either preparation to the wound.
Note Calendula tincture will sting strongly, but it has a greater antiseptic action.

Herb Aloe vera (*Aloe vera*, p. 64)
Remedy Cleanse the wound with the gel and cover with a dressing soaked in gel. Change frequently.

Herb Witch hazel (*Hamamelis virginiana*, p. 106)
Remedy Apply distilled witch hazel (available over the counter) to the affected area 2–3 times a day.

Healing wounds

Herbs Comfrey (*Symphytum officinale*, p. 142), aloe vera (*Aloe vera*, p. 64)
Remedy Apply comfrey ointment at the edges of the wound or, once a scab has formed, use a comfrey poultice. Use aloe vera gel to cleanse the wound (see left).
Caution Do not use comfrey on an open wound.

Bruises

Herbs Arnica (*Arnica montana*, p. 176), witch hazel (*Hamamelis virginiana*, p. 106)
Remedy Apply arnica ointment to bruises and swellings 2–3 times a day, or use distilled witch hazel, as above.
Caution Do not use arnica on broken skin.

Cold sores, chicken pox, shingles, & warts

Herbal medicine can help all these viral infections that affect the skin.

Cold sores are caused by the herpes simplex virus, and usually occur when the body has an infection or has been exposed to sunshine or wind. Tiny blisters form, mainly around the nostrils and lips.

Shingles and chicken pox are the result of a similar virus, causing sores to form all over the body. Shingles are a sign that the nervous system is run down and open to infection, so herbs that support the nerves and the immune system as a whole are as important as ones that work topically.

Warts, caused by the papilloma virus, can be difficult to clear. With persistence, the remedies here are often effective.

General cautions Always consult a professional practitioner if you have, or suspect you have, shingles. Take professional advice if you notice a sudden change to a wart.

Cold sores, chicken pox, & shingles

Herbs Echinacea (*Echinacea* spp., p. 96), St. John's wort (*Hypericum perforatum*, p. 110)
Remedies Take ½ tsp of tincture of either herb with water 2–3 times a day. Alternatively, take echinacea tablets or capsules, or make an infusion of St. John's wort and drink up to ¾ cup (150 ml) a day.

Herbs Garlic (*Allium sativum*, p. 63), ginger (*Zingiber officinale*, p. 159), lemon (*Citrus limon*, p. 86)
Remedy (Internal) Eat 1–2 cloves of garlic and 1–2 slices (1 g) of fresh ginger a day.
Remedy (External) Apply either fresh ginger, half a clove of garlic, or lemon juice to unopened cold sores, shingles, or pockmarks up to 6 times a day.

Herb Lemon balm (*Melissa officinalis*, p. 117)
Remedy (Internal) Make an infusion and drink up to 3 cups (750 ml) a day.
Remedy (External) Make a lotion by infusing 1½ tbsp of fresh or 3 tsp of dried leaves in ¾ cup (150 ml) of water for 10 minutes. Strain and dab onto spots 3–5 times a day.

Warts

Herb Aloe vera (*Aloe vera*, p. 64)
Remedy Apply the gel directly to the wart 2–3 times a day for up to 3 months.

Herb Arborvitae (*Thuja occidentalis*, p. 286)
Remedy Apply neat tincture to the wart 1–2 times a day for up to 3 months.

Fungal skin infections, including athlete's foot

Fungal skin infections are easily picked up through physical contact, and can be hard to clear. Athlete's foot is a fungus (tinea) that grows in the skin between and under the toes, causing it to split and peel away. This itchy, sore condition can be difficult to treat at home.

Self-help

Keep feet dry and clean and do not wear synthetic socks or tightly fitting shoes.

General remedies

Herb Comfrey (*Symphytum officinale*, p. 142)
Remedy Make a poultice and firmly apply to the affected area for 1–2 hours each day.
Caution Do not use comfrey on broken skin.

Herbs Tea tree (*Melaleuca alternifolia*, p. 116), clove (*Eugenia caryophyllata*, p. 101), calendula (*Calendula officinalis*, p. 77), thyme (*Thymus vulgaris*, p. 147)
Remedy Mix 5 drops of tea tree, clove, or thyme essential oil with 1 tsp of calendula ointment. Apply 1–2 times a day.
Caution Do not use thyme oil during pregnancy.

Herb Garlic (*Allium sativum*, p. 63)
Remedy Rub on ½ clove 2–3 times a day.

Athlete's foot

Herbs Turmeric (*Curcuma longa*, p. 94), calendula (*Calendula officinalis*, p. 77)
Remedy Mix ½ tsp of turmeric powder with 3 tsp (15 ml) of calendula ointment. Rub in between and under the toes each day.

Acne & boils

Acne and boils are the result of local infection, hormonal imbalance, or internal toxicity, which cause inflammation of the hair follicles and, with acne, sebaceous glands. They should be treated on the surface of the skin and internally.

Acne generally occurs during the teenage years and results in whiteheads, pustules, and cysts, usually on the face and back.

Boils are large, pus-filled areas of skin. They either disperse or burst in a week. As boils are often the body's way of expelling toxins, recurrent boils may indicate a weakened immune system. They can also suggest diabetes or a deep-seated bacterial infection.

Herbs such as tea tree and garlic are antiseptic and antibiotic. Calendula and comfrey promote healing, and comfrey helps to mend scarring.

Self-help
Increase intake of vitamin C and garlic.
General caution Do not squeeze or burst boils or acne pimples as the infection may spread. Seek professional advice for recurrent boils.

External remedies
Herbs Tea tree (*Melaleuca alternifolia*, p. 116), clove (*Eugenia caryophyllata*, p. 101), garlic (*Allium sativum*, p. 63)
Remedy Dab 1 drop of neat tea tree or clove essential oil onto the pus-filled head of a boil or pimple twice a day. Alternatively, cut a clove of garlic in half and rub over the area twice a day.

Herb Calendula (*Calendula officinalis*, p. 77)
Remedy Apply ointment or cream, or dab undiluted tincture on to the pus-filled area twice a day.

Herb Comfrey (*Symphytum officinale*, p. 142)
Remedy Apply comfrey ointment or cream to the pus-filled area twice a day.
Caution Do not use comfrey on broken skin.

Herb Lemon (*Citrus limon*, p. 86)
Remedy Dab pure lemon juice onto the pus-filled area, or dilute 1 tsp of lemon juice with 1 tbsp of water and use as a skin wash twice a day.

Herbs Slippery elm (*Ulmus rubra*, p. 149), calendula (*Calendula officinalis*, p. 77), myrrh (*Commiphora myrrha*, p. 86), echinacea (*Echinacea* spp., p. 96)
Remedy Mix 1 level tsp of slippery elm powder with sufficient calendula, myrrh, or echinacea tincture to make a thick, smooth paste. Place on and around the boil, and bandage securely.

Remove after 1–2 hours.
Note This remedy is useful for drawing splinters.

Internal remedies
Herbs Dandelion (*Taraxacum officinale*, p. 145), burdock (*Arctium lappa*, p. 69)
Remedy Make a decoction using 5 g of burdock root and 10 g of dandelion root with 3 cups (750 ml) of water. Divide into 3 doses and drink during the day.

Herb Echinacea (*Echinacea* spp., p. 96)
Remedy Take echinacea tablets or capsules, or make a decoction of 10 g of root to 3 cups (750 ml) of water and drink during the day.

Digestive disorders

Everyone falls prey to certain digestive problems and, for those with weak or unsettled digestion, life can be miserable. Poor digestive health usually results from insufficient digestive secretions, infections (such as gastroenteritis), disordered gut bacteria, stress, and anxiety. Herbal medicines can improve the complex functioning of the digestive system, helping to relieve acidity, nausea, and bloating. Eating simple, wholesome food can be beneficial, but it is difficult to generalize about diet. Some conditions may require fasting, while in other cases, a certain type of food might need to be avoided.

Seek immediate professional advice for:

- Difficulty in swallowing
- Severe pain
- Vomiting blood
- Blood in the stool

Important note For continuing or recurrent digestive problems, seek professional advice to determine the cause.

Stomachache
Cramping pain is a sign that the stomach and intestines are sore and irritated. This is normally due to poor digestion, excessive nervous tension, food poisoning, or infection. Stomachache may occur on its own or lead to vomiting and diarrhea (in which case, use the remedies on p. 316). Garlic and calendula are antiviral and will help clear digestive infections. Relaxing herbs, such as German chamomile and cramp bark, relieve stomach spasm. For maximum benefit, they are mixed with carminative herbs to help relieve gas.
General cautions Seek professional advice if stomach pain is severe or recurrent. All species of mint (*Mentha* spp.) are unsuitable for children under 5.

Stomach spasm
Relaxing herbs German chamomile (*Chamomilla recutita*, p. 82), lemon balm (*Melissa officinalis*, p. 117), cramp bark (*Viburnum opulus*, p. 154)
Carminative herbs Anise (*Pimpinella anisum*, p. 256), fennel (*Foeniculum vulgare*, p. 217), mint (*Mentha* spp., pp. 240–241), angelica (*Angelica archangelica*, p. 172)
Remedy Mix 3 parts of a relaxing herb to 1 part of a carminative herb and make an infusion. (For the carminative herbs, use fennel seeds, aniseed, mint leaves, or angelica root.) Drink up to 3 cups (750 ml) a day.

Digestive infections
Herb Garlic (*Allium sativum*, p. 63)
Remedy Eat 1–2 fresh cloves a day.

Herb Calendula (*Calendula officinalis*, p. 77)
Remedy Infuse 2 tsp of herb in 3 cups (750 ml) of water and drink up to 3 cups a day.

Herbs Yarrow (*Achillea millefolium*, p. 60), peppermint (*Mentha x piperita*, p. 118), catnip (*Nepeta cataria*, p. 246)
Remedy Mix equal parts of each herb. Make an infusion of 2 tsp of mixture to ¾ cup (150 ml) of water. Drink 1¼ cups (300 ml) a day.
Caution Do not take yarrow in pregnancy.

Before taking any herbal remedies, see pages 300 & 308–309

Nausea & vomiting, including motion sickness

Nausea and vomiting can occur for various reasons, including food poisoning, infections, fever, migraine, stress, or emotional problems, as well as motion sickness. For short-term conditions, there are many herbs that reduce or relieve the unpleasant, empty, gnawing symptoms of nausea and vomiting. Most of the herbs listed are also very useful for motion sickness.

Ginger, in particular, and other close relatives such as galangal and turmeric, are widely used for nausea and vomiting. They help to "warm" and settle the digestion.

Chiretta strengthens weak digestion and relieves nausea.

Lemon is an excellent cleansing remedy for weak and sluggish digestion. If you are pregnant, or suspect you may be pregnant, see *Morning Sickness*, p. 327, before taking any of these remedies.

General caution Seek professional advice if nausea is severe or is recurrent. All types or species of mint (*Mentha* spp.) are unsuitable for children under 5.

Nausea & motion sickness

Herbs Ginger (*Zingiber officinale*, p. 159), galangal (*Alpinia officinarum*, p. 169), turmeric (*Curcuma longa*, p. 94)

Remedy Make an infusion with one of the herbs listed using about 1–2 slices (½g) of fresh root or ¼–½ tsp of dried, powdered, or grated root to ¾ cup (150ml) of water. Use the fresh root if possible. Infuse for at least 5 minutes and sip while hot. Drink up to 3 cups (750ml) a day. Add 1–2 cloves (*Eugenia caryophyllata*, p. 101) if desired.

Option Use the remedy under *Nausea with Headache*.

Tip For motion sickness, take the infusion in a flask or chew crystallized ginger.

Weak digestion

Herbs Chiretta (*Swertia chirata*, p. 283), centaury (*Erythraea centaurium*, p. 211)

Remedy Take 2–4 drops of one of the tinctures on the tongue each hour.

Herb Lemon (*Citrus limon*, p. 86)

Remedy Drink the freshly squeezed juice of a lemon, neat or diluted, each morning.

Nausea due to emotional problems

Herb Lemon balm (*Melissa officinalis*, p. 117)

Remedy Make an infusion with the dried herb or use 2 tsp of fresh herb per ¾ cup (150ml) of water. Drink up to 3 cups (750ml) a day.

Vomiting with dizziness & vertigo

Herb Black horehound (*Ballota nigra*, p. 180)

Remedy Make an infusion and drink up to 3 cups (750ml) a day.

Caution Seek professional advice if symptoms do not immediately improve.

Nausea with headache

Herbs Peppermint (*Mentha × piperita*, p. 118), pennyroyal (*Mentha pulegium*, p. 241), *bo he* (*Mentha haplocalyx*, p. 240)

Remedy Make an infusion with 1 level tsp of one herb per ¾ cup (150ml) of water. Drink up to 2⅓–3 cups (600–750ml) a day.

Other uses This remedy combats abdominal fullness and helps improve the appetite and digestion.

Caution Do not give these herbs to children under 5. Do not take pennyroyal during pregnancy.

Loss of appetite & vomiting

Herb Codonopsis (*Codonopsis pilosula*, p. 87)

Remedy Make a decoction and sip 2½ tbsp (50ml) every 2–3 hours until the vomiting stops or the dose has been taken over 2 days.

Other uses For anorexia, add 5g of licorice (*Glycyrrhiza glabra*, p. 105).

Caution Do not take licorice during pregnancy.

Gas & bloating

Gas and bloating are common digestive problems. As a preventative, take bitter herbs, such as centaury and gentian, which improve digestion. Infusions of aromatic plants such as fennel, cardamom, anise, lemon verbena, or peppermint are effective remedies. All the herbs listed under *General Remedies* can be combined by adjusting the measurements of each herb using the same proportion to water.

General cautions Bitters are generally unsuitable and unpalatable for children under 5. All types or species of mint (*Mentha* spp.) are unsuitable for children under 5.

Protection & prevention

Herbs Centaury (*Erythraea centaurium*, p. 211), gentian (*Gentiana lutea*, p. 103)

Remedy Take 5–10 drops of tincture 3 times a day with water.

General remedies

Herbs Fennel (*Foeniculum vulgare*, p. 217), anise (*Pimpinella anisum*, p. 256)

Remedy Make an infusion with ¼–½ tsp of fennel or anise seeds per ¾ cup (150ml) of water and drink up to 3 cups (750ml) a day.

Herb Cardamom (*Elettaria cardamomum*, p. 97)

Remedy Make an infusion with the crushed seeds of 2 cardamoms per ¾ cup (150ml) of water. Drink up to 3 cups (750ml) a day.

Herb Lemon verbena (*Lippia citriodora*, p. 228)

Remedy Make an infusion using 1 tsp of dried or 2 tsp of fresh leaves per 1 cup (150ml) of water and take up to 3 cups (750ml) a day.

Herb Peppermint (*Mentha × piperita*, p. 118)

Remedy Make an infusion and drink up to 3 cups (750ml) a day. (See *General cautions*.)

Mouth ulcers & gum problems

Many astringent herbs can be used to treat mouth ulcers and tighten up weak gums and loose teeth. Sage is particularly effective as it also disinfects the mouth. Myrrh tincture will sting but it will also increase the rate of healing.

General remedies

Herb Myrrh (*Commiphora myrrha*, p. 89)

Remedy Dab neat tincture onto mouth ulcers and infected gums once every hour.

Herb Sage (*Salvia officinalis*, p. 135)

Remedy Use an infusion as a mouthwash, or rub gums with leaves or powder.

Mouth & tongue ulcers

Herbs Myrrh (*Commiphora myrrha*, p. 89), echinacea (*Echinacea* spp., p. 96), licorice (*Glycyrrhiza glabra*, p. 105)

Remedy Mix equal parts of the tinctures and apply neat or diluted (1 part tincture to 5 parts water) every hour.

Constipation & diarrhea

Herbs help both constipation and diarrhea by gently restoring normal bowel function. Constipation often results from insufficient intake of fruit, vegetables, and whole grains, while diarrhea is usually caused by intestinal infection or inflammation, such as food poisoning. Irritable bowel syndrome gives rise to alternating bouts of constipation and diarrhea, and spastic constipation results from tension and muscle spasm in the colon.

Herbs

Dandelion root, licorice, and yellow dock are mild laxatives.

Senna is a strong laxative and should only be taken when other herbs have failed.

Psyllium seeds and husks cleanse the colon and encourage normal bowel habits.

Cramp bark has antispasmodic properties and can help spastic constipation.

Agrimony, bael, bistort, and black catechu are astringent herbs that dry and tighten the bowel lining. Only take in the short term, as they impair absorption of food. They are taken mixed with soothing, demulcent herbs, such as psyllium or marshmallow, for diarrhea.

Diet for constipation

Fruit acts as a gentle laxative within the large intestine. Eat plenty of fresh fruit each day, such as figs (*Ficus carica*, p. 216), apples, or tamarind (*Tamarindus indica*, p. 284), which also counter vomiting, gas, and indigestion.

General caution Seek professional advice for persistent constipation or diarrhea.

Constipation

Herbs Yellow dock (*Rumex crispus*, p. 273), Chinese rhubarb (*Rheum palmatum*, p. 130)

Remedy Make a decoction using 1 tsp of either herb to ¾ cup (150 ml) of water. Take last thing at night.

Note Yellow dock is one of the mildest laxatives and should be tried first. If this has no effect, take a single dose of Chinese rhubarb each day. This has a stronger action than yellow dock.

Cautions Do not take Chinese rhubarb or yellow dock during pregnancy.

Persistent constipation

Herbs Dandelion (*Taraxacum officinale*, p. 145), licorice (*Glycyrrhiza glabra*, p. 105), yellow dock (*Rumex crispus*, p. 273)

Remedy 1 Make a decoction using 20 g of dandelion root to 3 cups (750 ml) of water and drink each day, or use the ground root to make an infusion and drink 1⅔–2⅓ cups (450–600 ml) a day.

Remedy 2 Mix 3 tsp of dandelion root and yellow dock and 1 tsp of licorice. Use the mixture to make a decoction with 3 cups (750 ml) of water and drink ¾–1¼ cups (150–300 ml) a day.

Cautions Do not take yellow dock or licorice during pregnancy.

Herbs Senna (*Cassia senna*, p. 80), ginger (*Zingiber officinale*, p. 159)

Remedy Steep 3–6 senna pods and 2–3 slices (1 g) of fresh ginger in ¾ cup (150 ml) of warm water. Alternatively, take senna tablets. Take either preparation for up to 10 days.

Note This is the strongest laxative listed.

Cautions Take for up to 10 days at a time. During pregnancy, take on advice of a health care practitioner. Do not give to children under 5.

Spastic constipation

Herb Cramp bark (*Viburnum opulus*, p. 154)

Remedy Make a decoction using 15 g of the root to 3 cups (750 ml) of water and take ¾–1¼ cups (150–300 ml) a day or take 2 tsp of tincture with water once per day.

Diarrhea

Herbs Agrimony (*Agrimonia eupatoria*, p. 165), sage (*Salvia officinalis*, p. 135), bael (*Aegle marmelos*, p. 164), bistort (*Polygonum bistorta*, p. 261), black catechu (*Acacia catechu*, p. 278)

Remedy The above herbs are listed in ascending order of astringency. Make a decoction using 1 heaping tsp of one herb to 1 cup (225 ml) of water and simmer for 15–20 minutes. Take up to 1⅔ cups (450 ml) a day for no longer than 3 days.

Note If using bistort or black catechu (the most astringent herbs), mix with demulcents such as psyllium seeds (*Plantago* spp., p. 128) or marsh mallow root (*Althaea officinalis*, p. 169). Add 1 tsp, plus a pinch of peppermint (*Mentha* x *piperita*, p. 114) or other mint (*Mentha* spp., pp. 240–241), per 1 cup (225 ml) of decoction.

Cautions Do not take for more than 3 days at a time and do not take again for 3 days. If there is no improvement, seek professional advice. Do not take sage in pregnancy. Do not give mint to children under 5.

Chronic diarrhea & irritable bowel syndrome

Herb Psyllium (*Plantago* spp., p. 128)

Remedy Take 1 heaping tsp of seeds and husks with at least ¾ cup (150 ml) of water, 2–3 times daily, or mix with food and then drink at least ¾ cup (150 ml) of water. Seeds may be soaked in cool water overnight before taking.

Acidity & indigestion

Indigestion, caused by too much acid production, suggests a poor or inappropriate diet. To coat the inner lining of the stomach and intestines and protect them from excess acidity, take slippery elm, arrowroot, or Iceland moss, which are sticky, mucilaginous herbs when soaked in water. Meadowsweet strengthens the lining of the stomach and reduces acidic symptoms, while German chamomile is amazingly versatile for a number of gastrointestinal problems.

Diet

Cut out acidic foods, such as oranges, red meat, spinach, and tomatoes, as well as alcohol and tobacco if possible.

General remedies

Herbs Slippery elm (*Ulmus rubra*, p. 149), arrowroot (*Maranta arundinacea*, p. 239), Iceland moss (*Cetraria islandica*, p. 190)

Remedy 1 Make an infusion with 2 heaping tsp of one of the herbs to ½ cup (100 ml) of water. Leave for 15 minutes. Take ½ cup (100 ml) up to 4 times a day.

Remedy 2 Make slippery elm "food" by mixing 1 heaping tsp of powder and 3 tsp of cold water. Stir in 1 cup (250 ml) of boiling water. Add a pinch of cinnamon (*Cinnamomum* spp., p. 85) or nutmeg (*Myristica fragrans*, p. 11) to taste. Take 1 cup (250 ml) 3 times a day.

Herbs Fennel (*Foeniculum vulgare*, p. 217), galbanum (*Ferula gummosa*, p. 216), anise (*Pimpinella anisum*, p. 256), or any one of the *Nausea & Vomiting* herbs listed on p. 316.

Remedy Make an infusion using 1 heaping tsp of fennel or anise seeds, or galbanum herb, to 3 cups (750 ml) of water. Drink during the day.

Indigestion, abdominal pain, bloating, & hiccups

Herb German chamomile (*Chamomilla recutita*, p. 82)

Remedy Make an infusion in a covered container. Drink up to 3 cups (750 ml) a day.

Acidity with gastritis

Herb Meadowsweet (*Filipendula ulmaria*, p. 102)

Remedy Make an infusion with the flowering tops. Drink up to 3 cups (750 ml) a day.

Before taking any herbal remedies, see pages 300 & 308–309

Nerve & stress-related problems

Most of us have little opportunity to escape from daily pressures, and consequently the nervous system is unable to recover its natural vitality. Long-term stress can lead to anxiety, nervousness, depression, insomnia, palpitations, and irritability. Herbal medicines can be wonderfully effective for nourishing the nervous system, calming and relaxing the mind, and gently stimulating or sedating the body. Headaches and migraine respond well to treatment with herbs, as can conditions directly affecting the nerves, such as neuralgia.

Seek immediate professional advice for:

- Severe nerve, chest, or head pain
- Headache or pain that does not improve within 48 hours despite self-medication
- Loss of sensation or loss of movement
- Double vision
- Severe depression

Anxiety, depression, & tension

Many people have experienced lack of well-being and feelings of powerlessness that develop as stress, anxiety, and tension take hold. There is no instant answer, but a remarkable number of herbs can reduce these symptoms, and, by supporting the nervous system, gradually restore health.

Lemon balm, skullcap, and damiana are all calming herbs that ease physical tension and help maintain a balanced mental and emotional state. Lemon balm alleviates stress-related digestive problems, skullcap combats panic attacks, and damiana acts as a gentle "pick-me-up."

Valerian has tranquilizing qualities.

Ginseng and Siberian ginseng are excellent for coping with stressful events such as competitive sports, examinations, or moving a household.

Ashwagandha is a supportive tonic herb, strengthening and encouraging recovery from long-term stress or chronic illness.

Lifestyle

When emotionally stressed, it is important to eat well, exercise regularly, and allow time for relaxation. Yoga and Tai Chi can be particularly helpful.

General remedies

Herbs Lemon balm (*Melissa officinalis*, p. 117), damiana (*Turnera diffusa*, p. 148), skullcap (*Scutellaria lateriflora*, p. 139)
Remedy Make an infusion using one of the herbs. Drink up to 2⅓ cups (600 ml) a day.

Herb St. John's wort (*Hypericum perforatum*, p. 110)
Remedy Take tablets or make an infusion and drink up to 2⅓ cups (600 ml) a day.
Note This remedy may take 2–3 weeks before there is a noticeable effect.

Digestive problems due to stress
Herb Lemon balm (*Melissa officinalis*, p. 117)
Remedy Make an infusion with a handful of fresh leaves and ¾ cup (150 ml) water, or make an infusion with the dried herb. Drink up to 3 cups (750 ml) a day, or add the daily dose to a bath.
Note This remedy also calms palpitations and encourages sleep.

Panic attacks & headaches
Herb Skullcap (*Scutellaria lateriflora*, p. 139)
Remedy Make an infusion and drink up to 3 cups (750 ml) a day.

Chronic anxiety & hyperactivity
Herb Valerian (*Valeriana officinalis*, p. 152)
Remedy Take 10 drops of tincture in water every hour for up to 2 weeks at a time.

Nervous exhaustion, muscle tension, & headaches
Herb Codonopsis (*Codonopsis pilosula*, p. 87)
Remedy Make a decoction and drink in equal doses during the day, or cook up to 25 g of the root a day in a soup or stew.

Short-term stress
Herbs Ginseng (*Panax ginseng*, p. 123), Siberian ginseng (*Eleutherococcus senticosus*, p. 94).
Remedy Either take ginseng tablets, chew 0.5–1 g of root a day, or use it in cooking. Alternatively take 1–2 g of Siberian ginseng capsules up to twice day.
Cautions Do not take for more than 6 weeks at a time. Do not give to children under 12. Do not take during pregnancy. Avoid drinks that contain caffeine.

Long-term stress & convalescence
Herb Ashwagandha (*Withania somnifera*, p. 156)
Remedy Make a decoction using 3 g of root to ¾ cup (150 ml) of water and take during the day, or chew the same amount of root.

Neuralgia (Nerve pain)

Neuralgia is the pain caused by an irritated, damaged, or trapped nerve. It usually occurs in brief, severe bouts and can be felt shooting along the nerve. Although it is difficult to treat, the following remedies may bring relief to minor problems. St. John's wort is analgesic and antiviral, helping to relieve sciatica (pain caused by a trapped spinal nerve) and head pain. Cloves have an anesthetic effect, and peppermint eases pain. Try also the St. John's wort oil rub (see *Back Pain*, p. 323).

General caution Seek professional advice if there is fever or swelling of the gums with toothache.

General remedies

Herbs St. John's wort (*Hypericum perforatum*, p. 110), lavender (*Lavandula officinalis*, p. 112), clove (*Eugenia caryophyllata*, p. 101)
Remedy Apply neat St. John's wort infused oil to painful areas, or add 20 drops each of clove and lavender essential oil to 2 tbsp plus 2 tsp (50 ml) of St. John's wort infused oil and then apply every 2–3 hours as required.

Herb Peppermint (*Mentha x piperita*, p. 118)
Remedy Make an infusion with 25 g of herb to 3 cups (750 ml) of water and bathe the affected area. Alternatively, dilute 20 drops of essential oil in 2 tbsp plus 2 tsp (50 ml) of carrier oil and gently massage into the painful area.
Caution Do not use on children under 5.

Head pain
Herb Clove (*Eugenia caryophyllata*, p. 101)
Remedy Mix ½ tsp of powder with water to make a thick paste and apply to the head.

Toothache

Herb Clove (*Eugenia caryophyllata*, p. 101)
Remedy Chew a clove or rub 1–2 drops of neat essential oil onto the affected tooth 2–3 times a day for up to 3 days.

Headaches & migraine

Headaches and migraine can be very debilitating, especially when they occur frequently.

Headaches are caused by many factors, such as toothache, neck tension, eyestrain, and hangovers. It is important to diagnose and treat the underlying cause, which could mean visiting a dentist, optician, or osteopath in the first instance. Herbal medicine can be very helpful for headaches, although choosing the right herbs can be difficult. The following remedies contain relaxing herbs that alleviate headaches triggered by stress as well as other more specific factors. Lavender is soothing, while vervain is a tonic and relaxing herb for nervous exhaustion. Peppermint is effective for headaches that are linked to indigestion.

Migraine is a more specific problem. The remedies aim both to prevent the onset of a migraine as well as treat the symptoms.

Hangovers are not a nerve problem in a direct sense, but they should be treated in the same way as any other type of mild poisoning that requires detoxification and headache relief. Make sure you also drink plenty of water.

General caution For migraine or recurrent headaches, consult a professional practitioner to diagnose and treat the underlying cause.

General remedy

Herb Lavender (*Lavandula officinalis*, p. 112)
Remedy Rub a few drops of neat essential oil on the temples.

Tension & sinus headaches

Herb Linden (*Tilia spp.*, p. 286)
Remedy Make an infusion using 1 heaping tsp of linden to ¾ cup (150 ml) of water, or use teabags. Drink up to 3 cups (750 ml) a day.

Nervous exhaustion & overactivity

Herbs Vervain (*Verbena officinalis*, p. 153), valerian (*Valeriana officinalis*, p. 152)
Remedy Make an infusion of vervain and drink up to 2¼ cups a day. Alternatively, mix ½ tsp of each tincture and take with water up to 3 times a day.
Caution Do not take vervain during pregnancy.

Digestive headaches & biliousness

Herbs Peppermint (*Mentha x piperita*, p. 118), pennyroyal (*Mentha pulegium*, p. 241)

Remedy Make an infusion of either herb in a covered container, using a teabag, a small handful of fresh leaves, or 1 level tsp of dried herb per ¾ cup (150 ml) of water. Drink up to 3 cups (750 ml) a day for up to 1 week, or up to 2⅓ cups (600 ml) a day if taking for 2–3 weeks.
Cautions Do not give to children under 5. Do not take pennyroyal during pregnancy.

Migraine prevention

Herb Feverfew (*Tanacetum parthenium*, p. 144)
Remedy At the first sign of an impending attack, take tablets or 10 drops of tincture with water. Alternatively, place a fresh leaf between slices of bread and eat as a sandwich.
Cautions Do not give to children under 12. Do not take in pregnancy.

Migraine

Herb Skullcap (*Scutellaria lateriflora*, p. 139)
Remedy Make an infusion using 1 heaping tsp of herb to ¾ cup (150 ml) of water. Drink up to 3 cups (750 ml) a day.

Herb Rosemary (*Rosmarinus officinalis*, p. 132)
Remedy Make an infusion using 1 level tsp of herb per ¾ cup (150 ml) of water and take up to 2⅓ cups (600 ml) each day.

Detoxification for hangover

Herb Dandelion (*Taraxacum officinale*, p. 145)
Remedy Make a decoction using 15 g of root to 3 cups (750 ml) of water. Take the decoction in small quantities at frequent intervals throughout the day.

Insomnia

Difficulty in sleeping affects everyone at one time or another. Herbs can provide a safe and gentle solution to this problem.

Sedative herbs such as German chamomile, linden, lavender, hops, and passionflower are relaxing and, unlike some herbs, are most likely to be effective against insomnia when taken at night. Hops are excellent when the mind refuses to "switch off."

Stimulant herbs are effective when the body suffers from nervous exhaustion and feels, paradoxically, too tired for sleep. Oats and ginseng encourage a good night's sleep, especially for people suffering from nervous tension and fatigue.

Herbal sleeping pills, containing combinations of valerian, hops, passionflower, and similar herbs, are often helpful in overcoming mild sleep problems and in reducing feelings of anxiety and stress.

General remedies

Herbs German chamomile (*Chamomilla recutita*, p. 82), linden (*Tilia spp.*, p. 286), lavender (*Lavandula officinalis*, p. 112), passionflower (*Passiflora incarnata*, p. 124)
Remedy The above herbs are listed in ascending order of strength. Start with the weakest, German chamomile, and if it does not help, try the next strongest. Make an infusion in a covered container using 1–2 heaping tsp per ¾ cup (150 ml) of water. Take prior to sleeping. Alternatively, take 1 tsp of tincture with water up to 3 times a night.

Herbs Valerian (*Valeriana officinalis*, p. 152), hops (*Humulus lupulus*, p. 108), passionflower (*Passiflora incarnata*, p. 124)
Remedy 1 Take tablets containing one or more of the herbs.
Remedy 2 Make a sachet with dried hops (see p. 108) and place inside your pillow.
Caution Do not take hops internally if feeling low or depressed.

Overactive mind

Herb Hops (*Humulus lupulus*, p. 108)
Remedy Take the tincture with water at night. Start with 10 drops up to a maximum of 40 drops each night.
Caution Do not take hops internally if feeling low or depressed.

Poor sleep & nervous exhaustion

Herb Oats (*Avena sativa*, p. 179)
Remedy Eat oats daily, for example as a hot cereal, and take 1 tsp of oat straw tincture with water 3 times a day.

Herbs Ashwagandha (*Withania somnifera*, p. 156), Siberian ginseng (*Eleutherococcus senticosus*, p. 98)
Remedy Take 1–2 g of ashwagandha or Siberian ginseng up to 3 times a day. Either chew the root, or cook it in a soup. Alternatively, take tablets.
Cautions Avoid taking caffeine while taking ashwagandha and Siberian ginseng. Do not take Siberian ginseng for more than 6 weeks at a time. Do not take during pregnancy. Do not give to children under 12.

Before taking any herbal remedies, see pages 300 & 308–309

Respiratory tract problems

The respiratory system stretches from the lining of the eyes and sinuses to the base of the lungs, and is constantly exposed to dust, dirt, and organisms in the air. It is no surprise that in our ever more polluted world we often face problems such as sinus congestion and asthma. Herbal remedies aim to protect the linings of the eyes, ears, sinuses, nose, and throat, as well as the respiratory "tree" of the lungs by countering infection, clearing congestion, soothing the mucous membranes, and relieving inflammation or allergy.

Seek immediate professional advice for:

- Difficulty in breathing or chest pain
- Cough that lasts for more than 2 weeks
- Severe pain in the respiratory tract
- Coughing up blood
- Fever of 102°F (39°C) or more
- Heavy nosebleed lasting longer than 1 hour

Coughs & bronchitis

The act of coughing is usually a reaction to irritant particles in the bronchial tubes. It is worthwhile to consider the type of cough you have and where it is centered. Herbal remedies can then be chosen to work effectively to clear or ease the cough.
Productive chest coughs may produce white, yellow, or green phlegm.
Unproductive coughs are dry and irritant and often take a long time to clear.
Bronchitis occurs when the lining of the lungs' airways becomes inflamed, resulting in a chest cough, possible breathlessness, and a raised temperature. Use both an external and an internal remedy.
Herbs Thyme is an effective antiseptic for the whole system. Licorice acts as a soothing expectorant for persistent coughs and makes any remedy more palatable. Take plenty of garlic to fight bronchitis.
General caution Seek professional advice if a cough lasts for more than 1 week without a cold or infection.

General remedies
Herb Thyme (*Thymus vulgaris*, p. 147)
Remedy Take 3 cups (750 ml) of infusion a day.

Dry coughs in the throat & chest
Herbs Balm of Gilead (*Populus* x *candicans*, p. 262), thyme (*Thymus vulgaris*, p. 147), licorice (*Glycyrrhiza glabra*, p. 105)
Remedy Make an infusion using equal parts of thyme, balm of Gilead buds, and licorice powder. Take ⅓ cup (75 ml) 6 times a day, or mix equal parts of each tincture and take 1 tsp up to 5 times a day with water. Reduce the dosage as the cough eases.
Cautions Seek professional advice if no improvement occurs after 1 week. Do not take licorice if pregnant.

Chest coughs & bronchitis
Herbs Elecampane (*Inula helenium*, p. 111), eucalyptus (*Eucalyptus globulus*, p. 100), licorice (*Glycyrrhiza glabra*, p. 105)
Remedy (Internal) Make a decoction of elecampane and take 1¼–1⅔ cups (300–450 ml) a day. Add 5 g licorice powder to improve flavor.
Note For acute bronchitis and coughs, add 5 g of eucalyptus leaf to the decoction.
Caution Do not take elecampane during pregnancy.

Herbs Echinacea (*Echinacea* spp., p. 96), garlic (*Allium sativum*, p. 63)
Remedy (Internal) Take ½ tsp of echinacea tincture with water 2–3 times a day, or take tablets. In addition, eat 2 garlic cloves daily.

Herbs Thyme (*Thymus vulgaris*, p. 147), cajuput (*Melaleuca leucadendron*, p. 240), eucalyptus (*Eucalyptus globulus*, p. 100)
Remedy (External) Mix 5 drops each of eucalyptus and thyme essential oils with 2 tsp of olive or sunflower oil. Massage over the chest and back, up to twice a day. Alternatively, burn 5–10 drops of one of the oils in a burner for 30 minutes.
Caution Do not apply thyme oil during pregnancy.

Nosebleeds

Many herbs are reputed to stop nosebleeds, and most are effective. Using an herb as snuff is a traditional way of staunching a nosebleed.
Caution If the nosebleed continues for some hours or is very heavy, seek immediate professional advice.

Prevention of nosebleeds
Herbs Eyebright (*Euphrasia* spp., p. 214), nettle (*Urtica dioica*, p. 150)
Remedy Make an infusion using 25 g of either herb to 3 cups of water. Take up to 2½ cups a day.

Nosebleeds
Herb Wild geranium (*Geranium maculatum*, p. 221)
Remedy First, pinch the nostrils and tilt back the head. Then sniff ½ tsp of the powdered herb.

Eye problems
Rather than treating the eyes themselves, these remedies benefit the mucous tissue lining the eyes, which is contiguous with the nose and throat. Problems affecting the linings of the eyes often respond well to local treatment with herbal remedies, but care must be taken not to irritate the eyes with particles of herbs left in the lotion.

Sore & tired eyes
Herbs German chamomile (*Chamomilla recutita*, p. 82), ju hua (*Chrysanthemum* x *morifolium*, p. 83)
Remedy Make a compress by infusing a German chamomile teabag, or make a poultice with 15 g of either herb to 1 cup (250 ml) of water. Cool, squeeze out the excess, and place the teabag or poultice over the eye.

Conjunctivitis
Herbs Eyebright (*Euphrasia officinalis*, p. 214), cornflower (*Centaurea cyanus*, p. 189)
Remedy Make an infusion with either herb and strain. When warm (not hot), put in an eyebath and bathe eyes well. Use no more than twice a day.
Caution Seek professional advice if there is no improvement in 3–4 days.

Colds, flu, & fevers

The common cold, with which most of us are only too familiar, is a viral infection normally affecting the nose and throat. Flu is considerably more debilitating and may include fever, headache, muscular pain, nausea, and vomiting. Both have a habit of striking when we are stressed or run down. Herbal home treatment is especially suitable for these familiar "self-limiting" ailments since it enables us to make life more comfortable, control fever, and improve the body's recovery rate.

Garlic, ginger, and lemon combine to create the classic flu remedy that can also be used to relieve colds, sore throats, and tonsillitis.

Ginger, cinnamon, cloves, and cayenne have heating properties and stimulate sweating. This helps to lower the body's temperature during fever.

Elderberry and yarrow are antiviral, stimulate sweating, and astringe the mucous membranes of the nose and throat, reducing the production of mucus.

Elecampane and cayenne are particularly helpful for respiratory infections.

Wormwood and gentian are bitter herbs that cool the body and combat high fever.

Diet
For all these problems, eat lightly. Fruit and vegetables are best, the latter perhaps in a soup. Avoid greasy, fatty, sugar-rich food and dairy products.

Self-help
Reduce fever and temperature by washing with cool or cold water and drinking plenty of liquid, especially when sweating.

General cautions Remember that in the very young and very old, even a common cold can develop into pneumonia. Always seek professional advice if symptoms persist or suddenly get worse.

General remedies
Herbs Garlic (*Allium sativum*, p. 63), ginger (*Zingiber officinale*, p. 159), lemon (*Citrus limon*, p. 86)
Remedy Crush a medium-size garlic clove, grate a similarly sized piece of fresh ginger, and squeeze the juice from 1 lemon. Mix together with 1 tsp of honey. Add ¾ cup (150 ml) of warm water and stir. Drink up to 1⅔ cups (450 ml) a day while symptoms last.

Herbs Thyme (*Thymus vulgaris*, p. 147), boneset (*Eupatorium perfoliatum*, p. 213)
Remedy Make an infusion using ½ tsp of each herb with ¾ cup (150 ml) of water and then drink 1⅔–2⅓ cups (450–600 ml) a day.
Note This remedy is very effective if thick green mucus and nasal congestion occur.

Colds
Herbs Lemon (*Citrus limon*, p. 86), cinnamon (*Cinnamomum* spp., p. 85)
Remedy Drink the freshly squeezed juice of 1 lemon, neat or diluted in warm water.
Option Add 1 tsp of honey to the juice and ½ tsp of cinnamon powder.

Herb Ginger (*Zingiber officinale*, p. 159)
Remedy Infuse 2–3 slices (1 g) of fresh ginger with ¾ cup (150 ml) of water for 5 minutes. Take up to 3 cups (750 ml) a day.

Herbs Elderberry (*Sambucus nigra*, p. 136), lemon (*Citrus limon*, p. 86)
Remedy Take 1 tsp (5 ml) of elderberry tincture or extract in warm water up to 3 times a day. Add in freshly squeezed juice from half a lemon.

High fever
Herbs Yarrow (*Achillea millefolium*, p. 60), meadowsweet (*Filipendula ulmaria*, p. 102), cayenne (*Capsicum frutescens*, p. 79)
Remedy Make an infusion using 1 tsp each of yarrow and meadowsweet, with a pinch of cayenne, to ¾ cup (150 ml) of water. Brew for 5 minutes and drink hot. Take up to 2⅓ cups (600 ml) a day.
Options Add 1 or 2 of the following herbs: 2–3 cloves (*Eugenia caryophyllata*, p. 101), ½ tsp of powdered or grated fresh ginger (*Zingiber officinale*, p. 159), ½ tsp of chopped or powdered cinnamon bark (*Cinnamomum* spp., p. 85), 1–2 crushed cardamom seeds (*Elettaria cardamomum*, p. 97), 2–3 crushed peppercorns (*Piper nigrum*, p. 258).
Caution Do not take yarrow during pregnancy.

Herbs Wormwood (*Artemisia absinthium*, p. 70), gentian (*Gentiana lutea*, p. 103)
Remedy Take 10 drops of either tincture with water 3 times a day in addition to the above remedy.
Caution Do not take wormwood in pregnancy.

Mild fever
Herbs Yarrow (*Achillea millefolium*, p. 60), elderberry (*Sambucus nigra*, p. 136)
Remedy Make an infusion with ½ tsp of each herb in ⅓ cup (100 ml) water. Brew for 10 minutes and drink up to 2⅓ cups (600 ml) a day.
Caution Do not take yarrow during pregnancy.

Herb Onion (*Allium cepa*, p. 168)
Remedy Bake a large onion at 400°F (200°C) for 40 minutes. Remove, and mix the juice with an equal amount of honey. Take 1–2 tsp an hour up to 8 times a day.

Flu with muscle aches & pains
Herbs Thyme (*Thymus vulgaris*, p. 147), lemon balm (*Melissa officinalis*, p. 117), elderflower (*Sambucus nigra*, p. 136)
Remedy Make an infusion using 5 g of each herb to 3 cups (750 ml) of water. Brew for 10 minutes and drink up to 3 cups (750 ml) a day.

Herb Echinacea (*Echinacea* spp., p. 96)
Remedy Take tablets or capsules, or up to ½ tsp of tincture with water twice a day. Alternatively, make a decoction with 5 g of root to 3 cups (750 ml) of water and then drink 1¼–2⅓ cups (300–600 ml) a day.

Sore throats & tonsillitis

The garlic, ginger, and lemon mixture listed under *General Remedies for Colds, Flu, & Fevers* (see above) can alleviate the symptoms of both sore throats and tonsillitis. The brave can slowly chew a clove of garlic; sage and echinacea are also strongly antiseptic. All these herbs will relieve symptoms and aid a speedy recovery.

General caution Always seek professional advice and treatment for children under 5 suffering from tonsillitis.

Sore throats
Herbs Tamarind (*Tamarindus indica*, p. 284), lemon (*Citrus limon*, p. 86)
Remedy Gargle with either a decoction of tamarind fruit or 1 tbsp (20 ml) of lemon juice, either neat or diluted in warm water.

Herbs Rosemary (*Rosmarinus officinalis*, p. 132), sage (*Salvia officinalis*, p. 135), myrrh (*Commiphora myrrha*, p. 89), echinacea (*Echinacea* spp., p. 96)
Remedy 1 Dilute 1 tsp of equal parts of all tinctures in 5 tsp of warm water and gargle. Swallow the mixture (except if pregnant).
Remedy 2 Make a sage infusion, brew for 10 minutes, and allow to cool a little. Gargle, then swallow. Add 1 tsp (5 ml) of vinegar and 1 tsp of honey to strengthen its action.
Caution Do not swallow sage during pregnancy.

Tonsillitis
Herbs Echinacea (*Echinacea* spp., p. 96), all herbs listed under *Sore Throats*
Remedy Take echinacea (see *Flu with Muscle Aches & Pains* above), or use one of the gargles listed under *Sore Throats*.
Caution Seek professional advice if there is no improvement after 2 days.

Before taking any herbal remedies, see pages 300 & 308–309

Congestion, sinus problems, & earache

Excessive nasal congestion is not always easy to treat and suggests poor air quality, inappropriate diet, or an allergy. The shape of the nose and sinuses (the air-filled cavities in the bones around the nose) can also play a role in this condition. Sinuses can become blocked with fluid, causing painful pressure. Earache may be caused by local infection—in which case garlic is particularly effective—or congestion. Lavender is helpful in soothing the pain of all types of earache.

Diet

As a first step, reduce foods thought to increase mucus production, such as dairy, eggs, fried and fatty food, sugar, and refined carbohydrates, such as white flour, as well as alcohol.
General caution Seek professional advice for earache, especially in children.

General remedy

Herb Eucalyptus (*Eucalyptus globulus*, p. 100)
Remedy Make a steam inhalation by infusing 15 g of herb, or put 5–10 drops of essential oil in 3 cups (750 ml) water. Inhale for 10 minutes.

Allergic states with excessive nasal mucus, such as hay fever

Herb German chamomile (*Chamomilla recutita*, p. 82)
Remedy Make a steam inhalation by infusing 15 g of herb, or put 5–10 drops of essential oil in 3 cups (750 ml) water. Inhale for 10 minutes.

Earache

Herb Lavender (*Lavandula officinalis*, p. 112)
Remedy Place 2 drops of essential oil on a cotton ball and plug into the ear.

Earache caused by infection

Herb Garlic (*Allium sativum*, p. 63)

Remedy Break open a garlic oil capsule, place 2 drops on a cotton ball, and plug into the affected ear. Alternatively, crush a large clove of garlic and soak in 1 tbsp of sunflower or olive oil for at least 24 hours. Strain the oil and warm it to body temperature. Then place 2 drops on a cotton ball and plug into the ear.

Earache due to chronic congestion

Herbs Echinacea (*Echinacea* spp., p. 96), thyme (*Thymus vulgaris*, p. 147), marsh mallow (*Althaea officinalis*, p. 169), elderflower (*Sambucus nigra*, p. 136)
Remedy Mix equal parts of each tincture and take 1 tsp 3 times a day with water.

Copious liquid mucus & sinus congestion

See *Allergic Rhinitis*, p. 310.

Sinus headaches

See *Tension & Sinus Headaches*, p. 319.

Musculoskeletal problems

Whether caused by accident, sports injury, or simple wear and tear, musculoskeletal problems can lead to a significant deterioration in quality of life. Manipulation is often the primary treatment, but herbal remedies can reduce pain and inflammation, relax muscles, detoxify the body, and speed up the rate of healing. External treatments soothe back muscles and joints, and sprained or sore limbs. Persevering with the simple home treatments given below can bring about a marked improvement of many problems.

Seek immediate professional advice for:

- Severe pain
- Significant or sudden joint swelling
- Broken or suspected broken bones
- Any injury that may need an X-ray

Caution Only give external remedies to children. Seek professional advice before giving internal remedies to them.

Sprains & fractures

Minor damaged areas benefit from herbs such as arnica and comfrey, which soothe bruising and speed up the healing process. Apply as soon as possible after treatment.
General caution Always seek professional treatment for broken bones, fractures, and severe sprains.

Sprains

Herb Arnica (*Arnica montana*, p. 176)
Remedy Apply ointment or cream to the damaged area and gently massage into the skin at least 3 times a day.

Caution Do not use arnica on broken skin.

Fractures

Herb Comfrey (*Symphytum officinale*, p. 142)
Remedy Gently apply ointment, cream or infused oil to the area at least 3 times a day.
Caution Do not use comfrey on broken skin.

Muscle aches & cramps

Muscle aches and cramps are entirely normal, particularly after strenuous activity, and the pain should lessen in time. Meanwhile, rubs and ointments containing soothing herbs, such as arnica, thyme, and cramp bark, can alleviate aching muscles.

Rheumatism is a general term for muscle or joint pain and stiffness, and the remedies listed here and under *Joint Pain & Stiffness*, p. 323, are appropriate for this condition.

Tired & aching muscles

Herb Arnica (*Arnica montana*, p. 176)
Remedy Apply cream or ointment.
Caution Do not use arnica on broken skin.

Herbs Thyme (*Thymus vulgaris*, p. 147), rosemary (*Rosmarinus officinalis*, p. 132)
Remedy Make an infusion with 25 g of one herb to 3 cups (750 ml) water. Brew for 10 minutes, strain into a bath, and soak for 20 minutes.

Cramps & muscle spasms

Herb Cramp bark (*Viburnum opulus*, p. 154)
Remedy (internal) Take 1 tsp of tincture with water up to 3 times a day. (external) Rub neat tincture firmly into the affected area.

Joint pain & stiffness, including arthritis & gout

The most common ailment characterized by joint pain and stiffness is arthritis, which is caused by inflammation of the joints. Aging or wear and tear may be the cause, but some arthritic conditions, and other joint problems such as gout, are due to the buildup of waste products in the joints.
Devil's claw is anti-inflammatory, relieving swollen and inflamed joints.
Lemon juice reduces acidity in the body. White willow relieves inflammation and pain and, when combined with other herbs, can lead to significant improvement in mild to moderate arthritis.
Meadowsweet and celery combine well to reduce acidity. All the herbal remedies here can be safely taken for 1–2 months.

Self-help

Improving posture, managing anxiety, and using herbal remedies to help the body eliminate toxins can all help control these conditions. Avoid acid-forming foods such as red meat, spinach, tomatoes, and oranges. Regular (but not excessive) exercise is beneficial, as is a relaxed, positive attitude.
General cautions For severe arthritis, consult a professional practitioner. Do not take devil's claw, black cohosh, or celery seed during pregnancy.

Arthritis & inflamed joints

Herb Devil's claw (*Harpagophytum procumbens*, p. 107)
Remedy Take tablets (see *General cautions*).

Herb Lemon (*Citrus limon*, p. 86)
Remedy Squeeze the juice from a lemon and drink neat or diluted in water each morning.

Herb White willow (*Salix alba*, p. 133)
Remedy Take tablets, or make a decoction using 10 g of root to 3 cups (750 ml) water. Take in 3 doses over 1–2 days as required.

Herbs Devil's claw (*Harpagophytum procumbens*, p. 107), celery (*Apium graveolens*, p. 68), white willow (*Salix alba*, p. 133)
Remedy Make a decoction with 8 g of each herb to 3 cups (750 ml) of water, divide into 4 doses, and take 2–3 doses a day; or mix equal parts of the tinctures and take 1 tsp with water 3 times a day (see *General cautions*).

Option If arthritis develops during menopause, replace devil's claw with 8 g of black cohosh (*Cimicifuga racemosa*, p. 61)

Herb Deadly nightshade (*Atropa belladonna*, p. 73)
Remedy Apply belladonna bandages in addition to one of the above remedies.

Arthritis associated with acid indigestion or peptic ulcer

Herbs Meadowsweet (*Filipendula ulmaria*, p. 102), celery (*Apium graveolens*, p. 68)
Remedy Make an infusion with meadowsweet and drink up to 3 cups (750 ml) a day, or mix 2 parts meadowsweet tincture with 1 part celery tincture and take ½ tsp with water 2–3 times a day (refer to *General cautions*).

Stiff & aching joints

Herbs St. John's wort (*Hypericum perforatum*, p. 110), comfrey (*Symphytum officinale*, p. 142), lavender (*Lavandula officinalis*, p. 112)
Remedy Mix 2½ tbsp of St. John's wort or comfrey infused oil with 20–40 drops of lavender essential oil and gently massage into the affected area.
Option Try the rub containing St. John's wort infused oil under *General Remedies* for *Back Pain* below.

Gout

Herb Celery (*Apium graveolens*, p. 68)
Remedy Take tablets, or make a decoction with the seeds. Divide into 3 doses and drink during the day or add 25 g of seeds to food per day (see *General cautions*).

Back pain

Above all, back problems require specialist attention and plenty of rest. Herbal remedies contribute to overall improvement by alleviating pain and muscle tension, and helping to make life more comfortable.
Cramp bark and prickly ash are warming, relaxing herbs, which, when rubbed into the affected area, help to "unknot" taut muscles.
Lavender and St. John's wort are useful herbs when nervous tension is contributing to the problem.
Devil's claw and cramp bark have effective anti-inflammatory properties and help reduce swollen joints.
Passionflower encourages sleep, particularly when back pain is accompanied by nervous tension.
Sciatica (a painful condition caused by a trapped spinal nerve) and neuralgia can both be relieved by using an external rub containing St. John's wort infused oil.

General cautions Back problems need specialist care. For chronic or severe back pain, seek the advice of a professional practitioner to gain the most benefit from herbal medicine.

General remedies

Herbs Cramp bark (*Viburnum opulus*, p. 154), prickly ash (*Zanthoxylum americanum*, p. 157)
Remedy Make a decoction using 15 g of cramp bark and 5 g of prickly ash bark to 3 cups (750 ml) of water. Strain and rub into the affected area, or use 1 tbsp of tincture and apply in the same way.
Note Use especially for tense neck and lumbar regions.

Herb Thyme (*Thymus vulgaris*, p. 147)
Remedy Make an infusion using 25 g of herb to 3 cups (750 ml) of water and strain into a bath. Soak for 20 minutes.

Herbs St. John's wort (*Hypericum perforatum*, p. 110), lavender (*Lavandula officinalis*, p. 112), pepper (*Piper nigrum*, p. 258), cramp bark (*Viburnum opulus*, p. 154)
Remedy Take 2 tbsp of sunflower oil or St. John's wort infused oil, add 20 drops of lavender essential oil, 10 drops each of rosemary and pepper essential oil, and 1 tsp of cramp bark tincture. Shake and rub into tense areas, either after a bath or having first warmed the area with a hot towel.
Other uses Use for sciatica and other back problems that cause neuralgia, as well as for stiff joints and chronic muscle ache.

Back pain due to joint inflammation

Herbs White willow (*Salix alba*, p. 133), cramp bark (*Viburnum opulus*, p. 154), devil's claw (*Harpagophytum procumbens*, p. 107)
Remedy Mix equal parts of each root and make a decoction. Divide into 6 doses and take over 2 days. If there is no improvement after 7 days, divide the decoction into 3 doses and take daily for up to a week.
Caution Do not take devil's claw during pregnancy.

Sleeplessness due to backache

Herbs Passionflower (*Passiflora incarnata*, p. 124), valerian (*Valeriana officinalis*, p. 152), cramp bark (*Viburnum opulus*, p. 154)
Remedy Make a decoction using 8 g each of passionflower, valerian, and cramp bark to 3 cups (750 ml) of water and drink ¾–1¼ cup (150–300 ml) at night (the decoction is sufficient for 2 days).

Before taking any herbal remedies, see pages 300 & 308–309

Urinary & fungal infections

Infections signal that the body's resistance to disease has become weakened, particularly if they are long-lasting or recurrent. Minor infections affecting the kidneys and urinary system are common and, despite being hard to shake off, can be treated by boosting the body's natural defenses. Fungal infections can also be difficult to clear and may require professional treatment, although herbs such as garlic (*Allium sativum*, p. 63) and tea tree (*Melaleuca alternifolia*, p. 116) are strongly antifungal. If the infection is chronic, it is necessary to support the immune system as a whole, with herbs such as echinacea (*Echinacea* spp., p. 96).

Seek immediate professional advice for:

- Infections that show no signs of improvement, or deteriorate after taking a herbal remedy
- Temperatures above 102°F (39°C)
- Pain in the kidneys
- Blood in the urine

Urinary infections

Cystitis (an infection of the bladder and urinary tubules) can be a serious problem if it spreads to the kidneys. Mild cystitis and other urinary infections can be cured with a mixture of antiseptic herbs such as buchu and soothing herbs such as marsh mallow. Taking echinacea or garlic at the same time improves the body's resistance to infection. Bilberry or cranberry, which are from the same genus, are excellent for urinary infections.
General cautions Seek immediate professional help if cystitis is severe or recurrent, or if there is blood in the urine or pain around the kidneys or small of the back.

General remedies

Herbs Buchu (*Barosma betulina*, p. 75), corn silk (*Zea mays*, p. 158), marsh mallow (*Althaea officinalis*, p. 169)
Remedy Make an infusion with 5 g of each herb to 3 cups (750 ml) of water. Divide into 4 doses and drink throughout the day.
Option Substitute juniper (*Juniperus communis*, p. 229) or goldenrod (*Solidago virgaurea*, p. 280) for buchu.
Caution Do not take juniper or buchu during pregnancy.

Herbs Bilberry (*Vaccinium myrtillus*, p. 151)
Remedy Make a decoction of the berries and drink 1²/₃–2¹/₃ cups (450–600 ml) a day.
Tip Cranberry juice may be substituted for bilberry decoction.

Herbs Garlic (*Allium sativum*, p. 63), echinacea (*Echinacea* spp., p. 96)
Remedy Take either or both herbs in capsule or tablet form.
Note Take in addition to other remedies.

Fungal infections

Fungal infections are common and can be hard to treat. Vaginal yeast infection is increasingly found as a side effect of conventional antibiotic treatment. Calendula is helpful for treating this troublesome condition. Candidiasis (accelerated growth of *Candida albicans*, a yeast-like organism within the gut) can cause considerable problems, but mild cases may be helped with antiseptic and antifungal herbs, such as garlic. All types of fungal infections can be helped with herbs that boost the immune system, such as echinacea, as well as by applying an external remedy to the affected area.

Diet

Diet is an important factor when treating fungal problems. Cut out or reduce intake of bread, alcohol, and other foods containing yeast or sugar.

Self-help

Candidiasis sufferers can take probiotic capsules or live yogurt to help the growth of beneficial bacteria in the intestines. For yeast infection, live yogurt can be inserted into the vagina.
General caution Seek professional advice for candidiasis, as it is often a difficult condition to treat.

General remedies

Herbs Echinacea (*Echinacea* spp., p. 96), thyme (*Thymus vulgaris*, p. 147)
Remedy Mix 2 parts echinacea tincture to 1 part thyme tincture and take 1 tsp twice a day with water.

Herbs Garlic (*Allium sativum*, p. 63)
Remedy Take 1–2 garlic cloves a day, crushed and swallowed with water or mixed with food.

Vaginal yeast infection

Herbs Calendula (*Calendula officinalis*, p. 77)
Remedy Make an infusion and allow to cool. Strain and use as a douche or wash.
Option Add the infusion to a bath and soak for 20 minutes.
Herbs Tea tree (*Melaleuca alternifolia*, p. 116)
Remedy Use pessaries or place 1–2 drops of essential oil diluted with 3 drops of olive oil on a tampon and insert into the vagina (this may sting). Remove after 2–3 hours and only use once a day.
Caution During pregnancy, use these pessaries and tampons only with professional advice.

Oral thrush

Herbs Licorice (*Glycyrrhiza glabra*, p. 105), myrrh (*Commiphora myrrha*, p. 89), echinacea (*Echinacea* spp., p. 96)
Remedy Mix equal parts of the tincture of each herb. Take 1 tsp as a mouthwash with water every 3–4 hours, as required.

Candidiasis

Herbs Olive leaf (*Olea europaea* p. 121), calendula (*Calendula officinalis*, p. 77), thyme (*Thymus vulgaris*, p. 147)
Remedy Make an infusion with 8 g of each herb to 3 cups (750 ml) water and drink 1¼–1²/₃ cups (300–450 ml) each day.

Herbs Pau d'Arco (*Tabebuia* spp., p. 143)
Remedy Make a decoction with 12 g bark to 3 cups (750 ml) of water. Divide into 3–4 doses and drink throughout the day. Alternatively, take capsules or ½ tsp of tincture with water up to 3 times a day.

Fungal skin infections, including athlete's foot

See p. 314.

Reproductive & menstrual problems

Women have always tended to use herbal medicine more than men, traditionally in their role as healers in the home and now, in part, due to the proven effects of many herbs on the reproductive system. Herbs such as wild yam contain constituents similar to the female sex hormones, estrogen and progesterone, which can help regulate the menstrual cycle, increase or decrease fertility, and support the body through menopause. Common menstrual problems, such as cramps, premenstrual syndrome, and heavy bleeding, respond well to self-treatment. However, chronic conditions or infertility in either women or men require professional attention.

Seek immediate professional advice for:

- Severe pain in the abdomen or pelvis
- Significant or sudden change in menstruation, such as prolonged, heavy, or irregular periods

Important note For the best treatment, consult an herbalist. Seek professional advice before taking a remedy if you believe that you may be pregnant. See *Pregnancy*, p. 327.

Menstrual Problems

The menstrual cycle can be disturbed for many reasons, most of them relating to hormonal imbalances. Other causes include stress, too much or too little exercise, weight problems, food sensitivity or allergy, steroids, the contraceptive pill, chronic illness, vitamin and mineral deficiency, and even excess caffeine, alcohol, or smoking. To determine the underlying cause, it is important to consult a professional practitioner.

Taking remedies for menstrual problems. The remedies listed should all be taken at the appropriate point in the cycle for 2–3 cycles.

The normal menstrual cycle lasts about 28 days. If this cycle varies greatly from one period to another without reason, it could be termed irregular.

Premenstrual syndrome (PMS) and period pain have many causes and are experienced at some stage by most people. Breast tenderness, sore nipples, and fluid retention are common symptoms.

Heavy periods can result in anemia. If your period lasts longer than 5 days or if you have to change your protection every 2 hours, your periods may be too heavy. Nettle (*Urtica dioica*, p. 150) is an excellent tonic, especially for heavy bleeding, as it contains more iron than spinach and can be eaten as a nourishing vegetable.

Self-help

Combine herbal remedies with a diet high in fresh vegetables and fruit, and low in fatty foods, sugar, and alcohol. Try not to smoke. Regular exercise, particularly of the waist and pelvis, is helpful, as is a relaxed attitude to life. All reproductive problems will benefit from this simple approach.

General caution For any chronic menstrual problem, it is wise to seek professional attention, especially if your periods are very heavy or painful.

Irregular cycle

Herb Chaste tree (*Vitex agnus-castus*, p. 155)
Remedy Take tablets, or take 30–40 drops (1.5–2 ml) of tincture with water each morning on waking for at least 2 months.

Herb Motherwort (*Leonurus cardiaca*, p. 232)
Remedy Make an infusion and take ¾–1¼ cups (150–300 ml) a day for up to 3 monthly cycles.
Caution Do not take if menstrual bleeding is heavy.

Premenstrual syndrome

Herb Vervain (*Verbena officinalis*, p. 153), linden (*Tilia* spp., p. 286)
Remedy (Internal) Make an infusion using either herb (or an equal mix of both) and drink up to 3 cups (750 ml) throughout the day.

Herb Valerian (*Valeriana officinalis*, p. 148)
Remedy (Internal) Take tablets containing valerian, or take 20–40 drops of tincture with water up to 5 times a day.

Herb Rosemary (*Rosmarinus officinalis*, p. 132)
Remedy (External) Make an infusion with 1 tbsp of dried or 2 tbsp of fresh leaves to 1 quart (liter) of water and strain into a warm bath each morning. Alternatively, add 5–10 drops of essential oil to a bath.
Note Also try the chaste tree remedy under Irregular Cycle above.

Breast tenderness & sore nipples

Herb German chamomile (*Chamomilla recutita*, p. 82)
Remedy Make a compress with an infusion of 50 g of herb and 1 cup (250 ml) of water. Place gently over the breasts. Repeat as often as required to achieve relief.

Herb Calendula (*Calendula officinalis*, p. 77)
Remedy Apply ointment to the nipples. If breast-feeding, wipe off the ointment before feeding.

Fluid retention

Herb Dandelion (*Taraxacum officinale*, p. 145)
Remedy Make an infusion with the leaves and drink up to 1⅔ cups (450 ml) a day.

Heavy menstrual bleeding

Herb *Chuang xiong* (*Ligusticum wallichii*), white peony (*Paeonia lactiflora*, p. 122), dong quai (*Angelica sinensis*, p. 67), rehmannia (*Rehmannia glutinosa*, p. 270)
Remedy Mix equal parts of each root and make a decoction using 15 g of the mixture to 3 cups (750 ml) of water. Drink in 3 equal doses throughout the day.
Note Any of these herbs will help, but they are best together, in which form they are known as *Four Things Soup*.

Herb Shepherd's purse (*Capsella bursa-pastoris*, p. 186), nettle (*Urtica dioica*, p. 150)
Remedy Make an infusion using 7.5 g of each herb (or 15 g of shepherd's purse only) to 3 cups (750 ml) of water. Divide into 3–4 doses and drink throughout the day.

Before taking any herbal remedies, see pages 300 & 308–309

Period pain

Flavor the decoctions with 1 heaping tsp of caraway seeds (*Carum carvi*, p. 187). Mix before decocting.

Herb Wild yam (*Dioscorea villosa*, p. 95), cramp bark (*Viburnum opulus*, p. 154), black haw (*Viburnum prunifolium*, p. 291)
Remedy Make a decoction using 15 g of herb to 3 cups (750 ml) of water. Sip small amounts during the day; or take 2 tsp of tincture with water 3–4 times a day for up to 3 days, then reduce the dose to 1 tsp a day for 5 days, or take tablets.

Herb White peony (*Paeonia lactiflora*, p. 122)
Remedy Make a decoction using 20 g of root to 3 cups (750 ml) of water. Sip this throughout the day.

Fertility problems in women

Although much more research is needed, herbal medicine does appear to increase fertility in women who are trying to conceive, especially if the problem is related to hormonal imbalances, age, or the amount of mucus produced by the cervix. Where there appears to be no physical problem preventing conception, for example a blocked fallopian tube, ovarian cysts, or internal scarring, herbal medicines are well worth trying. Diet, exercise, and lifestyle may also play a significant role in improving fertility.

Aiding conception

Herb Chaste tree (*Vitex agnus-castus*, p. 155)
Remedy Take tablets or take 20–40 drops of tincture with water each morning for a maximum of 3 months at a time.

Herb *Dong quai* (*Angelica sinensis*, p. 67)
Remedy Take tablets or make a decoction using 12 g of root to 3 cups (750 ml) of water and drink each day for up to 3 months.
Caution Discontinue if you become pregnant.

Low sex drive

Herb Schisandra (*Schisandra chinensis*, p. 137)
Remedy Soak 5 g (a small handful) of berries in water overnight. Strain the berries and make a decoction with 1 cup (250 ml) of water. Brew for 15 minutes and take the dose each day.

Herb Shatavari (*Asparagus racemosus*, p. 178)
Remedy Take 1 tsp of tincture twice a day with water.

Fertility problems in men

Impotence in men is a common problem, and herbal medicine has been used throughout history to help restore healthy sexual function.

A low sperm count, which is a common cause of infertility, is often related to lifestyle and general state of health.
Saw palmetto is a tonic herb that increases stamina. It benefits the male sexual organs and is reputed to increase potency.
Ashwagandha is an all-around tonic that is not as stimulating as ginseng, but is nonetheless helpful in restoring normal vitality after a long-term illness or stress.

General vitality

Herb Ashwagandha (*Withania somnifera*, p. 156)
Remedy Take 2 g of the dried root a day, either by chewing it, or taking it in powder form mixed with honey and, if required, water. Take for up to 6 weeks.

Impotence & premature ejaculation

Herb Ginseng (*Panax ginseng*, p. 123)
Remedy Take 0.5–1 g up to 3 times a day for 6 weeks at a time, either by chewing the root, cooking it in a soup or stew, or taking it in tablet form.
Note Ginseng is the best-known remedy for this condition. However, schisandra (*Schisandra chinensis*, p. 137) berries also benefit male sexuality. Take as listed above in *Fertility Problems in Women* under *Low Sex Drive* for up to 6 weeks.
Caution Do not take caffeine while taking ginseng.

Herb Saw palmetto (*Serenoa repens*, p. 140)
Remedy Take ½ tsp of tincture with water up to 3 times a day for up to 6 weeks.
Note Saw palmetto is also an excellent remedy for symptoms associated with an enlarged prostate.

Menopausal problems

Menopause is defined as the cessation of menstruation. It usually takes place between the ages of 45 and 55. After two years without having a period, you can be sure that the "change of life" has occurred.

Both estrogen and progesterone levels decline during menopause despite opinion to the contrary. Herbs such as chaste tree, which have a progesterogenic effect, are as important as those that support estrogen levels, since both hormones appear to help maintain bone density, reducing the risk of osteoporosis.

Maintaining vitality is important during menopause, since many problems result as much from being run-down and tired, as from hormonal changes. If you feel low and exhausted, some of these remedies may help to raise vitality and spirits. St. John's wort is an excellent medicine for depression.

Hot flashes and night sweats are principally caused by hormonal changes. However, nervous exhaustion increases the occurrence of these conditions.
General caution Seek professional advice if there is prolonged or irregular menstrual bleeding.

Decreased estrogen & progesterone levels

Herb Chaste tree (*Vitex agnus-castus*, p. 155)
Remedy Take tablets, or 20–40 drops of tincture with water each morning.

Herb Shatavari (*Asparagus racemosus*, p. 178)
Remedy Take ½ tsp of tincture 2–3 times daily with water.

Herb Black cohosh (*Cimicifuga racemosa*, p. 61)
Remedy Take tablets, or take 25 drops of tincture with water 3 times a day.
Option Black cohosh combines well with sage. Mix equal parts of each tincture and take 30–40 drops (1.5–2 ml) with water 3 times a day.

Depression & decreased vitality

Herb St. John's wort (*Hypericum perforatum*, p. 110)
Remedy Take ½ tsp of tincture with water 3 times a day.

Herb Oats (*Avena sativa*, p. 179)
Remedy Eat 25–50 g of oats as a breakfast cereal, or with other food.
Option In addition, make an infusion with oat straw. Divide into 3 doses and drink throughout the day.

Hot flashes & night sweats

Herb Sage (*Salvia officinalis*, p. 135)
Remedy Make an infusion and drink 1⅔ cups (450 ml), either during the day, or mainly at night, if this is when the problem chiefly occurs.

Herbs White willow (*Salix alba*, p. 133), black cohosh (*Cimicifuga racemosa*, p. 61)
Remedy Take one of the above herbs in tablet form, or take 1 tsp of tincture with water at night.

Herb White peony (*Paeonia lactiflora*, p. 122)
Remedy Make a decoction with 20 g root to 3 cups (750 ml) of water. Sip throughout the day.

Pregnancy

Although in many cultures herbs have traditionally been taken throughout pregnancy, it is wise to take herbs medicinally only when essential. Some herbs such as German chamomile (*Chamomilla recutita*, p. 82), linden (*Tilia* spp., p. 286), and corn silk (*Zea mays*, p. 158) are very useful and can be taken safely for 2–3 weeks at a time during pregnancy. Other herbs should be avoided altogether, as they have constituents that stimulate the muscles of the uterus and, in large doses, could cause a miscarriage. It is safe to continue using herbs in cooking throughout pregnancy.

Seek immediate professional advice for:

- Prolonged nausea causing an inability to eat properly and frequent vomiting leading to dehydration
- Frequent urination lasting for more than 3 days (or with pain after 2 days)
- Breast pain with swollen glands under the arms or fever
- Fluid retention that has not reduced after 3 days

Maintaining vitality

Pregnancy is a time of great change for the body. Many minor ailments can be relieved by homemade herbal remedies.

Morning sickness (sensations of nausea) need not be restricted to the morning. Generally starting in the 4th–6th week and lasting until the 14th–16th week, morning sickness has many causes, including hormone fluctuations, low blood pressure, low sugar levels, food allergies, poor diet, and stress.

Edema (fluid retention and bloating) is extremely common during pregnancy. Water seeps from the blood vessels into the surrounding tissue, causing puffiness. The ankles and calves are mostly affected.

Constipation often occurs as pregnancy develops. Pressure increases on the lower bowel, impeding circulation.

Heartburn (pain in the center of the chest) may also be caused by increased pressure within the body.

Stretch marks sometimes appear as the body swells. They can be minimized by rubbing aloe vera gel or olive oil into the skin to maintain its elasticity.

Childbirth can be helped by drinking raspberry leaf tea, a traditional remedy that prepares the uterine muscles for labor and giving birth.

Herbs during pregnancy

- For the first 3 months avoid all herbal remedies, including essential oils, unless professionally prescribed.
- The following herbs are particularly dangerous and should on no account be taken during pregnancy: blue cohosh (*Caulophyllum thalictroides*, p. 188), goldenseal (*Hydrastis canadensis*, p. 109), juniper (*Juniperus communis*, p. 229), pennyroyal (*Mentha pulegium*, p. 241), yarrow (*Achillea millefolium*, p. 60), and therapeutic doses of sage (*Salvia officinalis*, p. 135).

Morning sickness & nausea

The following remedies are an exception and can be taken during the first 3 months of pregnancy.
Herb German chamomile (*Chamomilla recutita*, p. 82)
Remedy Make an infusion in a covered container. Sip small quantities during the day. Do not drink more than 3 cups (750 ml) a day.

Herb Ginger (*Zingiber officinale*, p. 159)
Remedy Make an infusion with ½–1 tsp of grated fresh ginger per ¾ cup (150 ml) of water. Sip small amounts frequently throughout the day, rather than drinking ¾ cup (150 ml) at a time. Take a maximum of 1⅔ cups (450 ml) a day.

Herb Fennel (*Foeniculum vulgare*, p. 217)
Remedy Make an infusion with ½ tsp of seeds per ¾ cup (150 ml) of water and then drink up to 1⅔ cups (450 ml) a day.

Edema

Herb Corn silk (*Zea mays*, p. 158)
Remedy Make an infusion and drink up to 3 cups (750 ml) a day.

Constipation

Herbs Psyllium (*Plantago* spp., p. 128), flaxseed (*Linum usitatissimum*, p. 113)
Remedy Take 1–2 tsp of either of the seeds with a large glass of water each day or soak them in cold water overnight before taking.
Note Eat more dried fruit, especially figs.

Heartburn

Herb Meadowsweet (*Filipendula ulmaria*, p. 102)
Remedy Make an infusion and drink ¾–1¼ cup (150–300 ml) a day.

Headache & nervous tension

Herb Linden (*Tilia* spp., p. 286)
Remedy Make an infusion and drink 1⅔–2⅓ cups (450–600 ml) a day.

Preparing for childbirth

Herb Raspberry (*Rubus idaeus*, p. 272)
Remedy Make an infusion using 1 tsp of the chopped fresh or dried leaf per ¾ cup (150 ml) of water. Brew for 5–6 minutes and drink ¾–1 cup (150–300 ml) a day during the last 10 weeks of pregnancy.
Cautions Do not leave the infusion to brew for more than 5–6 minutes. Do not take until the last 10 weeks of pregnancy.

Stretch marks

Herbs Aloe vera (*Aloe vera*, p. 64), olive (*Olea europaea*, p. 121)
Remedy Rub aloe vera gel over the affected areas or massage olive oil firmly into the skin 1–2 times a day.

Poor sleep

See *Insomnia* (the German chamomile, linden, lavender, and passionflower remedy under *General Remedies*), p. 319.

Anemia & high blood pressure

See *Circulatory Problems*, p. 311.

Hemorrhoids & varicose veins

See *Varicose veins & hemorrhoids*, p. 312 and *Constipation & diarrhea*, p. 317.

Backache

See *Back pain*, p. 323.

Vaginal yeast infections

See *Fungal Infections*, p. 324.

Healing after childbirth

See *Cleansing wounds & Healing wounds*, p. 314.

Before taking any herbal remedies, see pages 300 & 308–309

Infants & children

The following herbs are considered particularly suitable for children, easing symptoms and speeding recovery. Most of the remedies are best given as infusions, and can be given in a bottle. Infusions can be flavored with honey (see *Cautions* right) or maple syrup if necessary, but they are better given unsweetened. The dosages given are for 1–6-year-olds, but they can be adjusted to suit other age groups (see below). Many of the remedies listed in other sections are also suitable for babies and children; herbs that are not appropriate are clearly identified (see p. 309 for dosage requirements before administering any adult remedies).

Seek immediate professional advice for:

- Severe diarrhea or vomiting; a temperature of 102°F (39°C); fever with convulsions; breathing difficulties; unusual drowsiness; high-pitched crying

Cautions Do not give babies under 6 months any medicine without professional advice. Do not give honey to children under 1 year as in rare cases it can cause food poisoning.

General ailments

Infants and children are susceptible to a wide array of ailments.

Digestive upsets that result in diarrhea and constipation can be the result of food intolerance or allergy in infants, especially when foods such as dairy are being introduced into the diet. Other minor digestive upsets due to infection or inflammation can cause loss of appetite.

Colic is a spasm of the gut causing cramping pain in the abdomen. It usually occurs during the first 3 months of life, particularly after feeding in the evening, when the digestion may not be working so well.

Diaper rash occurs when urine, moisture, and irritants in the diaper cause the baby's skin to become red, sore, and damp. It's essential to clean the baby thoroughly at each diaper change. Ensure that cloth diapers are thoroughly rinsed, avoid leaving a wet, chafing diaper on the baby, and remove the diaper completely whenever possible.

Cradle cap is a thick yellow-brown encrustation on the baby's scalp, caused by overactivity of the sebum oil glands.

Headaches, colds, catarrh, and chesty coughs are common problems in childhood and often respond well to herbal treatment.

Insomnia is a common childhood problem even though children require more sleep than adults and should sleep with ease. Overexcitement, teething, a wet diaper, or being too hot or cold may interfere with sleep patterns. Herbs such as linden will encourage a relaxed night's sleep.

Dosage *The dosages on this page are for 1–6-year-olds. For other ages, adapt as follows:*
6–12 months old—⅓ dose
7–12 years old—1½ dose
To adapt remedies from elsewhere in the book for children, see p. 309.

Digestive upsets, gas, & colic

The following infusions are suitable for infants over 6 months. For those under 6 months, the infusions can be taken by breastfeeding parents.
Herb Ginger (*Zingiber officinale*, p. 159)
Remedy Give ¼ level tsp of powder with ¼ cup (75 ml) of hot water 1–2 times a day.

Herb German chamomile (*Chamomilla recutita*, p. 82)
Remedy Make an infusion with 1 level tsp to ¾ cup (150 ml) of water. Give up to 1⅔ cups (450 ml) a day.

Herbs Anise (*Pimpinella anisum*, p. 256), fennel (*Foeniculum vulgare*, p. 217)
Remedy Make an infusion with 1 level tsp of either of the seeds to ¾ cup (150 ml) of water. Give up to 1 cup (300 ml) a day.

Herb Slippery elm (*Ulmus rubra*, p. 149)
Remedy Mix 1 tsp of powder with hot water to make a paste, then blend with cold or warm water as required and flavor with honey, cinnamon, or maple syrup. Give up to 50 g powder in doses during the day.

Constipation
Herbs Flaxseed (*Linum usitatissimum*, p. 113), slippery elm (*Ulmus rubra*, p. 149)
Remedy Give 1 tsp of flaxseed or slippery elm with a large glass of water each day.

Diarrhea
Herbs Agrimony (*Agrimonia eupatoria*, p. 165), common plantain (*Plantago major*, p. 258)
Remedy Make an infusion using 15 g of either herb to ½ liter of water and give up to 1¼ cup (300 ml) each day.

Diaper rash & inflamed skin rashes
Herb Chickweed (*Stellaria media*, p. 282)
Remedy Apply ointment 1–2 times a day.

Herb Calendula (*Calendula officinalis*, p. 77)
Remedy Make an infusion with 1 level tsp of each herb to ¾ cup (150 ml) of water. Give ¾–1¼ cup (150–300 ml) a day.
Note For diaper rash, the ointment is best.

Cradle cap
Herb Olive (*Olea europaea*, p. 121)
Remedy Apply olive oil to the area 1–2 times a day.

Colds, congestion, & chest coughs
Herb Thyme (*Thymus vulgaris*, p. 147)
Remedy Make an infusion with 1 level tsp herb to ¾ cup (150 ml) of water. Give ⅔–1 cup a day.

Herbs Elderberry (*Sambucus nigra*, p. 136), pelargonium (*Pelargonium sidoides*, p. 125), thyme (*Thymus vulgaris*, p. 147)
Remedy Make an infusion with 1 level tsp thyme leaves to ⅔ cup of water. Give ⅔–1 cup a day.
Remedy Give elderberry or pelargonium extract, as recommended by practitioner or supplier.

Earache
Herb Garlic (*Allium sativum*, p. 63)
Remedy Break open a garlic oil capsule, put 1 drop on a cotton ball, and plug into the ear.

Teething
Herbs German chamomile (*Chamomilla recutita*, p. 82), slippery elm (*Ulmus rubra*, p. 149)
Remedy Give German chamomile infusion (see *Digestive Upsets*) or make a paste from slippery elm powder and the infusion, and rub on the gums.

Difficulty in sleeping
Herbs German chamomile (*Chamomilla recutita*, p. 82), linden (*Tilia* spp., p. 286)
Remedy Make an infusion using either herb and give ¾–1¼ cups (150–300 ml) before bedtime.

Older adults

Traditionally, as we age, the "fire" or *qi* within us glows less brightly and our vitality slowly weakens. Many herbal medicines are ideally suited to treating the health problems that begin when people reach their late fifties, such as circulatory problems, weak digestion, and poor memory. The herbs recommended here can help to maintain good health, preventing or reducing the severity of symptoms that are often accepted as an inevitable consequence of aging. Self-treatment for other problems often experienced later in life, such as arthritis, is suggested in earlier sections.

Important note

- If taking conventional medication, tell your doctor if you intend to take an herbal remedy. This is especially important for the elderly.
- All remedies on this page need to be taken continuously for up to 3 months.
- If you are over 70 years of age, take ¾ of the stated dose for remedies given on other pages in this book.

Maintaining vitality

Many herbs help to maintain vitality.
Thyme is a much underrated herb. Recent research has discovered that it has antiaging and tonic properties that maintain vitality and reduce the chance of catching colds, flu, and other respiratory infections.
Ashwagandha is a tonic, calming herb that may slow the aging process. It is particularly suited to aid recovery from long-term illness.
Ginseng is well known as a remedy that supports vitality and resistance to stress and infection in older people.
Rhodiola has similar tonic, restorative properties to ashwagandha and ginseng, but enhances mental performance and has a mild antidepressant activity.

General remedy
Herb Thyme (*Thymus vulgaris*, p. 147)
Remedy Make a standard infusion. Take 1¼–1⅔ cups (300–450 ml) a day.

Stress or convalescence
Herb Ashwagandha (*Withania somnifera*, p. 156)
Remedy Take 1 g of the root 2–3 times a day, either by chewing it or chopping it and mixing with a little water.
Herb Ginseng (*Panax ginseng*, p. 123)
Remedy Take 1 g 1–2 times a day for up to 3 months. Chew the fresh or dried root, cook it in a soup, or take in tablet form.
Caution Do not take caffeine while taking ginseng.
Option If ginseng is too stimulating, take 3 g of codonopsis (*Codonopsis pilosula*, p. 87) a day in the same way as ginseng. This has a milder, but nonetheless tonic and strengthening, effect.

Nervous exhaustion & stress
Herb Oats (*Avena sativa*, p. 179)
Remedy Eat 25 g of oats each day (for example, as a hot cereal). Alternatively, take ½ tsp of the tincture twice a day.
Herb Rhodiola (*Rhodiola rosea*, p. 131)
Remedy Take ½ tsp (2.5 ml) of tincture 2–3 times a day or as recommended by supplier.

General conditions

Conditions that arise through aging need patient, long-term treatment.
Ginkgo is the oldest tree on the planet. Its leaves maintain good circulation to the head and brain, improving memory, concentration, and energy levels. Evidence suggests it may reduce the risk of a stroke.
Gotu kola has significant anti-inflammatory activity, for example in arthritis, but is also a tonic that helps to protect the nervous system and to maintain memory and cognition.
Garlic has great value as a long-term dietary supplement, helping to maintain healthy circulation, balance blood-sugar levels, reduce high blood pressure and fat levels in the blood, and improve resistance to infection, especially bronchitis.
Rehmannia, a Chinese tonic herb with strengthening and mildly stimulant properties, appears to lower blood pressure and blood fat levels. It is suitable for people who have a weak liver and metabolism.
Gentian, a bitter herb, helps the absorption of food by maintaining digestive secretions, which diminish with age.

Failing memory & concentration
Herb Ginkgo (*Ginkgo biloba*, p. 104)
Remedy Take ginkgo tablets. These need to be taken regularly for at least 3 months.
Herb Gotu kola (*Centella asiatica*, p. 81)
Remedy Take tablets or ½ tsp tincture twice a day.

Poor circulation & high blood pressure
Herb Garlic (*Allium sativum*, p. 63)
Remedy Take 1–2 raw cloves a day with food, or take garlic tablets or capsules on a regular basis.
Herb Buckwheat (*Fagopyrum esculentum*, p. 215)
Remedy Make a standard infusion and drink up to 1¼ cup (300 ml) a day.

Chronic infections
Herbs Garlic (*Allium sativum*, p. 63), echinacea (*Echinacea* spp., p. 96)
Remedy Take 1–2 raw cloves of garlic each day with food, or take either herb in tablet or capsule form on a regular basis.

Weakened liver & metabolism
Herb Rehmannia (*Rehmannia glutinosa*, p. 270)
Remedy Chew 5 g of root 1–3 times a day, or make a decoction with 5 g of root to 1 cup (250 ml) of water and take 1–3 times a day.

Weakened digestion
Herb Gentian (*Gentiana lutea*, p. 103)
Remedy Take 5–10 drops of tincture with water about 30 minutes before eating, 3 times a day.
Caution Do not take gentian if you suffer from acid indigestion or a peptic ulcer.

Arthritic pain & rheumatism
See *Joint Pain & Stiffness, Including Arthritis & Gout*, p. 323.
Note Take one of the remedies for a maximum of 2–3 weeks. If there is no improvement, consult an herbal practitioner.

Before taking any herbal remedies, see pages 300 & 308–309

Consulting an herbal practitioner

Many common health problems, such as colds and indigestion, do not require a professional consultation and can be successfully treated using herbs at home. However, persistent or more serious ailments, such as stomach ulcers and shingles, can be difficult or dangerous to treat on one's own and need the advice and treatment of a qualified herbal practitioner or naturopath.

What does herbal medicine treat best?

It is difficult to state exactly which ailments best respond to herbal medicine, since almost no research has been undertaken with this question in mind. Nevertheless, the experience of herbal practitioners and their patients suggests that many chronic and some acute illnesses readily improve with herbal medicine. Conditions that are commonly treated by herbalists include allergies, arthritis, chronic or frequent infections, circulatory problems, liver disease, menstrual and gynecological problems, skin disorders, and stress-related complaints such as headaches, insomnia, and palpitations.

Choosing a practitioner

Herbal practitioners tend to treat ill health more effectively as they gain greater experience. Anyone with a serious illness, such as rheumatoid arthritis or cancer, should seek an experienced practitioner. Nevertheless, herbalists newly launched into practice often bring a more flexible approach to treatment, having the time and enthusiasm for patients that may be lacking in their more senior counterparts. That said, a trusting relationship is as important as the treatment itself—always find a practitioner in whom you feel confident. The best way to find an herbalist is by recommendation, or by looking on the websites of the herbal organizations listed on this page.

The Consultation

On visiting an herbalist you should be made to feel welcome, receiving an attentive and sympathetic ear. The first consultation takes about an hour, so there is ample time for the practitioner to gain a rounded view of your health problems and life as a whole.

You will probably be asked about family traits, diet, lifestyle, levels of stress, and any particular anxieties that you may have. If appropriate, a physical examination will take place, and the practitioner will explain as far as possible what is wrong and how much improvement can be expected. Clinical tests may include urine analysis or measuring hemoglobin levels from a drop of blood. The herbalist will then recommend appropriate treatment, usually involving an herbal prescription, dietary advice, and a suggested exercise regimen. If you are already undergoing conventional treatment, the herbalist will advise you on its compatibility with herbal medicine and, if necessary, devise a program to discontinue pharmaceutical medicines gradually.

Subsequent consultations generally last about 30 minutes and are likely to take place every 4 to 6 weeks for a period of 3 months. This, of course, may vary, depending on the nature of the treatment.

Safety of herbs

Although herbal medicine is extremely safe, the fact that it is natural does not necessarily mean it is harmless. The best guarantee against poor treatment is to consult a well-trained practitioner who belongs to a recognized professional association and prescribes high-quality herbal medicines.

Professional training

Traditionally, herbalists learned their craft by apprenticeship. Nicholas Culpeper (1616–1654), for example, was apprenticed to an apothecary for 10 years. Today, herbal practitioners are generally trained at a college or university, acquiring their clinical skills in herbal and, in some cases, hospital clinics. The curriculum typically includes an in-depth study of medical sciences, such as physiology, pathology, pharmacology, and botany, as well as what can be called the herbal sciences, *materia medica*, nutrition, and therapeutics. Modern training attempts to honor and retain the best of traditional herbal medicine, while incorporating the insights of contemporary medical science and research.

Herbalism worldwide

Western medical herbalism is the traditional form of herbal medicine practiced in Britain. However, the Chinese and Ayurvedic traditions, among others, are becoming more popular and are raising their standards of training. If you wish to consult a Chinese or Ayurvedic herbalist, it is strongly recommended that you select a member of the associations listed on this page.

The regulation of medical herbalism varies considerably around the world. In the Far East, practitioners and hospitals routinely offer herbal medicine, acupuncture, and other traditional healing practices alongside Western conventional medicine. In the US, the leading practitioner organization is the American Herbalists Guild.

Herbal practitioners in continental Europe are known as phytotherapists, and are usually conventional medical practitioners who have studied plant medicine at the postgraduate level.

In Australia, the National Herbalists' Association of Australia (NHAA) is the leading professional body of herbal practitioners.

In many parts of the world, herbal medicine is unregulated. In this situation, it is wise to be cautious and, as far as possible, to find a practitioner based on personal recommendation.

Herbal practitioner organizations

This list is made up of recommended herbal practitioner organizations active in the US and Canada.

UNITED STATES

American Herbalists Guild
www.americanherbalistsguild.com
American Association of Naturopathic Physicians
www.naturopathic.org
National Certification Commission for Acupuncture and Oriental Medicine (NCCAOM)
https://mx.nccaom.org/FindAPractitioner
National Ayurvedic Medical Association
www.ayurvedanama.org
California College of Ayurveda
www.ayurvedacollege.com/resources/Ayurveda-practitioner-CAS

CANADA

The Canadian Herbalist's Association of British Columbia
www.chaofbc.ca
Ontario Herbalists Association
www.herbalists.on.ca

Useful websites

Herbalist organizations
See p. 330 for a list of herbalist organizations.

Finding an herbal practitioner
Use the American Herbalists Guild's Find an Herbalist National Locator Service to find AHG professional members in your area.
www.americanherbalistsguild.com/ member-profiles

American Herbalists Guild regional chapters
AHG chapters bring herbal communities together to share their love of herbs, and to provide support for the important work of clinical herbalism all over the country. Each chapter is unique, reflecting the needs and interests of their community. Check this list to see whether there is chapter in your area.
www.americanherbalistsguild.com/ ahg-chapters

Herbal education
There are a plethora of educational options in the US and Canada, ranging from introductory to postgraduate level. The best guide to this richness can be found at the AHG listing:
www.americanherbalistsguild.com/ school-profiles

A characteristic of the north American herbal world is the wonderful range of herb schools established by herbalists around the country. Many are listed by the AHG, but an example is the following:

California School of Herbal Studies
www.cshs.com

Degree courses
A number of universities now offer degree courses at various levels.
For example:

Maryland University of Integrative Health
www.muih.edu

Offers a Master of Science in Therapeutic Herbalism

Bastyr University
www.bastyr.edu/academics/areas-study/ bs-major-herbal-sciences

The flagship school of naturopathic medicine offers a well-respected Bachelor of Science degree with a Major in Herbal Sciences.

Online and distance learning
Many online and correspondence courses are offered by herbal teachers.
For example:

Sage Mountain
Rosemary Gladstar
www.sagemountain.com

Center for Herbal Studies
David Winston
www.herbalstudies.net

Foundations in Herbal Medicine
Tieraona Low Dog, MD
drlowdog.com

East West School of Planetary Herbology
Michael and Leslie Tierra
www.planetherbs.com

The School of Natural Healing
Dr. John R. Christopher MH
www.snh.cc

Northeast School of Botanical Medicine
7Song
www.7song.com

Herbal suppliers
Mountain Rose Herbs
The most comprehensive North American supplier of all things herbal
www.mountainroseherbs.com

Frontier Co-op
Member-owned supplier of herbs, spices, foods, and more since 1976
www.frontiercoop.com

Floracopeia
Suppliers of essential oils and flower essences
www.floracopeia.com

Starwest Botanicals
One of the largest suppliers of organic herbs in the United States
www.starwest-botanicals.com

Verditas Botanicals
Suppliers of 100 percent organic essential oils
verditasbotanicals.com

Simplers Botanicals
A leading source of therapeutic-quality, certified organic essential oils and herbal extracts
https://simplers.com

Neal's Yard
A world leader of natural health and beauty, supplying essential oils and herbal remedies
https://us.nyrorganic.com/shop/corp/

Equipment suppliers
An excellent guide with links to herbal medicine making supplies can be found at:
www.livingawareness.com/medicine-making-resources/

Mountain Rose Herbs is also a comprehensive equipment supplier:
www.mountainroseherbs.com

Buying herbal medicines

What should you look for when buying herbal medicines? It is usually most convenient to buy capsules, tablets, essential oils, pessaries, and perhaps tinctures, and to make up your own infusions, decoctions, and syrups (see p. 301 and p. 303).

- Buy from a reputable herb store, staffed by people knowledgeable about herbal medicines.
- Only buy herbs online from established herbal suppliers.
- Buy organic herbs and products where available.

Buying dried herbs
Dried herbs are generally available from herbal suppliers. Buying from shops is preferable to buying online because the herbs can be examined before purchasing. However, it is possible some online companies may supply fresher herbs due to higher turnover. To gain the best medicinal effect, good-quality produce is essential. Shop around and bear in mind the following points before buying:

- Herbs should not be stored in clear glass jars or in direct sunlight, as this causes oxidation, which affects their efficacy.
- Good-quality aromatic herbs should have a distinct scent and taste.
- Check for signs of infestation due to poor drying techniques, or adulteration. This can sometimes be recognized by the presence of dried grass or other non-medicinal material in the jar.
- Herbs lose their color as they age. Look for bright material that has been well dried and stored, and that is not too old. Calendula flowers (*Calendula officinalis*, p. 77) that are a vivid yellow/orange color are likely to make good medicine. If they have been sitting on a shelf for 18 months, they will probably look drab and pale.

Buying herbal products
When buying products such as capsules, tablets, essential oils, pessaries, and tinctures, always check the label on the jar or packet. If it does not do the following, do not buy it:

- Name all constituents of the product
- State the recommended daily dosage
- State the weight of each capsule or tablet, or volume of bottle
- List the weight of each constituent of a capsule, tablet, etc.
- List the ratio of herb in the product (for example, 1:3, meaning 1 part herb to 3 parts liquid).

Glossary

Many plant constituents and their actions are explained in How Medicinal Plants Work, pp. 10–16.

Medical

Abortifacient Causes abortion

Adaptogenic Helps the body adapt to stress and supports normal function

Anabolic Promotes tissue growth

Analgesic Reduces pain

Anaphrodisiac Inhibits libido and sexual activity

Anesthetic Numbs perception of external sensations

Anorexia Lack of appetite

Anthelmintic Expels or destroys parasitic worms

Anthraquinones Irritate the intestinal wall causing a bowel movement

Antibiotic Destroys or inhibits microorganisms

Anticoagulant Prevents blood clotting

Antifungal Combats fungal infections

Anti-inflammatory Reduces inflammation

Antimicrobial Destroys or inhibits micro-organisms

Antioxidant Prevents oxidation and breakdown of tissues

Antiseptic Destroys or inhibits microorganisms that cause infection

Antispasmodic Relieves muscle spasm, or reduces muscle tone

Antitussive Soothes and relieves coughing

Aperient Mild laxative

Aphrodisiac Excites libido and sexual activity

Aseptic Free from contamination by harmful bacteria, viruses or other microorganisms

Astringent Tightens mucous membranes and skin, reducing secretions and bleeding from abrasions

Autonomic nervous system Part of the nervous system responsible for the control of bodily functions that are not consciously directed, e.g. sweating, beating of the heart

Ayurveda Traditional Indian system of medicine, (see pp. 40–43)

Bitter Stimulates secretions of saliva and digestive juices, increasing appetite

Carcinogenic Causes cancer

Cardiotonic Improves heart function

Carminative Relieves digestive gas and indigestion

Carrier oil Oil such as wheatgerm, to which essential oils are added in order to dilute them for use

Cathartic A drastic purgative

Circulatory stimulant Increases blood flow, usually to a given area, e.g. hands and feet

Colic Abdominal pain produced by strong contractions of intestines or bladder

Compress A cloth pad soaked in a hot or cold herbal extract and applied to the skin

Counterirritant Superficial irritant used to relieve more deep-seated pain or discomfort

Cream A mixture of water and fat or oil that blends with the skin

Decoction Water-based preparation of bark, roots, berries, or seeds simmered in boiling water

Demulcent Coats, soothes, and protects body surfaces such as the gastric mucous membranes

Depurative Detoxifying agent

Detoxification The process of aiding removal of toxins and waste products from the body

Diaphoretic Induces sweating

Diuretic Stimulates urine flow

Doctrine of Signatures Theory that the appearance of a plant reveals its medicinal properties

Eclectic Popular system of herbal medicine in 19th- and early 20th-century North America

Edema Fluid retention

Elixir A liquid herbal preparation with a pleasant taste, due to the addition of honey or sugar

Emetic Causes vomiting

Emmenagogue Stimulates menstrual flow

Emollient Softens or soothes the skin

Essential oil Distillation of volatile oils derived from aromatic plants

Estrogenic With a similar action to estrogen in the body, supporting and maintaining the female reproductive organs

Expectorant Stimulates coughing and helps clear phlegm from the throat and chest

Febrifuge Reduces fever

Fixed oil A nonvolatile oil (plant constituent). An oil produced by hot or cold infusion (preparation)

Galenical A medicine, in a standard formula, prepared from plants

Hallucinogenic Causes visions or hallucinations

Hemostatic Stops or reduces bleeding

Hepatic Affects the liver

Hepatoprotective Protects the liver

Humor An important body fluid in traditional European or Indian medicine, (see p. 36)

Hypertension High blood pressure

Hypnotic Induces sleep

Hypoglycemic Lowers blood glucose levels

Hypotension Low blood pressure

Immune stimulant Stimulates the body's immune defenses to counter infection

Infusion Water-based preparation in which flowers, leaves or stems are brewed in a similar way to tea

Inhalation Breathing of medicinally infused steam or liquid through the nasal passages

Intermittent fever A fever that recurs regularly, e.g. malaria

Laxative Promotes evacuation of the bowels

Liniment External medication applied by rubbing

Mydriatic Dilates the pupil of the eye

Narcotic Causes drowsiness or stupor and relieves pain

Nervine Restores the nerves; relaxes the nervous system

Neuralgia Pain resulting from irritation or inflammation of a nerve

Ointment A blend of fats or oils that form a protective layer over the skin

Oxytocic Induces contractions of the uterus

Parasiticide Kills parasites

Parasympathetic nervous system Part of the nervous system involved in vegetative functions, especially digestion

Pectoral Acts on the lungs

Photosensitive Heightened sensitivity to sunlight

Physiomedicalism 19th- and 20th-century American and British system of herbal medicine

Poultice Herbal preparation usually applied hot to affected area to alleviate pain and reduce swelling

Prostaglandins Chemicals in plants and the human body that have a hormonal action affecting a wide range of conditions including pain and inflammation

Purgative A very strong laxative

Qi Vital energy force in Chinese philosophy, (see p. 26)

Rubefacient Stimulates blood flow to skin, causing reddening and warming

Sedative Reduces activity and nervous excitement

Simple An herb used on its own

Spasmolytic Relaxes muscles

Steroids Active chemicals, of animal and plant origin, with powerful hormonal actions

Stimulant Increases rate of activity and nervous excitement

Stomachic Eases stomach pain or increases stomach activity

Styptic Stops bleeding when applied topically

Sympathetic nervous system Part of the nervous system involved in maintaining arousal, alertness, and muscle tone

Systemic Affecting the body as a whole rather than individual organs

Terpenes Molecules that form the base of most constituents of volatile oils

Tincture Plant medicine prepared by macerating herb in water and alcohol

Tonic Exerts a restorative or nourishing action on the body

Tonify Strengthens and restores body systems

Topical Application of herbal remedy to body surface

Vasoconstrictor Contracts and narrows blood vessels

Vasodilator Relaxes and widens blood vessels

Vermifuge Expels intestinal worms

Volatile oil Plant constituent distilled to produce essential oil

Vulnerary Heals wounds

Yin and yang Complementary opposites in Chinese philosophy, (see pp. 44–46)

Botanical

Aerial parts Parts of plant growing above ground

Annual Plant that completes its life cycle in a year

Aril Secondary covering over the seed in certain plants

Aromatic Plant with high levels of volatile oil

Axil Upper angle formed by leaf stem and supporting stem or branch

Basal leaves Leaves growing from the base of the stem

Biennial Plant that completes its life cycle in 2 years, generally flowering in the second year

Capsule Dry fruit that splits open when ripe to scatter seeds

Composite flowers Flowers made up of usually 2 types of tiny florets, disk and ray; some have disk florets only

Compound Leaves or flowers made up of many individual small flowers or leaflets

Cordate Having heart-shaped leaves

Corm Bulblike, underground storage organ formed by a swollen stem base

Corolla Collective term for the petals of a flower

Deciduous Plant that sheds leaves each year

Dioecious Species with male and female parts on separate plants

Herbaceous Plant that dies down at the end of the growing season

Insectivorous Plant that traps and digests insects and other small animals

Lanceolate Lance-shaped

Latex Milky fluid found in various plants and trees

Panicle A branched cluster of flowers on stalks in a pyramid-shaped arrangement

Perennial Plant that lives for at least 3 seasons

Pinnate A compound leaf with leaflets growing in 2 rows on each side of its mid-rib

Rhizome Underground storage stem

Stamen Male fertilizing organ of a flowering plant

Stigma Female organ of a flower

Succulent Plant with thick, fleshy leaves and/or stems

Trifoliate Plant with 3 leaves or leaflets

Tuber Thickened part of underground stem

Umbel Umbrella-like arrangement of flowers with all flower stems arising from the same point

Whorl Ring of leaves or flowers radiating out horizontally from a central point

Wildcrafting Harvesting herbs from the wild

Bibliography

This selected listing of references is provided as a guide to those interested in learning more about the history, science and present-day practice of herbal medicine.

Herbal medicine

Allen, D. & Hatfield, G.
Medicinal Plants in Folk Tradition
(USA, Timber Press, 2004)

Barker, J.
The Medicinal Flora of Britain and Northwestern Europe
(UK, Winter Press, 2001)

Barnes, J., Anderson, L. A., & Phillipson, J. D.
Herbal Medicines
(UK, Pharmaceutical Press, 2007)

Bartram, T.
Encyclopaedia of Herbal Medicine
(UK, British Herbal Medicine Association, 1995)

Bensky, D. & Gamble, A.
Chinese Herbal Medicine Materia Medica
(USA, Eastland Press, 1993)

Bone, K.
Clinical Guide to Blending Liquid Herbs
(UK, Churchill Livingstone, 2003)

Bone, K.
Functional Herbal Therapy
(UK, Aeon, 2021)

Bown, D.
The Royal Horticultural Society Encyclopedia of Herbs & Their Uses
(UK, Dorling Kindersley, 1995)

Bradley, P. (ed.)
British Herbal Compendium
(UK, British Herbal Medicine Association, 1992)

Bremness, L.
Herbs
(UK, Dorling Kindersley, 1994)

Brice-Ytsma, H.
Herbal Medicine in Treating Gynaecological Conditions: Herbs, Hormones, Pre-Menstrual Syndrome and Menopause
(UK, Aeon, 2020)

British Herbal Medicine Association
British Herbal Pharmacopoeia
(UK, British Herbal Medicine Association, 1983)

Bruneton, J.
Pharmacognosy and Phytochemistry of Medicinal Plants
(UK, Intercept, 1995)

Bruton-Seal, J. & Seal, M.
Hedgerow Medicine
(UK, Merlin Unwin Books, 2008)

Chevallier, A.
Herbal First Aid
(UK, Amberwood, 1993)

Chevallier, A.
Herbal Remedies
(UK, Dorling Kindersley, 2007)

Chevallier, A.
Hypericum: Natural Antidepressant and More
(UK, Souvenir Press, 1999)

Duke, J
Anti-ageing prescriptions
(UK, Rodale, 2003)

Duke, J.
The Green Pharmacy
(USA, Rodale Press, 1997)

Easley, T. and Horne, S.
Modern Herbal Dispensatory: A Medicine-Making Guide
(US, North Atlantic Books, 2016)

Erasmus, U.
Fats That Heal, Fats That Kill
(Canada, Alive, 1993)

Felter, J. & Lloyd, J.
King's American Dispensatory
(USA, Eclectic Medical, 1983)

Fulder, S.
The Book of Ginseng
(USA, Arts Press, 1993)

Fulder, S.
Ginger, The Ultimate Home Remedy
(UK, Souvenir Press, 1993)

Grieve, M. (ed. Leyel, C. F.)
A Modern Herbal (free download available)
(UK, Penguin, 1980)

Hoffman, D.
Holistic Herbal: A Safe and Practical Guide to Making and Using Herbal Remedies (4th ed.)
(UK, Thorsons 2003)

Lis-Balchin, M.
Aromatherapy Science
(UK, Pharmaceutical Press, 2006)

Low, T.
Wild Herbs of Australia and New Zealand
(Australia, Angus & Robertson, 1985)

Martindale, W.
The Extra Pharmacopoeia (26th ed.)
(UK, The Pharmaceutical Press, 1972)

Mills, S.
The Essential Book of Herbal Medicine
(UK, Penguin, 1991)

Mills, S. and Bone, K.
The Essential Guide to Herbal Safety
(UK, Churchill Livingstone Elsevier, 2005)

Mills, S. and Bone, K.
Principles and Practice of Phytotherapy (2nd ed.)
(UK, Churchill Livingstone Elsevier, 2013)

Murray, M.
The Healing Power of Herbs
(USA, Prima, 1995)

Ody, P.
The Complete Medicinal Herbal
(UK, Dorling Kindersley, 1993)

Price, S. & Price, L.
Aromatherapy and Health Professionals (4th ed.)
(UK, Churchill Livingstone, 2011)

Priest, A. W. & Priest, L. R.
Herbal Medication
(UK, Fowler, 1984)

Rogers, C.
The Woman's Guide to Herbal Medicine
(UK, Hamish Hamilton, 1995)

Romanucci-Ross, L., et al
The Anthropology of Medicine: from Culture to Method
(USA, Bergin & Garvey, 1983)

Schauenberg, P. & Paris, F.
Guide to Medicinal Plants
(UK, Lutterworth Press, 1977)

Schultes, R. & Raffauf, R.
The Healing Forest
(USA, Dioscorides Press, 1990)

de Sloover, J. & Goossens, M.
Wild Herbs, a Field Guide
(UK, David & Charles, 1981)

Stargrove, M., Treasure, J. & McKee, D. L.
Herb, Nutrient, and Drug Interactions: Clinical Implications and Therapeutic Strategies
(UK, Mosby Elsevier, 2008)

Stobart, A.
The Medicinal Forest Garden Handbook
(UK, Permanent Publications, 2020)

Svoboda, R.
Ayurveda: Life, Health and Longevity
(UK, Arkana, 1992)

Talalaj, S. & Czechowicz, A.
Herbal Remedies, Harmful and Beneficial Effects
(Australia, Hill of Content, 1989)

Trease, C. & Evans, W.
Pharmacognosy (13th ed.)
(UK, Ballière Tindall, 1989)

Uphof, J.
Dictionary of Economic Plants
(UK, Wheldon & Wesley, 1970)

Valnet, J.
The Practice of Aromatherapy
(UK, C. W. Daniel, 1980)

Wagner, H. et al. (ed.)
Economic and Medicinal Plant Research (vols. 1–5)
(UK, Sangam, 1993)

Warrier, P. et al. (ed.)
Indian Medicinal Plants (vols. 1–5)
(UK, Sangam, 1993)

Weiss, W.
Herbal Medicine
(UK, Arcanum, 1988)

Williamson, E.
Potters Herbal Cyclopaedia
(UK, C. W. Daniel, 2003)

History of herbal medicine

Bruton-Seal, J. & Seal, M.
Herbalist's Bible: John Parkinson's Lost Classic Rediscovered, The
(UK, Merlin Unwin Books, 2014)

Culpeper, N.
The English Physitian Enlarged
(UK, George Sawbridge, 1653)

Gerard, J.
The Herball or General History of Plants
(UK, John North, 1597)

Griggs, B.
New Green Pharmacy
(UK, Vermilion, 1997)

Gunther, R.
The Greek Herbal of Dioscorides
(UK, Oxford University Press, 1934)

Hoizey, D. & Hoizey, M. J.
A History of Chinese Herbal Medicine
(UK, Edinburgh University Press, 1993)

K'Eogh, J. (ed. Scott, M.)
An Irish Herbal
(UK, Aquarian Press, 1986)

Larre, C.
The Way of Heaven (Neijing suwen)
(UK, Monkey Press, 1994)

Lloyd, G. (ed.)
Hippocratic Writings
(UK, Penguin, 1978)

Manniche, L.
An Ancient Egyptian Herbal
(UK, British Museum Publications, 1989)

Pliny the Elder (ed. Healey, J.)
Natural History: A Selection
(UK, Penguin, 1991)

Porter, R.
The Greatest Benefit to Mankind
(UK, Harper Collins, 1997)

Swinburne Clymer, R.
Nature's Healing Agents
(USA, The Humanitarian Society, 1973)

Tobyn, G., Denham, A. & Whitelegg, M.
The Western Herbal Tradition: 2000 Years of Medicinal Plant Knowledge
(UK, Churchill Livingstone, 2010)

Unschuld, P.
Medicine in China
(UK, University of California Press, 1985)

Vogel, V.
American Indian Medicine
(UK, University of Oklahoma Press, 1970)

Journals

Australian Journal of Medical Herbalism
British Medical Journal
Canadian Journal of Herbalism
Herbalgram
Journal of Alternative and Complementary Medicine
Journal of Ethnopharmacology
Journal of Herbal Medicine
Lancet
New Scientist
Phytomedicines
Planta Medica
Review of Aromatic and Medicinal Plants

Index

Bold page numbers refer to main plant entries in Key medicinal plants and Other medicinal plants. Ailments for which there is a self-help treatment are in bold.

Index of herbs by ailment

This index includes a wide range of ailments, listing key herbs used to treat each one. Page numbers in **bold** denote a self-help use.

Acknowledgments

Author's acknowledgments
Without the unfailing good humor and commitment of the team at Dorling Kindersley this book would not have been possible. My sincere and heartfelt thanks to Penny Warren, Valerie Horn, Spencer Holbrook, Christa Weil and Rosie Pearson. The responsibility for faults or omissions in this encyclopedia is entirely mine, though I have been greatly helped in compiling sections of this book by Anne McIntyre MNIMH, Noel Rigby MNHAA and Eve Rogans MRTCM. Many other fellow medical herbalists and colleagues have contributed in discussion or ideas, whether knowingly or not, to the writing of this book. The list cannot be exhaustive but in particular I would like to thank Richard Adams MNIMH, Celia Bell PhD, Christopher Hedley MNIMH, Michael McIntyre FNIMH, Ellis Snitcher MD, Christine Steward MNIMH, Midge Whitelegg PhD MNIMH and John Wilkinson PhD. Above all, I am indebted to those who kept the fires of herbal medicine burning in the mostly chill and dispiriting winds of the mid-twentieth century. Without their commitment and love for herbal medicine, the current renaissance in plant medicine would not be taking place. Lastly, to Maria, Leon and Tamara for whom I have had so little time while writing, my deepest thanks for your patience, love and understanding.

For the 2016 edition
For this revised edition, DK staff have (as always) proved themselves to be efficient, helpful, and gentle (but accurate) in their critical comments. In particular, I want to thank Toby Mann, for his thoughtful and skillful input during the editorial process, and Lisa Dyer for steering the project to a successful conclusion. I would also like to thank Julie Bruton-Seal, Kofi Busia, Nikki Darrell, Jill Davies and Rowan Hamilton, who all (in different ways) made essential contributions to this new edition.

Publisher's acknowledgments
DK would like in particular to thank Ruth Midgley for her editorial expertise and Colin Nicholls MNIMH for his expert advice and knowledge. Many thanks also to Tracey Beresford, Polly Boyd, Joanna Chisholm, Charlotte Evans, Fay Franklin, Fred Gill, Nell Graville, Constance Novis, Frank Ritter, Blanche Sibbald, Linda Sonntag and Clare Stewart for editorial assistance; to Tracey Clarke who contributed to the original design and to Maxine Chung for design assistance; to Zoë Saunders for modeling; to Raquel Leis and Ana Pedro for help with finding plants; and to Kathie Gill for the index. Dorling Kindersley are particularly grateful to Duncan Ross of Poyntzfield Herb Nursery for photographing plants in the Himalayas; to Fiona Crumley and the staff of the Chelsea Physic Garden for their invaluable advice and to Dr. Yongfeng Wang at Aston University and Dr. Y. Wong at Hosten University, who helped track down and verify elusive Chinese herbs. Many thanks also to Jacqueline Horn, Professor Shouming Zhong of East-West Herbs; Noel Rigby and Woods & Woods in Australia; Neal's Yard in Covent Garden; Anthony Lymon-Dixon of Arne Herbs; Hambledon Herbs and Iden Croft Herbs of Kent.

Grateful thanks also to Deni Bown, and to James Morley and the staff of the Royal Botanic Gardens Kew for their expertise. Also: University of Oklahoma Press, University of California Press and Arkana.

For the 2016 edition
DK would like to thank Jane Simmonds for proofreading, Marie Lorimer for preparing the index, Karen Constanti and Philippa Nash for design assistance, Alastair Laing for editorial advice and support, and Vanessa Hamilton for additional illustrations.

For the 2023 edition
I am indebted to an ever-expanding number of people, who have helped and enabled me to write what I hope has become, over the years, an increasingly measured, accurate, and useful introduction to herbal medicine. Without them, the book would either not exist or would be "thin gruel," lacking the many detailed insights given to me by teachers, colleagues, patients, and staff at DK. In particular, I would like to thank Kerry Bone and Simon Mills, whose books, writings, and teaching on professional Western herbal medicine have inspired a generation of herbalists and underpin much of what is written here. I would also like to give my sincere thanks to the team at DK, especially, Sophie Blackman and Zara Anvari, for creating a fresh, contemporary look for the book and making the writing and editorial process almost pain-free.

Publisher's acknowledgments
DK would like to thank Francesco Piscitelli for proofreading the book; Ruth Ellis for providing the indexes; Ruth Jenkinson for shooting the herbs on the cover; Christine Keilty for sourcing the props for the photo shoot; Andrew Pinder for his illustrations; and Sarah Smithies for picture research.

2001 edition team
Project Editor Jennifer Jones, **Art Editor** Karen Sawyer, **Editor** Lesley Riley, **Picture Researcher** Louise Thomas, **Category Publisher** Mary-Clare Jerram, **Art Director** Tracy Killick, **Production** Bethan Blase

Encyclopedia of Herbal Medicine reissue, ISBN 9780241229446; picture credits
The publisher would like to thank the following for their kind permission to reproduce their photographs:
(Key: a-above; b-bottom; c-center; f-far; l-left; r-right; t-top)

123RF.com: Natalia Pauk 131cra; **A–Z Botanical Collection Ltd:** Pallava Bagla 84tla, Chris Martin Bahr: 289tra, Pam Collins: 234c; **AF Fotografie:** 52; **Alamy Images:** 125cla, Album 56, Classic Image 20, Carole Drake 125cr, Jenny Gu 115bl, imageBROKER 54, 298, Hamza Khan 25, Nature Picture Library 222, Christopher Nicholson 31, Panther Media GmbH 239, pumkinpie 97cla, Matyas Rehak 217bl, robertharding 41, Inga Spence 127bl, C J Wheeler 147cla, WILDLIFE GmbH 125cr, 217tr, Wirestock, Inc. 213br; **American Museum of Natural History:** Heather Angel: 125tl; **Deni Bown:** 98bl,

111tl, 119tl, 122bl, 126tl, 218tr, 231c, 239br, 283br; **Bridgeman Images:** Granger 22, Heini Schneebeli 26; **By Permission of the British Library:** 23r; **Neil Campbell Sharp:** 124bl, Alain Compost: 101bl, Dennis Green: 152tl, Dr. Eckart Pott: 154bl, Hans Reinhard: 73tl, 90bl, 112tl; **Dorling Kindersley:** Hampton Court Flower Show 227tl, RHS Wisley 188tr, 224, 226tl; **Dreamstime.com:** Aleksandramoslavac 200br, AnnaEvere 35, Argenlant 240, Oksana Byelikova 48, Oksana Byelikova 230, Amphawan Chanunph 153bl, Chernetskay 121cr, Clearvista 267tl, Halpand 108cla, Montree Lakchit 78cb, Lianem 134cla, Volha Lukyanchy 231, Marinodenisenko 157, Sandy Matzen 34, Werner Meidinger 33, Neosiam 66bl, Marina Novosad 154clb, Ovydyborets 78cr, Manfred Ruckszi 110bl, Diamantis Seitanidi 132bl, Jill Shepherd 235bc, Sommai Sommai 66cb, Chalermchai Thaisamrong 66cr, Herman Vlad 104bl, Whiskybottle 182, Whiskybottle 241, Nicolette Wollenti 206; **Mary Evans Picture Library:** Wolf: 271; © **Steven Foster 1996:** 72bl, 80bl, 99tl, 123tl, 140tl, 143tl; **GAP Photos:** 53, Thomas Alamy 70cla, Thomas Alamy 176, Dave Bevan 128bl, Mark Bolton 121bl, 308, Christa Brand 39, Jonathan Buckley 55, Keith Burdett 32, Keith Burdett 50, Keith Burdett 167, Liz Every 57, Liz Every 131cla, John Glover 60cla, Sonia Hunt 113bl, Ernie Janes 203bl, Andrea Jones 76cla, Fiona McLeod 166tc, Jonathan Need 38, Nova Photo Graphik 51, 69cla, 118bl, 163br, 164tr, 195tc, 265clb, 270, Jerry Pavia 63cla, Howard Rice 18, 106cla, J S Sira 274, Friedrich Strauss 142cla, Friedrich Strauss 253, Visions 242, Richard Wareham 78bl, Dave Zubraski 27, 194; **Garden Picture Library:** J.S. Sira: 62bl; **Getty Images:** Corbis Documentary/Scott Smith 11, tinglee1631 238br; **Getty Images/iStock:** 136cla, Jetapura Vinuben Arvindbha 74bl, cinoby 280tc, Yves Dery 199, Elenathewise 44, ErikAgar 95cla, ma-no 28, marilyna 43, msk.nina 78c, rootstocks 254, sayhmog 215, tc397 83bl, ThamKC 67cra, tottoto 258, James Wagstaff 211, wichaiphoto 245; **Robert Harding Picture Library:** 284; **Holt Studios International:** Nigel Cattlin: 84tl, 158tl, 237tl, Bob Gibbons: 70tl, 105tl, Primrose Peacock: 188l; **Tim Low:** 116tl; **Marianne Majerus Garden Images:** Bennet Smith 67cla; **The Metropolitan Museum of Art:** Gift of Mr. and Mrs. Klaus G. Perls, 1991 49; **Oxford Scientific Library:** G.I. Bernard: 107bl, Sally Birch: 117bl, Deni Bown: 64bl, 68bl, 82tl, 120tl, 135tl, 157tl, 208tl, Jack Dermid: 266, Geoff Kidd: 150tl, Avril Ramage: 79tl; **Photo Researchers Inc./ National Audubon Society** / Alvin E. Staffan: 149bl; **Photos Horticultural Picture Library:** 86tl, 146bl; **Premaphotos:** 148tl; **Scala/Duomo Anagni:** 21; **Science Photo Library:** New York Public Library Picture Collection 36, Geoff Tompkinson 30; **Shutterstock.com:** Frank Gebauer 17, Kristina Ismulyani 40, Nancy Ayumi Kunihir 200tc, Vladimir Melnik 89cla, myboys.me 44, NOPPHARAT539 92cla, pakn 94bl, Starover Sibiriak 102cla, Svetlana Zhukova 85bl; **Harry Smith Collection:** 141bl, 100tl, **Tony Stone Worldwide:** Jacques Jangoux: 184tl; **Wikipedia:** Discott 75tl.
All other images © Dorling Kindersley
For further information see: www.dkimages.com

DK | Penguin Random House

THIS EDITION

DK UK
Senior Editor Sophie Blackman
Senior Designer Glenda Fisher
Editor Emma Hill
Senior US Editor Megan Douglass
US Consultant David Hoffman
Designer Tessa Bindloss
Senior Production Editor Tony Phipps
Senior Production Controller Stephanie McConnell
Jacket & Sales Material Coordinator Jasmin Lennie
Jacket Designer Glenda Fisher
Senior Acquisitions Editor Zara Anvari
Editorial Manager Ruth O'Rourke
Managing Art Editor Marianne Markham
Art Director Maxine Pedliham
Publishing Director Katie Cowan

DK INDIA
DTP Coordinator Pushpak Tyagi
DTP Designers Manish Upreti, Nityanand Kumar, Vijay Kandwal
Production Manager Pankaj Sharma
DTP Coordinator Pushpak Tyagi
Freelance Editor Rishi Bryan

FIRST EDITION

Project Editor Penny Warren
Editors Valerie Horn, Christa Weil
Senior Editor Rosie Pearson
Senior Art Editor Spencer Holbrook
Designers Robert Ford, Jeremy Butcher, Rachana Devidayal
Picture Researcher Jo Walton
Illustrator Gillie Newman
Main Photographers Andy Crawford, Steve Gorton
Managing Editor Susannah Marriott
Managing Art Editor Toni Kay
DTP Designer Karen Ruane
Production Antony Heller

This American Edition, 2023
First American Edition, 1996
Published in the United States by DK Publishing
1745 Broadway, 20th Floor, New York, NY 10019

A catalog record for this book
is available from the Library of Congress.
ISBN 978-0-7440-8179-4

DK books are available at special discounts when purchased
in bulk for sales promotions, premiums, fund-raising, or educational use.
For details, contact: DK Publishing Special Markets,
1745 Broadway, 20th Floor, New York, NY 10019
SpecialSales@dk.com

Printed and bound in Malaysia

For the curious
www.dk.com

IMPORTANT NOTICE
Do not try self-diagnosis or attempt self-treatment for serious or long-term problems without first consulting a qualified medical herbalist or medical practitioner as appropriate. Do not take any herb without first checking the cautions in the relevant herb entry (see pp. 58–293) and the Essential Information on pp. 308–309. Do not exceed any dosages recommended. Always consult a professional practitioner if symptoms persist. If taking prescribed medicines, seek professional medical advice before using herbal remedies. Take care to correctly identify plants and do not harvest restricted or banned species. So far as the author is aware, the information given is correct and up to date as of December 2022. Practice, laws, and regulations all change, and the reader should obtain up-to-date professional advice on any such issues. In addition, this book contains general information on growing cannabis, which is a controlled substance in North America and throughout much of the world. As the use and cultivation of cannabis and its derivative products can carry heavy penalties, you should research your local laws before using the information in this book. The author and the publisher expressly disclaim any liability, loss, or risk, personal or otherwise, which is incurred as a consequence, directly or indirectly, of the use and application of any of the contents of this book.